# CLINICAL MANUAL OF GYNECOLOGY

## NOTICE

Medicine is an ever-changing science. As new research and clinical experience broaden our knowledge, changes in treatment and drug therapy are required. The editors and the publisher of this work have checked with sources believed to be reliable in their efforts to provide information that is complete and generally in accord with the standards accepted at the time of publication. However, in view of the possibility of human error or changes in medical sciences, neither the editors nor the publisher nor any other party who has been involved in the preparation or publication of this work warrants that the information contained herein is in every respect accurate or complete, and they are not responsible for any errors or omissions or for the results obtained from use of such information. Readers are encouraged to confirm the information contained herein with other sources. For example and in particular, readers are advised to check the product information sheet included in the package of each drug they plan to administer to be certain that the information contained in this book is accurate and that changes have not been made in the recommended dose or in the contraindications for administration. This recommendation is of particular importance in connection with new or infrequently used drugs.

# CLINICAL MANUAL OF GYNECOLOGY

## SECOND EDITION

**Editors**
Thomas G. Stovall, MD
Robert L. Summitt, Jr., MD
Charles R. B. Beckmann, MD, MHPE
Frank W. Ling, MD

Department of Obstetrics and Gynecology
University of Tennessee
College of Medicine
Memphis, Tennessee

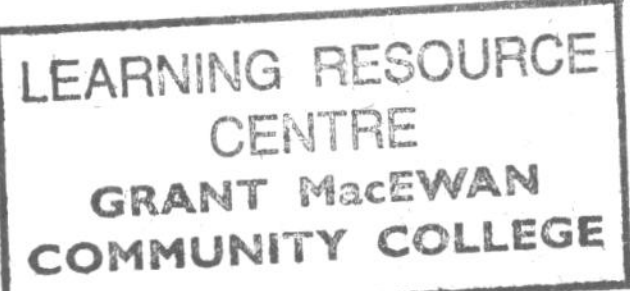


**McGraw-Hill, Inc.**
**Health Professions Division**

New York St. Louis San Francisco Auckland Bogotá
Caracas Lisbon London Madrid Mexico Milan Montreal
New Delhi Paris San Juan Singapore Sydney Tokyo Toronto

CLINICAL MANUAL OF GYNECOLOGY



12345678910 DOCDOC 98765432

ISBN 0-07-105389-1

This book was set in Optima by TSI Graphics.
The editors were Edward M. Bolger and Muza Navrozov;
the production supervisor was Clare B. Stanley;
the cover was designed by Marsha Cohen/Parallelogram.
R. R. Donnelley & Sons Company was printer and binder.

**Library of Congress Cataloging-in-Publication Data**

Clinical Manual of Gynecology./edited by Thomas G. Stovall . . . [et al.]—2nd ed.
p. cm.
Includes bibliographical references.
Includes index.
ISBN 0-07-105389-1
1. Gynecology—handbooks, manuals, etc. I. Stovall, Thomas G.
II. Series.
[DNLM: 1. Genital Diseases, Female—handbooks. WP 39 C641]
RG110.C55 1992
618.1—dc20
DNLM/DLC
for Library of Congress 90-7949
CIP

# Contents

Contributors ix

Foreword xii
*Joe Leigh Simpson*

Preface xiii

Part I: GENERAL CARE OF THE PATIENT

1. History and Physical Examination 3
*Charles R. B. Beckmann*
*Frank W. Ling*
*Barbara M. Barzansky*
*Barbara F. Sharf*
*Daniel L. Clarke-Pearson*

2. Care of the Hospitalized Patient 14
*Roger P. Smith*
*Barbara M. Barzansky*

3. Shock in the Gynecologic Patient 23
*Irvin K. Stone*
*Patrick Duff*

Part II: GENERAL GYNECOLOGY

4. Diseases of the Breast 49
*William H. Hindle*
*Frank W. Ling*

5. Benign Diseases of the Vulva 66
*John R. Musich*
*Thomas G. Stovall*

6. Benign Diseases of the Cervix and Vagina 80
*Jessica L. Thomason*
*Janine A. James*
*Frederik F. Broekhuizen*

7. Benign Diseases of the Uterus—Leiomyoma Uteri and the Hysterectomy 91
*Paula A. Hillard*

8. Benign Diseases of the Ovaries and Fallopian Tubes 116
*Guy I. Benrubi*

9. Pelvic Relaxation 128
*Bertram H. Buxton*
*Robert L. Summitt, Jr.*

10. Gynecologic Urology 144
*Robert L. Summitt, Jr.*
*John O. L. DeLancey*
*Thomas E. Elkins*

11. Abortion 164
*Stephen R. Carr*
*Thomas G. Stovall*
*Charles R. B. Beckmann*

12. Ectopic Pregnancy 185
*Thomas G. Stovall*
*Charles R. B. Beckmann*

13. Gynecologic Problems in Children 206
*David Muram*

14. Pelvic Pain and Dysmenorrhea 218
*Roger P. Smith*

15. Premenstrual Syndrome 238
*Joyce M. Vargyas*
*Frank W. Ling*

16. Sexual Problems 251
*Domeena Renshaw*

17. Contraception and Sterilization 263
*John C. Jarrett*
*George M. Ryan, Jr.*

18. Sexual Assault 289
*Charles R. B. Beckmann*
*Linda L. Groetzinger*
*Sylvia Lessman*
*Michael L. Bolos*

19. Sexually Transmitted Diseases and Pelvic Inflammatory Disease 314
*Jessica L. Thomason*
*Janine A. James*
*Frederik F. Broekhuizen*

## Part III: GYNECOLOGIC ENDOCRINOLOGY AND INFERTILITY

20. Amenorrhea and Hyperprolactinemia 335
*Eldon D. Schriock*

21. Anovulation and Dysfunctional Uterine Bleeding 350
*Paul G. Stumpf*

22. Menopause and the Climacteric 359
*Vivian Lewis*

23. Hirsutism, Defeminization, and Virilization 376
*Gretajo Northrop*

24. Normal and Abnormal Sexual Differentiation and Development 401
*Ira M. Rosenthal*

25. Infertility 424
*William L. Gentry*
*John E. Buster*

26. Endometriosis 444
*Steven J. Ory*

## Part IV: GYNECOLOGIC ONCOLOGY

27. Vulvar Dysplasia and Carcinoma 459
*Daniel L. Clarke-Pearson*

28. Vaginal Dysplasia and Carcinoma 474
*Daniel L. Clarke-Pearson*

29. Carcinoma of the Cervix 486
*Guy I. Benrubi*

30. Carcinoma of the Uterus 502
*Guy I. Benrubi*

31. Carcinoma of the Fallopian Tube 520
*Guy I. Benrubi*

32. Carcinoma of the Ovary 524
*Guy I. Benrubi*

33. Gestational Trophoblastic Disease 543
*John R. Lurain III*

## Part V: AMBULATORY GYNECOLOGY

34. Common Office Gynecologic Procedures 559
*Robert L. Summitt, Jr.*
*Thomas G. Stovall*
*Charles R. B. Beckmann*

35. Differential Diagnosis by Presentation 575
*W. Kirkland Ruffin*
*Thomas G. Stovall*
*Frank W. Ling*
*Robert L. Summitt, Jr.*

## Appendix A

Drug Therapy in Gynecology 603
*Rebecca Rogers*

## Appendix B

Antibiotic Therapy in Gynecology 621
*Rebecca Rogers*

**Index** **633**

# Contributors*

**Barbara M. Barzansky, PhD** [1,2]
Assistant Director of Division of Undergraduate Medical Education
The American Medical Association
Chicago, Ill

**Charles R. B. Beckmann, MD, MHPE** [1,11,12,18,34]
Associate Professor and Head, Medical Education Research
Department of OB/GYN
University of Tennessee, Memphis
Memphis, Tenn

**Guy I. Benrubi, MD** [8,29,30,31,32]
Associate Professor
Division of Gynecologic Oncology
University Hospital of Jacksonville
Jacksonville, Fla

**Michael L. Bolos** [18]
Attorney
Shorewood, Ill

**Frederik F. Broekhuizen, MD** [6,19]
Associate Professor
Department of OB/GYN
University of Wisconsin Medical School
Sinai Samaritan Medical Center
Milwaukee, Wis

**John E. Buster, MD** [25]
Professor and Director
Division of Reproductive Endocrinology and Infertility
Department of OB/GYN
University of Tennessee, Memphis
Memphis, Tenn

**Bertram H. Buxton, MD** [9]
Professor Emeritus
Department of OB/GYN, Division of Gynecology
University of Tennessee, Memphis
Memphis, Tenn

**Stephen R. Carr, MD** [11]
Assistant Professor
Maternal Fetal Medicine
Department of OB/GYN
Women & Infants Hospital of Rhode Island
Providence, RI

**Daniel L. Clarke-Pearson, MD** [1,27,28]
Professor and Head, Division of Gynecologic Oncology
Department of OB/GYN
Duke Medical Center
Duke S. Hospital
Durham, NC

**John O. L. DeLancey, MD** [10]
Assistant Professor
Department of OB/GYN
Division of Gynecology
University of Michigan
Ann Arbor, Mich

**Patrick Duff, MD** [3]
Professor, Department of OB/GYN
University of Florida, College of Medicine
Division of Maternal Fetal Medicine
Gainesville, Fla

*The numbers in brackets following the contributor name refer to chapter(s) authored or co-authored by the contributor.

**Thomas E. Elkins, MD** [10]
Assistant Professor and Chief
Department of OB/GYN, Division of Gynecology
University of Michigan Medical Center
Women's Hospital
Ann Arbor, Mich

**William L. Gentry, MD** [25]
Reproductive Endocrinologist
Department of OB/GYN
Methodist Center for Reproduction and Transplantation Immunology
Greenwood, Ill

**Linda L. Groetzinger, MSW** [18]
Clinical Assistant Professor of Medical Social Work
University of Illinois Medical Center
Chicago, Ill

**Paula A. Hillard, MD** [7]
Assistant Professor of OB/GYN
Department of OB/GYN
University of Cincinnati Medical Center
Cincinnati, Ohio

**William H. Hindle, MD** [4]
Director, Breast Diagnostic Center
Department of OB/GYN
Women's Hospital
LAC/USC Medical Center
Associate Clinical Professor
University of Southern California School of Medicine
Los Angeles, Calif

**Janine A. James, MD** [6,19]
Assistant Professor
Department of OB/GYN
University of Wisconsin Medical School
Sinai Samaritan Medical Center
Mt. Sinai Campus
Milwaukee, Wis

**John C. Jarrett, MD** [17]
Director, In Vitro Fertilization
Indianapolis Fertility Clinic
Indianapolis, Ind

**Sylvia Lessman, MSW** [18]
Irvine, Calif

**Vivian Lewis, MD** [22]
Director of Reproductive Endocrinology
Department of OB/GYN
University of Rochester
Rochester, NY

**Frank W. Ling, MD** [1,4,15,35]
Associate Professor and Director
Division of Gynecology
Department of OB/GYN
University of Tennessee, Memphis
Memphis, Tenn

**John R. Lurain III, MD** [33]
Professor
Department of OB/GYN
Northwestern University School of Medicine
Chicago, Ill

**David Muram, MD** [13]
Associate Professor
Chief, Section of Pediatric and Adolescent Gynecology
Department of OB/GYN
University of Tennessee, Memphis
Memphis, Tenn

**John R. Musich, MD** [5]
Chairman, Department of OB/GYN
William Beaumont Hospital
Royal Oak, Mich

**Gretajo Northrop, MD** [23]
Associate Professor
Department of Medicine and OB/GYN
Rush Medical College
Chicago, Ill

**Steven J. Ory, MD** [26]
Assistant Professor
Department of OB/GYN
Mayo Medical School
Rochester, Minn

**Domeena Renshaw, MD** [16]
Professor and Director
Department of Psychiatry/Sexual Dysfunction Clinic
Loyola University Stritch School of Medicine
Maywood, Ill

**Rebecca Rogers, PharmD** [App. A,B]
Assistant Professor
Clinical Pharmacy
University of Tennessee, Memphis
Memphis, Tenn

**Ira M. Rosenthal, MD** [24]
Clinical Professor of Pediatrics
Department of Pediatrics
Section of Pediatrics Endocrinology
Wyler Children's Hospital
Chicago, Ill

**W. Kirkland Ruffin, MD** [35]
Lieutenant Commander and Chairman
Department of General Surgery
Millington Naval Hospital
Millington, Tenn

**George M. Ryan, Jr., MD** [17]
Professor
Department of OB/GYN
University of Tennessee, Memphis
Memphis, Tenn

**Eldon D. Schriock, MD** [20]
Assistant Clinical Professor
Department of OB/GYN
University of California, College of Medicine, San Francisco
San Francisco, Calif

**Barbara F. Sharf, MD** [1]
Associate Professor
Department of Medical Education
University of Illinois
Chicago, Ill

**Roger P. Smith, MD** [2,14]
Associate Professor/Chief
Department of OB/GYN, Division of General OB/GYN
Medical College of Georgia
Augusta, Ga

**Irvin K. Stone, MD** [3]
Associate Professor and Director
Department of OB/GYN, Division of Gynecology
University of Florida College of Medicine
Gainesville, Fla

**Thomas G. Stovall, MD** [5,11,12,34,35]
Assistant Professor
Department of OB/GYN, Division of Gynecology
University of Tennessee, Memphis
Memphis, Tenn

**Paul G. Stumpf, MD** [21]
Project Director
Department of OB/GYN
Jersey Shore Medical Center
Neptune, NJ

**Robert L. Summitt, Jr., MD** [9,10,34,35]
Assistant Professor
Department of OB/GYN, Division of Gynecology
University of Tennessee, Memphis
Memphis, Tenn

**Jessica L. Thomason, MD** [6,19]
Professor and Chief
Division of Infectious Diseases
Department of OB/GYN
Sinai Samaritan Medical Center
Milwaukee, Wis

**Joyce M. Vargyas, MD** [15]
Associate Director
Department of Reproductive Endocrinology
Institute of Medicine for Reproductive Health
Los Angeles, Calif

# Foreword

Gynecology in the 1990s is an exciting specialty, pivotal to almost all of medicine. Indeed, women comprise half of the population, and particularly in younger women gynecologic problems are never far from the horizon. Conversely, gynecological disorders interact with a host of disorders from other medical disciplines—psychiatry, internal medicine, general surgery, and pediatrics. The age groups of gynecologic concerns extend from the neonatal to the geriatric years. Even if physicians did not accept the pivotal role of gynecology, patients would remind us. Gynecological problems are the current darlings of the media—contraception, infection and AIDS, infertility, menopause. Moreover, today's patients are not only desirably well informed but often demanding.

Concomitant to the increased interest in gynecology by the public and the medical profession alike has been marked advances in the scientific basis and thus clinical characterization and treatment for gynecological disorders. In previous decades, gynecological disorders received relatively little scientific attention, perhaps because the specialty as a whole did not emphasize academic pursuits. This inevitably meant that gynecological diseases imparted to many the comfortable, albeit not satisfying, air of immutability. Not so at present. The host of new scientific advances and new clinical investigations means new and better diagnostic and treatment modalities.

Yet these advances are not without responsibilities. Every physician wants to offer his or her best effort. Keeping up with gynecologic advances is enervating, especially for the student, physician-in-training and the nongynecologist. Although existing texts are lucid and accurate, they often prove laborious to the uninitiated and to those pressed to refresh one's memory concerning a disease manifested by a patient in the next room. In particular, exhaustive gynecologic texts are not realistic to the nongynecologist.

The editors of *Clinical Manual of Gynecology* have addressed the above dilemmas in this crisp volume. As a group, they are complete gynecologists. As individuals, they represent expertise in sub-specialties of pelvic surgery, urogynecology, medical education, and psychosomatic medicine. Contributors complement the editors' expertise, representing still other areas of gynecology. Throughout the volume the reader is provided with the essential scientific basis for understanding current diagnostic criteria and treatment.

This manual is easy to read, yet eschews overly simplistic approaches. *Clinical Manual of Gynecology* should find a place on the shelves (and pockets of white coats!) of students, house officers, and attending physicians.

Joe Leigh Simpson, MD
Faculty Professor and Chairman
University of Tennessee, Memphis

# Preface

Here is a guide for the clinician who is involved with the health care of women. For this revised edition we have updated the information to reflect current practice and to emphasize the immediacy and practical nature of the content. Its outline format and pocket size are designed for maximum usability and accessibility. We believe that residents, staff, and faculty of obstetrics and gynecology, medicine, surgery, emergency medicine, and family medicine will find this text useful. Each chapter was written with the practical management of gynecologic patients as a primary focus. A thorough review of pathophysiology and complete differentials are not included, but we have attempted to provide information that is needed from a practical standpoint. We believe that this balance of information will be helpful.

This work is the result of the efforts of many authors, who have worked numerous hours on their contributions. We wish to thank our secretaries, Martha Mitchum and Ruthe Brady, for their input into manuscript preparation. In addition, we wish to give praise to Jill Keir and Nat Russo for their editorial advice and help with production.

We welcome your feedback on this work as we look to continually improve its quality and practicality.

We wish to dedicate this book to our wives, Donna, Peggy, Claudia, and Janis, and to our children, Elliott, Elizabeth, David, Katherine, Mandy, and Trevor.

# Part I

# General Care of the Patient

# CHAPTER 1

# History and Physical Examination

**Charles R. B. Beckmann**
**Frank W. Ling**
**Barbara M. Barzansky**
**Barbara F. Sharf**
**Daniel L. Clarke-Pearson**

Interacting with the patient in a confident personal manner will allow for a relaxed examination and a professional future relationship. The history and physical examination is important not only to obtain information, but also to allow opportunity to develop a professional rapport with the patient.

**I. Initial interaction with the patient**

- **A. Setting.** A private setting is important for history taking. Good eye contact and communication in addition to having the clinician seated at the same level as the patient is essential.
- **B. Greetings and getting started.** Greeting with a handshake is mannerly yet demonstrates warmth. Using surnames is best, although some clinicians find it useful to ask the patient how she would like to be addressed. "How may I help you today?" is an example of a useful neutral question. Taking notes while interviewing the patient is not a distraction if preceded by an explanatory statement.
- **C. Personal or embarrassing topics.** Many issues (such as sexually transmitted diseases) may evoke strong emotional responses. Such responses can be avoided in most cases by an explanatory preamble such as: "I must ask some questions which are quite personal. I am not doing so to pry into your private life. I am just seeking the information I need to provide you with the best health care." Such a preamble is not needed in all cases.

**II. History**

- **A. The chief complaint** is the reason for the patient's visit. It should be presented in proper chronological sequence.
- **B. Menstrual history**
  1. **Menarche** is the age at which menses began. The first few menses may be quite irregular in character.
  2. **Menstrual history** includes the duration, frequency of, and interval between menstrual periods. The last menstrual peri-

od (LMP) is dated from the first day of the last normal menses. Any intermenstrual bleeding or contact bleeding should be noted. Menstrual flow can be estimated by the number of pads or tampons used during menses or the size of menstrual clots if passed. Menstrual pain is abnormal when it interferes with normal daily activities. Perimenstrual symptoms (e.g., fluid retention, anxiety) should be noted.

3. **The climacteric** includes irregularity in menstrual frequency and duration often associated with hot flashes, mood changes, and dry mucous membranes. A history of hormonal or psychoactive medications is important. Surgical or medical oophorectomy should be noted.
4. **Postmenopausal bleeding** (bleeding 6 months after cessation of menses) should be documented or stated as a pertinent negative.

C. **Obstetric history** includes the number of pregnancies (gravidity) and outcomes of each (parity) and is abbreviated by:

Gravida (G) **a** Para (P) **b c d e**

where: a = Number of pregnancies; b = Number of term pregnancies; c = Number of preterm pregnancies; d = Number of abortions (spontaneous or induced) and ectopic pregnancies; e = Number of living children. Specific information about each listing above should be included.

D. **Gynecologic history**

1. **Breast history** should include previous or existing breast disease, history of breast feeding, the use of breast self-examination techniques, previous mammography or breast biopsy, and a family history of breast cancer.
2. **Previous gynecologic surgery.** Questions should include type of surgery, for what reason, when, where, and by whom, and results. Surgical records should be obtained.
3. **Infectious diseases.** Vaginitis and other diseases local to the vagina should be reviewed as to the characteristics, frequency, duration and treatment. Past history of sexually transmitted diseases should be documented including episodes of pelvic inflammatory disease (PID).
4. **A history of infertility** should include questions about previous diseases or surgery that may affect fertility, previous pregnancies, and duration of time in which pregnancy has been attempted (but not achieved).
5. **Diethylstilbestrol (DES)** use by the patient's mother during her pregnancy should be noted.

E. **Sexual/contraceptive history**

1. **Sexual history.** Data to be elicited should include:
   a. Age at first intercourse
   b. The patient's present sexual partner(s) and their sex
   c. Types of sexual practices
   d. Level of satisfaction with their sex lives
2. **Contraceptive history** should include the contraceptive method currently used, the reason for its choice, when

begun, any problems or complications, and the patient's and her partner's satisfaction with the method. Previous contraceptive methods should also be noted.

3. **Child and adult sexual abuse and assault**. Inquiry about past or present sexual abuse or assault should be made of all patients, especially those with recurrent nonspecific gynecological complaints, nonsomatic sexual dysfunction, and unusually phobic responses to gynecologic health care.

## III. Physical examination

A. **General principles**. The patient should be asked to empty her bladder and to don the gown provided.

1. **Assistance**. An assistant must be present for the pelvic examination to assist in the preparation of specimens and as a chaperone. A chaperone is important in these litigious times for the genital examination of any patient.
2. **Explanation of procedures to the patient**. Procedures should be thoroughly explained to the patient before they are performed. Such explanation decreases anxiety and helps the patient to relax.

B. **Generalized written report format**. Organs and potentially pathologic findings (such as masses, discharges, lesions, etc.), should be described as appropriate: color, consistency, shape, size, tenderness, mobility, odor, relationship to other structures, and anatomic location.

1. Breast
2. Abdomen
3. Pelvic examination
   a. Vulva
   b. Clitoris
   c. Bartholin's, urethral, and Skene's glands
   d. Vagina
   e. Cervix. Pap smear or cultures performed should be noted
   f. Uterus
   g. Adnexa
   h. Rectovaginal. A stool guaiac test should be performed

## IV. Breast examination. See Figure 1.1

A. **Inspection** is done with the patient's arms at her side and then raised over her head. Tumors may distort the relationships of the breast's support tissues so that these movements disrupt the shape, contour, or symmetry of the breast.

B. **Palpation.** The breasts are also palpated with the patient's arms at her side and then raised over her head in the sitting and then supine positions. Palpation should be done using the flat of the fingers and not the tips. A spiral pattern is described over each breast so as to uniformly cover all of the breast tissue, including that of the axillary tail. If nodules are found, their size, shape, consistency, mobility, tenderness, and location should be noted.

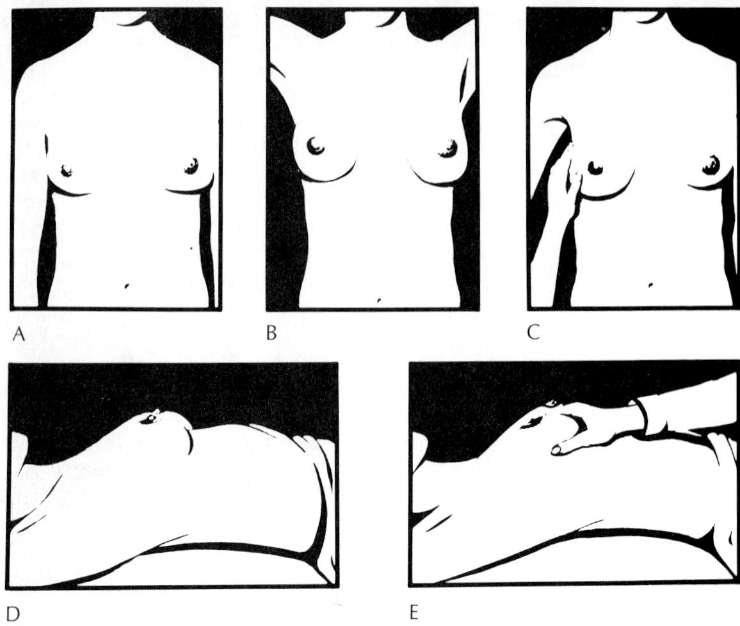


FIGURE 1.1. The breast examination. (A and B) Inspection of the breast with arms at rest and raised. (C) Palpation of the axilla with the arm in slight extension. (D and E) Positions for palpation of the outer and inner halves of the breast.

Gentle pressure inward and then upward at the sides of the areola should be applied to express any fluid present. If fluid is expressed, it should be sent for culture and sensitivity and cytopathology.

C. **Breast self-examination (BSE).** All women should be instructed in BSE and encouraged to do so monthly, usually a week after the menses when the breasts are not tender or more nodular as they are in the menstrual time. The technique is a simplified version of the physician's examination. The patient should lie with a towel or pillow under her shoulder so that the breast lies flat on the chest. Examination should be done starting at the nipple and moving outward in ever-widening circles until all the breast has been palpated. The right hand is used to examine the left breast and the left, the right breast. The patient is told to use the flat of her fingers rather than the tips. A similar examination while showering or bathing is also useful. The patient should then be instructed to stand in front of a mirror, examining her breasts for swelling, bumps, dimples, and irregularities on the skin or breast contour, first with her arms at her sides and then with them raised over her head with her hands clasped. The patient should be instructed to look for changes, not to try to duplicate the physician's examination, and to report any changes as soon as they are noticed.

V. **Pelvic examination — procedure.** Ask the patient to sit at the edge of the examining table. Place an opened draping sheet over the patient's knees unless she requests otherwise.

A. **Positioning and patient preparation**

1. **Patient positioning**

a. **Helping the patient assume the lithotomy position.** The examining table's head should be raised 30°. The patient should be asked to lie back, place her heels in the stirrups, and move down to the end of the table until her buttocks are at the edge of the table.

b. **Draping** should cover the legs yet not obstruct the clinician's view. Some patients may prefer no drape.

2. **Position of examination light.** The lamp should be positioned in the front of the clinician's chest at the level of the perineum so that the light is directed on the perineum (Fig. 1.2).

B. **Gloving.** Both hands should be gloved; there should be minimal contact with equipment after gloves are doned. A clean glove should be used on the hand used for the rectovaginal examination.

C. **Inspection and examination of the external genitalia**

1. **Initial maneuvers and general principles.** After telling the patient you are going to touch her, place the back of your

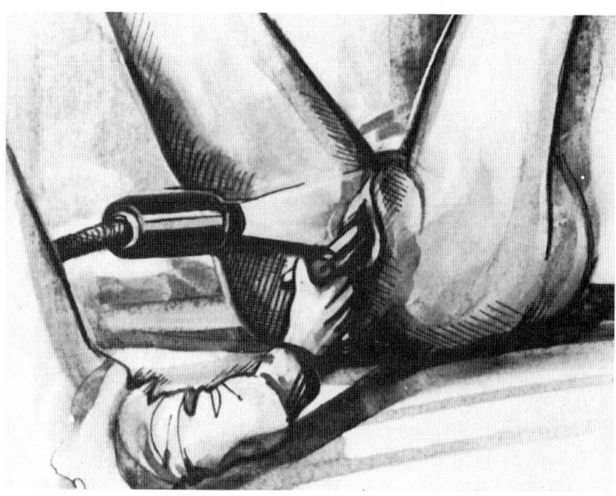

FIGURE 1.2. Position of light for speculum examination.

hands on the patient's lower inner thigh and thereafter quickly move to sequential inspection and palpation of the external genitalia.

2. **Examination of specific structures of the external genitalia**
   a. **Mons.** Inspect the mons for lesions, parasites, and evidence of irritation.
   b. **Clitoris.**
   c. **Labium majus and minus.** Inspect the introitus, the urethral opening, and the areas of the urethral and Skene's glands. Palpate the Bartholin's gland area between a finger in the vagina and the thumb.
   d. **Rectum and perirectal area.**

**D. Speculum examination**

1. **Speculum selection and preparation.** The narrow blades of the Pederson speculum work well for most nulliparous women, whereas parous women can accommodate a medium Graves speculum which has wider blades. Large specula are available for patients with pelvic relaxation (Fig. 1.3). Pediatric specula are usually reserved for young children or patients with vaginal stenosis (Fig. 1.4). The speculum should be warmed before use.
2. **Insertion of the speculum and visualization of the cervix** (see Fig. 1.5).

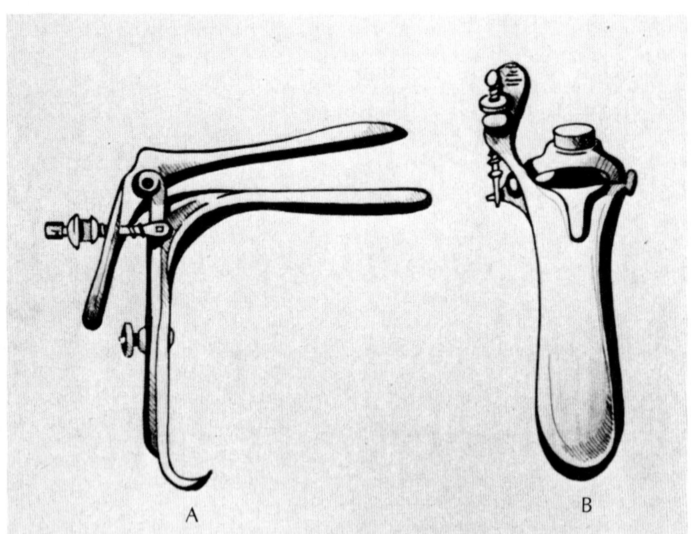


FIGURE 1.3. Adult-sized specula. (A) Medium Graves speculum. (B) Medium Pederson speculum.

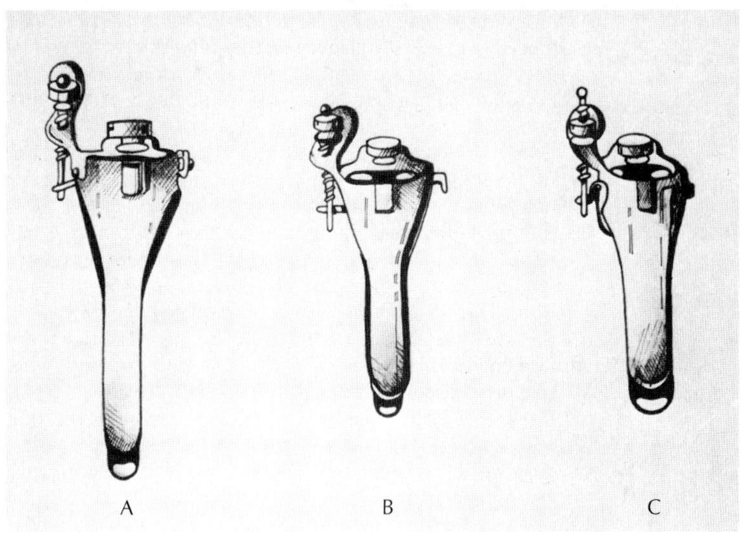


FIGURE 1.4. Pediatric specula. (A) Pediatric Pederson speculum. (B) Pediatric Graves speculum. (C) Pediatric Pederson speculum with extra-narrow blades.

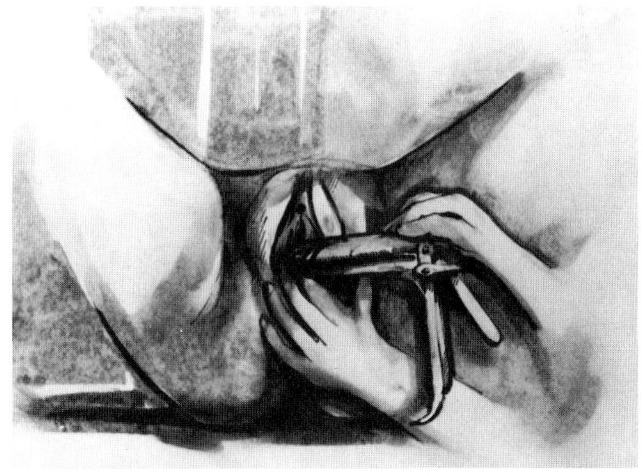

FIGURE 1.5. Speculum insertion.

a. Hold the speculum by the handle with the blades completely closed. Moistening the speculum with water may help with insertion. Lubricants, which may contaminate specimens that are collected, should be avoided.
b. The introitus is opened by gentle downward pressure on the perineum. The speculum is inserted at about a 45° angle from the horizontal. The speculum should pass the full length of the vagina with little resistance. Care should be taken not to put pressure on the sensitive structures superior to the speculum.
c. The cervix will move into view between the blades of the speculum as it is opened. The speculum is then locked into the open position. The patient should be reassured that sensations of the need to urinate are from the speculum. Failure to find the cervix may result from not having the speculum inserted far enough or by withdrawing the speculum slightly as the speculum is opened.
d. For most patients, the speculum is opened sufficiently by use of the upper thumb screw. More space may be obtained, if needed, by expanding the vertical distance between the blades by use of the thumb screw on the speculum handle.
e. After speculum placement, inspect the cervix and vaginal walls. Obtain a Papanicolaou's (PAP) smear and cultures for sexually transmitted diseases if needed. (see obtaining the PAP smear section, VI)

3. **Speculum withdrawal and inspection of the vaginal walls.** After telling the patient that the speculum is to be removed, open the blades slightly to avoid catching the cervix between the blades. The speculum is withdrawn slowly to allow inspection of the vaginal walls. As the end of the speculum blades approach the introitus, there should be no pressure on the thumb hinge so that the speculum blades do not hit the sensitive vaginal, urethral, and clitoral tissues.

E. **Bimanual examination**

1. **General procedures.** Two fingers are inserted into the vagina until they are in the posterior fornix behind and below the cervix. Use a sufficient amount of lubricant to facilitate examination. Additional space may be found by downward distention of the perineum, but never upward pressure which will cause pain by crushing tissue against the pubic arch. Many clinicians find it useful to rest the elbow of the vaginal hand on the leg or knee.
2. **Examination of the pelvic organs**
   a. **The cervix** should be examined for its size, shape, position, mobility, and the presence or absence of tenderness or mass lesions.

b. **The uterus** is evaluated for its size, shape, consistency, configuration, and mobility, as well as masses or tenderness and for position (anteversion, midposition, retroversion, anteflexion, retroflexion).

c. **The adnexae** are palpated to assess the ovaries, fallopian tubes, and support structures. Examination begins by placing the vaginal fingers to the side of the cervix deep in the lateral fornix. The abdominal hand is moved to the same position over the adnexae. The adnexae are palpated by upward pressure for the vaginal fingers and downward pressure from the abdominal fingers. Adnexal structures are evaluated for size, shape, consistency, configuration, mobility, and tenderness, as well as for masses. The ovaries are palpable in the normal menstrual woman about one-half of the time and are not normally palpable in postmenopausal women in whom a palpable mass requires further evaluation. Excessive pressure on the ovaries should be avoided, as it will cause pain.

**F. Rectovaginal examination** allows evaluation of the posterior aspect of the pelvic structures. A pelvic examination without the rectovaginal component is incomplete. Because the rectovaginal examination is not comfortable, an explanation of the importance of the examination is appropriate. The steps of the procedure are:

1. Don a new glove with a liberal supply of lubricant.
2. Insert the second finger into the rectal canal, first at about a 45° angle for about 1 to 2 cm, then downward. This maneuver allows the finger to follow the anatomic course of the rectal canal.
3. The index finger is then inserted into the vagina and both fingers are inserted until the pelvic structures are palpable.
4. Palpation of the pelvic structures is then accomplished as in their vaginal palpation. Palpate the uterosacral ligaments to determine if they are symmetrical, smooth, and nontender or if they are nodular, slack, or thickened. The rectal canal is evaluated as in any rectal examination with particular attention to the integrity and function of the rectal sphincter.
5. A guaiac determination is made from fecal material collected on the rectal finger.

## VI. The PAP smear

### A. Obtaining the PAP smear

1. **Specimens** are collected from the exocervix and endocervix which allows full evaluation of the transformation zone.

   a. **The exocervical sample** is obtained by rotating a wooden or plastic spatula around the exocervix (see Fig. 1.6). The spatula is then lightly pressed onto a premarked slide which is immediately fixed (Fig. 1.7).

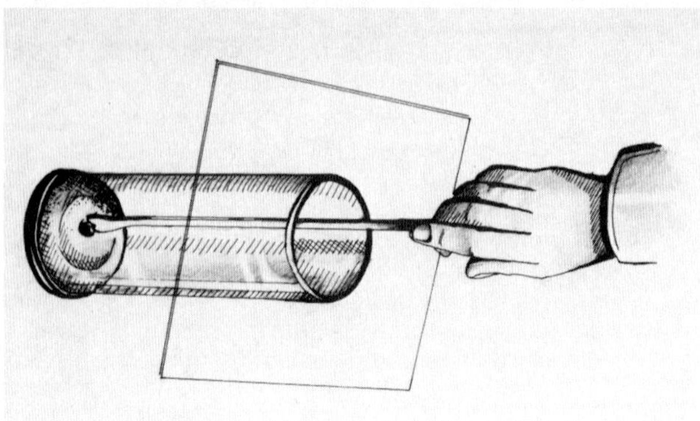

FIGURE 1.6. Obtaining the exocervical specimen is done by gently twirling a wooden spatula a few revolutions on the outer portion of the cervix.

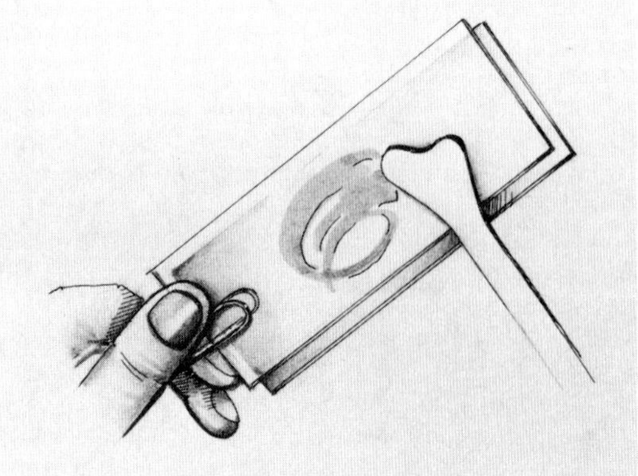

FIGURE 1.7. Placing the Papanicolaou (PAP) specimen onto the glass slide. The wooden spatula is gently pressed against the glass slide so that the material is transferred to the glass slide with minimal damage.

   b. **The endocervical sample** is obtained in a similar manner using the traditional moistened cotton swab or by using one of the newer brush-type sampling devices.
   c. **The vaginal sample.** A vaginal lesion or the vaginal wall of a patient exposed to diethylstilbestrol in utero is sampled by scraping the lesion with a second spatula, fixing the specimen immediately after it is obtained.
2. **Fixing and handling the specimens.** Immediate fixation is important to avoid air drying artifacts that may compromise cytopathologic evaluation. Lubricating gel and talcum powder should be avoided as they cause distortion and reduce

the quality of PAP smears. Slides left in air longer than 10 seconds demonstrate a high incidence of such artifacts.

## BIBLIOGRAPHY

Beckmann CRB, Clarke-Pearson D, Evenhouse R. A reusable plastic training model for teaching PAP smear technique. Am J Obstet Gynecol. 1987; 157:259–260.

# CHAPTER 2

# Care of the Hospitalized Patient

**Roger P. Smith**
**Barbara M. Barzansky**

The almost sacred trust placed in the physician by the patient requires more than just caring for the specific disease process at hand. It requires a total commitment to the well-being of the patient. The physician must maintain effective treatment of their disease, while protecting them from further physical, emotional, and financial harm through the application of knowledge, skills, compassion, and understanding.

In the hospital setting the patient's life is under the physician's control. Most of the time, care will be dictated by the condition necessitating hospital admission. This dictates much of the care the patient receives but does not relieve the obligation for care in the broader sense. Attention to detail and the needs of the patient in ways other than the disease at hand is constantly required.

**I. Routine admitting orders** will vary according to the patient's condition, disease process, and planned procedures. It is best to write orders in a specific sequence so that nothing is inadvertently omitted. One such sequence is as follows:

- **A.** Vital signs
- **B.** Activity
- **C.** Nursing (special care)
- **D.** Diet
- **E.** Intravenous fluids
- **F.** Fluid intake and output
- **G.** Special medications
- **H.** Sleep and other routine medications
- **I.** Diagnostic examinations
- **J.** Laboratory studies

**A. Vital signs** (pulse, respirations, blood pressure, temperature) should be ordered based upon the condition of the patient. Acutely ill patients require frequent assessment (q15 min, q30 min, q1 h, q2 h). Patients admitted for elective or preoperative evaluation may have evaluations made less frequently. The use of a b.i.d., t.i.d. (usually q shift) or q.i.d. schedule will prevent the patient from being awakened during the night.

B. **Activity.** Unrestricted activity (up ad lib) is appropriate for most patients before surgery or for those whose condition does not warrant special restrictions. Restrictions such as bed rest (with or without bathroom privileges) or special bed positions (such as semi-Fowler's or Trendelenburg positions) are specified in this section of the orders.

C. **Nursing.** This section contains special requests of the nursing staff regarding such matters as wound care, catheter drainage and care, skin care, and so on.

D. **Diet.** A regular (general) diet is appropriate for most patients except when the patient's condition, pending surgical procedures, or specialized tests (radiographic) are planned. Patients should be restricted to nothing by mouth (NPO) for at least 8 to 12 hours prior to surgical procedures. For some radiographic procedures or where eventual surgery involving the bowel is anticipated, a clear liquid diet should be specified. Special diets such as restricted sodium, diabetic or calorie controlled diets may be required. Consultation with a dietitian should be considered when in doubt.

E. **Intravenous fluids.** Patients requiring parenteral medications (e.g., antibiotics) or who are unable to eat (e.g., immediately postop) will require intravenous fluids. The rate of administration will depend on the patient's ability to take p.o. nutrition. The choice of fluid will depend on the patient's clinical situation and overall medical status.

F. **Fluid intake and output.** The recording of fluid intake and output is important to the management of the acutely ill or postoperative patient. The frequency of recording should be specified. Special instructions about notification in case of variance from expected output must be specific (e.g., notify if urinary output is less than 25 cc per hour, notify service if nasogastric [NG] suction > 100 mL/h).

G. **Special medications.** In addition to therapeutic medications dictated by the patient's condition, any medications that the patient is taking at the time of admission to the hospital must be reordered. Careful reevaluation of the need for these medications, possible interactions with new medications, and possible interference with planned tests and procedures are all required. Even if the patient has brought medication with her (and the hospital allows patients to keep bedside medication) each medication the patient will be taking must be written out in the orders, complete with dosage, route, and frequency.

H. **Sleep and other routine medications.** Medications for the comfort of the patient (analgesics, hypnotics, laxatives) should be specified.

I. **Diagnostic examinations.** Radiographic or other special studies (e.g., proctoscopy, sonography, electrocardiogram [ECG], electroencephalogram, pulmonary function) should be specified. The sequence of these examinations should be considered and specified when necessary (an intravenous pyelogram [IVP] should not immediately follow an upper gastrointestinal study, but the reverse can often be done).

J. **Laboratory studies.** Both routine admission studies as required by the individual hospital and those laboratory studies mandated by the patient's diagnosis and condition must be written out. It is wise to list those studies that have been carried out during the process of admission to avoid duplication (e.g., complete blood count [CBC] — Done).

II. **Preoperative considerations.** For surgery patients, several considerations are necessary before the patient may safely be moved to the operating room. These steps may be carried out rapidly in cases of acute distress, or may require several days of hospital care before all the necessary preparations are complete. These steps follow.

   A. Determining the appropriate procedure(s)
   B. Preoperative evaluations
   C. Informed consent
   D. Preoperative note
   E. Preoperative preparation and orders

A. **Determining the appropriate procedure(s)**. For elective surgery the procedure usually has been determined in the outpatient setting before the patient's admission. Prior to the procedure reevaluating the plan, including the total care of the patient is advised. Is the procedure necessary (other management options)? Is it the best one for the patient? Are there alternative procedures that fit the patients' needs better (hysterectomy vs. tubal ligation)? Are there other procedures that should be done before the planned one (diagnostic laparoscopy prior to planning tubal surgery), at the same time (excision of a nevus), or after (special dietary consultation)? Most often these questions will not alter the planned course of operative management, but this reevaluation will insure that the most efficient, appropriate, and safest care is given.

B. **Preoperative evaluations** can be classified as:

   1. **Laboratory data.** Most hospitals have policies that dictate the minimum laboratory studies acceptable before surgery of any type. This generally consists of a complete blood count and urinalysis. Some require screening chemical profiles including electrolytes, blood urea nitrogen (BUN) creatinine, direct and/or indirect bilirubin, alkaline phosphatase, SGOT, SGPT, or others. Additional tests such as prothrombin time (PT), partial thromboplastin time (PTT), platelet count, radio plasma reagin (RPR) and blood typing may be required. Even if these are not required, they should be strongly considered based upon the patient's history (the use of diuretics that depress potassium, malnutrition, substance abuse) and condition (bleeding, ascites). Additional tests may be indicated by the general history the

patient provides (e.g., a history of thyroid disease might engender such tests as triiodothyronine ($T_3$), thyroxine ($T_4$), and thyrotropin (TSH).

2. **Imaging.** Most hospitals require a recent chest x-ray prior to surgery. Additional imaging with x-ray, tomography, ultrasound, or magnetic imaging may be required for complete preoperative evaluation.
3. **Organ system function.** Evaluation of the cardiac and pulmonary systems is required for all patients undergoing surgery and anesthesia. Any patient over the age of 35 or those with a history of cardiopulmonary disease should have an ECG prior to surgery. Pulmonary function studies should be carried out in any patient where compromise of pulmonary function either exists prior to surgery (kyphoscoliosis, chronic lung disease) or can be anticipated based upon the procedure planned (upper abdominal incision). Smokers should be advised to stop smoking 2 to 4 weeks in advance of their procedure and all patients undergoing major procedures will benefit by being acquainted with incentive spirometry prior to surgery. The function of other organ systems (renal, hepatic) should be evaluated as indicated by history and physical findings.
4. **Consultation(s)** with the anesthesiologist responsible for the care of the patient in the operating room is required. This allows the anesthesiologist to be familiar with the patient and the procedure planned. Many anesthesiologists prefer to write their own preoperative medication orders. Additional consultations for evaluation or management should be dictated by the patient's individual needs.

C. **Informed consent.** All surgery (and many invasive tests) require the patient's informed consent be given. This is not only a legal and moral obligation, but an important opportunity for patient education and improved rapport. Each institution will have its own consent form but all embody the same basic information. The final consent should indicate that the physician has discussed the planned procedure in enough detail to allow an "informed" decision regarding the procedure. This discussion should be in words that the patient can understand, should include the alternatives available, the expected outcome, and foreseeable complications. It should be balanced in its discussion of advantages and complications so as to neither frighten unnecessarily nor engender complacency. Adequate allowance for questions must be made and noted in the consent. Appropriate elements of the informed consent include:

1. Indications for a procedure (including the condition being treated).
2. Risks and benefits of the proposed procedure.
3. Alternative procedures or treatments with their risks and benefits.

4. Expected outcome of treatment.
5. Length of treatment, hospitalization or disability.

D. **A preoperative note** organizes and documents the preparation of surgery. The note should contain:
1. Preoperative diagnosis
2. Planned procedure
3. Planned anesthetic
4. Surgeon(s)
5. Preoperative laboratory findings
6. Preoperative imaging findings
7. Status of blood and/or special equipment

E. **Preoperative preparation and orders** will vary with the type and site of surgery and the condition of the patient. They will usually contain the following elements:
1. **Diet.** NPO after midnight for all patients. Specialized diets prior to that time as dictated by other needs (clear liquid if bowel surgery is possible, diabetic, etc.).
2. **Patient preparation** (often known as "shave and prep"). This should include any preparations necessary for the following:
   a. **Operative area.** It is not generally recommended that the operative area be routinely shaved. If hair removal is necessary for the area of incision, it should be done through the use of a depilatory (when possible) or clipping immediately prior to surgery. Washing the surgical area with an antiseptic soap the night before surgery has been advocated, however, the value of this has not been proven.
   b. **Bowel.** For most procedures mechanical cleansing of the colon with tap water enemas prior to surgery is all that is required. For procedures where bowel surgery is likely, a more thorough catharsis and antibiotic bowel preparation is advisable.
   c. **Vagina.** Vaginal cleansing with a povidone-iodine (Betadine®) douche has been suggested prior to vaginal surgery. Efficacy in reducing infection is lacking, but in the absence of contraindications (hypersensitivity), it is probably safe.
   d. **Bladder.** For all procedures have the patient void on call to the operating room. When a catheter is required, it may be inserted once the patient is asleep in the operating room.
3. **Preoperative medication** orders generally fall into the categories of:
   a. **Hypnotics.** A good night's sleep prior to surgery is desireable and should be insured with the use of a hypnotic, if not ordered by the anesthesia consultant. Drugs such as flurazepam hydrochloride (Dalmane®) 30 mg, triazolam (Halcion®) 0.25 mg, or secobarbital (Seconal®) 100 mg may be used. The order is best writ-

ten for a specific time (e.g., give medication at 11 P.M.) rather than as a p.r.n.

b. **Sedatives.** If not ordered by the anesthesiologist, sedation with the combination of meperidine (Demerol®) 50 mg, hydroxyzine (Vistaril®) 25 mg, and atropine 0.4 mg given on call to the operating room is recommended.

c. **Prophylaxis.** For potentially contaminated cases, including those involving opening the vagina to the peritoneum, antibiotic prophylaxis on call to the operating room has been proven effective in reducing infections. For the patient at risk for thrombo-embolic complications, prophylaxis with "mini-dose" heparin should be considered preoperatively (5000 U subcutaneous [SQ] b.i.d.).

d. **Therapeutic medications** that require maintenance during the operative procedure (insulin, dilantin, digitalis) must be specified along with any alteration in the dose or route of administration.

4. **Preoperative laboratory and blood** studies required prior to surgery should be specified along with any special instructions concerning the time of the test or disposition of the results. For patients with significant anemia or for any procedure where there is a good possibility of more than 500 mL of blood loss, type and cross matching of blood (packed cells) is indicated (usually 2 to 6 U depending upon the procedure planned). For any patient with a hemoglobin of less than 10 g or a hematocrit of less than 30%, preoperative transfusion should be strongly considered. Because of the risks associated with transfusion, autologous blood donation or donation by designated donors should be considered where possible.

## III. Postoperative considerations

**A. Postoperative note.** Immediately following surgery, a postoperative note and orders are required. The postoperative note should include the following information:

1. Preoperative diagnosis
2. Postoperative diagnosis
3. Procedure
4. Surgeon assistant(s)
5. Anesthesia
6. Findings
7. Fluids given during the case
8. Tubes and drains
9. Estimated blood loss
10. Complications
11. Disposition and condition of patient

With respect to the patient's long-term care, the "procedure" and "findings" sections are most important. Both need to be recorded in detail to provide all the information needed for future care. The findings section is often left out or is incomplete. A complete statement of findings is one mark of the superior surgeon.

**B. Postoperative orders.** Following a surgical procedure all previous orders are suspended, therefore, postoperative orders must include not only those orders specific to the immediate postoperative care required, but also any preoperative orders that are to be continued. The format of postoperative orders will be similar to that of admitting orders, but with slight additions:

1. Vital signs
2. Activity
3. Nursing (special care)
4. Diet
5. Fluid intake and output
6. Intravenous fluids
7. Pain medications
8. Sleep and other routine medications
9. Special medications
10. Respiratory care
11. Laboratory studies

1. **Vital signs** (pulse, respirations, blood pressure (BP), temperature) should be ordered based upon the condition of the patient. The frequency of these observations is generally decreased as the patient awakens from the procedure (q15 min in recovery room, q30 min × 2, then q1 h × 2, then q4 h after the patients returns to the floor). If the physician is to be notified for any abnormal findings, they should be specified here (notify physician if BP < 100/60 or pulse > 100 beats/min).
2. **Activity.** Bed rest is usually indicated until the patient is fully awake after minor procedures. For more major procedures, early progressively increasing activity should be ordered as consistent with the patient's condition.
3. **Nursing.** Special orders regarding catheter or drain care, patient positioning and so on must be specified. Additional requests (such as for excessive wound drainage) should be indicated here.
4. **Diet.** For patients who have undergone minor surgery, a return to a general diet when awake is generally appropriate. For patients who have had major surgery, especially when the bowel has been handled to any degree, the diet may be gradually advanced as tolerated, beginning on the second postoperative day (if bowel sounds are present).
5. **Fluid intake and output.** The frequency of recording should be specified. Special instructions about notification in case of variance from expected output must be specific (notify service if urinary output is less than 25 cc/h, notify service if NG suction > 100 mL/h).

6. **Intravenous fluids.** For normal postoperative maintenance dextrose 5% in Ringer's lactate at a rate of 125 mL/h will generally be sufficient. The rate and character of the fluids must be modified based on operative blood loss, fluid loss from nasogastric suction, drains, or "third spacing" (ileus, edema) and the patient's cardiopulmonary and renal status.
7. **Pain medications.** Analgesics in appropriate amounts, routes and frequencies must be provided to allow postoperative pain relief. Studies indicate improved analgesia are given early in the postoperative period and continued on a regular basis to avoid the development of significant discomfort (meperidine [Demerol] 75 mg IM q3 h p.r.n., morphine sulfate 10 mg IM q3 h p.r.n.).
8. **Sleep and other routine medications.** Hypnotics, laxatives, and any preoperative medications that are to be resumed after surgery must be reordered.
9. **Special medications.** Antibiotics, anticoagulants, sedatives, medications for nausea, or other specific medications.
10. **Respiratory care.** For at least the first 24 hours after surgery, some form of respiratory care is appropriate. This may range from encouragement (turn, cough, and deep breath q2 h, incentive spirometry q4 h) to supportive (e.g., intermittent positive pressure breathing with ultrasonic nebulizer × 15 min q4 h).
11. **Laboratory studies.** Postoperative laboratory studies to monitor the patient's status and response to the procedure should be specified along with the time the test is desired and any special instructions regarding the reporting of the results (CBC in A.M.—call results to floor).

C. **Postoperative rounds** should be made at least daily with appropriate notations in the medical record indicating attention to:
   1. Review of chart and objective data
   2. Patient complaints and observations
   3. Physical findings
   4. Treatment plan

1. **Review of chart and objective data.** Frequent review of the chart records of vital signs, intake and output, nursing notes, and returning laboratory results will often identify significant changes. Many physicians ignore the nursing notes, but in so doing miss important information provided by the health-care team member who spends the most time with the patient and is therefore most likely to notice important details that may affect the care of the patient.
2. **Patient complaints and observations** should include the location and character of pain, the presence of vaginal or wound drainage, bowel movements or the passage of flatus, difficulty or pain on voiding, productive cough, or how oral intake has been tolerated.

3. **Physical findings.** These should include pertinent negative findings as well as any positive ones. Notations about the character of lung sounds, presence of bowel sounds, degree of softness or tenderness of the abdomen, presence of calf swelling, condition of the dressing, and so on, have great significance.
4. **Treatment plan.** Notations about planned management is not only important as an aid to formulating your thoughts, but also serves as an alert to important changes in management for others who may care for the patient.

# CHAPTER 3

# Shock in the Gynecologic Patient

**Irvin K. Stone (Hemorrhagic Shock)**
**Patrick Duff (Septic Shock)**

Shock is a hemodynamic disorder characterized by diminished perfusion of vital organ systems, resulting in tissue hypoxia and, ultimately, anoxia and acidosis. The three most common causes of shock are hypovolemia (hemorrhagic shock), myocardial infarction, and sepsis. This chapter will review hypovolemic and septic shock.

## HEMORRHAGIC SHOCK

Hemorrhagic shock is a state of diminished organ perfusion resulting from profuse blood loss. Depending upon the degree of blood loss and subsequent lack of perfusion, organ malfunction may be transient or permanent. The female reproduction tract, although accustomed to repetitive episodes of minor blood loss, may be the source of life-threatening hemorrhage. The gynecologic surgeon must be prepared to deal with this event in a timely efficient manner. Although reversal of the perfusion disorder is of primary importance, correction of the inciting event usually requires surgical intervention. Therefore, hemorrhagic shock should be considered primarily a surgical disorder.

The function and anatomy of the pelvic organs predispose them to excessive blood loss. Of primary importance is the extensive system of anastomosing vessels in the pelvis. These anastomoses allow collateral circulation within and between three major vascular networks.

1. Lumbar-iliolumbar arteries
2. Middle sacral-lateral sacral arteries
3. Superior rectal-middle rectal arteries

In addition, the valveless portal vein can shunt blood into the pelvis by the inferior mesenteric and superior rectal veins. Because of this extensive collateral circulation, minor disruptions in vessel integrity may result in significant blood loss.

**I. Etiology.** Hemorrhagic shock originating in the lower reproductive tract usually is secondary to trauma. In the upper genital tract ectopic pregnancy and neoplastic processes are the most common causes of hemorrhage. Iatrogenic hemorrhagic shock may result from unintentional trauma (e.g., uterine perforation or vessel injury during surgery) or intentional trauma (e.g., radical surgery). Shock may occur intraoperatively or postoperatively. In the latter instance, it may be due to inadequate blood replacement or continued blood loss from the operative field.

**II. Pathophysiology.** Symptoms of acute blood loss are a function of the amount of blood lost and the body's ability to compensate for hypovolemia. When hemorrhage occurs, pressure-sensitive baroreceptors in the aortic arch transmit impulses to the hypothalamic sympathetic centers. These, in turn, initiate release of epinephrine from the adrenal gland and norepinephrine from postganglionic nerve endings. In response to these compounds, vasoconstriction of the cutaneous and splanchnic beds occurs and heart rate and myocardial contractility increase. Precapillary and postcapillary vasoconstriction results in decreased capillary hydrostatic pressure and impaired tissue perfusion.

Hemorrhagic shock may be divided into four classes. The clinical manifestations associated with each class of hemorrhagic shock are summarized in Table 3.1.

**A. Class I hemorrhage.** With mild hemorrhage of less than 750 cc, autoregulatory mechanisms suffice to maintain organ perfusion, providing that the hemorrhage is controlled. Symptoms

**Table 3.1. Classification of Hemorrhagic Shock**

| ITEM | CLASS I | CLASS II | CLASS III | CLASS IV |
|---|---|---|---|---|
| Blood loss (mL) | up to 750 | 750–1500 | 1500–2000 | 2000 or more |
| Blood loss (%BV) | up to 15 | 15–30 | 30–40 | 40 or more |
| Pulse rate | < 100 | > 100 | > 120 | 140 or higher |
| Blood pressure (mm Hg) | Normal | Normal | Moderately decreased | Severely decreased |
| Pulse pressure (mm Hg) | Normal or increased | Mildly decreased | Moderately decreased | Severely decreased |
| Capillary refill test | Normal | Positive | Positive | Positive |
| Respiratory rate | 14–20 (normal) | 20–30 | 30–40 | > 35 |
| Urine output (mL/hr) | 30 or more | 20–30 | 5–15 | Negligible |
| CNS–mental status | Slightly anxious | Mildly anxious | Anxious and confused | Confused—lethargic |

Adapted with permission from the American College of Surgeons Committee on Trauma. Advanced Trauma Life Support (ATLS™) Student Manual. Tacoma, Wash: American College of Surgeons; 1988.

are usually referred to the organ associated with the blood loss (e.g., vulvar pain associated with hematoma formation, peritoneal irritation associated with a leaking ectopic pregnancy). Heart rate is increased, but blood pressure (BP) usually is normal. Capillary blanching, created by compressing the patient's fingernail, promptly resolves when compression ceases.

**B. Class II hemorrhage.** With blood loss of 1000 to 1250 mL, sustained catecholamine release will cause increased peripheral vasoconstriction. This will be reflected in a decrease in pulse pressure. The time for capillary refill is increased.

**C. Class III hemorrhage.** If blood loss is 1500 to 1800 mL, and replacement is not adequate, decreased tissue perfusion results in the development of systemic lactic acidosis. In response to declining pH, the precapillary arterioles relax, but the postcapillary venules remain constricted. This, in turn, results in increased hydrostatic pressure in the capillary beds. Intravascular fluid extravasates into the interstitial space, and SBP decreases. Renal blood flow decreases, and the renin–angiotensin system is activated. At this point, if volume replacement is not adequate, autoregulatory mechanisms no longer are effective in maintaining hemodynamic stability.

**D. Class IV hemorrhage.** Massive blood loss exceeding 2000 mL ultimately will result in a severe systemic metabolic lactic acidosis. Cellular integrity is lost, and irreversible vasomotor collapse occurs. Disseminated intravascular coagulation is a frequent complication of end-stage shock.

## III. Management

**A. Oxygenation and ventilation.** Patients in shock are hypoxic and, accordingly, should receive supplemental oxygen. The mode of oxygen delivery should be determined by the patient's level of consciousness. For the conscious patient, oxygen should be administered by face mask at 6 to 8 L/min. Intubation and mechanical ventilation will be necessary for the unconscious patient.

**B. Fluid resuscitation**

**1. Procedure**

a. A large-bore intravenous catheter (14–16 gauge) should be inserted peripherally in the forearm or antecubital fossa. In cases of severe shock, two sites of venous access should be secured.

b. If necessary to obtain venous access, a cutdown should be performed. Except in unusual circumstances, catheterization of the subclavian or internal jugular vein should be reserved for hemodynamic monitoring and should not be used for fluid replacement. At the time that the intravenous catheters are placed, blood should be obtained for hematocrit determination, coagulation profile, and type and crossmatch.

c. As a general rule, 3 cc of crystalloid should be administered for every 1 cc of blood loss. Ringer's lactate or normal saline are the preferred fluids for initial volume expansion. The speed with which fluid is infused should be based upon the volume of estimated blood loss and the promptness of the hemodynamic response to intravascular repletion. Administer fluids in small increments of 200 mL/10 min. Modify the rate of replacement in accordance with assessment of BP, pulse rate, urine output, and sensorium.

2. **Patient response.** Patients with minimal-to-moderate blood loss usually will become hemodynamically stable with crystalloid replacement alone. Transfusion may not be necessary unless further blood loss is anticipated.

C. **Blood transfusion.** If stabilization is not accomplished with crystalloid or if initial stabilization is followed by subsequent deterioration in the patient's condition, transfusion is indicated. Once infusion of blood products is begun, crystalloid replacement should be reduced proportionately to avoid volume overload.

1. **Crossmatching.** The response to crystalloid administration determines the extent to which crossmatching can be accomplished. With life-threatening hemorrhage, type-specific blood (compatible ABO and rhesus type) is used if the patient's type is known. If this is not available, O-negative blood should be used. If crystalloids stabilize the patient, complete crossmatching then can be accomplished.

2. **Choice of blood products**

a. Whenever possible, component therapy using **packed** red blood cells is preferred. To decrease the number of units of transfused red cells, use of a cell saver to recycle intraperitoneal blood should be considered.

b. When massive transfusion is required, dilution of platelets can occur. When the platelet count decreases to the range of 20 000 to 30 000 $mm^3$, coagulation may be seriously impaired. If severe thrombocytopenia develops, **platelet transfusions** should be administered. If depletion of other coagulation factors is documented and the coagulation profile is abnormal, **fresh frozen plasma** is also indicated. In general, once more than 6 U of blood have been transfused, 1 U of fresh frozen plasma should be administered for each subsequent 2 U of red cells.

D. **Hemodynamic monitoring.** The decision to insert a central monitoring catheter should be based upon the degree of blood loss and the medical condition of the patient. In deciding to implement invasive hemodynamic monitoring, the physician should be certain that potential benefits clearly outweigh the risk of complications such as infection, thromboembolism, pneumothorax, and hemothorax. As a general rule, if the patient's hemodynamic status does not stabilize within 30 minutes of the time that fluid resuscitation is initiated, invasive monitoring should be implemented. Central monitoring is of paramount importance in patients who have pre-existing cardiovascular or renal compromise

1. **Monitoring of central venous pressure.** In young healthy patients with significant blood loss, the central venous pressure (CVP) is useful in managing fluid replacement. Access can be obtained by catheterization through the antecubital, subclavian, or internal jugular vein. In patients with hypovolemic shock, CVP should be maintained in the range of 5 to 12 cm $H_2O$.
2. **Monitoring of pulmonary capillary wedge pressure.** CVP measurements are sensitive to rapid infusions of fluid, malposition of the catheter, pneumothorax, and application of the pneumatic antishock garment. Moreover, in the presence of myocardial failure, CVP may not be an accurate reflection of left ventricular preload. Therefore, right heart catheterization, rather than CVP monitoring, is the only reliable means of measuring and adjusting fluid replacement in these situations. In this clinical setting myocardial function will be maximized when pulmonary capillary wedge pressure (PCWP) is 10 to 12 mm Hg.

E. **Pneumatic antishock garments.** The antishock garment may be of great value in the initial management of hemorrhage. The device elevates BP and improves tissue perfusion primarily by increasing ventricular afterload. It also decreases the diameter of the pelvic vessels, thus reducing blood flow and circumferential tension and thereby minimizing endothelial disruption and enhancing clot formation (Fig. 3.1).

1. **Indications/contraindications.** The garment should be applied if SBP is less than 80 mm Hg or if the pressure is between 80 and 100 mm Hg and the patient is acutely symptomatic. The only absolute contraindication to use of the device in gynecologic patients is congestive heart failure.
2. **Inflation procedure**
   a. Place the patient in the supine position and apply the shock garment. Set the valves for the leg sections in the "open" position.
   b. Use the foot pump to begin inflation of the leg sections.
   c. Monitor the patient's BP continuously during inflation of the leg sections. Discontinue inflation when the patient's SBP increases to the range of 80 to 100 mm Hg and tissue perfusion begins to improve. The maximum inflation pressure is 104 mm Hg. Once the desired change in BP has been achieved, set the inflation control valves in the "closed" position.

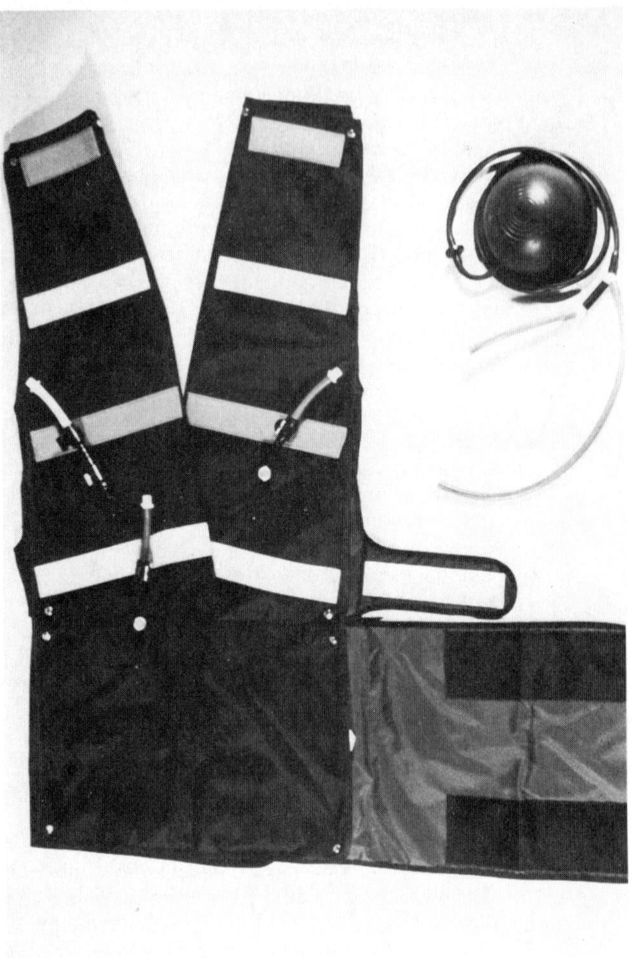

FIGURE 3.1. Photograph of the pneumatic antishock garment. Separate, color-coded tubes connect each leg section and the abdominal section to the foot pump. Individual inflation control valves allow the separate sections to be inflated and deflated independently.

d. Once the leg sections are inflated, set the abdominal valve to the "open" position. Use the foot pump to inflate this section, discontinuing inflation as BP is restored to normal and pelvic hemorrhage is controlled.

3. **Deflation procedure.** Deflation of the antishock device should be gradual, starting with the abdominal compart-

ment. Deflation should proceed until the SBP decreases by 5 mm Hg, at which time additional intravenous fluid should be infused until BP is stable. If surgical intervention is planned, deflation of the abdominal compartment should be deferred until after induction of anesthesia. The leg compartments may remain inflated during surgery. When the leg compartments are deflated, the serum lactic acid concentration may increase, but this usually does not cause a major clinical problem.

F. **Arterial embolization.** In selected patients, hemorrhage may be controlled by embolizing pelvic vessels with particulate matter such as gelfoam. This procedure allows selective occlusion of a single bleeding vessel or nonselective occlusion of the hypogastric artery. Consideration should be given to this procedure in the patient whose medical condition places her at significant operative risk from more invasive surgical efforts to control bleeding. However, it should be attempted only in medical centers where experienced radiologists have a thorough understanding of the anatomy of the pelvic vasculature.

G. **Surgical intervention.** Once fluid resuscitation has been initiated, preparations should be made for surgery to control the source of bleeding.

1. **Hypogastric artery ligation** should be used to control hemorrhage when a specific bleeding site cannot be identified or when fertility may be lost if a more radical procedure such as hysterectomy is performed. The operation requires that the retroperitoneal space be dissected to expose both hypogastric arteries. The vessels should be isolated and doubly ligated just distal to the first posterior division.
2. **Ligation of ovarian vessels.** The collateral circulation in the pelvis is extensive, and bleeding may continue despite ligation of the hypogastric arteries. In patients who wish to preserve fertility, the next step in management should be ligation of the ovarian vessels at the level of the infundibulopelvic ligament.
3. **Uterine artery ligation** controls bleeding of uterine origin and is primarily used in the treatment of postpartum hemorrhage secondary to uterine atony. Because this is one of the easiest procedures to perform, it is often the first maneuver in attempting to surgically control postpartum bleeding. Bilateral ligation is performed at the junction of the cervix and corpus uteri, including a portion of the lateral cervix in each bite.
4. **Hysterectomy.** If ligation of the hypogastric, ovarian and/or uterine arteries fails to control hemorrhage, hysterectomy may be necessary as a life-saving measure. Once the uterus has been removed, if bleeding in the region of the vaginal cuff cannot be controlled, consideration should be

given to insertion of a Logothetopulos pack to compress vessels for a period of 24 to 48 hours. The pack then may be removed vaginally. Pressure packs may be necessary in the rare patient with uncontrollable bleeding from the presacral or the superior gluteal vasculature. To maintain pressure, it may be necessary to close abdominal fascia around appropriately placed in-dwelling clamps. Removal of these devices and packs can be attempted in 48 to 72 hours.

5. **Topical hemostatic agents.** The local application of microfibrillar collagen at the time of surgery may be of value in controlling hemorrhage from small vessels. However, every effort should be made to directly ligate or coagulate bleeding vessels.

## SEPTIC SHOCK

Septic shock is the third most common cause of shock in the United States. It is responsible for 20 000 to 60 000 deaths annually. The mortality associated with this disorder is as high as 50% to 80%, with respiratory failure the most common immediate cause of death. Genital tract surgery and pelvic infection are two of the major factors that predispose to septic shock.

### I. Predisposing factors

#### A. Nonsurgical factors

1. Septic shock occurs almost exclusively in hospitalized patients. Patients at particular risk for developing septic shock include elderly individuals who have chronic debilitating diseases such as cirrhosis, disseminated malignancies, and immunodeficiency disorders. Patients receiving immunosuppressive drugs, cytotoxic agents, and parenteral hyperalimentation also are uniquely susceptible to serious infection and subsequent septic shock.
2. In gynecologic patients who do not have underlying malignancies, the principal disorders that are associated with septic shock are septic abortion, acute pyelonephritis, postoperative pelvic infection, acute salpingitis, and pelvic abscess. Fortunately, less than 5% of individuals with these conditions will develop the life-threatening complication of septic shock.

**B. Surgical factors.** Multiorgan trauma and surgery of the biliary, urinary, intestinal, or genital tract predispose even the healthy patient to increased risk of sepsis.

**II. Mortality.** The prognosis in septic shock is dependent upon the severity of the patient's underlying illness. Patients who have rapidly fatal diseases such as a hematologic malignancy or an advanced solid tumor have a mortality rate that exceeds 80%. Patients with less serious, but ultimately fatal illnesses, have a mortality rate in the range of 40% to 50%. Immunocompetent patients without serious underlying illnesses have a much better prognosis. In these individuals, the mortality associated with septic shock is approximately 15%. The majority of gynecologic patients who develop septic shock are among the group of patients with the best prognosis.

**III. Microbiology.** Any microorganism capable of infecting a human host can cause septic shock. In most instances, however, the microorganisms responsible for sepsis are part of the patient's endogenous flora. Of particular importance are the aerobic Gram-negative bacilli. Thirty percent to 50% of cases of septic shock are caused by *Escherichia coli*. Twenty percent to 30% are the result of infections caused by *Klebsiella, Enterobacter,* and *Serratia* organisms. Ten percent of cases are due to *Pseudomonas aeruginosa* infections, and a similar percentage are due to infections caused by *Proteus* and *Providencia* sp. *Pseudomonas* infections are particularly likely to occur in immunosuppressed patients. The remaining cases of septic shock are caused by Gram-positive aerobic bacteria, anaerobic Gram-negative bacilli, viruses, rickettsia, and fungi. In approximately 16% of patients, septic shock is caused by multiple organisms.

**IV. Pathophysiology.** Although still not completely understood, the pathophysiology of shock due to Gram-negative bacteremia has been investigated extensively, and it will be used as the basis for the following discussion. The cell wall of Gram-negative bacteria contains a complex lipopolysaccharide which is termed endotoxin. This substance is released into the host's circulation at the time of the bacterium's death. Once in the bloodstream, endotoxin initiates the intricate series of pathophysiologic derangements summarized in Figure 3.2.

**A. Activation of the coagulation cascade**

1. One of the first effects of endotoxin is direct activation of Hageman Factor (XII) which, in turn, initiates the intrinsic clotting cascade. Hageman Factor also directly activates Factor VII and thereby stimulates the extrinsic coagulation pathway. Activation of the coagulation system leads to concurrent activation of the fibrinolytic system. Plasmin then acts upon Hageman Factor to produce substances termed prekallikrein activators. These compounds activate prekallikrein to form kallikrein, which, in turn, causes conversion of plasminogen to plasmin and also directly activates Hageman Factor. The net result of these events is enhanced coagulation and accelerated fibrinolysis.
2. Another major effect of kallikrein activation is the production of inflammatory mediators such as hydrogen peroxide, oxygen- and hydroxy-free radicals, and bradykinin. These agents cause intense inflammatory injury.

**B. Activation of the complement system.** Endotoxin also activates the complement cascade. Activation occurs through the classic pathway, the alternate (properdin) pathway, and through direct

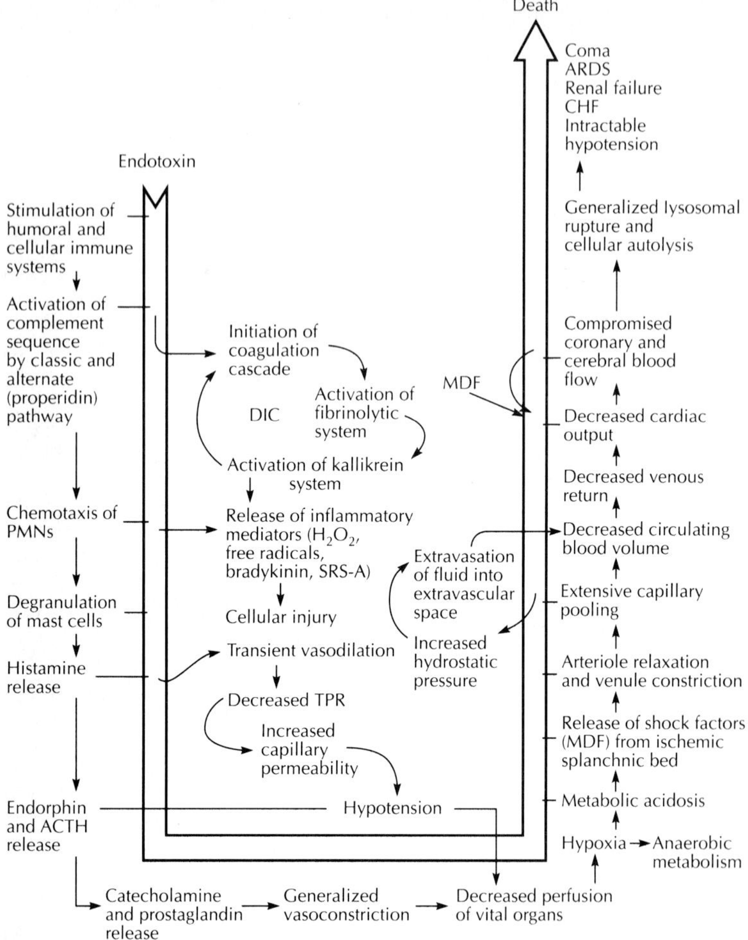


FIGURE 3.2. The pathophysiology of septic shock. ARDS = adult respiratory distress syndrome; CHF = congestive heart failure; DIC = disseminated intravascular coagulation; MDF = myocardial depressant factor; TPR = total peripheral resistance; PMN = polymorphonuclear leukocytes; ACTH = corticotropin. From Duff P, Gibbs RS. Maternal sepsis. In: Berkowitz RL, ed. Critical Care of the Obstetric Patient. Churchill-Livingstone: New York; 1983. Reprinted with permission.

stimulation of the first component of complement. There are three major effects of complement activation.

1. C5a and C5,6,7 complex interact to promote migration of neutrophils into injured tissue.

2. Neutrophils release leukotrienes (slow reacting substance of anaphylaxis) which cause vasoconstriction and increased vascular permeability in the postcapillary venules and exert an additional chemotactic effect on neutrophils. Neutrophils then release other inflammatory mediators such as hydrolytic enzymes and superoxides.
3. C3a and C5a interact to cause degranulation of mast cells and release of histamine. Histamine release has several major pathophysiologic effects:
   a. Disruption of endothelial integrity
   b. Increase in capillary permeability
   c. Vasodilation
   d. Hypotension
4. In response to this initial state of hypotension, there is an increase in the host's heart rate and cardiac output. Even in this hyperdynamic state of shock, however, myocardial contractility is abnormal. Recent investigations have demonstrated segmental and global ventricular wall dysfunction in patients with septic shock.

C. **Activation of sympathetic nervous system.** The initial state of vasodilation and decreased peripheral resistance usually is transient. As sepsis evolves, there is intense activation of the sympathetic nervous system. The principal biologic effect of this sympathetic discharge is generalized vasoconstriction. Vasoconstriction is intensified by the local effects of prostaglandins released from injured endothelial tissue. The most serious effect of generalized vasoconstriction is diminution in perfusion of vital organs, ultimately resulting in severe systemic metabolic acidosis. Subsequently, there is a visible change in circulatory hemodynamics, marked by relaxation of smooth muscle in the wall of arterioles and constriction of smooth muscle in the wall of venules. This process results in extensive pooling of blood in capillary beds, increased hydrostatic pressure, and transudation of intravascular fluid into the extravascular space. Capillary pooling also causes a decrease in circulating blood volume and a decrease in venous return to the heart. Ultimately, there is a corresponding decrease in cardiac output and systemic BP.

D. **Other factors impairing myocardial contractility.** Two other factors also appear to contribute to impaired myocardial contractility.
   1. Shock results in release of beta endorphins from the pituitary gland. Endorphins lower BP, decrease heart rate, and depress myocardial contractility.
   2. In addition, preliminary laboratory and clinical investigations indicate that, in shock, the pancreas releases a substance termed myocardial depressant factor. The most important effects of myocardial depressant factor are depression of myocardial contractility, stimulation of vaso-

constriction within the splanchnic vasculature, and depression of neutrophil and monocyte phagocytosis.

**E. Pulmonary dysfunction.** Endotoxemia also causes profound derangements in respiratory physiology. As indicated in Figure 3.3, endotoxin directly damages the endothelium of the pulmonary vasculature. Platelets adhere to fragments of exposed collagen and activate the coagulation cascade, resulting in stasis of blood flow in the pulmonary microcirculation. Platelets and endothelial cells also release prostaglandins, which intensify pulmonary vasoconstriction. The net effect of these disturbances is impairment of pulmonary perfusion, ischemia, and further vasoconstriction.

In response to endothelial injury, the complement system is activated, and phagocytic cells are attracted to the area of tissue damage. Phagocytes, in turn, release chemicals that inten-

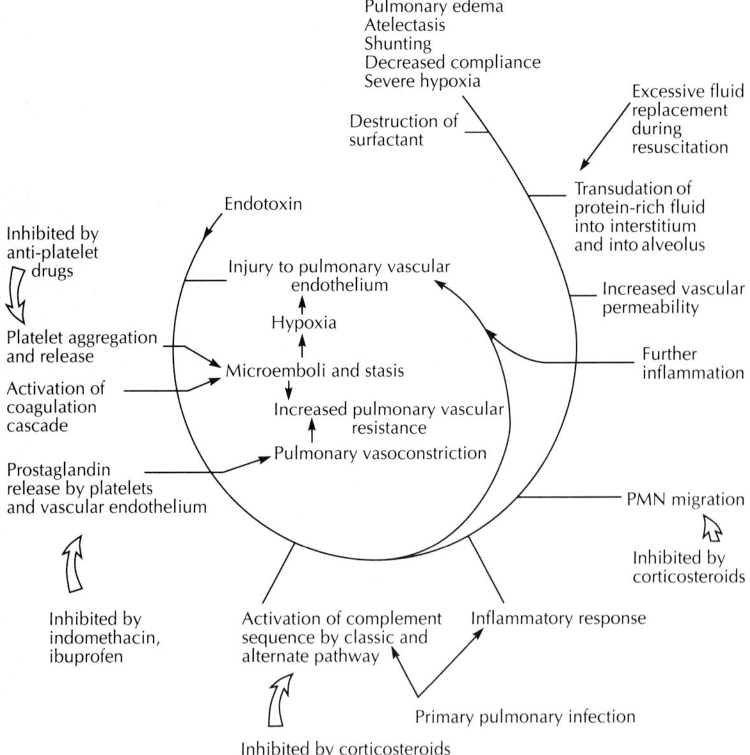


FIGURE 3.3. The pathophysiology of respiratory dysfunction in septic shock. PMN = polymorphonuclear leukocytes. From Duff P, Gibbs RS. Maternal sepsis. In Berkowitz RL ed. Critical Care of the Obstetric Patient. Churchill-Livingstone: New York; 1983. Reprinted with permission.

sify the inflammatory process. Capillary permeability increases, and protein-rich fluid transudes into the interstitium and alveoli. The functional consequence of these events is atelectasis, perfusion-ventilation imbalance, decreased compliance, interstitial and intra-alveolar edema, severe hypoxemia, pulmonary hypertension, and, ultimately, respiratory failure.

F. **Other effects of endotoxin**

1. Endotoxin adheres to the cell membrane of circulating neutrophils and monocytes, causing these cells to be removed from the circulation by reticuloendothelial cells in the spleen. Therefore, neutropenia may be present early in the shock state. As cell-mediated immunity is activated, however, rebound leukocytosis usually ensues. This rebound effect, of course, does not occur in immunosuppressed patients, who are precisely those at greatest risk for developing septic shock.
2. Endotoxin also exerts a prominent effect on the temperature-regulating center of the hypothalamus. In the early phase of sepsis, hypothermia often is present. Subsequently, however, most patients develop a temperature elevation. The febrile response is enhanced by release of endogenous pyrogen from neutrophils.

## V. Clinical manifestations

A. **Signs and symptoms.** The earliest manifestations of septic shock are restlessness, anxiety, disorientation, and temperature instability. In addition, nausea and vomiting are common symptoms. The most prominent pathophysiologic changes are those affecting the cardiovascular system. Early evidence of septic shock may include tachycardia and hypotension, with subsequent biventricular failure and cardiac arrhythmia. Fifty percent of patients with septic shock develop the adult respiratory distress syndrome (ARDS). The usual clinical signs of ARDS are tachypnea, dyspnea, stridor, and central cyanosis. Other common findings in patients with septic shock include hematuria, pyuria, oliguria, jaundice, nausea, vomiting, and hemorrhage secondary to disseminated intravascular coagulation.

B. **Physical examination** of the chest in patients with ARDS typically reveals dullness to percussion, decreased tactile and vocal fremitus, diminished breath sounds, and rales. Additional physical findings such as costovertebral angle tenderness, wound infection, pelvic mass, uterine and adnexal tenderness, and peritonitis may be present, depending upon the primary site of infection.

## VI. Differential diagnosis.

The principal disorders that must be considered in the differential diagnosis of septic shock are:

A. Cardiogenic shock

B. Hypovolemic shock

C. Pulmonary embolism
D. Cardiac tamponade
E. Aortic dissection
F. Hemorrhagic pancreatitis
G. Diabetic ketoacidosis.

## VII. Diagnosis

A. **Laboratory studies.** Table 3.2 lists the laboratory studies that are of value in the evaluation of the patient with suspected septic shock.

B. **Culture.** In addition to these laboratory tests, microbiologic cultures of blood and other sites are essential in establishing the diagnosis of sepsis and in determining the primary site of infection. The following is a brief list of appropriate cultures.

1. Urine Gram stain and culture obtained aseptically from a bladder catheter
2. Sputum culture and Gram stain
3. Aerobic and anaerobic blood cultures—two sets
4. Blood culture for fungal organisms, especially if patient is immunosuppressed or receiving hyperalimentation
5. Culture of operative site, wound, or abscess cavity when appropriate

C. **Radiographic studies**

1. **Chest x-ray** is helpful in detecting the presence of pneumonia, pulmonary edema, and ARDS.
2. **Abdominal x-ray** is of value in diagnosing intestinal obstruction or perforated viscus.

**Table 3.2. Laboratory Evaluation of Patients with Suspected Septic Shock**

| LABORATORY TEST | RESULT |
|---|---|
| White blood cell count | Initially decreased, then increased |
| Hematocrit | Variable |
| Platelet count | Decreased |
| Fibrin degradation products | Increased |
| Fibrinogen | Usually decreased |
| Prothrombin time, partial thromboplastin time | Prolonged |
| Arterial pH | Initially increased, then decreased |
| Arterial $pO_2$ | Usually decreased |
| Arterial $pCO_2$ | Usually decreased |
| Serum $HCO_3$ | Usually decreased |
| Blood urea nitrogen | Increased |
| Serum creatinine | Increased |
| Bilirubin | Increased |
| Transaminases | Increased |
| Alkaline phosphatase | Increased |
| Serum glucose | Variable |

3. **Intravenous pyelography** may identify intraparenchymal or perinephric abscess, ureteral fistula, or ureteral injury.
4. **Computerized tomography, MRI and ultrasonography** can delineate a pelvic or abdominal abscess.

D. **Hemodynamic monitoring** also is of importance in establishing the diagnosis of septic shock. **Electrocardiography** is indicated to exclude the diagnosis of myocardial infarction and to detect cardiac arrhythmias. **Right heart catheterization** studies are particularly valuable in distinguishing between septic shock and cardiogenic or hypovolemic shock.

## VIII. Management

### A. Correction of hemodynamic derangements

1. **Hemodynamic monitoring**
   a. An **arterial catheter** should be inserted to monitor blood pressure and arterial oxygenation.
   b. A **bladder catheter** should be placed to measure urine output accurately.
   c. **Right heart catheterization** should be performed to evaluate cardiac function and to monitor fluid resuscitation.
2. **Fluid resuscitation**
   a. Fluid resuscitation with crystalloids should be initiated while hemodynamic monitors are being placed. Adequate venous access should be obtained to administer fluids as well as medications. Plasma deficits should be corrected by infusion of isotonic crystalloids, such as normal saline or lactated Ringer's solution, or colloid solutions, such as albumin or plasmanate.
   b. If the patient has experienced acute blood loss, blood transfusion may be initiated simultaneously with volume replacement.
   c. **Initial fluid replacement** should occur in small increments of 150 to 200 cc infused over 10 minutes. Adjustments in the rate of infusion should be based upon changes in BP, pulse, jugular venous pressure, and urine output. Continued restoration of intravascular volume should be guided by direct measurement of PCWP. The optimal PCWP in septic shock is approximately 12 mm Hg.
3. **Pneumatic antishock garment** (see pulmonary dysfunction section, IV-E). While fluid resuscitation is being initiated, application of the pneumatic antishock garment may result in immediate improvement in cardiac function and tissue perfusion. Early use of the antishock garment may decrease the amount of fluid needed for resuscitation, thereby reducing the risk of iatrogenic pulmonary edema. The

pneumatic unit should be deflated gradually as normal perfusion pressure is re-established by intravenous fluid administration.

4. **Vasopressors.** If the measures outlined above fail to restore adequate tissue perfusion, vasopressor therapy is indicated.
   a. **Dopamine or dobutamine** are the preferred agents in septic shock. These drugs increase myocardial contractility and heart rate without causing a disproportionate increase in myocardial oxygen consumption. They stimulate dopaminergic receptors in the renal, mesenteric, coronary, and cerebral vasculature and cause vasodilation. Unlike pure beta agonists, they cause vasoconstriction in skeletal muscle. Their net effect, then, is to preserve blood flow to vital organs.
   b. **Administration.** Dopamine and dobutamine must be administered by continuous intravenous infusion. The usual starting dose for both agents is 2 to 5 μg/kg/min. The infusion should be increased slowly until the desired hemodynamic response is achieved. In doses exceeding 15 to 20 μg/kg/min, the drugs will stimulate alpha receptors and cause sustained decrease in tissue perfusion.
5. **Digitalization.** In patients with overt heart failure, digitalization should be accomplished by administering a loading dose of 0.75 mg digoxin in three divided doses, 4 to 6 hours apart. The loading dose is followed by a daily maintenance dose that sustains a therapeutic serum digoxin concentration of 0.5 to 2.5 ng/mL. The usual maintenance dose will be in the range of 0.25 to 0.375 mg/d.
6. **Naloxone.** Endogenous beta-endophins released in septic shock cause decreased heart rate, decreased myocardial contractility, and decreased systemic BP. Preliminary studies have demonstrated that the hypotensive and cardiodepressant effect of beta-endorphins can be reversed by administration of naloxone. Dosage of naloxone has ranged from 0.01 mg/kg to 0.4 mg/kg. Administration of naloxone should be reserved for those patients whose hypotension has been refractory to the measures outlined above.
7. **Intra-aortic balloon counterpulsation.** A final treatment modality that should be considered in patients with refractory hypotension is intra-aortic balloon counterpulsation. The beneficial effects of the aortic balloon are increased diastolic BP, increased coronary blood flow, decreased afterload, increased cardiac output, and increased left ventricular stroke work index. The patients most likely to respond favorably to this therapy are those who have low cardiac output states. Experience with this treatment is too

limited however to justify routine use in septic shock.

**B. Treatment of infection**

**1. Antibiotic therapy**

a. **Standard regimen.** Although it is not the only acceptable regimen, the antibiotic combination of penicillin (5 000 000 U q6 h), gentamicin or tobramycin (1.5 mg/kg q8 h), and clindamycin (900 mg q8 h) will provide effective coverage for virtually all the organisms that may be responsible for septic shock in gynecologic patients. Metronidazole (500 mg q6 h) is an acceptable alternative to clindamycin in this clinical setting. Aztreonam (2g q8h) can be substituted for gentamicin or tobramycin if there is concern about the patient's renal function.

b. **Alternate regimens.** In certain situations, different antibiotic combinations may be indicated:

(1) **Patients with *Staphylococcus aureus*** infection should be treated with the standard regimen (a. above) but with substitution of a semi-synthetic penicillin such as nafcillin (1 g q4 h or 2 g q6 h) for penicillin.

(2) **Patients with systemic fungal infections** should be treated with antifungal agents such as amphotericin B or miconazole.

(a) The dosage of **amphotericin B** will vary according to the individual tolerance of each patient. Treatment usually is initiated at a single daily dose of 0.25 mg/kg and increased gradually to a maximum daily dose of 1.0 mg/kg or an alternate-day dose of 1.5 mg/kg. Each dose should be administered slowly by intravenous infusion over a period of approximately 6 hours. The recommended concentration for intravenous infusion is 0.1 mg/kg.

(b) The intravenous dose of **miconazole** varies according to the specific fungal organism that must be treated. The usual dose for treatment of systemic candidiasis is 200 to 600 mg q8 h.

(3) **Immunosuppressed neutropenic patients with *Pseudomonas* infection** should be treated with amikacin (7.5 mg/kg q12 h) plus an extended-spectrum penicillin such as mezlocillin or piperacillin (4 g q6 h) or ticarcillin-clavulanic acid (3.1 g q6 h).

(4) **Immunocompromised patients with *Pneumocystis carinii* infection** should be treated with trimethoprim-sulfamethoxazole. The appropriate dosage is 20 mg/kg/d of trimethoprim and 100

mg/kg/d of sulfamethoxazole in four divided oral doses. Recent studies have demonstrated that pentamidine, administered by inhalation, is also effective for this purpose.

2. **Surgery.** In addition to antibiotic therapy, elimination of the source of infection may require surgery, for example, to drain an abscess, to remove infected products of conception, or to extirpate grossly contaminated pelvic organs. Surgical intervention, in fact, may be the single most important step in stabilization of the critically ill patient. Definitive surgical therapy should not be delayed simply because the patient appears to respond initially to fluid resuscitation.

C. **Evaluation and support of the respiratory system.** The most common cause of death in patients with septic shock is respiratory failure. Twenty-five percent to 50% of patients with septic shock will develop ARDS, and 80% to 90% of these individuals will die. Therefore, a major objective in the management of the critically ill patient is prevention of respiratory failure.

1. Administer oxygen as needed through a face mask.
2. Monitor arterial blood gases frequently.
3. Avoid excessive fluid administration by closely monitoring intake and output.
4. Initiate mechanical ventilation with a volume-cycled respirator at the earliest manifestation of respiratory failure. Although the list below is not all-inclusive, the following conditions usually warrant institution of mechanical ventilation.
   a. Patient exhaustion
   b. Inability to manage the patient's respiratory secretions by more conservative means
   c. Progressive retention of $CO_2$ ($pCO_2 > 55–60$ mm Hg)
   d. Persistent hypoxemia ($pO_2 < 50$ mm Hg) despite maximal delivery of oxygen by face mask
   e. Progressive decrease in vital capacity to less than approximately 1.5 L

D. **Corticosteroids.** Because of significant complications and potential adverse effects, the use of corticosteroids in patients with septic shock is highly controversial. Included is a comparison of beneficial and adverse effects of corticosteroid use.

1. **Beneficial effects of corticosteroids.** The potential beneficial effects of corticosteroids include:
   a. Positive inotropy
   b. Peripheral and central vasodilation
   c. Enhancement of gluconeogenesis
   d. Inhibition of beta-endorphin secretion
   e. Shift in the oxygen dissociation curve to enhance oxygen release to the tissue
   f. Inhibition of inflammation

2. **Complications.** These beneficial effects are offset, however, by several serious complications. Major sequelae such as gastrointestinal bleeding, hyperosmolality, hyperglycemia, and acute psychosis occur in approximately 6% of patients receiving corticosteriods. Of even greater importance are the effects of corticosteroids on immune surveillance. These agents inhibit neutrophil mobilization and chemotaxis, decrease the efficiency of intracellular bacterial killing, and impair lymphocyte and monocyte function. These effects may be particularly life-threatening in patients who survive the initial shock state but then succumb to multiorgan failure resulting from uncontrolled infection.
3. Because of these serious adverse sequelae, we no longer recommend use of corticosteroids for treatment of septic shock.

E. **Other supportive measures**
1. Avoid wide fluctuations in body temperature, because thermal instability aggravates cardiovascular dysfunction.
2. In immunosuppressed patients with infections caused by *Pseudomonas* organisms, consider transfusion of compatible white cells.

IX. **Disseminated intravascular coagulation (DIC)** occurs in approximately 25% to 30% of patients who have septic shock. Several mechanisms appear to be responsible for the development of DIC in patients who have severe infections. The net effect of these processes is massive depletion of coagulation factors which then predisposes the patient to uncontrolled hemorrhage.

A. **Pathophysiology**
1. Endotoxin directly damages vascular endothelium. Platelets adhere to sites of endothelial injury and release several substances (adenosine diphosphate, adenosine triphosphate, calcium, acid hydrolases, cathepsins, thromboxane $A_2$, and phospholipids) which casue vasoconstriction and additional platelet aggregation, and directly activate the intrinsic clotting cascade.
2. Endothelial injury also results in release of substances rich in thromboplastic activity which activate the extrinsic coagulation cascade.
3. Endotoxin directly activates Hageman Factor (XII) which initiates the intrinsic coagulation cascade. Hageman Factor also activates Factor VII which, in turn, initiates the extrinsic cascade.
4. Activation of the coagulation cascade leads to activation of the fibrinolytic system. The subsequent formation of fibrin degradation products has an additional anticoagulant effect.

5. Activation of the fibrinolytic system activates the kallikrein system which, in turn, directly stimulates the intrinsic coagulation system.

B. **Diagnosis** of DIC should be considered when the patient experiences prolonged bleeding from a venipuncture site or surgical incision or develops profuse spontaneous bleeding from the urinary, gastrointestinal, or genital tract.
   1. The simplest bedside laboratory test for confirming the diagnosis is observation of a red-stoppered tube of blood. Failure of the specimen to clot within 5 to 7 minutes usually is indicative of a coagulopathy.
   2. Demonstration of a prolonged bleeding time, decreased platelet count, decreased fibrinogen concentration, and elevation in the concentration of fibrin degradation products also is of value in establishing the diagnosis of DIC. In addition, the prothombin time and partial thromboplastin time will be abnormally prolonged in the presence of a severe coagulopathy.

C. **Treatment**
   1. The primary objective in treatment of DIC is elimination of the underlying cause (e.g., sepsis).
   2. Deficiencies in coagulation factors must be corrected by infusion of specific blood components.
      a. Thrombocytopenia should be corrected by administration of **platelet concentrates.** Treatment should be initiated with 4 to 6 U; additional units should be infused as necessary to keep the platelet count at a level $>$ 50 000 $mm^3$.
      b. Deficits in fibrinogen should be corrected by administration of **cryoprecipitate** which also is an excellent source of factors VIII and XIII. Cryoprecipitate should be administered in a sufficient volume to maintain the fibrinogen concentration above 100 mg/dL. Administration of a single unit of cryoprecipitate will raise the serum fibrinogen level 10 mg/dL. Routine dosages range from 8 to 12 U.
      c. Deficiencies in other coagulation factors are best corrected by administration of **fresh frozen plasma** or **fresh whole blood.** Fresh frozen plasma should be infused in small increments of 1 to 2 U until coagulation abnormalities are corrected and hemorrhage is controlled.

## X. Toxic shock syndrome

A. **Etiology.** This potentially fatal systemic disorder is caused by toxins produced by *Staphylococcus aureus.*

B. **Pathogenesis.** There is a similarity between the pathophysiology of toxic shock syndrome and that of gram-negative septic shock. Three preconditions are necessary for the occurrence of toxic shock syndrome:

1. Infection or colonization with *S. aureus*
2. Production of toxic shock toxin by the organism
3. Presence of a portal of entry for toxin to enter systemic circulation

C. In addition to the highly publicized relation to absorbent tampons, conditions associated with toxic shock include (selected list):
1. Surgical wound infections
   a. Exploratory laparotomy
   b. Tubal ligation
   c. Dilation and curettage
   d. Hysterectomy
   e. Bladder suspension
   f. Urethral suspension
2. Nonsurgical focal infections
   a. Cellulitis
   b. Subcutaneous abscesses
   c. Mastitis
   d. Infected insect bite
3. Postpartum cases
   a. Vaginal delivery
   b. Spontaneous abortion
   c. Cesarean section
   d. Vaginal delivery with transmission to the neonate
4. Nonmenstrual vaginal conditions
   a. Vaginal infections
   b. Use of the diaphragm or contraceptive sponge
   c. Pelvic inflammatory disease
   d. Vulvovaginal steroid cream

D. **Case definition**
1. Fever—temperature > 38.9°C, 102°F
2. Rash—diffuse macular, erythema
3. Desquamation—1 to 2 weeks after onset of illness
4. Hypotension—systolic < 90 mm Hg or orthostatic dizziness
5. Negative blood, pharyngeal, or cerebrospinal fluid culture
6. Involvement of three or more of the following organ systems:
   a. Gastrointestinal (vomiting, diarrhea)
   b. Muscular (mylagia or creatine phosphokinase [CPK] at least twice expected values)
   c. Mucous membrane inflammation (vaginal, oropharyngeal, conjunctional)
   d. Renal (BUN or creatinine at least twice normal or ≥ 5 WBC/hpf on microscopic urinalysis)
   e. Hepatic (total bilirubin, SGOT, SGPT at least twice normal).
   f. Hematologic (platelets ≤ 100 000/mm$^3$)
   g. CNS—disorientation or altered sensorium

- h. Cardiopulmonary
  - (1) RDS
  - (2) Pulmonary edema
  - (3) New onset of second and third degree heart block
  - (4) Myocarditis

7. Negative serologic tests for measles, leptospirosis, Rocky Mountain Spotted Fever

**E. Signs and symptoms**

1. Most common findings
   - a. Fever > 38.9°F
   - b. Hypotension
   - c. Diffuse rash
2. Other findings
   - a. Erythematous pharyngitis, inflamed genitalia, conjunctivitis
   - b. Myalgias and arthralgias
   - c. Headache, confusion, agitation, decreased mentation
   - d. Nausea, vomiting, diarrhea

**F. Differential diagnosis**

1. Other exanthems
   - a. Kawasaki's disease
   - b. Scarlet fever (streptococcal and staphylococcal)
   - c. Rocky Mountain Spotted Fever
   - d. Viral diseases
   - e. Leptospirosis
   - f. Bullous impetigo
   - g. Rubella and rubeola
   - h. Meningococcemia
   - i. Erythema multiforme
   - j. Acute rheumatic fever
2. Gastrointestinal illnesses
   - a. Staphylococcal food poisoning
   - b. Pancreatitis
   - c. Appendicitis
   - d. Gastroenteritis
   - e. Dysentery
3. Miscellaneous disorders
   - a. Systemic lupus erythematosus
   - b. Hemolytic uremic syndrome
   - c. Pelvic inflammatory disease
   - d. Stevens-Johnson syndrome
   - e. Acute pyelonephritis
   - f. Legionnaire's disease
   - g. Septic shock
   - h. Reye's syndrome
   - i. Tularemia
   - j. Tick typhus
   - k. Rhabdomyolysis

**G. Prevention**

1. Prompt medical and surgical treatment of localized suppurative staphylococcal infections.
2. Minimize use of tampons, particularly "superabsorbent" tampons
3. Patients with history of toxic shock should not resume use of tampons until *S. aureus* has been eliminated from the lower genital tract

## BIBLIOGRAPHY

Aeder M, Crowe J, Rhodes R, Shuck J, Wolf W: Technical limitations in the rapid infusion of I.V. fluids. Ann Emerg Med. 1985; 14:307.

American College of Surgeons Committee on Trauma Advanced Trauma Life Support (ATLS™) Student Manual. Tacoma, Wash: American College of Surgeons; 1988.

Blaisdell FW. Controversy in shock research: The role of steroids in septic shock. Circ Shoc. 1981; 8:673.

Broome CV. Epidemiology of toxic shock syndrome in the United States: Overview. Rev Infect Dis. 1989; 11:S14.

Brotman S, Soderstrom C, Oster-Granite M, Cisternino S, Browner B, Cowley RA. Management of severe bleeding in fractures of the pelvis. Surg Gynecol Obstet. 1981; 153:823.

Bruni FD, Komwatara P, Soulsby ME, Hess ML: Endotoxin and myocardial failure: Role of the myofibril and venous return. Am J Physiol. 1978; 235:H150.

Cavanaugh D, Knuppel RA, Shepherd JH, Anderson R, Rao PS. Septic shock and the obstetrician/gynecologist. South Med J. 1982; 75:809.

Duff P. Management of septic shock in the pelvic surgery patient. Infect Surg. Feb 1985; 101–116.

Eskridge RA. Septic shock. Crit Care Q. 1980; 2:55.

Faden AI, Holaday JW. Opiate antagonists: A role in the treatment of hypovolemic shock. Science. 1979; 205:317.

Freid MA, Vosti KL. The importance of underlying disease in patients with gram-negative bacteremia. Arch Intern Med. 1968; 121:418.

Holaday JW, Faden AI. Naloxone reversal of endotoxin hypotension suggests role of endorphins in shock. Nature. 1978; 275:450.

Kaplan RL, Sahn SA, Petty TL. Incidence and outcome of the respiratory distress syndrome in gram-negative sepsis. Arch Intern Med. 1979; 139:867.

Kreger BE, Craven DE, Carling PC. Gram negative bacteremia. III and IV. Am J Med. 1980; 68:332.

Lefer AM. Role of a myocardial depressant factor in shock states. Mod Concepts Cardiocasc Dis. 1973; 42:59.

Maclean L. Shock, a century of progress. Ann Surg. 1985; 201:407.

Ordog G, Wasserberger J, Blasubramanium S. Coagulation abnormalities in traumatic shock. Ann Emerg Med. 1985; 14:650.

Raffa J, Trunkey DD. Myocardial depression in sepsis. J Trauma. 1978; 18:617.

Reingold, AL, Shards KN, Dan BB, Broome CV. Toxic-shock not associated with menstruation. A review of 54 cases. Lancet. 1982; i:1.

Schumer W. Steroids in the treatment of clinical septic shock. Ann Surg. 1976; 184:333.

Sheagren JN. Septic shock and corticosteroids. N Eng J Med. 1981; 305:456.

Waeckerle JF. Antishock garments. Crit Care Q. 1980; 2:15.

# Part II

# General Gynecology

# CHAPTER 4

# Diseases of the Breast

**William H. Hindle**
**Frank W. Ling**

Fear of breast cancer is one of the major reasons women consult physicians. Twenty-five percent of women consult their physicians about breast lumps. More than 60% of women have palpable lumpiness in their breasts. The physician must therefore be familiar not only with diagnosis and treatment of benign and malignant breast lesions, but also with the need for patient education and monitoring of health status as it relates to the breast.

The glandular tissue of the breast is formed from modified sweat glands organized in about 20 lobes between the superficial and deep layers of pectoral fascia (Fig. 4.1). There are more lobes in the upper outer quadrants, resulting in a more solid consistency in those areas. Each lobe has a single duct draining to the nipple. Fibrous bands (Cooper's ligaments) attach the skin to the superficial fascia (Fig. 4.2). The lymphatic drainage of the breasts is primarily to the axilla with transpectoral, internal mammary, and infra- and supraclavicular adjacent pathways.

The breasts are endocrine target organs that respond to cyclic estrogen and progesterone with ductal proliferation, increased vascularity and fluid retention. The cyclic proliferation and involution associated with menstruation is not uniform throughout the breast (Fig. 4.3). During pregnancy, with the stimulation of placental lactogen, prolactin and human chorionic gonadotropin, the ductal epithelium proliferates, the ducts dilate and the alveolar cells enlarge. After delivery, prolactin stimulates the alveolar cells to secrete milk.

The initial section of this chapter will focus on malignant breast disease with particular emphasis on detection. Benign breast lesions will be discussed at the end of the chapter.

## BREAST CANCER

### I. Incidence (1990)

The lifetime risk for developing breast cancer is one in ten for women in the United States. There are more than 142 000 new

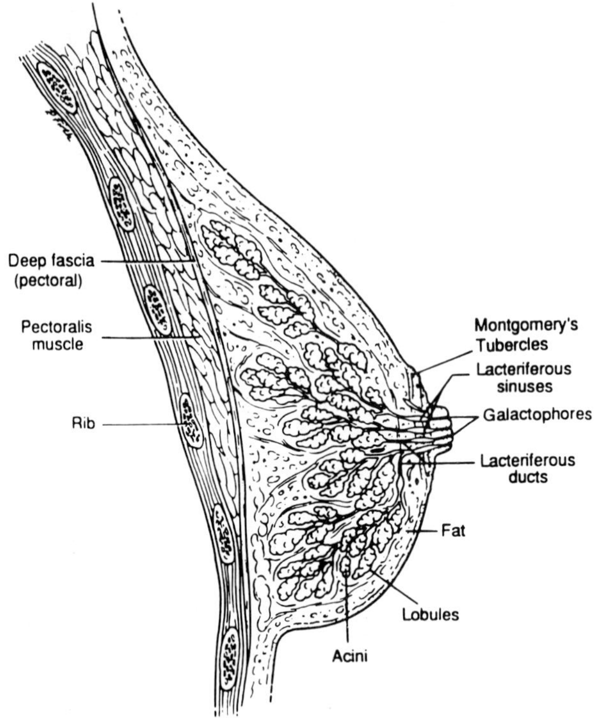


FIGURE 4.1. Diagrammatic anatomy of the female breast.

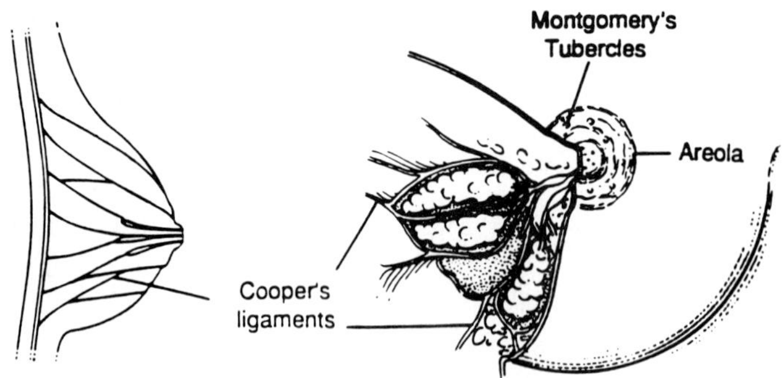


FIGURE 4.2. Diagrammatic representation of Cooper's ligaments of the breast.

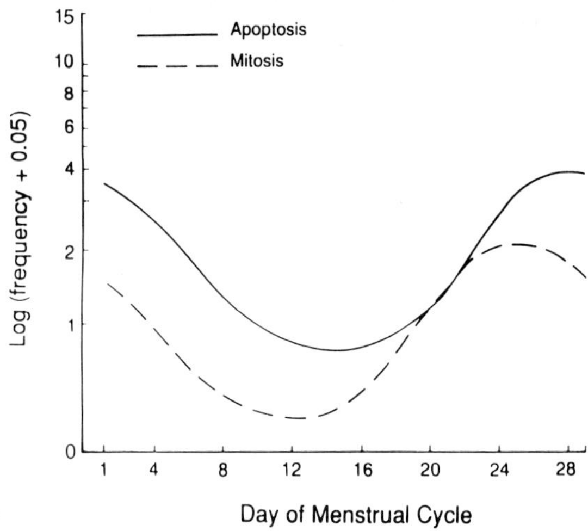


FIGURE 4.3. Logarithmic analysis of the frequency of mitosis and cell fragmentation (apoptosis) in the ductal epithelium of the human breast plotted against the day of the menstrual cycle showing high level of mitotic activity during the luteal phase. Adapted from Ferguson DJ, Anderson TJ. Morphological evaluation of cell turnover in relation to menstrual cycle in the "resting" human breast. Br J Cancer. 1981; 44:177–181.

cases of breast cancer annually and it is the most common cancer in U.S. women. Breast cancer accounts for over 29% of the malignancies in women. Cancer of the breast is rare in women under 25 years of age with 95% of cases occurring in women over age 30. The age specific incidence rate increases with progressive age (Fig. 4.4).

## II. Morbidity and mortality

**A. Morbidity.** Significant morbidity typically relates to side effects or complications of therapy. The two primary modes of therapy are surgery and radiation.

**B. Mortality.** Breast cancer accounts for 18% of cancer deaths. Over 43 000 women a year die from breast cancer in the United States.

## III. Etiology and risk factors

Although a specific cause is not known, several risk factors have been identified.

**A. Previous breast cancer.** There is a fivefold increased risk of breast cancer developing in the remaining breast.

**B. Family history.** There is increased risk with a history of breast cancer in a first degree relative (mother or sister), especially if they have had bilateral breast cancer and particularly if it was premenopausal in onset. A woman with an affected first degree

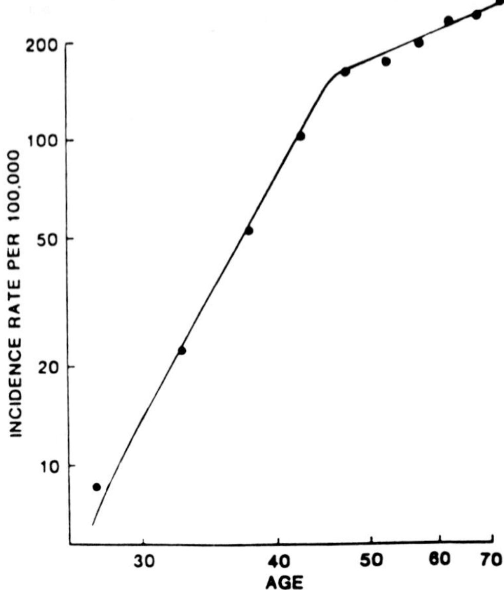


FIGURE 4.4. Incidence of breast cancer vs. age (United States white women 1969–1971). Adapted from Henderson BE, Ross KR, Pike MC. Breast neoplasia. In: Mishell DR Jr, ed. Menopause: Physiology and Pharmacology. Chicago: Year Book Medical; 1987:263–274.

relative has a risk of 2.3, whereas the risk for a woman with an affected second degree relative is 1.5. The sister of a patient with bilateral breast cancer diagnosed after 50 years of age has a relative risk of 5.0 and if the disease is diagnosed before 40 years of age, the relative risk increases to 10.5.

C. **Menstrual history.** There is increased risk if menarche occurs before age 11 or after age 14. Menopause after the age of 55 and menstrual history of more than 35 years duration are associated with a threefold to fourfold increased risk of breast cancer.

D. **Pregnancy.** There is no increased risk with pregnancy. Nulliparous women have a threefold increased risk of breast cancer, and there is increased risk if the first child is born after age 30.

E. **Obesity.** There is a slight increased risk associated with obesity.

F. **Nonrisk factors.** Contrary to widely held misconceptions, oral contraceptives (Fig. 4.5), exogenous estrogen treatment, cigarette smoking, and alcohol consumption have not been consistently shown to increase the risk of breast cancer.

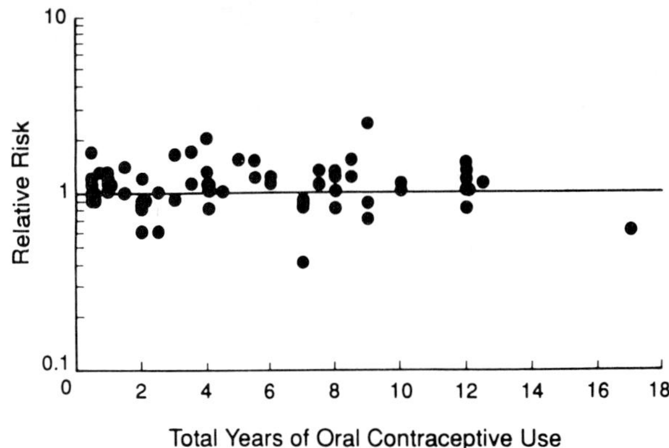


FIGURE 4.5. Analysis of the relative breast cancer risk in women less than 60 years of age with prior oral contraceptive use reported in 17 studies. Adapted from Schlesseman JJ. Cancer of the breast in reproductive tract in relation to use of oral contraception. Contraception. 1989; 40:1–38.

## IV. Pathophysiology/tumor spread

A. **Local spread.** The tumor spreads directly into the surrounding breast tissue, eventually invading deep into the pectoralis muscle or involving the skin.

B. **Lymphatic spread.** Approximately one-half of patients have axillary node involvement at the time of diagnosis of palpable cancers. The second most common site of lymphatic spread is the internal mammary chain. Axillary node involvement is related to tumor size rather than tumor location within the breast.

C. **Hematogenous spread.** Blood-borne metastases occur primarily in bones, the lungs, and the liver but can involve the adrenal glands, thyroid, peritoneum, ovaries, brain, uterus, and pleura.

## V. Diagnosis

### A. History and physical examination findings

1. **Breast mass or "lump."** Breast cancer is most commonly found by the patient or physician as a painless, usually freely mobile mass in the breast. Eighty-five percent of breast cancers are infiltrating ductal carcinomas which often induce a fibrotic response and therefore can present as stony hard masses. Malignant masses do not change with menstruation.

2. **Nipple discharge** is a nonspecific finding with manipulation of the nipple; as many as 80% of premenopausal women can have some elicited milky nipple discharge.

However, cancer may be accompanied by either a bloody or serous spontaneous nipple discharge. Intraductal papillomas are the most common cause of spontaneous bloody nipple discharge. Ductal ectasia can cause greenish nipple discharge. All spontaneous nipple discharges should be evaluated, especially those which are bloody, red-tinged, or serous.

3. **Breast asymmetry.** Patients may complain of breast asymmetry. This asymmetry may be caused by an anatomic distortion from a growing carcinoma or from a benign tumor.
4. **Skin changes.** By direct extension or involvement of Cooper's ligaments, advanced cancer can cause skin retraction, dimpling and/or nipple retraction. Lymphatic blockage can cause lymphedema and skin thickening resulting in the classic "peau d'orange" appearance. Dilated superficial veins and ultimately skin ulceration are seen with advanced breast cancer.
5. **Changes with metastatic disease** can include bone pain, weight loss dyspnea, or other cachectic systemic manifestation.

B. **Clinical breast examination.** Examination of the breast should follow a thorough, consistent, and systematic method of inspection and palpation. Educating the patient in the technique of breast self-examination (BSE) should be done at the same time.

1. **Inspection and palpation with the patient sitting on the examining table:**
   a. Inspect for symmetry, contour, and vascular pattern variations.
   b. Inspect the skin, noting:
      (1) Irritation
      (2) Discoloration
      (3) Retraction
      (4) Dimpling
      (5) Edema
   c. Have the patient place her arms above her head and then on her hips. This allows the physician to better visualize deformities. This is the optimum position in which to examine the axillae for adenopathy. Fifty percent of axillary metastases are "missed" during preoperative palpation of the axilla.
   d. Palpate the supraclavicular areas, although this rarely reveals metastatic disease unless positive nodes are present in the axilla.
2. **Inspection and palpation with the patient lying supine:**
   a. Inspect the breast and skin as in the upright position.
   b. Note nipple retraction or discharge.

c. Palpate the breast tissue, axilla, supraclavicular region, and adjacent chest wall.
   (1) A pillow or towel under the back may aid in palpation.
   (2) Palpate using the finger pads (not the finger tips) of the first three fingers, using firm, gentle pressure in small circular motion with varying degrees of pressure. Follow a vertical strip pattern, covering the entire anterior chest wall.
   (3) A dominant mass is a distinct three-dimensional lesion readily distinguishable from adjoining breast tissue. All dominant masses must be investigated.
   (4) Description of any abnormalities should be noted on a drawing and labelled right and/or left.

**C. BSE.** As many as 90% of breast cancers are first found by the patient herself. Because of early detection, women practicing regular BSE are diagnosed with an earlier stage of cancer and are less likely to have positive lymph nodes. The 5-year survival rate of women who develop breast cancer is greater in women who have done thorough, regular BSE.

Patients should be instructed in the same systematic method of inspection and palpation used in the physician's examination. The patient should be asked to demonstrate the technique of BSE to a physician or nurse at the time of her annual physical exam. The physician or nurse can then offer further instruction and re-enforcement as indicated. Demonstration models of lumps are effective in teaching BSE. In menstruating women, the optimum time to do a BSE is 5 days after cessation of menstruation. Nonmenstruating or irregularly menstruating women should do BSE on a calendar basis, such as the first of each month.

1. **Inspection and palpation in the shower:**
   a. Examine when skin is wet; the hands will glide over the skin more easily and smaller lumps can be felt.
   b. Use the flat of the fingers over every part of the breast.
   c. Use the right hand to examine the left breast and vice versa.
2. **Inspection in front of a mirror:**
   a. Look at the breasts with arms at the sides.
   b. Raise arms overhead. Look for changes in contour, dimpling of skin, swelling, or change in the nipple.
   c. Rest palms on hips and press down firmly to flex chest muscles. Look for changes.
3. **Palpation lying down:**
   a. To examine the right breast, place a folded towel or pillow under the right shoulder. Place the right hand behind head.

b. Use the left hand, flat parts of the fingers, to make small circular motions to cover the entire area of the breast, including the nipple. A ridge of firm tissue in the lower curve of the breast is normal.
c. Repeat the same palpation for the left breast.
d. Gently squeeze the nipple of each breast between the thumb and index finger. Clear or bloody discharge should be reported to the doctor.

**D. Diagnostic procedures**

1. **Mammography** is essential to the evaluation of all breast masses. As a screening procedure mammography is the only technique that will consistently detect tumors less than 1 cm in diameter. Women with nonpalpable cancers detected by mammography, who are properly treated, have a 90% 5-year survival. Mammography is diagnostic in more than 80% of palpable malignant breast lesions. Mammography can detect multiple lesions, lesions of the contralateral breast, and enlarged nodes. The common malignant lesions usually have a stellate appearance with irregular borders and can contain clustered irregular microcalcifications that are associated with malignancy in about 25% of cases. A "negative" mammogram does not rule out cancer. Radiation for current mammography screening is less than 0.05 rad per film using low dose screening fast film. The radiation risk is minimal.
   a. Indications for mammography:
      (1) Dominant palpable mass
      (2) Persistent spontaneous nonmilky nipple discharge
      (3) Mass reported by patient, but not palpable by physician
   b. Screening recommendations for asymptomatic women:
      (1) A "baseline" mammogram for all women between the ages of 35 and 40 years
      (2) Every 1 to 2 years for women 40 to 49 years old
      (3) Annual mammogram for women over 50 years old
      (4) Annual mammogram for all high-risk women: for example, mother or sister with breast cancer or a patient with previous breast cancer
2. **Breast aspiration cytology.** Fine-needle aspiration of breast masses for cytology is cost-effective, efficient, and accurate for both benign and malignant diagnoses. Local anesthetic is not necessary. Breast fine-needle aspiration for cytology is performed with a three-finger control syringe or pistol syringe holder and a 22-gauge needle with a clear plastic hub (Fig. 4.6). The cellular material obtained by aspiration is within the bore of the needle and

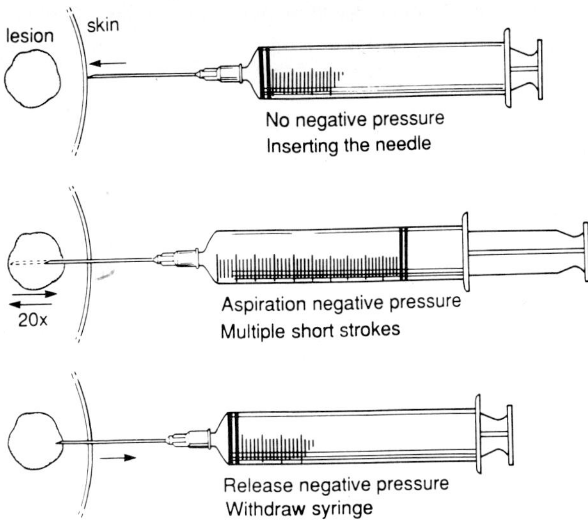


FIGURE 4.6. Technique of fine needle aspiration for cytology of solid breast masses.

is then ejected onto a slide and smeared, fixed, and stained in a similar manner to a Papanicolau (PAP) smear. The procedure is no more painful than a venipuncture. It provides a cytologic diagnosis in more than 80% of palpable breast cancers. False-positives are rare. If an adequate epithelial cell sample is obtained, there should be less than 10% false-negatives. In some cases no epithelial cells will be found and a specific cytologic diagnosis cannot be made. In these cases, open biopsy is necessary. When an adequate cell sample is obtained and the findings correlate with palpation and mammography, breast aspiration cytology by fine-needle aspiration approaches 99% accuracy for both benign and malignant palpable masses. The cytologic interpretation must be made by a cytopathologist trained and experienced in evaluating cellular aspirates of the breast. The results can be obtained rapidly and an anxious patient can be told her specific cytologic diagnosis and expeditious treatment arranged. Hematoma formation may be seen as a false-positive on a subsequent mammogram. Therefore, a mammogram should be done prior to or at least 2 weeks after aspiration.

3. **Aspiration of cysts.** Aspiration of dominant breast masses differentiates cysts from solid masses. When nonbloody fluid is obtained and a cystic mass completely "clears" by aspiration, no further treatment is required. Any aspirated

bloody fluid should be examined cytologically. Cysts with residual masses should have an open biopsy. Follow-up (e.g., in 1 month and 3 months) is essential to evaluate recurrent cysts.

4. **Evaluation of nipple discharge.** Cytologic evaluation of nipple discharge has little clinical value due to the high rate of false-negatives and false-positives. Only 3% of invasive breast cancers have associated nipple discharge. Bloody nipple discharge from a single nipple duct is from intraductal papillomas in 75% of cases.
5. **Open biopsy** is the definitive step in determining if a breast mass is malignant. This surgical procedure is usually done under local anesthesia on an outpatient basis. Open biopsy is diagnostic in more than 99% of cases. Nonpalpable lesions demonstrated on mammography require radiograph-directed needle localization just prior to the scheduled biopsy. A circumareolar incision is made (or one following Langhan's skin lines). Strict hemostasis should be maintained but not usually with cautery, because cautery can be painful. Sharp excision, rather than stretching and exerting undue pressure, minimizes pain. The closure consists of absorbable subcuticular stitches. Drains are not routinely used. More than 25% of biopsies in women over 50 years of age are positive for cancer. Indications for open biopsy:
   a. A persistent undiagnosed three-dimensional mass
   b. Suspicious mammography
   c. Serosanguineous nipple discharge
   d. Nipple elevation/retraction
   e. Skin changes such as edema, erythema, or induration
6. **Estrogen and progesterone receptor analysis.** This assay requires 0.5 g of tissue and should be performed on all cancers. The tissue must be frozen within 10 minutes for accurate analysis. Alternately, immunocytochemical stains of fine-needle aspirates are available for receptor assays.

## VI. Treatment

### A. Staging

Several systems for staging breast cancer have been proposed. Clinical staging as proposed by the American Joint Committee on Cancer includes:

1. Stage I—Tumor less than 2 cm in diameter, nodes not involved, no distant metastasis
2. Stage II—Tumor less than 5 cm in diameter, nodes not fixed, no distant metastasis
3. Stage III—Tumor greater than 5 cm, or invading skin or

attached to chest wall, or with supraclavicular nodes, no distant metastasis

4. Stage IV—Distant metastasis

B. **Surgical treatment**

1. **Modified radical mastectomy** with axillary node dissection is the standard treatment. Unlike the Halstead radical mastectomy, the pectoralis major muscle is left intact. Complications include decreased arm range of motion, pain, skin slough, and wound infection.
2. **Lumpectomy** (partial mastectomy, segmental mastectomy) with adjuvant radiation therapy can be used for small tumors < 5 cm (Fig. 4.7). Because only the tumor and a clear margin of tissue is removed surgically, the cosmetic outcome is improved. Complications of radiation are uncommon but include edema of the arm, pneumonitis, and lung fibrosis. Axillary lymph node dissection is done for staging and prognosis and is not associated with greater long-term survival.

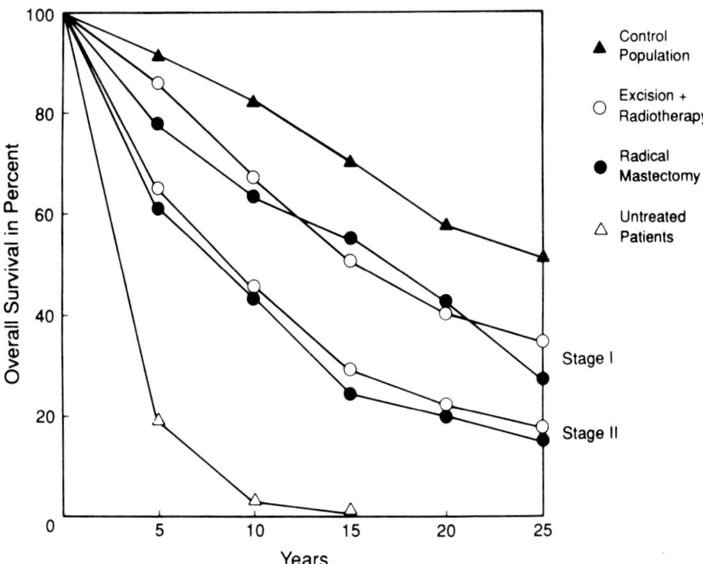


FIGURE 4.7. Comparison of overall survival, and survival of untreated breast cancer patients and women treated by breast conserving surgery (lumpectomy, radiation therapy, axillary lymph node dissection) and radical mastectomy (and lymph node dissection), for stage I and stage II breast cancer. Adapted from Vorherr H. Radiosensitivity of in situ carcinoma of the breast. Lancet. 1985; ii:282.

3. **Radical (Halstead) mastectomy** is rarely indicated. It involves resection of the entire breast along with pectoralis major and minor muscles, and axillary contents. The long-term survival is no better than with modified radical mastectomy.
4. **Breast reconstructive surgery,** immediate or delayed, should be available to all patients who desire it and whose general condition and cancer stage are appropriate for reconstruction.

C. **Radiation therapy's** primary usefulness is for local recurrence (60% of recurrences are local) and bone involvement. The routine use of radiation therapy after surgery in patients with positive axillary nodes successfully decreases local recurrence but does not alter long-term survival. Adjuvant radiation therapy is used as initial therapy in conjunction with lumpectomy. The complications such as arm edema and weakness occur usually in less than 3% of cases.

D. **Chemotherapy**
1. Premenopausal women with positive nodes have improved survival if adjuvant chemotherapy is used.
2. Combinations of drugs are more effective than single agents. The most popular combination is cyclophosphamide (Cytoxan), methotrexate, and 5-fluorouracil.
3. Complications include hair loss, leukopenia, sterility, amenorrhea, nausea, and malaise.
4. Except for cancer smaller than 1.0 cm, all breast cancer diagnosed in premenopausal women should be considered for adjuvant chemotherapy.

E. **Hormone manipulation**
1. The primary role of hormone manipulation is in advanced disease. The response is temporary and partial.
   a. Premenopausal women have a lower incidence of estrogen receptors (30%) than postmenopausal women (60%).
   b. The response is approximately 50% if estrogen receptors are positive, but only 10% if they are negative.
   c. If both estrogen and progesterone receptors are present, the response approaches 80%.
2. Oophorectomy induces response in less than 30% of premenopausal women.
3. Tamoxifen, 10 mg b.i.d., is the drug of choice when metastatic axillary nodes are present and the tumor is estrogen receptor positive.
4. Megestrol acetate, diethystilbestrol, and androgen therapy are still used, but are being replaced by other medications such as tamoxifen.

F. **Alternate adjuvant therapy**
Recent studies indicate a significant disease-free prolongation in a portion of node negative women (premenopausal and

postmenopausal) treated with adjuvant hormonal (tamoxifen) therapy or chemotherapy.

G. **Follow-up**

1. The patient should be seen every 3 months for a year, every 6 months for 5 years, and yearly thereafter.
2. Annual mammography of the remaining breast is mandatory.
3. The patient should have an annual chest x-ray in most cases.

H. **Psychological support**

1. This can be offered through hospital support groups or The American Cancer Society's "Reach to Recovery" groups.
2. The patient should be encouraged to have a positive self-image.
3. The sexual partner should be counseled as to his or her feelings and how to cope with them.

## VII. Prognosis

A. **Survival**

1. Stage I—85% 5-year survival
2. Stage II—65% 5-year survival
3. Stage III—40% 5-year survival
4. Stage IV—10% 5-year survival

B. **Survival factors.** The involvement of the axillary lymph nodes is the single most important prognostic factor (Fig. 4.8). Patients with negative axillary nodes have a 75% 5-year survival and 65% 10-year survival. Figures for patients with positive nodes are 45% and 25%, respectively. The more nodes that are involved, the poorer the prognosis.

C. **Recurrence.** In all stages, most recurrences occur within two years, but breast cancer can recur anytime up to 20 or even 30 years after initial treatment.

D. **Diet.** Breast cancer seems to be associated with diets high in meats, dairy products, vegetable oil, and animal fat, and low in fiber. Women with breast cancer should be encouraged to eat a diet high in grains, vegetables, fruits and fibers, and low in fats.

## VIII. Breast cancer and pregnancy

A. **Incidence.** Breast engorgement, particularly during lactation, makes detection of breast masses more difficult. Breast cancer occurs in less than 1 in 3000 pregnancies, comprising less than 3% of all breast cancers.

B. **Diagnosis** using fine-needle aspiration or open biopsy should be performed on any suspicious mass.

C. **Treatment** should proceed as with a nonpregnant patient. Lumpectomy with adjuvant chemotherapy is usually not an appropriate choice for an ongoing pregnancy. A patient with

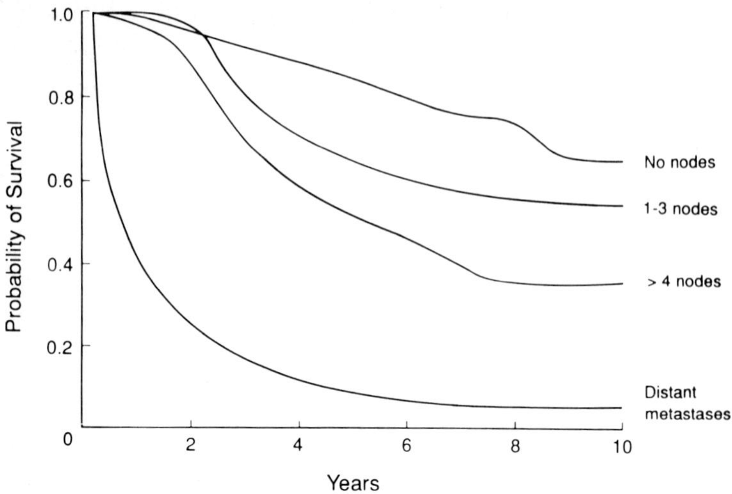


FIGURE 4.8. Comparison of Duke University statistics of survival of breast cancer patients treated by conventional surgery with variable lymph node involvement and distant metastasis. Adapted from McCarty KS Jr. Effects of progesterone on the breast. Int Proc J. 1989; 1(1):169–173.

breast cancer and positive nodes early in pregnancy may elect abortion because of the risk of chemotherapy to the fetus. Late in pregnancy, chemotherapy should be delayed until postpartum.

**D. Prognosis.** Stage-for-stage, the prognosis is similar to the nonpregnant patient. After initial treatment, if there is no evidence of persistent or recurrent disease, there is no documented reason to recommend against subsequent pregnancy, although most oncologists advise waiting at least two years.

## BENIGN BREAST DISEASE

In addition to diagnosing and/or ruling out malignant breast lesions, the physician should be familiar with common benign breast disorders: how they present and how best to manage them.

### I. Fibrocystic breasts

**A. Incidence.** It is the most common breast condition, occurring in more than 50% of women. Unless exogenous estrogens are given postmenopausally, symptoms cease when ovarian function ceases.

**B. Signs and symptoms**

1. Cyclic bilateral breast pain, which is accentuated premenstrually, is the typical history.
2. The breast tissue is tender with easily palpable multiple small cysts or "lumps" of varying sizes.

### C. Treatment

1. Fine-needle aspiration (FNA) of cysts, which is performed for diagnosis, is therapeutic for benign cysts and may well relieve localized pain.
2. Open biopsy should be performed if:
   a. The fluid is bloody
   b. There is a residual mass after aspiration
   c. The cyst recurs
3. Dietary alterations including avoiding salt and eliminating tobacco, caffeine, and methylxanthines, can decrease tenderness and lumpiness in selected patients. The results are not predictable and do not have a proven scientific basis using prospective controlled studies, yet many patients have some improvement with this form of therapy.
4. Diuretics such as hydrochlorothiazide 25 to 50 mg/d for 7 to 10 days prior to menstruation in conjunction with a low salt diet can help.
5. Danazol 200 mg b.i.d. is 80% effective in the long-term treatment of severe cases.
6. Bromocriptine can be given 5 mg daily for cases that do not respond to danazol.
7. Vitamin E (400–800 IU/d) has been useful in selected patients.
8. In rare circumstances, mastectomy is performed because of intractable pain unrelieved by medical therapy.

## II. Fibroadenoma

A. **Incidence.** Fibroadenomas are the most common benign tumors in the female breast. They occur most commonly in 20- to 30-year-old women. They may be stimulated by pregnancy and usually regress at the menopause.

B. **Signs and symptoms.** They typically present as single, nontender, freely mobile firm masses.

C. **Treatment.** Surgical excision usually under local anesthesia is the definitive treatment. Alternately, they can be diagnosed cytologically by FNA and subsequently followed carefully.

## III. Intraductal papilloma

A. **Incidence.** They may occur at any time during adulthood, although they tend to occur around the time of menopause.

B. **Signs and symptoms.** The patient typically presents with a bloody, serous, or turbid spontaneous nipple discharge, usually with no associated palpable mass.

C. **Treatment.** Direct palpation of a particular "trigger point" on the breast can elicit nipple discharge. This can direct the surgeon in performing an excisional biopsy under local anesthesia. Galactography (ductography) can usually precisely identify the location of the lesion.

## IV. Mammary duct ectasia

A. **Incidence.** This typically occurs in a woman's fifth decade. The subareolar ducts are dilated and filled with old dried breast secretions.

B. **Signs and symptoms.** The patient can complain of spontaneous nipple discharge, pain, and tenderness. The discharge is usually thick and green. The nipple may retract and the axillary nodes may be enlarged, thus simulating cancer.

C. **Treatment.** Excisional biopsy confirms the diagnosis. No further treatment is necessary.

## V. Fat necrosis.

This is usually caused by trauma, although often the initial incident may go unrecognized. A hard, irregular mass may be associated with retraction or dimpling of the overlying skin and can simulate cancer. The treatment is excision biopsy.

## VI. Breast abscess.

The area of infection is edematous, erythematous, warm, and tender. They are often multilocular. They occur most often during pregnancy or lactation. If nursing, the patient should be encouraged to continue and be offered antibiotics, for example, dicloxacillin, 250 mg q.i.d. This should cure the vast majority of cases. Infrequently, aspiration drainage of pus by an 18-gauge needle using local anesthesia is necessary. If resistant or too far advanced, drainage under general anesthesia may be necessary in some cases. Cultures most commonly grow out *Staphylococcus aureus.*

## BIBLIOGRAPHY


Azzarelli A, Guzzon A, Pilotti S, Quaglivolo V, Bono A, Dipietro S. Accuracy of breast cancer diagnosis by physical, radiologic, and cytologic combined examinations. Tumor. 1983; 2:137.

Donegan WL, Spratt JS. Cancer of the Breast. 3rd ed. Philadelphia, Pa: WB Saunders; 1988.

Harris JR, Hellman S, Henderson IC, Kinne DW. Breast Disease. Philadelphia, Pa: JB Lippincott; 1987.

Hindle W, Navin J. Breast aspiration cytology: A neglected gynecologic procedure. Am J Obstet Gynecol. 1983; 146:482.

Hindle WH. Breast Disease for Gynecologists. E Norwalk, Conn: Appleton & Lang; 1990.

Kline TS, Kline IK. Breast: Guides to Clinical Aspiration Biopsy. New York: Igaku-Shoin; 1989.

Kopans DB. Breast Imaging. Philadelphia, Pa: JB Lippincott; 1989.

Limited surgery and radiotherapy for early breast cancer—special report. N Eng J Med. 1985; 21:1365.

Lippman ME, Lichter AS, Danfort DN, Jr. Diagnosis and Management of Breast Cancer. Philadelphia, Pa: WB Saunders; 1988.

Marchant DJ. Breast disease. Clin Obstet Gynecol. 1982; 25:351.

Rodes N. Impact of breast cancer screening on survival: A 5 to 10 year followup study. Cancer. 1986; 57:581.

Rosemond G, Maier WP, Brobyn TJ. Needle aspiration of breast cysts. Surg Gynecol Obstet. 1969; 128:351.

Tabar L, Dean PB. Teaching Atlas of Mammography. 2nd Revised ed. Thieme Medical Pubs, 1985.

Weitheimer MP, Costanza ME, Dodson TF, D'orsi CD, Pastides H, Zepha JG. Increasing the effort toward breast cancer detection. JAMA. 1986; 255:1311.

Wilson RE, Donegan WL, Mettlin C, Natarajan N, Smart CR, Murphy GP. 1982 National survey of carcinoma of the breast in the United States by the American College of Surgeons. Surg Gynecol Obstet. 1984; 159:309.

Winchester DP, Sener S, Immerman S, Blum M. A systematic approach to the evaluation and management of breast masses. Cancer. 1983; 51:2535.

# CHAPTER 5

# Benign Diseases of the Vulva

**John R. Musich**
**Thomas G. Stovall**

Vulvar diseases are some of the most common gynecologic problems. Occupying the female genitalia from the mons pubis to the rectum and bordered by the lateral portions of the labia majora, the vulva can exhibit many variations of normal anatomy while being host to multiple symptomatic and asymptomatic pathologic conditions. Developmental anomalies or abnormalities, such as Müllerian tract agenesis or duplication, clitoral hypertrophy, imperforate hymen, ureteral epispadias or hypospadias, are possible but infrequently seen. Instead, most vulvar disorders occur because this region is in large part an organ of skin and, like skin elsewhere, can manifest inflammatory, vascular, dermatologic, dystrophic, cystic, and both benign and malignant neoplastic changes. A complete discussion of all vulvar disorders is beyond the scope of this chapter. For detailed reviews the reader is referred to the cited Bibliography section. This chapter considers only the vulvar infectious diseases and dystrophies most commonly seen in clinical practice.

## VULVAR INFECTIOUS DISEASE

Of the important infectious diseases that affect the vulva, herpes and syphilis are discussed in other chapters. To be presented in this chapter are the remaining vulvar infections that confront the practitioner with varying frequency: candidiasis (moniliasis), chancroid, granuloma inguinale, lymphogranuloma venereum, condyloma acuminata, Bartholin's duct abscess, and pediculosis pubis.

I. **Incidence of vulvar infections.** Candidiasis is one of the most common vulvar disorders seen in everyday practice. Usually manifested in conjunction with monilial vaginitis, it causes clinical problems for millions of women annually. In reproductive age women, condyloma acuminata occurs very frequently, while pediculosis pubis (pubic lice) is a frequent infestation usually seen in adolescent women. Abscesses of Bartholin's duct are seen frequently in a time epidemic for sexually transmitted diseases. Granuloma inguinale, lymphogranuloma venereum and chancroid are infrequently seen in the United States, usually in indigent female populations.

**II. Morbidity and mortality of vulvar infections.** Except for the uncommon cases of severe vulvar disfigurement caused by condyloma acuminata, chancroid, granuloma inguinale or lymphogranuloma venereum, vulvar infectious diseases are not usually thought of in terms of morbidity as much as they are in terms of aggravating local symptoms and social embarrassment. These diseases are rarely associated with mortality.

**III. Candidiasis** is caused by the fungus *Candida albicans* and is frequently referred to as yeast or monilial infections. *C. albicans* is a normal inhabitant of the vaginal flora, and in primary vulvar infections the vagina is usually the source of the vulvar spread. The vulva is the most common mucocutaneous surface infected by this organism. Candidiasis is one of the most common vulvar disorders seen in everyday practice. Pregnancy, diabetes mellitus, oral contraceptive use, antibiotic therapy, Trichomonas vaginitis, and cutaneous injury to the vagina or vulva are the most common inciting circumstances associated with symptomatic vulvar candidiasis.

**A. Diagnosis**

1. **Clinical presentation.** The diagnosis of vulvar candidiasis is usually made solely by observing its classic gross appearance in a patient with compatible symptoms.
   a. Candidiasis is nearly always associated with vulvar pruritus; indeed, a complaint of vulvovaginal itching should always be considered candidiasis until proven otherwise. Rarely, vulvar candidiasis is an isolated entity and is more commonly an associated infection with candida vaginitis.
   b. Candidiasis is characterized by a yellow-white curdlike vaginal discharge often forming plaquelike lesions on the ectocervix and vaginal walls. It causes labial inflammation with edematous, tender, weeping areas induced by intense scratching and subsequent cracking or fissure formation of the affected vulvar skin. The infection frequently spreads to the lateral labia majora, perianal mucosa, and genitocrural areas of the inner thighs.
   c. If in a chronic phase, candidiasis may be present as a dry, scaling lesion with a slightly elevated, reddened margin, or if moist, with a diffuse grayish surface glaze.
2. **Laboratory findings.** The diagnosis of candidiasis on the basis of signs and symptoms is confirmed by identification of budding and pseudomycelia formation on either microscopic examination of a Papanicolaou (PAP) smear or of a potassium hydroxide (KOH)-treated microscopic wet

preparation of the discharge. Culture methods are available but rarely indicated.

**B. Management**

1. The primary treatment for candidiasis is usually with one of the following specific antifungal preparations, all of which are satisfactory treatments:
   a. Nystatin (Mycostatin)—daily vaginal suppository application for 1 week.
   b. Miconazole (Monistat)—daily application for 3 days to 1 week of either vaginal cream or vaginal suppository. A Monistat dual-pack is available, which comes with three vaginal suppositories with Monistat cream for vulvar application.
   c. Terconazole (Terazol)—daily vaginal suppository application for 3 days.
   d. Clotrimazole (Gyne-Lotrimin, Mycelex-G)—two tablets or cream vaginally combined with external application daily vaginally for 3 to 7 days.
   e. Butoconazole (Femstat)—daily application of cream for 3 days.
2. A combination of intravaginal and vulvar treatment is required. A cream should be used for external application. This is usually applied once or twice daily depending on symptom severity.
3. The traditional 7-day regimen has been shown to be no more effective than the newer 3-day treatment course.
4. In certain cases with particularly bothersome vulvar inflammation, Nystatin therapy plus triamcinolone (Mycolog) cream (applied externally to the vulva twice a day in a thin film) will be beneficial.
5. Other adjunctive measures described that may or may not be beneficial include an acidifying cleansing vaginal douche with 2 tablespoons of vinegar in a quart of water (daily for 3–5 days), wearing cotton undergarments rather than heat and moisture-retaining synthetic fabrics, yeast-free diet and the use of condoms by the sex partner to prevent reinfection by an asymptomatic male carrier, particularly during the course of antifungal therapy.
6. **Underlying medical problems,** including poorly controlled diabetes, intercurrent infections, exogenous obesity, and immunosuppression, must be treated to affect a lasting cure of candidiasis.
7. **Recurrent or chronic candidiasis**
   a. The use of ketoconazole (400 mg daily) or nystatin tablets (500 000 U daily or twice daily) have been reported. A 50% recurrence rate following drug discontinuation along with liver toxicity when using ketocanazole are bothersome problems.
   b. Other therapies include painting the vagina with 1%

gentian violet or 600 mg boric acid suppository twice daily.

c. Prophylactic treatment for 1 or 2 days at the beginning of each menses has also been successful in some patients with cyclic symptomatology.

**IV. Chancroid** is caused by *Hemophilus ducreyi*, a small gram-negative bacillus. It is sexually transmitted and is actually seen more frequently in men than women (ratio of about 10:1).

**A. Diagnosis**

1. **Clinical presentation.** Most diagnostic confusion involves distinguishing chancroid (soft painful chancre) from primary syphilis (hard painless chancre), herpes genitalis, granuloma inguinale, and lymphogranuloma venereum. Chancroid usually involves the urethra, posterior fourchette, and the vestibular mucosa bounded by the labia minora. After a 3 to 5 day incubation period, the small single or multiple pustules erode to form shallow, soft, strikingly painful, malodorous ulcers, which may become confluent and have virtually no induration. Ipsilateral inguinal lymphadenopathy occurs in 40% to 50% of patients.
2. **Diagnostic procedures.** The lesion has no characteristic histologic features, although stained smears (Gram, Giemsa, Wright) obtained from the undersurface of the ragged edges of the ulcers exhibiting chains of gram-negative rods may be helpful. Conclusive laboratory techniques for confirmation of chancroid are lacking. Antigen skin testing and complement-fixation studies are of questionable worth in a clinical setting.

**B. Management**

1. **Primary therapy.** Sulfa has long been the standard treatment of chancroid, although streptomycin or trimethoprim-sulfamethoxazole is preferred for treatment failures and may have a role as primary therapy. Treatment regimens include the following:
   a. Trimethoprim-sulfamethoxazole (Bactrim, Septra), 2 tablets per day p.o. for 14 days (each tablet contains 160 mg trimethoprim and 800 mg sulfamethoxazole).
   b. Tetracycline, 2 g/d p.o. for 14 days. Bacterial resistance has been reported, making trimethoprim-sulfamethoxazole the treatment of choice.
   c. Sulfisoxazole (Gantrisin), 4 g/d p.o. for 14 days.
   d. Streptomycin, 1 g/d IM for 6 days.
2. **Treatment during pregnancy for patients with sulfa allergy.** Erythromycin and cephalosporins are usually reserved for patients with sulfa allergies or in pregnancy. Treatment regimens include the following:

a. Erythromycin, 2 g/d p.o. in divided doses for 14 days.
b. Cephalothin (Keflin), 1 g IV q.i.d. for 5 days (inpatient regimen).

V. **Granuloma inguinale** is caused by *Calymmatobacterium (Donovania) granulomatis,* a gram-negative encapsulated bacillus. It is sexually transmitted.

A. **Diagnosis**

1. **Clinical presentation.** After an incubation period of 1 to 12 weeks, granuloma inguinale's clinical presentation differs from chancroid mainly in the extent of its vulvar involvement. Initially a reddened papule in the vestibular area, the lesion erodes and extends as a painless, irregular, ragged-edged ulcer with an erythematous, granular base. Local extension of the disease commonly involves the perineum, perirectal skin, genitocrural creases, and inguinal folds. Extension to the vagina and cervix is possible, as are oral lesions consequent to oral-genital contact. Lymphatic spread is uncommon but more likely to occur whenever secondary bacterial infection of the primary lesion occurs.
2. **Diagnostic procedures** are aided by the microscopic finding of Donovan bodies in a biopsy specimen from the lesion's margins. The Donovan body, a large mononuclear macrophage containing numerous clusters of the encapsulated *C. granulomatis* organism, is best seen in Giemsa or silver stains and is confirmatory of granuloma inguinale when present.
3. **Differential diagnosis.** As with most genital ulcers, the differential diagnosis includes chancroid, lymphogranuloma venereum, syphilis, and herpes. In addition, a vulvar carcinoma must be ruled out as granuloma inguinale and carcinoma may coexist.

B. **Management**

1. The treatment of choice is tetracycline, 2 g/d p.o. in divided doses for at least 14 days, or until a complete clinical response occurs with healing of the ulcerative lesion. Doxycycline 100 mg b.i.d. may also be used.
2. Other regimens include:
   a. Sulfonamides, 2 g/d p.o. in divided doses for 14 days.
   b. Streptomycin, 1 g/d IM for 7 days.
   c. Ampicillin, 2 g/d p.o. in divided doses for 14 days.
   d. Erythromycin, 2 g/d p.o. for 14 days.

VI. **Lymphogranuloma venereum** (LGV) is caused by *Chlamydia trachomatis,* an organism that shares properties of both bacteria and viruses and is therefore difficult to culture.

A. **Diagnosis**

1. **Clinical presentation.** After an incubation period of 4 to 21 days, LGV starts as a small vesicle or papule on the mucocutaneous surfaces of the vulva. The initial lesion may ulcerate but heals rapidly. In a few weeks, the patient will have a symptomatic inguinal lymphadenitis that is usually unilateral but may be bilateral. The enlarged, considerably tender inflammatory nodal mass (bubo) is covered by erythematous inguinal skin, that may become fixed to the underlying nodes. In severe cases, spread to surrounding inguinal and vulvar structures may occur, fluctuance may develop and destructive ulceration, drainage, scarring, and fistula formation may result in chronic vulvar disease. A classic sign of LGV is the double genitocrural fold or groove sign, which is a depression between groups of inflamed nodes.
2. **Diagnostic procedures** are dependent on obtaining the history of a healed precursor vulvar lesion followed by the symptomatic appearance of inguinal adenitis. Biopsy of the nodal lesions can be done, but the histologic appearance is not specific for LGV. Historically, a Frei test was done but is no longer used because of low sensitivity. Complement fixation is reliable and obtainable through most laboratories, as is monoclonal antibody test done on nodal aspirate. A titer of 1.64 is diagnostic.
3. **Differential diagnosis** includes chronic vulvar infectious disease, lymphoma, carcinoma with nodal metastases, granuloma inguinale and, when the perirectal areas are involved, ulcerative colitis must be considered.

B. **Management**

1. **Antibiotic.** Lymphogranuloma venereum is preferentially treated with sulfa or tetracycline regimens as described for chancroid and granuloma inguinale.
2. **Surgery.** Surgical drainage or aspiration of the bubo is frequently necessary to prevent further spread or sinus tract development.

VII. **Condyloma acuminata** is caused by the human papillomavirus (HPV) of the DNA-containing papovavirus group and is sexually transmitted. There is increasing evidence that a relationship exists between HPV and cervical intraepithelial neoplasia and cervical cancer.

A. **Diagnosis**

1. **Clinical presentation.** In its early stages, the lesion's growth is rarely appreciated, with patients usually presenting with a complaint of feeling a lump in her vulvar area. Pregnancy, sexual promiscuity, oral contraceptive usage, and persistent vaginitis may predispose to or stimulate their growth. As with all other sexually transmitted dis-

eases, condyloma acuminata is seen with increasing frequency today. It presents as a small, pink, soft papillomatous or warty lesion, predominantly in the periclitoral, vestibular, perineal, and perianal area. Lateral spread to the labia majora is uncommon, whereas spread to the vagina, cervix, and urethra is common. Confluence of many individual warts is frequently seen, giving the impression of a single, fleshy, proliferative lesion. Secondary infection, bleeding, and discharge are common. Predisposing factors for infection include immunosuppression, diabetes, pregnancy and local trauma.

2. **Diagnostic procedures.** Condyloma acuminata is one of the most frequently seen vulvar disorders, and for this reason its diagnosis is readily made by its classic appearance alone. Biopsy and histologic verification can be done but are unnecessary unless there is no response to therapy. Malignant changes are rarely seen, but in patients with atypical wartlike masses or those refractory to treatment, biopsy is mandatory. Over 50 subtypes of HPV have been identified. HPV 6, 11, 16, and 18 are the most common types in genital infections with types 16 and 18 associated with premalignant lesion.

B. **Management** must be individualized based on condyloma location, size, extent of disease, and whether the patient is pregnant.

1. **Medical therapy**
   a. **Topical podophyllin** (10% to 25%) in a benzoin base applied carefully to the lesion, with instructions to the patient to wash it off 4 to 6 hours later. Several applications once a week over a few weeks may be necessary, and care must be taken to avoid irritating normal mucosal surfaces with the podophyllin resin. Podophyllin is contraindicated in pregnancy.
   b. **Trichloroacetic acid** (TCA) has also proven effective. It is applied directly to the lesion(s) and does not require washing off later. Several applications per week may be necessary for resolution. It may be safely used in pregnancy also.
   c. **5-Fluorouracil (Efudex Cream).** A variety of regimens have been proposed. The cream may be applied to the vulvar area and left for 4-6 hours prior to being washed. This can be repeated two to three times a week for 4 to 12 weeks. The cream may be placed onto a tampon and placed into the vagina. It should be removed and a vaginal douche performed after 4-6 hours.
   d. **Immunotherapy.** Interferon A has been used but the treatment is generally disappointing and requires local wart injection three times a week for several weeks.

2. **Surgical therapy.** Cryotherapy, electrocautery, or laser therapy may be necessary in refractory cases or with very large lesions. Laser extirpation is probably the most effective of these modalities, performed by a gynecologic surgeon or dermatologist specially trained in laser surgery.
3. **Adjuvant therapy.** Treatment of sexual partners, the use of condoms to prevent reinfection as well as instruction in genital self-examination should be considered for all patients.

**VIII. Bartholin's duct abscess.** Bartholin's gland is an embryonic derivative of the urogenital sinus, which in the adult woman is located within the lower pole of the labium majus. The gland is composed of mucin-producing and excreting acini which open to the posterolateral vestibule just external to the hymenal ring through a transitional and squamous epithelium-lined duct. Cystic dilatation of the gland's duct due to obstruction is probably the most common finding in patients complaining of vulvar masses. Although obstetric or accidental trauma, congenital atresia, ductal epithelial hyperplasia, or inspissated mucus may cause the occlusion, most symptomatic Bartholin's duct cysts are clinically associated with infection and abscess formation. Although Bartholin's duct abscesses frequently harbor gonorrheal infection, organisms such as *Staphylococcus aureus, Streptococcus fecalis, Escherichia coli,* and *Pseudomonas* may also be etiologically involved.

**A. Diagnosis**

1. Diagnosis of Bartholin's duct abscess is readily made by its appearance. A normal Bartholin's gland and duct are nonpalpable, and any cystic swelling in the base of the labia majora almost certainly represents a cyst or abscess. These may range in diameter from 1 to 10 cm, may be asymptomatic, or may be painfully tender, particularly if due to infection.
2. The differential diagnosis of such a lesion includes lipomas, fibromas, hydroceles, accessory breast tissue, or hernias, but unlike duct cysts, these entities usually involve the upper portions of the labia majora and rarely extend into the area of the posterior fourchette. In women over 40 years, Bartholin's gland carcinoma should be considered, although it is rare.

**B. Management** of Bartholin's duct abscesses is dependent upon the suspected cause and symptoms. Many small ductal cysts are asymptomatic, do not interfere with intercourse or cause discomfort with walking, sitting, or activity, and may spontaneously wax or wane in size. Most cysts, however, are painful edematous abscesses that require prompt evaluation and treatment.

1. **Sitz baths.** If left alone, most ductal abscesses will eventually "point" and spontaneously rupture resulting in imme-

diate perineal relief. This process may be hastened with frequent warm water sitz baths.

2. **Incision and drainage.** If necessary, outpatient drainage can be achieved by simply incising the abscessed duct through the overlying, anesthetized, mucocutaneous vestibule. This incision and drainage will provide prompt relief but may not prevent recurrence. A Word catheter should be inserted for 7 to 14 days to facilitate drainage and formation of an epithelized outflow tract.
3. **Definitive surgical therapy**
   a. **Marsupialization** of the duct is performed during a time when the cyst is readily palpable but before spontaneous rupture occurs. Recurrence after a proper marsupialization is unlikely. The procedure, usually done under general anesthesia, consists of incising the abscess as in an incision and drainage, but instead of closing the wound, the ductal epithelium is sutured to the vaginal mucosa with a fine suture (e.g., 3-0 catgut). This will keep the wound open, allowing healing from the base of the cavity and thereby closure of the cavity. If marsupialization is planned for a patient over 40 years of age, a biopsy should be sent for histologic analysis at that time to rule out carcinoma.
   b. **Glandular excision** is the only definitive procedure. Total excision is infrequently indicated in a young woman, but in an older patient where carcinoma is a possibility, total excision may be necessary for histologic diagnosis.
4. **Antibiotic therapy and culturing.** Like other infected abscesses, the key to treatment of abscess of Bartholin's duct is surgical drainage. Although culturing the abscess fluid is not essential to management, it may be done. More than 80% of cultures from the cysts are sterile as are one-third of cultures from abscessed Bartholin's ducts. When cultures are positive, generally they reveal a mixed polymicrobic infection. Likewise, adequate drainage usually precludes the need for antibiotic therapy.

**IX. Pediculosis pubis** is caused by Phthirus pubis, commonly referred to as crabs. Pediculosis pubis may be spread by sexual intercourse or by contact with other infested body areas or inanimate objects (e.g., bedding, bed clothes, towels).

A. **Diagnosis.** The affected area always itches and may be reddened, either from irritation by the parasite or by chronic scratching. The diagnosis can usually be made by observing the insect near the pubic hair roots.

B. **Management.** Because eggs and/or larvae are usually present on the hair shafts, treatment must be aggressive and occasionally repeated. The recommended treatment is Kwell shampoo (lindane 1%) of the affected area and over the rest of the body, with repeat shampoo as needed. Those who have come in contact with the patient or bed clothes, etc., which the patient has used should also be examined. Bed clothing and other items should be thoroughly washed in very hot water with copious amounts of detergent to avoid recontamination. Adjuvant use of antihistamines to control itching that may persist after the organism has been cured is of benefit.

X. **Scabies** is a parasitic infection of *Sacroptes scabiei*. Unlike pediculosis pubis, the infection has no prediction for hair-bearing areas. The presenting symptom in these patients is itching in the pubic area secondary to allergic sensitization. Definitive diagnosis is made by scraping the skin with a needle and placing the crust onto a microscopic slide with a drop of oil. The treatment is the same for pediculosis pubis (crabs).

## VULVAR DYSTROPHIES

White and red lesions of the vulva have been the subject of numerous confusing reports in the medical literature. Much of the confusion has resulted from the inconsistent and variable terminology used to describe the many possible lesions that fall into this area of vulvar disease. In this section a simplified classification of the vulvar dystrophies, along with general management guidelines, is presented.

I. **Clinical considerations.** Vulvar dystrophies are common entities, particularly in women over 50 years of age. Although uniformly benign, they can cause significant morbidity, usually in the occurrence of intense pruritus that may result in disabling and persistent scratching and patient's fear over the possibility of cancer.

II. **Pathogenesis and pathophysiology.** Vulvar dystrophies of all types share a common histopathology, that of changes in the vulvar epithelium and underlying connective tissue that are probably secondary to the influences of chronic inflammation and irritation. In deviating from normal epithelium, vulvar skin will become dystrophic in one of two ways: either it becomes atrophic (thinned-out) or it becomes hypertrophic or hyperplastic (thickened). In either case, the wetness of the vulva will cause the superficial, and usually increased, keratin layer of the epithelium to become whitish or grayish in color. The thicker the keratin layer, the whiter the lesion becomes. Along with the response of the keratin to moisture, underlying connective tissue changes, such as relatively decreased vascularity, variable hyalinization, and loss of normal pigmentation, contribute to the pale white appearance of these lesions. These lesions also share a common symptomatic presentation, that of pruritus and burning. Malignant degeneration is uncommon (less than 1% to 2%) but must be considered in all cases.

**III. Diagnosis.** Biopsy is mandatory for all vulvar lesions and dystrophies that do not exhibit an obvious diagnostic appearance. In this way guesswork can be eliminated, malignancies will not be overlooked, and appropriate management will be afforded to the patient.

**IV. Classification.** Three items comprise the classification of vulvar dystrophies used in the selection of evaluation and management.

- **A.** Hyperplastic dystrophies
  - **1.** Hyperplastic without atypia
  - **2.** Hyperplastic atypia (mild, moderate, severe)
- **B.** Lichen sclerosis—atrophic dystrophies
- **C.** Mixed dystrophies
  - **1.** Lichen sclerosis with hyperplastic dystrophy
  - **2.** Without atypia
  - **3.** With atypia (mild, moderate, severe)

**V. Management**

- **A.** Hyperplastic dystrophies
  - **1. Clinical features.** All hyperplastic vulvar diseases, commonly referred to as leukoplakia, have a thickened epithelium that is characterized microscopically by hyperkeratosis (thickening of the keratin layer) and hypertrophy of the rete pegs (acanthosis). Hyperplastic dystrophies occur most often in postmenopausal women, although reproductive age occurrences are possible. The posterior fourchette, labia majora, lateral labia minora, and clitoral areas are the most common areas of involvement.
  - **2. Biopsy.** Because of pruritus and consequent scratching, the appearance of the lesion may be distorted, making biopsy essential to rule out atypical or malignant changes.
    - a. Biopsies may be taken by excisional or punch technique under local anesthesia.
    - b. Multiple biopsies may be necessary. Toluidine blue staining often aids in the selection of biopsy sites. After applying a 1% toluidine blue (aqueous) solution to the affected area and allowing it to dry, the vulva is rinsed with dilute acetic acid, usually 1%. Normal epithelium will be left stain-free, while the nuclei of abnormal superficial keratinized epithelium will take up the stain and indicate appropriate areas for biopsy.
  - **3. Treatment**
    - a. **Corticosteroids.** Primary treatment for the hyperplastic dystrophies consists of topical corticosteroids. Topical creams are preferred over ointments because of their lesser likelihood to trap heat and moisture. Twice-daily application of a thin film to the affected area should give results within 2 to 3 weeks, although thick lesions may require long-term therapy. Patients should be counseled regarding compliance with treatment and the need for longer treatment with larger lesions. Caution

must be exercised, however, as chronic application and overtreatment with steroids may result in atrophic changes and symptomatic worsening of the original problem. One of the following steroid preparations is recommended:

(1) Hydrocortisone 1%
(2) Fluocinonide (Lidex) 0.05%
(3) Fluocinolone acetonide (Synalar) 0.01%
(4) Triamcinolone acetonide (Aristocort, Kenalog) 0.1%
(5) Betamethasone valerate (Valisone) 0.1%

b. **Tranquilizers.** The adjunctive use of tranquilizer is sometimes helpful in the anxious patient or the patient with especially severe pruritus.

(1) Chlordiazepoxide hydrochloride (Librium), 15 to 40 mg p.o. daily divided into three or four doses, available in 5, 10, and 25 mg tablets.
(2) Diazepam (Valium), 4 to 40 mg p.o. daily in two to four divided doses, available in 2, 5, and 10 mg tablets.

c. **Antihistamines.** The adjunctive use of antihistaminics is also often helpful in the patient with especially severe pruritus.

(1) Diphenhydramine hydrochloride (Benadryl), 100 to 250 mg p.o. in divided doses, available in 25 and 50 mg capsules and an elixir at 12.5 mg per 5 mL.
(2) Hydroxyzine hydrochloride (Vistaril), 225 to 400 mg p.o. daily in divided doses, available in 25, 50, and 100 mg capsules.
(3) Hydroxyzine pamoate (Atarax), 225 to 400 mg p.o. daily in divided doses, available in 10, 25, 50, and 100 mg capsules, occasionally indicated.

d. **Burow's solution** (15% aluminum acetate in water) has a soothing effect. A warm sitz bath of Burow's solution can be used four to five times daily if needed to control pruritus.

**B. Lichen sclerosus.** Atrophic lesions of the vulva are the most common of the white dystrophies. Other terms used include: kraurosis vulvae, senile atrophy, atrophic vulvitis, atrophic leukoplakei, lichen planus atrophicus, and the popular lichen sclerosus et atrophicus (LS A). Patients with lichen sclerosus are not at an increased risk for developing vulvar carcinoma.

1. **Clinical features.** Similar in most clinical respects to the hyperplastic lesions, lichen sclerosus differs in one important aspect. Unlike the hyperplastic dystrophies, lesions with underlying atrophy may destroy the normal vulvar anatomy, causing dissolution of the labia minora, scarring together of the clitoris and periclitoral structures, and introi-

tal contracture. Atrophic dystrophies have a general appearance that is characterized by desiccation and thinning out of the affected areas. Histologically, hyperkeratosis is frequently present, but the diagnostic features are the relative loss of rete pegs and the homogeneous hyalinization of the subepidermal layers.

2. **Treatment**
   a. Primary therapy consists of topical testosterone three times daily for 4 to 6 weeks, after which the frequency of application may be decreased or stopped entirely. Because there are no commercial preparations, the pharmacy will have to be asked to make up a testosterone preparation in a neutral base, usually testosterone propionate 2% in a petroleum jelly base.
   b. A program of intermittent but continuing therapy is necessary for atrophic lesions, which are frequently recurrent compared to hyperplastic lesions.
   c. Patients should be counseled with regards to the chronic nature of this lesion as well as the need for compliance with therapy. This will help to avoid patient frustration with prolonged therapy.

C. **Mixed dystrophies**

1. **Clinical features and diagnosis.** Mixed hypertrophic–atrophic lesions are uncommon but demand continuing attention because of a greater tendency of atypia and malignant changes than either of the pure dystrophies. Because of their variable degrees of atrophic or hypertrophic involvement and tendency to atypia, mixed dystrophies require multiple-site biopsies to better define the pathology.
2. **Treatment** options depend on the extent of the predominant lesion.
   a. Hypertrophic: corticosteroid therapy followed by testosterone therapy.
   b. Lichen sclerosus: testosterone therapy followed by corticosteroid therapy.

## VULVODYNIA

I. **Definition.** Vulvodynia is defined as chronic vulvar discomfort, characterized by the patient's complaints of burning, stinging, irritation, or rawness.

II. **Clinical presentation**

A. Erythema of the vulvar and vestibular area may be present, but the lack of abnormal physical findings is the rule.

B. Most patients have suffered for many months and have seen numerous physicians without significant relief.

## III. Etiology

A. **Vestibular gland.** The significance of vestibular gland pain in the etiology is not known. In these patients pain is elicited when vestibular gland orifices are palpated with cotton-tipped applicators, and with intercourse. This entity may be the result of persistent infection, inflammation, or postinflammatory tissue damage, but histologically this is not seen.

B. **Papillomatosis,** small papillae-like structures, may be seen around the vulvar vestibule and posterior introitus in some patients. They may be normal or associated with a subclinical infection of human papillomavirus. This group of patients requires application of acetic acid, colposcopy, and directed biopsy.

**IV. Patient evaluation** should center around treatment of an infection, if one is found, colposcopy to evaluate papillomatosis and biopsy if colposcopy reveals a possible HPV component. The patient's fear of cancer should be put to rest, and use of potential allergens or irritants should be stopped.

**V. Treatment.** A definitive plan for treatment is not known, and therefore treatment must be individualized. Spontaneous remissions do occur. Steroids, nonsteroidal anti-inflammatory agents, antibiotics, and retinoid compounds are of little value. 5-fluorouracil applied two to three times per week for 6 to 12 weeks and acyclovir, 1200 mg daily for 3 months have been helpful in some patients. Topical anesthetic preparations (1% lidocaine gel) afford temporary relief. Laser ablation and surgical excision of the involved vestibule and hymen with mobilization and reapproximation of the vagina and perineum has met with success in 60% to 80% of patients. Alcohol injection is also of benefit in some patients, but like surgical excision should be a treatment of last resort.

## BIBLIOGRAPHY

Benson MD, Brown ER, Keith LG. Sexually transmitted diseases. Curr Probl Obstet Gynecol Fertil. 1985; 8(12):1.

Kaufman RH, Friedrich EG, eds. Vulvar disease. Clin Obstet Gynecol. 1985; 28:121.

Kaufman RH, Friedrich Jr. EG, Gardner HL, eds. Benign Diseases of the Vulva and Vagina. 3rd ed. Chicago: Year Book Medical; 1989.

Tovell HMM, Young AW, eds. Evaluation and management of diseases of the vulva. Clin Obstet Gynecol. 1978; 21:951.

# CHAPTER 6

# Benign Diseases of the Cervix and Vagina

**Jessica L. Thomason**
**Janine A. James**
**Frederik F. Broekhuizen**

Nonmalignant diseases of the vagina and cervix are frequent clinical problems. Symptoms of vaginitis are some of the most common complaints voiced by patients to their physician. Culturing the vagina to diagnose vaginitis is costly and the information gained is not usually helpful. In fact, results are often confusing and antibiotics are inappropriately administered, leading to a vicious cycle of iatrogenically produced yeast infections. Culturing the endocervix for sexually transmitted diseases (STDs) is useful when patient's vaginal secretions contain numerous white blood cells and do not contain vaginal pathogens such as trichomonads. However, the most accurate, reliable and inexpensive method to diagnose vaginitis is by microscopic examination of patient's vaginal secretions.

## VULVOVAGINITIS

Vulvovaginitis, or vulvar discomfort, is a common physical complaint of women, encompassing a range of problems from infectious diseases (e.g., bacterial vaginosis, candida vaginitis, trichomonas vaginitis, and gonorrhea), life-cycle dependent problems such as prepubertal vaginitis, atrophic vaginitis seen in postmenopausal women, and vulvar dystrophies. Proper therapy requires accurate diagnosis with an orderly approach.

### I. Vaginal discharge characteristics in the reproductive-aged patient

#### A. Discriminating characteristics of vaginal discharge

1. **Appearance** is a subjective characteristic. More objective criteria should be used in diagnosis.
   a. **Normal.** The appearance of a normal vaginal discharge is floccular. A normal discharge does not pool at the patient's introitus or posterior fourchette.
   b. **Abnormal.** A homogeneous discharge is abnormal and appears as a cup of milk that has been poured into the vaginal vault. Such discharges easily saturate a swab

and can be wiped from the vaginal walls. The presence of discharge at the introitus warrants evaluation.

2. **pH.** The normal pH of the vagina is 3.5 to 4.5.
3. **Odor.** The normal vaginal discharge does not have a foul or fishy odor.

B. **Nondiscriminating characteristics of vaginal discharge.** Neither the color of vaginal fluid nor the presence of bubbles in the discharge are characteristics pathognominic of pathological conditions.

C. **Diagnosis of vaginitis.** The etiology of a vaginal discharge is diagnosed by the characteristics outlined in Figure 6.1 and Table 6.1:

1. Assessing the pH of vaginal fluid using appropriate coloremetric paper. Obtain a sample of vaginal secretions from anterior or lateral vaginal walls on a dry swab and apply to pH paper. Do not sample the endocervix or posterior fornix

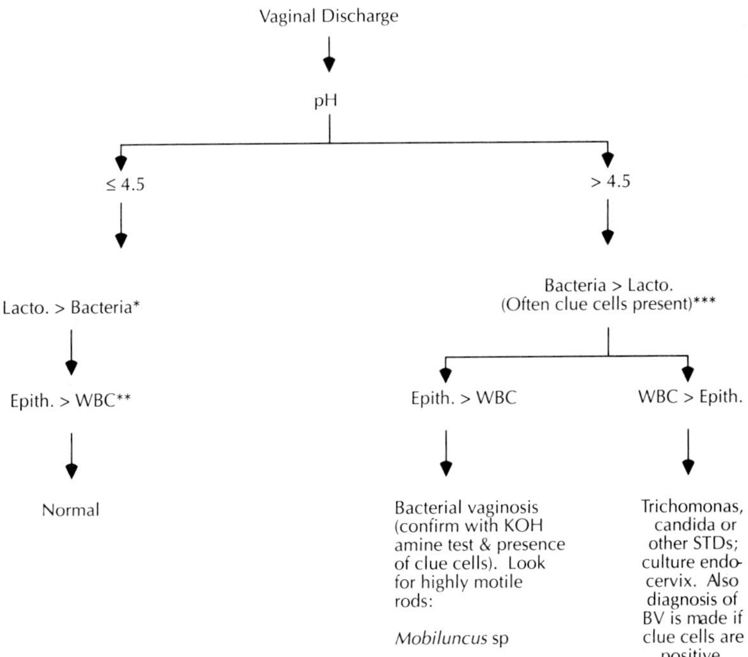


FIGURE 6.1. Work-up of the vaginal discharge. **Lactobacillus* sp > background bacteria. **Epithelial cells > white blood cells (WBC). ***All epithelial cells do not need to be "clue cells" for diagnosis. STDs = sexually transmitted diseases; GC = gonorrhea; BV = bacterial vaginosis; KOH = potassium hydroxide.

**Table 6.1. Differentiating Characteristics of Vaginitis in the Reproductive-Aged Woman***

| TEST OR FINDING | BACTERIAL VAGINOSIS | CANDIDA VAGINITIS | TRICHOMONAS VAGINITIS | OTHER STD (e.g., CHLAMYDIA, GONORRHEA, ETC.) |
|---|---|---|---|---|
| pH | $> 4,5$ | $< 4.5$ | $> 4.5$ | $< 4.5$ |
| KOH amine test | Positive | Negative | Positive if bacterial vaginosis also | Negative |
| *Lactobacillus* sp > background bacteria | No | Yes | Usually no | Yes |
| Epithelial cells > WBCs | Yes | No | No (many WBCs) | No (many WBCs) |
| Pathogens | No | Yeast buds and/or pseudohyphae | Trichomonads | No |
| Other characteristics | 50% have highly mobile curved bacteria (*Mobiluncus* sp) | Infection may show WBC $\geq$ epithelial cells | — | — |

*Assumes no "mixed" vaginitis.
STD = sexually transmitted disease; KOH = potassium hydroxide; WBC = white blood cell.

because the pH in these areas is normally high. A pH value greater than 4.5 is abnormal.

2. Obtain a sample of vaginal secretions with a premoistened swab from the lateral vaginal walls (avoid endocervical or cul-de-sac areas) for microscopic analysis.
3. A "fishy" or "foul" odor after mixing a drop of 10% potassium hydroxide (KOH) with the vaginal secretions is abnormal.

D. **Microscopic examination of vaginal fluid.** A "wet prep" sample for microscopic evaluation is obtained as above. The swabs are placed into two test tubes (12 × 75 mm) containing two drops of saline and KOH, respectively. Place one drop of each mixture on one microscope slide and cover each with a separate cover slip (22 × 22 mm). First scan 10 viewing fields with the 10X objective (10 × 10 [objective eyepiece] = 100 power). Second, look in more detail with the 40X objective (40 × 10 = 400 power) at 10 to 20 viewing fields for the following (all recommended for objective diagnostic criteria):

1. ***Lactobacillus*** sp. normally outnumber other background bacteria, otherwise the flora is abnormal. If uncertain about what *Lactobacillus* sp looks like, Gram stain the specimen. *Lactobacillus* sp appear as large gram-positive rods.
2. **Cellular content of the discharge.** Normally squamous epithelial cells outnumber white blood cells (WBCs). An inverted ratio suggests vaginitis secondary to trichomonads, gonorrhea, Chlamydia trachomatis, or other endocervical STDs.
3. **Clue cells** are epithelial cells that have their border obscured with bacteria. "Dirty" epithelial cells have bacteria located on the cells, not at the cell's border.
4. **Other vaginal pathogens** such as *Trichomonas* sp, *Mobiluncus* sp, and yeast hyphae may be identified.

## II. Bacterial vaginosis (BV).

Previously, BV was referred to as gardnerella vaginitis, nonspecific vaginitis, nonspecific vaginosis, anaerobic vaginosis, or *Corynebacterium* or *Haemophilus* vaginitis.

A. **Infective agent.** The exact etiology of the infection is unknown. Patients are characterized by having much higher concentrations of anaerobes per milliliter of vaginal fluid than normal patients. Recently a new anaerobe, *Mobiluncus* sp, has been associated with the disease. *Gardnerella vaginalis* was previously thought to be the etiologic agent of the disease, hence the previous name gardnerella vaginitis. This disease is not usually characterized by an inflammatory response with an increase in WBCs; therefore the name vaginosis instead of vaginitis.

B. **Incidence.** Bacterial vaginosis is the most common type of vaginitis found in women of reproductive age.

C. **Symptoms.** Most symptomatic patients complain of a foul or fishy odor and may have an increased amount of vaginal discharge. However, over 50% of patients may be entirely asymptomatic.

D. **Signs**
   1. **External signs.** If any signs are present, a homogeneous discharge may be noted at the introitus.
   2. **Vaginal signs.** A homogeneous discharge, that can be easily wiped from the vaginal walls, is often seen. This discharge looks as if a cup of milk had been poured into the vagina. The vaginal pH is >4.5 and the discharge has a foul, fishy odor.

E. **Microscopic diagnosis** (Fig. 6.1 and Table 6.1). Epithelial cells usually outnumber WBCs on the wet prep and background bacteria far outnumber the normally present *Lactobacillus* sp. In addition, in approximately half of patients, a highly motile curved bacterial rod (*Mobiluncus* sp) can be seen moving in a characteristic serpentine and corkscrew spinning pattern. Clue cells are prominent in this disease but not all epithelial cells have to be clue cells to make this diagnosis.

F. **Culture** of the vagina for *Gardnerella vaginalis* is expensive, and offers no useful clinical information. *Gardnerella vaginalis* can be isolated from 40% to 60% of all normal women. Thus, vaginal culture is not recommended.

G. **Therapy.** Approximately 50% of patients respond to metronidazole (Flagyl®, 250 mg p.o. b.i.d. for 10 days). Clindamycin 300 mg b.i.d. × 7 days is also a recommended treatment by the Centers for Disease Control.

H. **Recurrent infections.** Patients can effectively control the foul odor for short time periods by douching with vinegar or hydrogen peroxide. If retreatment with metronidazole is planned within 3 weeks of previous treatment, a WBC count is indicated because metronidazole can cause neutropenia. Treatment of the sexual partner should be considered.

I. **Treatment of sexual partner.** The frequency of recurrent infections suggests this disease may be transmitted sexually. Metronidazole, 500 mg b.i.d. × 7 days or clindamycin 300 mg b.i.d. × 7 days may be effective.

J. **Sequelae.** Studies indicate patients with BV during pregnancy have a higher incidence of premature rupture of the membranes, premature labor, postpartum endometritis, and chorioamnionitis. Gynecologic infectious sequelae include postsurgical cuff cellulitis after hysterectomy, mucopurulent cervicitis, laparoscopically proven pelvic inflammatory disease, and recurrent urinary tract infections.

III. **Candida vaginitis.** (Other names include "monilia" vaginitis, yeast vaginitis, and vaginal thrush.)

A. **Infective agent.** *Candida albicans* can be isolated in 90% of cases whereas other *Candida* sp account for the remainder.

B. **Incidence.** Candida vaginitis is the second most common type of vaginitis in reproductive-aged woman. It occurs frequently in the prepubertal, postmenopausal, and pregnant patient.

C. **Symptoms.** The hallmark of candida vaginitis is vulvar pruritus. Dysuria occurs only with severe disease.

D. **Physical signs**

1. **External signs.** Vulvar signs range from minimal to severe erythema with microulcerations. Severity of patients' symptoms do not correlate with physical signs of disease.
2. **Vaginal signs.** A classic "cottage cheese"-like discharge occurs in less than 10% of patients. A useful diagnostic sign is that of a sticky discharge attached to the vaginal walls or cervix. Most patients have a normal appearing discharge with a pH $\leq$ 4.5.

E. **Microscopic diagnosis** (Table 6.1). Microscopic examinations of wet preps, looking for pseudohyphae or yeast buds, are only 80% accurate. Therapy should not be withheld because of failure to demonstrate hyphae or buds when signs or symptoms of disease exist. The presence of yeast buds in symptomatic patients is a sign of infection. However, yeast buds in asymptomatic patients do not constitute diagnostic criteria of yeast vaginitis because buds may occur in 5% to 20% of normal patients.

F. **Therapy**

1. **Indications for therapy.** All symptomatic patients should be treated regardless of microscopic examination findings. Asymptomatic patients should be treated if pseudohyphae are seen.
2. **External creams/ointments.** Apply five to six times per day to the vulva.
   a. Nystatin
   b. Miconazole 2% derm cream
   c. Clotrimazole
   d. Amphotericin B, Fungisone 3%
   e. Boric acid, Borofax ointment 5%
   f. Ketoconazole
   g. Econazole
3. **Intravaginal creams**
   a. Miconazole (Monistat 7/Monistat 3)—the standard regimen is one applicator (5 g) nightly for either 3 or 7 nights.
   b. Clotrimazole (Gyne-Lotrimin, Mycelex-G1%)—the standard regimen is one applicator (5 g) nightly for 7 nights.
   c. Butoconazole (Femstat)—one applicator (5 g) daily for 3 nights.
   d. Terconazole (Terazol-7)—one applicator (5 g) daily for 7 nights.
4. **Intravaginal suppositories**
   a. Miconazole (Monistat 100 mg suppository daily × 7 days, or 200 mg daily × 3 days or 500 mg for a single application)

b. Clotrimazole (Gyne-Lotrimin; Mycelex)
   (1) Gyne-Lotrimin 100 mg—one tablet intravaginally for treatment.
   (2) Gyne-Lotrimin 500 mg—one tablet intravaginally as a single treatment.
   (3) Mycelex-G 100 mg—one tablet intravaginally for 7 nights.
   (4) Mycelex G 500 mg—one tablet intravaginally as a single dose.

c. Boric acid—one suppository nightly for 7 nights.

d. Nystatin (Nilstate, Mycostatin)—one tablet (100 000 U) daily for 14 days.

e. Terconazole (Terazol-3 80 mg)—one suppository intravaginally at bedtime for 3 consecutive days.

G. **Treatment of sexual partner.** Unnecessary except in recurrent disease. Colonization from the mouth and ejaculate can be treated with oral preparations (ketoconazole 200 mg tablet daily × 14 days).

H. **Recurrent infections.** Patients who experience three or more infections per year may be characterized as chronic or recurrent. Examination of patients for underlying medical diseases is needed. Rule out diabetes, collagen vascular diseases, and anemia. Often patients have evidence of human papillomavirus. Consider colposcopy in such patients. A 6-month trial with ketoconazole (oral tablets, 200 mg b.i.d. × 14 days then 100 mg daily for 6 months, or 200 mg b.i.d. for 5 days with the onset of menses for 6 months) may be helpful. Also, clotrimazole 500 mg per vagina after menses or 100 mg daily for 5 days per month has been found helpful.

## IV. Trichomonas vaginitis

A. **Infective agent.** The infecting organism is *Trichomonas vaginalis*, an anaerobic, flagellated protozoan.

B. **Incidence.** In private practice, the incidence of vaginal trichomonas infection is as low as 3%, but can be as high as 60% in STD clinics.

C. **Symptoms.** The most frequent symptom in acute infection is copious vaginal discharge. Pruritus as well as vulvar irritation is reported, although patients with chronic infection can be entirely asymptomatic. Postcoital bleeding occurs rarely.

D. **Signs**

1. **External signs** range from none to copious discharge.
2. **Vaginal signs.** Secretions are easily wiped from vaginal walls. Classic greenish, frothy discharge is found in less than 5% of patients. Rarely, punctate lesions seen on the cervix give a "strawberry"-like appearance. Concomitant bacterial vaginosis infection is frequently encountered. Erythema of the vagina may be noted in some cases.

E. **Microscopic diagnosis** (Table 6.1). Look for organisms with whip-like flagellae that are motile and slightly larger than WBCs. If secretions are allowed to sit or evaporate, the solution becomes hypertonic, resulting in immobilization of trichomonads. Dead or nonmotile trichomonads resemble WBCs and are difficult to distinguish. For accurate diagnosis, motility should be observed. Microscopic diagnosis is only 80% to 90% accurate but increases when more fields are viewed.

F. **Culture.** If microscopic diagnosis is negative, but clinical suspicion of infection is high, culture in a selective medium.

G. **Therapy.** The only drug available in the United States is metronidazole. Efficacy studies indicate a one-time 2 g oral dose of metronidazole is as effective as the 5- or 7-day regimen (500 mg b.i.d.) and has the added advantage of better patient compliance. There is no difference in the incidence of side effects between various regimens.

H. **Treatment of sexual partner.** Simultaneous therapy with metronidazole for sexual partners of all patients increases cure rates. However, the natural history of acute infections in males suggests 40% to 60% of men spontaneously clear the infection within 3 weeks if not re-exposed to disease. Condom therapy for males with oral treatment of women may be an option for some patients if multiple partners are involved. Most men are asymptomatic although infected.

I. **Recurrent disease.** Most recurrences in patients are secondary to reinfection or inadequate patient compliance with medication. Although "resistant" strains of *T. vaginalis* have been reported, occurrence in routine practice is rare.

## V. Prepubertal vaginitis

A. **Etiology.** There are many etiologies for prepubertal vaginitis:

1. **Candida vulvitis/vaginitis.** This is the most frequent cause in children. Usually the disease occurs secondary to poor perineal hygiene.
2. **Foreign bodies.** Toilet tissue, buttons, and safety pins are common objects found in the vaginal area.
3. **Infections.** Pinworms (*Enterobius vermicularis, T. vaginalis, Neisseria gonorrhea,* and *Chlamydia trachomatis* are the most frequent infectious organisms. Sexual abuse must be considered.
4. **Bacterial vaginosis** has been documented to occur in children. Sexual abuse history should be sought.
5. **Malignancy** of the genital tract is a rare cause of vaginal discharge in childhood.

B. **Symptoms.** Vulvar scratching or staining of underwear is often noted by the child's parent as the presenting symptom.

C. **Signs.** Vulvar erythema is often the only sign of disease. Depending upon the age of the child, examination under anesthesia may be necessary for completeness.

D. **Therapy** is directed to the etiology of the problem. After the vagina has been irrigated with saline, the vaginitis disappears. Candida infections may be treated with topical agents as previously discussed (see candida vaginitis section, III-F). Cultures of the pharynx, vagina, and rectum for STDs should be performed if sexual abuse is suspected. Rule out syphilis and human immunodeficiency virus (HIV) with blood studies in all cases of sexual abuse.

## VI. Postmenopausal vaginitis

A. **Etiology.** Sexually transmitted diseases, previously discussed causes of vaginitis in reproductive-aged woman, and atrophic vaginitis may cause symptoms in the postmenopausal woman.

B. **Atrophic vaginitis**

1. **Patient symptoms.** Mild pruritus, dyspareunia, and postcoital spotting may occur.
2. **Patient signs.** Signs of atrophy of the vulva with friable skin and a "tight" introitus may help to identify atrophic vaginitis. The vaginal mucosa appears pale, flat, and lacks normal moisture.
3. **Microscopic diagnosis.** The absence of vaginal pathogens and the presence of RBCs and WBCs on microscopic examination suggests the disease. Normally in the postmenopausal woman, *Lactobacillus* sp. are decreased.
4. **Therapy.** Application of local vaginal estrogen creams on a daily basis for 5 weeks followed by intravaginal application three to four times per week effect cure (e.g., Premarin vaginal cream; 1 g nightly). This disease reflects underlying permanent hormone status; therefore, the patient should know that the disease will return unless chronic intravaginal or oral hormonal therapy is used (see Chapter 22, Menopause and the Climacteric, Management Section, VII-A-3-d).

C. **Genital tract malignancy** should be ruled out in women presenting with pruritus, postcoital spotting, or vulvar irritation (see Chapter 22, Menopause and the Climacteric, and the chapters from the Gynecologic Oncology section for this anatomic area, Chapters 27, Vulvar Dysplasia and Carcinoma; 28, Vaginal Dysplasia and Carcinoma; and 29, Carcinoma of the Cervix, for the details of evaluation for malignancy).

# BENIGN VAGINAL LESIONS

## I. Congenital vaginal anomalies (see also Chapter 5, Benign Diseases of the Vulva)

A. **Atresia and agenesis** include total or partial vaginal absence, distal vs. proximal absence, imperforate hymen, and intersex conditions. Uterine and renal anomalies are frequently associated with vaginal lesions.

B. **Vaginal duplication.** Partial or complete duplication of the vagina is frequently seen presenting as a vaginal septum.

C. **Rare vaginal lesions.** Transverse vaginal septa and fistulae.

II. **Benign cystic vaginal lesions** occurring in the vagina are uncommon. They include mesonephric (Gartner's) duct cysts, paramesonephric duct cysts, mucoid cysts, Skene's gland cysts, endometriosis, adenosis, and urethral diverticulum. Cysts usually appear less than 2 cm in diameter or length and are usually asymptomatic.

A. **Diagnosis.** The location of the cysts helps to identify the type of cyst. For example, paramesonephric cysts occur throughout the vagina whereas mesonephric cysts occur more laterally.

B. **Treatment.** Usually no treatment is necessary. However, if infection or symptoms occur, surgical removal is performed.

III. **Benign noncystic vaginal lesions.** Solid nonmalignant lesions commonly encountered in the vagina include *Condyloma acuminata*, vaginal polyps, fibromas, and pigmented lesions.

A. **Diagnosis.** Biopsy of lesions under local anesthesia.

B. **Treatment** is tailored to the specific lesions diagnosed.

## BENIGN CERVICAL LESIONS

I. **Cystic and noncystic lesions**

A. **Congenital anomalies**

1. Lesions discussed under benign vaginal lesions may also occur involving the cervix (i.e., duplication, mesonephric duct cysts, etc.).

2. **Diethylstilbestrol (DES)-induced cervical lesions** are becoming less common as the use of DES during pregnancy is eliminated. In girls whose mothers were treated with DES, there is an increased risk of the development of vaginal adenosis (islands of glandular tissue lined by columnar epithelium). In these areas, there is an increased incidence of clear-cell adenocarcinoma of the vagina, and thus close observation is essential. Because malignant changes are uncommon prior to puberty, in the absence of symptoms, regular surveillance with cytology, coloposcopy, and pelvic examination may be postponed until menstruation is established. Digital vaginal and rectal examinations should also be performed, with follow-up examinations performed at least yearly. Ablation or excision should not be undertaken unless atypical epithelial changes are documented.

B. **Nabothian cysts** are small inclusions of mucus glandular elements covered by normal cervical epithelium. They are common, benign, and occur singularly or multiply. They require no treatment unless they become quite symptomatic.

C. **Cervical polyps** usually arise from the endocervix and are easily removed by outpatient excisional biopsy. Send specimens for pathological evaluation, although malignancy is rare.

D. **Cervical lacerations.** Obstetric lacerations of the cervix usually occur at 3 and 9 o'clock and require no therapy unless repeated pregnancy loss is part of the patient's history. These lacerations sometimes make obtaining adequate Papanicolaou (PAP) smears difficult.

E. **Ectropion and eversion** is a normal, dynamic, ongoing process whereby endocervical tissue extends into the portio and is slowly covered by squamous epithelium. No therapy is necessary.

F. **Condyloma acuminata.** Because of the association of condyloma with vulvar and cervical intraepithelial neoplasia, colposcopic inspection of the lower genital tract is required to determine the presence of dysplasia, carcinoma in situ, and invasive changes (see Chapter 5, Benign Diseases of the Vulva).

## BIBLIOGRAPHY

Bushell TE, Evans EG, Llewellyn PA, Meadon JD, Milne JD, Warnick DW. Prophylactic use of clotrimazol in recurrent vaginal candidosis. Antifungal Drugs. Ann NY Acad Sci. 1988; 544:558–560.

Kaufman RL, Friedrich EG, Gardner HL. Benign Diseases of the Vulva and Vagina. Chicago, Ill: Year Book Medical; 1989.

Sobel JD. Recurrent vulvovaginal candidiasis: A prospective study of the efficacy of maintenance ketoconazole therapy. N Eng J Med. 1986; 315:1455–1458.

Thomason JL, Gelbart SM. Trichomonas vaginalis. Obstet Gynecol. 1989; 74:536–541.

Thomason JL, Gelbart SM, Anderson RJ, Walt AK, Osypowski PJ, Broekhuizen FF. Statistical evaluation of diagnostic criteria for bacterial vaginosis. Am J Obstet Gynecol. 1990; 162:155–160.

Thomason JL, Gelbart SM, Broekhuizen FB. Advances in the understanding of bacterial vaginosis. J Reprod Med. 1989; 34:581–587.

Thomason JL, Gelbart SM, Scaglione NJ. Bacterial vaginosis. Contemp Obstet Gynecol. 1989; 34;21–26.

"Vulvovaginal Candidiasis" Symposium. Am J Obstet Gynecol. 1988; 158:985–1013.

# CHAPTER 7

# Benign Diseases of the Uterus—Leiomyoma Uteri and the Hysterectomy

**Paula A. Hillard**

## LEIOMYOMA UTERI

Uterine leiomyomata, myomas, or "fibroids" are by far the most common benign uterine tumor. Other benign uterine growths, such as uterine vascular tumors, are rare. The diagnosis of uterine leiomyomata is usually made on physical examination. They may be asymptomatic or cause a range of symptoms from abnormal uterine bleeding to pelvic pressure. The management is based on the primary symptoms and may include observation, myomectomy, or hysterectomy.

I. **Incidence.** Uterine leiomyomata are the most common tumors of the uterus, and are present in at least 20% of all women, more commonly in blacks than whites. Asymptomatic leiomyomata may be present in 40% to 50% of women over 40 years of age. Uterine leiomyomata may occur singly but are often multiple.

II. **Anatomic classification.** All uterine leiomyomata begin in an intramural (interstitial) location and cause distortion of the endometrial cavity and/or the serosal surface of the uterus as they grow.
   A. **Cervical leiomyomata** are located within the stroma of the cervix and may cause distortion of the uterine blood supply.
   B. **Submucous leiomyomata** (approximately 5% of all leiomyomata) produce distortion of the endometrial cavity with thinning or compression of the endometrium.
   C. **Pedunculated submucous leiomyomata** from the endometrial cavity may prolapse through the cervix into the vagina.
   D. **Subserous leiomyomata** are located just beneath the uterine visceral peritoneum, distorting the external uterine contour.
   E. **Pedunculated subserous leiomyomata** develop a stalk, or pedicle, and may be mistaken for ovarian masses.
   F. **Parasitic leiomyomata** develop from pedunculated subserous leiomyomata that have parasitized a blood supply from other intra-abdominal organs, commonly the omentum or mesentery, and have subsequently lost their uterine blood supply.

G. **Intraligamentous leiomyomata** lie within the anterior and posterior leaves of the broad ligament and may derive their primary vasculature from the vessels of the broad ligament.

## III. Morbidity and mortality

A. **Morbidity.** Although the majority of leiomyomata are asymptomatic, significant symptoms occur in some women with resultant economic, psychological, and physical sequelae.

B. **Mortality** from benign uterine leiomyomata is essentially zero, although other diagnoses with mortal potential may be obscured, delayed, or missed in the presence of leiomyomata. Such diagnoses include ovarian malignancy, sarcomatous changes with malignant degeneration of leiomyomata, and other uterine malignancies.

## IV. Etiology.

The etiology of uterine leiomyomata is unknown. Several studies have suggested that each leiomyoma arises from a single neoplastic cell within the smooth muscle of the myometrium.

A. **Hormonal responsiveness** and binding has been demonstrated in vitro. Clinical observations confirm that leiomyomata occur in reproductive age groups with potential for enlargement during pregnancy and regression after menopause. Two environmental factors affecting leiomyomata growth have been suggested:

1. Estrogen stimulation, either systemically or locally within the leiomyomas
2. Synergistic effects of elevation of growth hormone (GH) or human placental lactogen (HPL)

B. **Genetic factors** may predispose to leiomyomata in that incidence is three to nine times higher in blacks than in whites.

## V. Pathology

A. **Grossly,** uterine leiomyomata are discrete nodular tumors that vary in number and size. They may be microscopic or huge (a uterine weight of 74 lb has been reported). They may symmetrically enlarge the uterus or significantly distort the uterine contour. The consistency of the individual leiomyomata varies from hard and stony with a calcified leiomyoma, to soft with degeneration, although the usual consistency is described as firm or rubbery. Although they do not have a true capsule, the margins are blunt, noninfiltrating or pushing and are usually separated from the myometrium by a pseudocapsule of connective tissue allowing enucleation at surgery. There is usually one major vessel supplying each tumor. The cut surface is characteristically whorled.

B. **Degenerative pathologic changes** within the uterine leiomyoma are reported to occur in approximately two-thirds of all pathologic specimens. One study revealed no relationship between clinical presenting symptoms and type of degenerative changes, which include:

1. **Hyaline degeneration,** either localized or extensive, which is an almost invariable feature of uterine leiomyomata giving the tumor a soft, pale appearance on sectioning.
2. **Cystic degeneration** with liquefaction of hyalinized areas and the formation of cystic cavities.
3. **Calcification,** frequently occurring with leiomyomata in postmenopausal women.
4. **Infection and inflammation,** seen in submucous tumors with occasional formation of micro-abscesses.
5. **Necrosis and hemorrhage** related to impairment of blood supply, which may be secondary to torsion of a pedicle or may be associated with pregnancy. The term red degeneration reflects the dark red appearance similar to that of uncooked beef and is usually associated with pregnancy.
6. **Myxomatous degeneration** with a gelatinous appearance.
7. **Mucoid degeneration,** grossly similar to myxomatous changes.
8. **Fatty degeneration,** usually associated with hyaline changes.

C. **Microscopically,** uterine leiomyomata are composed of bundles of smooth muscle with a whorl-like pattern. Connective tissue forms a portion of the tumor and may predominate over the smooth muscle cells, resulting in the designation of fibromyoma. Although the term "fibroid" for these tumors is commonly used, it is not technically correct. The cellular characteristics include elongated cells with abundant eosinophilic cytoplasm. The nuclei are elongated, uniform, and cigar-shaped, with rare or absent mitotic figures.

D. **Leiomyomata with unusual histologic patterns** may occasionally be seen, with hypercellularity, slightly atypical or enlarged nuclei or giant cells.

1. **Cellular leiomyomata** characteristically have an increased density of cells as the predominant pattern. Mitotic figures are rare but must be carefully searched for to distinguish this tumor from a leiomyosarcoma.
2. Other unusual patterns include **epithelioid leiomyomata** composed of rounded cells arranged in cords or nests.
3. The term **symplastic leiomyoma** describes a smooth muscle tumor with multinucleated giant cells or those containing irregular and bizarre nuclei. The number of mitoses allows differentiation from leiomyosarcomata.

E. **Leiomyomata with unusual growth patterns** may invade blood vessels, extend from the uterus, or even rarely metastasize, but are considered to be benign.

1. The term **leiomyomata with vascular invasion** has been used to designate tumors with microscopically demonstrated vascular invasion occurring only within the leio-

myoma and without a significant number of mitotic figures. This finding is of no clinical significance, because the behavior of these tumors is benign.

2. **Intravenous leiomyomatosis** is defined as grossly visible extension of benign smooth muscle tumor into vessels, or growth of benign smooth muscle in vessels beyond the margins of a leiomyoma. Broad ligament and pelvic veins may be involved and extension into the heart has been reported. Clinically, cure of this tumor involves simple hysterectomy and removal of any extrauterine tumor. Pathologically, the differential diagnosis of this tumor includes benign metastasizing leiomyoma, low grade stromal sarcoma with vascular invasion (endolymphatic stromal myosis), high grade endometrial stromal sarcoma, leiomyosarcoma, and disseminated peritoneal leiomyomatosis.
3. **Benign metastasizing leiomyoma** from the uterus is a rare occurrence. The few documented cases of lymphatic, intra-abdominal, or pulmonary metastases have occurred in the setting of a previous surgical procedure, usually a dilation and curettage (D & C), or in the presence of pregnancy. Some of the "metastases" from this tumor associated with pregnancy have regressed after pregnancy, indicating hormonal support.
4. **Disseminated peritoneal leiomyomatosis** is rare and only a small number of cases of this tumor have been reported in which serosal or subperitoneal tissues contain tissue histologically resembling smooth muscle cells. Most of the patients were pregnant or recently pregnant, and the tumors were reported to be completely benign with spontaneous regression.

F. **Leiomyomata with an increased number of mitotic figures may occur**
   1. During pregnancy or in women receiving progestational agents, leiomyomata may show an increased mitotic activity.
   2. Leiomyomata undergoing necrosis may show a focal increase in mitotic activity.
   3. "Smooth muscle tumors of uncertain malignant potential" is a category that reveals that the dividing line between leiomyoma and leiomyosarcoma is not clear cut.

G. **Leiomyosarcoma** is a rare malignant neoplasm comprised of cells that have smooth muscle differentiation. Recent reports suggest that malignant degeneration of a preexisting leiomyoma is extremely rare. The typical patient is in her mid-50s. The primary presentation may be abnormal bleeding, although the majority of diagnoses are made only after microscopic examination of a uterus with suspected leiomyomata. Microscopically, the characteristics of uterine leiomyosarcomata generally include hypercellularity, cellular atypia, pleomorphism, and mitoses. Most authors accept the diagnosis of sarcoma in the presence of 10 or more mitoses per 10 high power fields. Therapy is primarily surgical, that is, hysterectomy. The role of pelvic radiation or adjuvant chemotherapy is not yet well-defined. Good prognostic signs have included premenopausal age, low mitotic count, origin in, and localization to a leiomyoma.

## VI. Differential diagnosis

The diagnosis of uterine leiomyomata is frequently made on the basis of the clinical findings of an enlarged, irregular uterus on pelvic examination. However, any tumor of the pelvis can potentially be confused with an enlarged uterus.

A. **Common conditions** that may be confused with uterine leiomyomata are as follows.
   1. Although usually obvious, a **full urinary bladder** may cause a "palpable mass" which disappears upon urination. Likewise, a full rectosigmoid may confuse the unwary examiner.
   2. Normal anatomic variants, such as a **sharply anteflexed or retroflexed uterus,** may be confused with a leiomyoma.
   3. **Pregnancy,** either in conjunction with small leiomyomata or by itself may make the differential diagnosis difficult.
   4. **Ovarian or adnexal masses** are probably the most common and potentially dangerous missed diagnoses and include:
      a. Functional cysts
      b. Inflammatory masses such as tubo-ovarian complexes or diverticular abscesses
      c. Neoplastic tumors including ovarian cancer

B. **Uncommon conditions** must also be excluded:
   1. **Pelvic kidney**
   2. **Carcinoma of the colon and rectum**
   3. **Retroperitoneal tumors**
   4. **Uterine sarcomata** or other malignant tumors. Whereas malignant uterine neoplasms are rare, this diagnostic possibility must be considered, especially in older women.

## VII. Diagnosis

A. **Signs and symptoms.** The majority of uterine leiomyomata are asymptomatic and are discovered on routine pelvic examinations. Only 20% to 50% of uterine leiomyomata are estimated to produce symptoms. These symptoms may be a primary complaint or may only be elicited by questioning. Caution must be used in concluding that leiomyomata are the sole causation of symptoms commonly associated with leiomyomata.
   1. **Abnormal uterine bleeding**
      a. Perhaps the most common symptom associated with uterine leiomyomata and one leading to surgical intervention, is menorrhagia. Reported series of patients

undergoing myomectomy reveal that 30% of the patients had menstrual abnormalities.

b. A number of different etiologic factors have been suggested, including ulceration over a submucosal tumor, anovulation, increased endometrial surface area, interference by leiomyomata with uterine contractility, and compression and obstruction of venous plexi with resultant dilation. None has been proven conclusively.

2. **Chronic pelvic pain** was noted as a preoperative symptom in approximately one-third of reported series of patients undergoing myomectomy. Chronic pain may be characterized as dysmenorrhea, dyspareunia, and pelvic pressure.
3. **Acute pelvic pain** may result from torsion of a pedunculated leiomyoma or infarction and degeneration.
4. **Urinary symptoms** may include:
   a. **Frequency,** resulting from extrinsic pressure on the bladder
   b. **Partial ureteral obstruction,** related to pressure at the pelvic brim by large tumors. Reports of the incidence of partial ureteral obstruction range from 1% to 75% of all leiomyomata, with most reports suggesting some degree of ureteral obstruction in 30% to 70% of those tumors above the pelvic brim. The location, size, and configuration of uterine leiomyomata and the presence of associated conditions such as endometriosis or pelvic inflammatory disease, obviously affect the reported incidence. Intraligamentous tumors may cause lateral and posterior displacement and subsequent compression against the bony pelvis. Ureteral compression on the right is three to four times as common as on the left, because the left ureter is protected by the sigmoid colon.
   c. Rarely **complete urethral obstruction occurs,** resulting from elevation of the base of the bladder by cervical or lower uterine leiomyomata with impingement on the region of the internal sphincter.
5. **Infertility**
   a. **Incidence.** Leiomyomata alone are an infrequent primary cause of infertility and have been reported as a sole cause in less than 3% of infertile patients. In review of myomectomies performed for all indications, a prior history of infertility was noted in 27%.
   b. **Postulated etiologies** of infertility include:
      (1) Interference with rhythmic uterine contractions after intercourse, resulting in impaired sperm transport
      (2) Distortion of the uterine cavity leading to an increased distance that sperm must travel

(3) Myometrial hypercontractility secondary to degeneration of leiomyomata
(4) Cornual location, distorting the tubal lumina
(5) Cervical location, impinging on the endocervical canal
(6) Endometrial ulceration or vascular alteration leading to improper implantation

6. **Pregnancy loss or complications**
   a. The **incidence** of problem pregnancies is low in women with leiomyomata, and many patients have uncomplicated pregnancies and deliveries. One study followed the size of uterine leiomyomata during pregnancy with ultrasound examinations and noted no demonstrable change in their size for 90% of the patients.
   b. **Reported pregnancy complications** associated with leiomyomata include an increased risk of:
      (1) Spontaneous abortion
      (2) Degeneration and pain
      (3) Interference with placental function
      (4) Premature labor or premature rupture of membranes
      (5) Soft tissue dystocia
      (6) Abnormal fetal presentation or position
      (7) Uterine inertia or postpartum hemorrhage
      (8) Postpartum endomyometritis
7. **Uncommon symptoms** associated with leiomyomata include:
   a. Rectosigmoid compression, with constipation or intestinal obstruction
   b. Prolapse of a pedunculated submucous tumor through the cervix, with associated severe cramping and subsequent ulceration and infection; uterine inversion has also been reported
   c. Venous stasis of the lower extremities and possible thrombophlebitis secondary to pelvic compression.
   d. Polycythemia
   e. Ascites

B. **Physical examination.** A complete pelvic examination, including rectovaginal examination and Papanicolaou (PAP) smear, should be performed. The size, shape, position, consistency, and mobility of the uterus and adnexae should be described.

C. **Laboratory evaluation and diagnostic procedures**
   1. **Routine studies**
      a. **Laboratory evaluation** in all women suspected of having uterine leiomyomata should include a complete blood count (CBC), sedimentation rate, pregnancy test, stool guaiac testing, and a PAP smear. If the diagnosis is in question, additional studies may be appropriate to confirm the clinical impression.

b. **Sounding and measuring the endometrial cavity** with a uterine sound or probe is a simple office technique that may help to confirm uterine enlargement with leiomyomata.

c. **Endometrial sampling** with an endometrial biopsy or D & C is mandatory in the presence of abnormal bleeding, in that an endometrial lesion—carcinoma or hyperplasia—may coexist with leiomyomata. Abnormal bleeding cannot be assumed to be due to leiomyomata.

d. An **intravenous pyelogram** (IVP) will demonstrate ureteral deviation, compression or dilatation in the presence of moderately large and laterally located fibroids, and may provide an indication for surgical intervention for otherwise asymptomatic leiomyomata.

**2. Additional studies**

a. **Radiographs,** such as an abdominal flat plate x-ray taken for other indications may reveal characteristic calcifications.

b. **Diagnostic laparoscopy** may prove valuable in distinguishing a laterally located or pedunculated leiomyoma from an ovarian tumor. Laparotomy can thus be avoided if the patient is otherwise asymptomatic.

c. **Hysteroscopy** provides direct evidence of submucous leiomyomata distorting the uterine cavity.

d. A **hysterosalpingogram** will indirectly demonstrate the contour of the endometrial cavity and any distortion or obstruction of the utero-tubal junction secondary to leiomyomata.

e. **Pelvic ultrasonography** may help document the dimensions and locations of uterine leiomyomata and will usually facilitate differentiation from adnexal pathology. When ultrasound examination reveals the kidneys in their proper location, it eliminates the possibility of a horseshoe or pelvic kidney, and can give some insight to possible ureteral compression if the calices appear dilated.

f. **Computerized tomography** is seldom indicated as a primary diagnostic procedure for leiomyomata.

g. **Magnetic resonance imaging** is a relatively new technique which may have some advantages over ultrasound for preoperatively localizing leiomyomata, although its major current disadvantage is its expense.

## VIII. Management

**A. Judicious patient observation and follow-up** is primarily indicated for uterine leiomyomata, with intervention reserved only for specific indications and symptoms.

1. **Explanation of pathology to the patient.** When small uterine irregularities are noted on pelvic examination in an asymptomatic woman, she should be informed of their presence and that the diagnosis is almost certainly a benign uterine growth — fibroids. Repeat examinations are necessary at regular intervals — 3 months initially and then every 6 months — to assure that the tumors are not growing rapidly. The patient should be informed of the approximate size of the leiomyomata, and of the possibility that symptoms related to the fibroids, such as abnormal uterine bleeding or pelvic pressure or pain, may develop and require treatment in the future.
2. **Documentation** of uterine size should be recorded in the patient's chart, and the location of the palpable leiomyomata described and diagramed. Ultrasound examination may aid in documenting uterine size.

**B. Surgical treatment**

1. **Indications for surgery.** Potential indications for surgical treatment require careful judgment and assessment of the degree of associated disability.
   a. **Abnormal uterine bleeding,** including menorrhagia or metrorrhagia, without other endometrial causes, is perhaps the most frequent indication for surgery. When bleeding from leiomyomata results in anemia, surgical intervention is warranted. Endometrial sampling is essential prior to surgical intervention in any women over 35 with leiomyomata and abnormal bleeding. A D&C, may not only have a transient therapeutic effect, but may also allow a perimenopausal woman to avoid major surgery. Abnormal endometrial findings should prompt treatment of that condition.
   b. **Pain** directly attributable to leiomyomata may be
      (1) Chronic with severe dysmenorrhea, dyspareunia, or lower abdominal pressure and/or pain
      (2) Acute, as in torsion of a pedunculated leiomyoma, infarction during pregnancy, or the "labor-like" pains of a pedunculated leiomyoma that is prolapsing through the cervix. Pain assessment is a subjective judgment. The degree of disability that a woman experiences should be quantitated in terms of requirement for pain medications, or frequency of missed work or alteration of activities.
   c. **Urinary symptoms,** including urinary frequency or urgency, acute urinary retention, or hydroureter and hydronephrosis may warrant intervention.
   d. **Inability to evaluate the adnexa** because of a laterally located leiomyoma, uterine size greater than 12 weeks, or the patient's obesity should prompt the use

of diagnostic procedures, including transvaginal ultrasonography or laparoscopy to avoid delaying the diagnosis of ovarian cancer or benign ovarian mass.

e. **Rapid enlargement of the uterus** during the premenopausal years, or any increase in uterine size in a postmenopausal woman, may result from a uterine sarcoma and is an indication for a further diagnostic work-up, with endometrial sampling prior to definitive surgery.

f. **Infertility.** The majority of women with leiomyomata will conceive and carry a pregnancy to term with no complications or problems, and thus a myomectomy should not be performed solely because of the presence of uterine leiomyoma without a demonstrated period of inability to conceive and a thorough infertility evaluation. For the small number (2% to 10%) of infertile women in whom leiomyomata are the only abnormal finding, myomectomy may be indicated.

g. **Enlarged uterine size alone** has been suggested as an indication for surgery, although there is no universal agreement as to what size warrants surgery. A uterus larger than 12 to 14 weeks in size is more likely to cause pressure symptoms or ureteral compression, or even abdominal girth enlargement or distortion that is bothersome to the patient. Size as sole indication for hysterectomy should be viewed with caution for women nearing the menopause, because leiomyomata are likely to decrease in size postmenopausally.

**2. Hysterectomy** is the definitive surgical management of symptomatic uterine leiomyomata. (See hysterectomy section, I).

a. The indication for abdominal hysterectomy is primarily the presence of other pelvic pathology.

b. Vaginal hysterectomy is indicated for small symptomatic leiomyomata in a mobile uterus that descends well. Technical concerns include the potential need for morcellation of large leiomyomata.

**3. Abdominal myomectomy**

a. **Indications for abdominal myomectomy** as an alternative to hysterectomy include a desire for childbearing and severely symptomatic leiomyomata in young women. Because of the possibility that the location or size of uterine leiomyomata may make myomectomy technically unfeasible, or that coexistent pathology may be found, the gynecologist should not promise to do a myomectomy, but must state that the final judgment will depend on intraoperative findings and that a hysterectomy may be necessary.

(1) In the small number of women in whom leiomyomata are found to be the sole cause of infer-

tility, recommendations have been made that myomectomy be restricted to intramural and submucous tumors 2 cm or greater in size, subserous tumors obstructing the tubal lumen, or pedunculated submucous leiomyomata.

(2) Recurrent pregnancy loss, not associated with other causes.

(3) Large and enlarging leiomyomata, greater than 10 to 12 week size, in women not currently interested in fertility but who ultimately desire fertility.

b. **Contraindications**

(1) Small asymptomatic uterine leiomyomata usually do not warrant a myomectomy,

(2) Abdominal myomectomy during pregnancy should be avoided whenever possible.

(3) In women past the childbearing years, the surgical risks dictate definitive management with hysterectomy rather than myomectomy.

c. **Techniques to minimize blood loss during myomectomy,** which may be considerably greater than that associated with hysterectomy, include:

(1) Rubber-shod clamps to occlude the uterine and/or ovarian vessels.

(2) The use of rubber catheter as a tourniquet occluding the uterine vessels by surrounding the lower uterine segment, with removal at 10-minute intervals to prevent ischemic damage or manual compression of the lower uterine segment.

(3) Injection of vasoconstrictive pharmacologic agents such as vasopressin or neosynephrine into the uterus to decrease bleeding at the incision sites.

(4) Careful planning of the uterine incision, with preference given to a vertical midline incision through which multiple leiomyomata may be removed.

(5) The preoperative use of gonadotropin-releasing hormone (GnRH) analogs (see medical therapy section, VIII-C).

(6) The use of electrocautery or laser.

d. **The prevention of postoperative adhesions** is important, and is facilitated by:

(1) Single vertical anterior uterine incision to minimize adhesions involving the tube and ovary.

(2) Removing posteriorally located leiomyomata through a fundal extension of the anterior incision.

(3) Transcavity enucleation of posteriorally located submucous tumors.
(4) Uterine serosal closure with small caliber non-reactive suture.
(5) Consideration of a uterine suspension for retroverted uterus.
(6) Intra-abdominal placement of dextran solution.
(7) Irrigation with heparinized ringer lactate solution.
(8) Avoid placing dry sponges or lap packs in the abdominal cavity.

e. **Vaginal delivery after successful myomectomy** is usually possible, although some authors have recommended cesarean delivery, particularly for patients in whom the endometrial cavity has been entered. Pregnancy rates following abdominal myomectomy for infertility have ranged from 10% to 89% in one series, with most reports suggesting that 40% to 50% of women are able to conceive. Uterine size prior to myomectomy may significantly affect success of myomectomy. Recurrence risk or growth of leiomyomata following myomectomy have ranged from 15% to 30%. Multiple leiomyomata in women younger than 35 have a greater risk of recurrence, in part because of the longer period of time before menopause.

4. **Vaginal myomectomy.** The primary indication for vaginal myomectomy is that of a prolapsed pedunculated submucous leiomyoma. Although a D&C will on occasion result in removal of a small pedunculated submucous leiomyoma prior to its prolapse, these tumors frequently cause heavy and prolonged bleeding, often leading to anemia, and are frequently necrotic and infected. Vaginal myomectomy with cross clamping and suture of the pedicle is preferable to a vaginal hysterectomy when the tumor is infected and necrotic. If multiple leiomyomata remain symptomatic after vaginal myomectomy, vaginal or abdominal hysterectomy can be performed at a later date with lower risk of infectious morbidity. In the event that the stalk proves too broad for a vaginal approach, abdominal hysterectomy may need to be performed.
5. **Laparoscopic myomectomy** with either laser or electrocautery excision or vaporization may result in less blood loss and maximal preservation of normal uterine tissue. Additional studies are necessary to define the role of laparoscopic myomectomy.
6. **Hysteroscopic resection of small submucous leiomyomata,** although dependent on the skill of the surgeon in a specialized technique with appropriate equipment, may offer benefits for a selected group of patients.

7. **Hysterectomy.** Definitive surgical management of symptomatic uterine leiomyomata (See section I on hysterectomy).

C. **Medical therapy**

1. **The use of GnRH agonists** results in a 40% to 60% decrease in uterine volume and induces amenorrhea. The hypoestrogenism resulting from treatment has been associated with a reversible bone loss if used for periods longer than 6 months and symptoms including hot flashes. Bone loss is not a problem for short treatment courses <6 months. The combination of (GnRH) agonist and low-dose hormonal replacement has been reported and effectively minimizes the hypoestrogenic effects as well as maintains fibroid size reduction. To date, experience with this form of therapy is limited. Regrowth of leiomyomata is experienced within a few months after agonist discontinuation in the vast majority of women treated, unless surgery is performed.
   a. Patients who may most benefit from this treatment include:
      (1) Women desiring fertility with large leiomyomata may undergo preoperative medical therapy prior to myomectomy.
      (2) Women with anemia may be treated to allow recovery of normal hemoglobin levels, minimizing the need for transfusion or allowing autologous blood donation prior to surgical management.
      (3) Women approaching menopause may be treated in an effort to avoid hysterectomy.
      (4) Women with large leiomyomata may be treated preoperatively to make vaginal hysterectomy, hysteroscopic resection or ablation, or laparoscopic destruction more feasible.
      (5) Women with medical contraindications to surgery may benefit.
2. **Hormonal therapy,** such as the use of progestational agents, may result in a small decrease in uterine size and amenorrhea, allowing an anemia to resolve with iron therapy prior to definitive surgery, but success with this modality is extremely limited and not curative.

## IX. Prognosis

A. **Contraceptive choices** for women with small asymptomatic uterine leiomyomata who choose to delay childbearing may be problematic. These women should be made aware that their leiomyomata may potentially enlarge and compromise future fertility. The use of combination oral contraceptive pills is not contraindicated with careful follow-up and examination of uterine size. Progestin-only pills may be another option. Intrauterine devices (IUDs) are contraindicated in the presence of submucous leiomyomata that distort the endometrial cavity.

B. **Pregnancy** for women with leiomyomata may range from easily achievable to ultimately unattainable. Many women with small leiomyomata escape clinical detection, as the incidence of leiomyomata during pregnancy has been reported to be only 1% to 3%. Pregnancy complications including premature labor, antepartum, and postpartum bleeding were noted to be increased when there was contact between the placental implantation site and the leiomyoma. Large uterine leiomyomata may be associated with an increased risk of spontaneous abortion, or leiomyomata may undergo degeneration, causing pain or even potentially obstructing labor. Pedunculated leiomyomata are more likely to undergo torsion during pregnancy. Breech and other abnormal fetal positions may result from leiomyomata.

C. **Menopause** results in regression of the size of the uterine leiomyomata. Perimenopausal women may thus benefit from medical therapy as temporizing management. Enlargement of uterine leiomyomata in a postmenopausal woman is cause for concern and requires surgical intervention. Postmenopausal bleeding may occur as a result of uterine leiomyomata, although it should be investigated thoroughly by endometrial biopsy and other techniques as discussed later in the text, to rule out significant pathology (see Chapter 30, Carcinoma of the Uterus).

## THE HYSTERECTOMY

### I. Incidence

A. **National.** Hysterectomy is the most frequently performed major surgical procedure in the United States. As such, and because of the significant impact in terms of economic, psychological, emotional, sexual, and medical factors, hysterectomy is the focus of much debate and controversy. In 1985, the National Center for Health Statistics estimated that 670 000 hysterectomies were performed. This corresponds to a rate of 6.9/1000 women or 8.6/1000 women with intact uteri. Between 1970 and 1980, the number and rate of hysterectomies increased to a maximum in 1975 and have subsequently declined toward 1971 levels. By age groupings, the greatest number of hysterectomies are performed on women of reproductive age (ages 15 — 44); the median age for women having a hysterectomy was 40.9 for the period 1965 to 1984.

B. **Regional variation.** Differences in hysterectomy rates are marked between individual communities, states, and geographic regions of the United States. In 1980, the rate per 100 000 population (women and men) was highest in the South and lowest in the Northeast. The reasons for these geographic differences are unclear and undoubtedly complex, but may reflect regional differences in uterine disease and differences in surgical practice.

C. **Race.** Between 70% and 75% of all hysterectomies performed between 1970 and 1978 were on white women. However, the rate of hysterectomy is higher for blacks than whites: 972/100 000 black women ages 15 to 44 vs. 777/100 000 white women in 1978. More recent data suggest that this difference may no longer exist.

D. **Vaginal vs. abdominal.** One-fourth of all hysterectomies for women between the ages of 15 and 44 are performed vaginally. Regionally, 33.3% of hysterectomies in the West are vaginal, whereas only 17% of hysterectomies in the Northeast are vaginal.

## II. Morbidity and mortality

A. **Complications.** As with any major surgical procedure, hysterectomy carries a risk of complications ranging from minor to the ultimate complication, death.

1. The overall incidence of all complications, major and minor, ranges from 25% to 50% in women undergoing hysterectomies.
2. Factors influencing risk include:
   a. Indications for surgery (serious pathology increases the risk)
   b. Age of the patient
   c. Underlying medical conditions
   d. Surgical approach (vaginal vs. abdominal)
   e. Surgical technique (such as the use of drains)
   f. Surgeon's experience, skill, and training
   g. Duration of procedure
   h. Use of prophylactic antibiotics
3. **Febrile morbidity** is defined as oral temperature of 38°C (100.4°F) or greater on any two postoperative days excluding the first 24 hours postoperatively, and includes fever due to urinary tract infection, pulmonary problems, wound and vaginal cuff infection.
   a. Febrile morbidity is the most frequent complication of hysterectomy with reported rates of up to 40/100 operations. In one study, no clear source of infection was identified for approximately one-half of the women experiencing febrile morbidity.
   b. The benefits of prophylactic antibiotics have been documented in numerous studies for women undergoing vaginal hysterectomy, with reduction of infectious morbidity and shorter hospital stays. The benefits for abdominal hysterectomies are less certain.
4. **Hemorrhage** as a complication of hysterectomy is frequent, although difficult to define because of the difficulties in clinical estimation of blood loss.

a. Rates of transfusion serve as a quantitative measure of hemorrhage and have been reported as approximately 1 in 10 overall, with abdominal hysterectomy associated with a rate of approximately 15/100 operations and vaginal hysterectomy 8 to 13/100 cases. Transfusion may in some instances have been necessitated by preexisting anemia.

b. Rates of hemorrhage are increased with:

(1) Complicated pelvic pathology, such as extensive adhesions from previous infection or endometriosis.

(2) Associated vaginal colporrhaphy.

5. **Unintended major surgery** may be necessary to control hemorrhage or repair injury to the bowel or urinary tract. Rates of ureteral injury range from 0.2 to 0.5/100 hysterectomies with bladder lacerations from 0.3 to 0.8/100 operations. This risk is reduced by constant surgical attention to the location of the ureters. Recognition of visceral injury and immediate appropriate repair is essential to uncomplicated healing.

6. **Other complications associated with hysterectomy** include urinary retention, pulmonary atelectasis, paralytic ileus, wound dehiscence, neuropathy, and deep venous thrombosis or thrombophlebitis.

7. **Length of hospital stay** for hysterectomy has declined since 1970 when it averaged slightly less than 10 days for both abdominal and vaginal hysterectomies. Since 1971, the average hospital stay for vaginal hysterectomy has been shorter than that for abdominal hysterectomy. Third party insurance plans that insist upon preadmission testing and prohibit hospital admission the day prior to surgery have already had an effect on average length of stay. In many locations, patients remain in the hospital after vaginal hysterectomy for 3 to 4 days and 4 to 5 days after abdominal hysterectomy.

B. **Late sequelae of hysterectomy** can include:

1. **Rehospitalization** for pelvic infection, abscess, hemorrhage, or thromboembolism.

2. The **residual ovary syndrome,** which involves pathology of adnexal tissues left in situ.

a. Symptoms and signs include pain, dyspareunia, and a cystic ovarian mass. Rates of reoperation for this problem vary from 1 to 4/100 hysterectomies. Findings at reoperation typically include extensive adhesions and cystic enlargement of the residual fallopian tube(s) and ovary(ies).

b. Prophylactic oophorectomy or removal of normal appearing and functioning ovaries at the time of hysterectomy has been recommended as a means of preventing both the residual ovary syndrome and ovarian malignancy. Many gynecologists recommend that a bilateral oophorectomy be performed along with a hysterectomy for all postmenopausal women, and for premenopausal women beyond a certain age (variously 40, 45, 50). The risk and benefits of such a procedure must be individually discussed with the patient, as well as the need for postoperative estrogen replacement therapy.

3. **The psychological impact** of a hysterectomy must be considered for each individual woman.
   a. **Common concerns** about hysterectomy include:
      (1) Loss of childbearing ability
      (2) Loss of menses
      (3) Loss of femininity or youth
      (4) Effects on aging and appearance
      (5) Loss of sexual desire
      (6) Lowered self-esteem
      (7) Loss of ability to achieve orgasm
      (8) Coitus feeling different/being less satisfying for her or her sexual partner
   b. **Rates of adverse emotional reactions** to hysterectomy are difficult to assess, in that many reports are of nonrandom populations that are small in number.
   c. **Postoperative depression and stress reaction** may occur, and if severe, psychiatric referral may be necessary. Risk factors for severe depression include:
      (1) Previous psychiatric problems, especially depression
      (2) Previous difficulty in coping with stress
      (3) Marital discord
      (4) Young age
      (5) Emergency hysterectomy
   d. **Measures to minimize adverse psychological reactions** include:
      (1) Assessing risk
      (2) Discussing surgery and dispelling misconceptions, including impact on sexual functioning
      (3) Involving partner/family
      (4) Postoperative explanation of surgical findings
      (5) Psychiatric referral if symptoms are severe or persist over 6 months

C. **Mortality**

1. The risk of **death from hysterectomy** is low, approaching 1 to 2/1000 hysterectomies. Causes and contributing factors include:
   a. Pulmonary embolus
   b. Myocardial infarction
   c. Cardiac arrest

d. Overwhelming sepsis
e. Stroke
f. Anesthetic complication

2. **Underlying disease processes** may contribute to hysterectomy associated deaths, including extensive malignancy, ruptured pelvic abscess, and obstetrical hemorrhage.

III. **Indications** for hysterectomy include both malignant and benign disease. Hysterectomies for benign disorders have been categorized as emergency and elective.

A. **Benign disorders**

1. **Emergency indications** include:
   a. Ruptured interstitial pregnancy with uterine damage
   b. Obstetric hemorrhage after failure of conservative treatment
   c. Uterine rupture or perforation
   d. Ruptured tubo-ovarian abscess
2. **Elective indications,** which include urgent and advisable conditions, are: (the first three indications account for over 50% of all hysterectomies for benign disease)
   a. Uterine leiomyomata
   b. Abnormal uterine bleeding (dysfunctional uterine bleeding [DUB])
   c. Symptomatic pelvic relaxation
   d. Pelvic pain
   e. Chronic pelvic inflammatory disease (PID) with adhesions
   f. Endometriosis

B. **Premalignant or localized invasive disease,** including:

1. Cervix—cervical intraepithelial neoplasia (CIN)
2. Endometrium—atypical endometrial hyperplasia
3. Adnexa—ovarian mass, ovarian or tubal neoplasia

C. **Questionable indications** include:

1. Sterilization
2. Purely elective or prophylactic
3. Premenstrual syndrome
4. A combination of questionable indications

D. **Inappropriate indications** include:

1. Abnormal PAP smear without further evaluation
2. Postmenopausal bleeding without further evaluation
3. Small asymptomatic uterine leiomyomata

IV. **"Unnecessary" hysterectomies.** The definition of "necessary" hysterectomy provokes disagreement among physicians. It is even more difficult to find agreement on a corresponding definition of "unnecessary" hysterectomy.

A. **The absence of pathology** has been cited as evidence that the hysterectomy was unnecessary. However, in a number of appropriate cases, no pathology may be found, including:

1. DUB—after failed attempts at conservative management or with resultant anemia
2. Symptomatic pelvic relaxation

B. **The presence of minimal pathology** does not prove that the hysterectomy was necessary, as in the case of small, asymptomatic uterine leiomyomata.

C. **The quality of life** of the individual woman is a consideration that is affected by her physical, mental, and emotional health. The degree of disability of an individual patient is not quantifiable. The effect of a gynecologic problem on the quality of an individual's life is a valid factor to consider along with other more objective findings.

D. **Second surgical opinions** are currently being mandated by various third party insurance plans in an effort to eliminate "unnecessary" hysterectomies. This strategy has the problem of lack of agreement among physicians about the degree of "necessity" of elective surgery. Quality of life factors and decision making by the patient herself further complicate the issue. When the patient herself requests the opinion of another physician, this request should be encouraged and respected.

V. **Preoperative radiographic studies.** There are few absolute rules with regards to the preoperative radiographic evaluation of patients prior to hysterectomy. However, some general guidelines can be outlined.

A. **Chest radiograph (CXR).** A CXR should be preformed in any patient over the age of 35 for evaluation of heart size, and lung disease. In addition, a CXR should be performed on all patients in whom the preoperative diagnosis is an ovarian mass to rule out metastatic disease.

B. **Mammography** should be done prior to any elective surgical procedure, in the patient age 40 or older if it hasn't been done within the previous 12 months, also any patient with a palpable breast abnormality should be evaluated with mammogram. Patients with an adnexal mass should be considered for mammography to evaluate the possibility of a primary breast carcinoma.

C. **IVP.** An IVP not only indicates renal function, but also kidney location, ureteral caliber and position. Patients with a history of genital or renal tract abnormality require preoperative IVP. Some surgeons obtain an IVP in all patients with an adnexal mass, and when broad ligament or cervical leiomyomata are present. This may not be necessary when ureteral exposure is obtained with retroperitoneal dissection in all cases.

D. **Barium enema (BE).** A BE is mandatory for any patient with rectal bleeding, or change in stool caliber. A BE should also be obtained in patients over 40 years of age with an adnexal mass to eliminate the possibility of a primary colon carcinoma metastatic to the ovary.

E. **Pelvic ultrasound.** A pelvic ultrasound is not needed prior to all hysterectomies. It can produce useful information on ovarian size and may be helpful in differentiating a primary uterine from ovarian neoplasm. Renal size and location may also be determined.

## VI. Preoperative patient education

A. A careful explanation of the reason for surgery is essential prior to any recommendations about treatment.
   1. The woman's familiarity with the disease process and medical sophistication should be assessed prior to a discussion that might prove to be condescending or excessively complex.
   2. Lay terminology should be used, when appropriate, rather than complicated medical terms, although the name of the abnormal condition (such as endometriosis) should be discussed and written down.
   3. Diagrams of involved pelvic anatomy are frequently helpful.

B. **Diagnostic studies** may be necessary to confirm the diagnosis, to rule out other pathology, or as preoperative testing. These studies are often done on an outpatient basis. The reasons for the tests and what will be done should be explained.

C. **Treatment alternatives** and options to hysterectomy, both surgical and nonsurgical, must be discussed and documented. These may include, depending on the patient's condition:
   1. Hormonal therapy including combination oral contraceptives, progestins, antigonadotropins, or GnRH agonists
   2. D & C
   3. Diagnostic and operative laparoscopy
   4. Laser lysis of adhesions
   5. Myomectomy
   6. Operative hysteroscopy
   7. Destruction of endometrium using electrocoagulation or laser ablation
   8. Sterilization with tubal ligation or vasectomy and other contraceptive alternatives
   9. More conservative abdominal procedures, such as unilateral oophorectomy or cystectomy
   10. Observation

D. **Benefits of the surgery** should be anticipated by the physician and the likelihood of a successful outcome should be addressed, although it must be made clear to the patient that because medicine and surgery are not exact sciences, no guarantees are possible. Benefits that the individual patient anticipates ultimately determine whether or not a hysterectomy is performed. These quality of life considerations are difficult to quantify, but may provide considerable motivation.

E. **Specific questions related to the planned surgery** should be discussed and written documentation made of the discussions:
   1. Urgency of the procedure (Does the hysterectomy need to be done next week, next month, in 6 months or only when or if symptoms become more severe?)
   2. Length of anticipated hospitalization
   3. Recommendations about the type of anesthesia
   4. The likelihood of transfusion and the possibility of family member or autologous donation
   5. Surgical approach—vaginal vs. abdominal and why
   6. Recommendations about associated surgery oophorectomy, colporrhaphy, appendectomy, urethral suspension
   7. Length of anticipated recovery period and extent of disability
   8. Discussion of indications for estrogen replacement therapy

F. **Potential surgical risks** of a hysterectomy should be discussed and put into perspective in terms of a qualitative and quantitative assessment of the degree of risk:
   1. Hemorrhage
   2. Infection
   3. Unintended major surgery
   4. Injury to bowel or bladder, or fistula
   5. Anesthetic complication
   6. Cardiac arrest

G. **The psychological and sexual impact** of hysterectomy is an important issue, and sufficient time must be allotted to deal with the individual woman's concerns and fears. Her partner should be encouraged to participate in the discussions and decision making. A second surgical opinion, if desired by the patient, should be encouraged. Through such processes of preoperative information sharing, counseling, and involvement with her physician, the individual woman can reach and give an informed decision and consent to undergo hysterectomy.

## VII. Surgical approach

A. The **choice between a vaginal and an abdominal hysterectomy** is influenced by:
   1. The surgeon's skill, experience, and preference
   2. The indications for the procedure
   3. Associated problems such as stress urinary incontinence, pelvic relaxation, or chronic pain
   4. The woman's preference
   5. Medical conditions such as morbid obesity, or previous back or hip surgery precluding stirrups
   6. Previous history of abdominal or pelvic surgery, including cesarean deliveries
   7. **Procedures that may be performed concurrently** and that may influence the choice of surgical approach, including:

a. **Oophorectomy**
   (1) The recommendation for oophorectomy at the time of hysterectomy is a decision and judgement that depends on:
      (a) The individual patient's age
      (b) The health of the patient's ovaries
      (c) The patient's family history of cancer
      (d) The patient's preferences
      (e) The biases of the surgeon
   (2) Before a decision to perform oophorectomy is made, consideration should be given to the value of ovarian hormone production.
      (a) **Estrogen.** Premature loss of estrogen may result in osteoporosis and a possible increased risk of coronary heart disease. If oophorectomy is performed, estrogen replacement therapy should be considered.
      (b) **Androgens** are receiving increased recognition for their role during the postmenopausal years in promoting health and well-being.
   (3) **Cancer prevention.** Twelve/1000 women in the United States over the age of 40 will develop ovarian cancer. If oophorectomy were performed at the time of hysterectomy for all women over the age of 45, some women would undergo an unnecessary procedure whereas others would not experience a subsequent cancer. The risk vs. benefits must be carefully weighed.

b. **Colporrhaphy**

c. **Appendectomy**

d. **Urethral suspension**

**B. Vaginal hysterectomy.** Public health analyses assessing savings in medical costs as a result of the reductions of hospital stay and morbidity associated with the vaginal approach support its use with prophylactic antibiotics for women of reproductive age for whom either approach is clinically appropriate.

1. **Advantages** of this approach include:
   a. Lack of abdominal scar
   b. Less disturbance of bowel function
   c. Earlier discharge following surgery
   d. More rapid recovery after discharge
2. **Indications** may include:
   a. Pelvic relaxation
   b. Abnormal uterine bleeding
   c. Small leiomyomata
   d. Massive obesity
   e. Cervical dysplasia
   f. Adenomyosis

3. **Relative contraindications**
   a. Concern about ovarian disease
   b. Obesity where the vagina is quite long
   c. Lack of uterine mobility and descent
   d. Uterine size greater than 12 weeks
   e. History of pelvic surgery
   f. History of pelvic infection
   g. Necessity of abdominal exploration
4. **Technique.** The vaginal hysterectomy technique developed by Heaney or its many modifications are used by most vaginal surgeons.
5. **Intraoperative complications** may include:
   a. Injury to the bladder, most commonly at the time of attempted entry into the peritoneal cavity
   b. Ureteral injury with placement of ligatures of clamps too far lateral to the uterine vessels
   c. A loss of control of the uppermost pedicle with retraction of the ovarian vessels and intra-abdominal bleeding

C. **Abdominal hysterectomy**
1. **Advantages** of the abdominal approach relate primarily to the ability to deal more easily with intra-abdominal and adnexal pathology, pelvic adhesions, and large uteri because of the increased exposure provided by the larger abdominal incision.
2. **Indications** for the abdominal approach may include:
   a. Large leiomyomata or mass lesions
   b. Pelvic inflammatory disease, either acute with abscess formation and lack of response to antibiotics, or chronic with pelvic adhesions
   c. Endometriosis
   d. Adnexal disease, specifically including possible ovarian neoplasia
   e. Pelvic pain
3. **Contraindications.** Few if any conditions are contraindications to abdominal hysterectomy, although if either approach is clinically applicable, the lower rates of morbidity and shorter hospital stay associated with vaginal hysterectomy would argue for the vaginal approach. Combined abdominal and vaginal procedures may be necessary when a colporrhaphy is indicated in the face of occasional conditions necessitating an abdominal hysterectomy.
4. **Technique**
   a. **Operative technique.** Descriptions of operative technique abound in surgical texts and atlases. Operative techniques are designed to minimize tissue trauma, risk of infection, and hemorrhage while removing the uterus with all due care and caution to avoid injury to the urinary tract and bowel.

b. **Intraoperative complications** may include:
   (1) **Injury to the ureter.** When ureteral involvement is anticipated or suspected adjacent to pelvic pathology, preoperative IVP or placement of ureteral catheters may prevent injury. Knowledge of pelvic anatomy, visualization, and palpation of the ureters at the time of surgery are essential. Anatomic sites of injury, in order of frequency:
      (a) Lateral to the uterine vessels
      (b) At the ureterovesical junction
      (c) At the base of the infundibulo-pelvic ligament at the pelvic brim
   (2) **Bladder injury,** which must be noted and correctly repaired to prevent fistulas
   (3) **Bowel injury**
   (4) **Hemorrhage.** The risk of hemorrhage is minimized by proper technique and knowledge of anatomy.

## BIBLIOGRAPHY

Buttram VC, Reiter RC. Uterine leiomyomata: Etiology, symptomatology, and management. Fertil Steril. 1981; 36:433–445.

Dicker RC, Greenspan JR, Strauss LT, Cowart MR, Scally MJ, Peterson HB, DeStefano F, Rubin GL, Ory HW. Complications of abdominal and vaginal hysterectomy among women of reproductive age in the United States. Am J Obstet Gynecol. 1982;144:841–848.

Easterday CL, Grimes DA, Riggs JA. Hysterectomy in the United States. Obstet Gynecol. 1983; 62:203–212.

Garcia CR, Cutler WB. Preservation of the ovary: A reevaluation. Fertil Steril. 1984;42:510–514.

Hendrickson MR, Kempson RL. Smooth Muscle Neoplasms. In: Surgical Pathology of the Uterine Corpus. Philadelphia, PA: WB Saunders; 1980.

Hysterectomies in the United States, 1965–84. DHHS Publication No. (PHS) 88-1753, December 1987.

Ingersoll FM, Malone LJ. Myomectomy: An alternative to hysterectomy. Arch Surg. 1970; 100:557–561.

Katz VL, Dotters DJ, Droegemueller W. Complications of uterine leiomyomas in pregnancy. Obstet Gynecol. 1989; 73:593–596.

Lee NC, Dicker RC, Rubin GL, Ory HW. Confirmation of the preoperative diagnoses for hysterectomy. Am J Obstet Gynecol. 1984;150:283–287.

Lifshitz S, Buchsbaum HJ. Urinary Tract Involvement by Benign and Malignant Gynecologic Disease. In: Buchsbaum HJ, Schmidt JD, eds. Gynecologic and Obstetric Urology. Philadelphia, PA: WB Saunders; 1978.

Maheux R, Guilloteau C, Lemay A, Bastide A, Fazekas ATA. Luteinizing hormone-releasing hormone agonist and uterine leiomyoma: A pilot study. Am J Obstet Gynecol. 1985; 152:1034–1038.

Marut EL. Etiology and pathophysiology of fibroid tumor disease: Diagnosis and current medical and surgical treatment alternatives. Obstet Gynecol Surv. 1989; 44:308–310.

McCarthy S. MR imaging of the uterus. Radiology. 1989; 171:321–322.

Mintz PD, Sullivan MF. Preoperative crossmatch ordering and blood use in elective hysterectomy. Obstet Gynecol. 1985; 65:389–92.

Persaud V, Arjoon PD. Uterine leiomyoma: Incidence of degenerative change and a correlation of associated symptoms. Obstet Gynecol. 1970; 35;432–436.

Polivy J. Psychological reactions to hysterectomy: A critical review. Am J Obstet Gynecol. 1974;118:417–426.

Porges RF. Changing indications for vaginal hysterectomy. Am J Obstet Gynecol. 1980;136:153–158.

Ranney B, Frederick I. The occasional need for myomectomy. Obstet Gynecol. 1979; 53:437–441.

Sandberg SI, Barnes BA, Weinstein MC, Braun P. Elective hysterectomy: Benefits, risks and costs. Med Care. 1985; 23:1067–85.

The determination of the necessity of gynecologic surgery. ACOG Statement of Policy, American College of Obstetricians and Gynecologists, May 7, 1977.

Thompson JD, Birch HW: Indications for hysterectomy. Clin Obstet Gynecol. 1981;24:1245–1258.

Winer-Muram HT, Muram D, Gillieson MS. Uterine myomas in pregnancy. J de L'Association Canadienne Des Radiologistes. 1984; 35:168–170.

CHAPTER 8

# Benign Diseases of the Ovaries and Fallopian Tubes

**Guy I. Benrubi**

## OVARY

Benign ovarian masses pose diagnostic and therapeutic dilemmas for the clinician because of somewhat contradictory goals. Although the clinician must diagnose and promptly treat possible malignancy, he must preserve fertility, often in young patients, and avoid procedures that carry inappropriate risks. A systematic approach to diagnosis and treatment avoids unnecessary surgery and morbidity.

### I. Incidence

A. **Functional cysts.** It is probable that every woman will have functional ovarian cysts during her reproductive life. Most of these will go undetected, but some will be discovered, either because they become symptomatic causing the patient to seek evaluation or they are discovered on routine physical examination.

B. **Benign neoplastic masses.** Approximately 80% of all ovarian neoplasia is benign. Thus, the lifetime risk of developing benign ovarian neoplasia by age 70 is approximately 3% to 4%.

### II. Morbidity and mortality

A. **Related to disease.** Benign ovarian tumors may grow to remarkably large size and then regress in size without adversely affecting the health of the patient. On the other hand, patients with preexisting conditions such as endometriosis or pelvic inflammatory disease may develop large ovarian masses with associated complications such as ureteral obstruction with subsequent renal impairment. Torsion of the ovary is a cause of acute abdomen, occurring almost exclusively in the presence of ovarian enlargement. There is also the theoretical potential of ovarian vein thrombosis and pulmonary embolus as an ovarian tumor increases in size and especially if torsion occurs. A bilateral ovarian process, even when benign, may lead to destruction of ovarian tissue and thus ovarian function.

B. **Related to the effects of surgery on fertility.** When surgical treatment is required, the patient is at risk for the formation of pelvic adhesions which may compromise future fertility. Frequently, an ovary or entire adnexa may have to be removed with a negative effect on fertility. Even when cystectomy instead of oophorectomy is performed, the function of the ovary and its blood supply can be compromised.

C. **Related to hormonal effects.** Any ovarian tumor, whether malignant or benign, whether arising from specialized stromal element or not, is potentially functional and can secrete estrogen. This can lead to end organ changes such as anovulation and endometrial cancer as a result, and to hyperplasia in postmenarchal women. Occasionally benign ovarian neoplasia may lead to low-grade endometrial cancer. In premenarchal patients, precocious puberty may be the result.

D. **Related to misdiagnosis.** Because the signs and symptoms of benign ovarian masses are so nonspecific, occasionally pelvic conditions that require immediate intervention may be mistakenly diagnosed as benign ovarian tumors. The most common problems are delay in the diagnosis of malignancy and misdiagnosis of ectopic pregnancy (although with the advent of sensitive radioimmunoassay of human chorionic gonadotropin [hCG] this is increasingly less common).

## III. Etiology

A. **Ovulation theory.** This theory of the etiology of benign ovarian neoplasia states that there is invagination of the capsular epithelium, after ovulation, into the stroma of the ovary. Under hormonal stimulation while in the stroma, this small epithelial inclusion cyst gives rise to ovarian epithelial tumors.

B. **Endocrine theory.** The capsular epithelium of the ovary is Mullerian in origin, and this tissue is responsive to hormones in the same manner Mullerian epithelium responds when present in the endometrium or in the fallopian tube. According to the endocrine theory, under certain "unbalanced" hormonal conditions, this may lead to neoplasia.

C. **Exogenous substances theory.** This theory suggests that irritants such as talc may be the initiating factors in benign and/or malignant ovarian neoplasia.

D. **Transformation theory.** In all probability, most ovarian cancers do not arise from preexisting benign ovarian neoplastic lesions in a process of cellular transformation. However, malignant degeneration in benign neoplasia is a possibility and has been documented.

## IV. Pathogenesis

A. **Functional cysts** are usually less than 6 cm in diameter, but on occasion 10 cm follicular cysts have been removed.

1. **Follicular cysts** may result when ovulation does not occur. They are lined by granulosa cells and theca cells. Often, the granulosa cells are compressed by the fluid in the cyst. When this happens they are termed "simple cysts" because pathologically they are indistinguishable from nonfollicular cysts. Depending on their make up some of these cysts are estrogen producers. Follicular cysts are gonadotropin dependent and therefore should spontaneously regress after menses.
2. **Corpus luteum cysts** form if the regression of the luteal cells in a corpus luteum is delayed. Bleeding may occur into the cyst cavity, or if it ruptures, into the peritoneum. This bleeding may at times be severe, and it may mimic a ruptured ectopic pregnancy.

B. **Benign neoplastic ovarian tumors.** The variety of benign neoplastic ovarian tumors is best understood if the different types of cells present in the ovary are used as a reference for their origin.

1. **Tumors of epithelial cell origin.** The capsular epithelium is Mullerian in origin and may develop epithelial ovarian neoplasia that corresponds to the type of epithelium found in the rest of the reproductive tract. Sixty percent to 70% of all ovarian neoplasia is epithelial in origin.
   a. **Serous cystadenoma.** Accounting for 25% of all benign ovarian neoplasms, serous cystadenomas are usually seen in patients between the ages of 30 and 40. Up to 20% of the time they occur bilaterally. Histologically, they occur in simple and papillary varieties, frequently exhibiting small calcified areas called psammoma bodies. Serous cystadenomas are one of the two most common ovarian neoplasms that occur in pregnancy. They correspond to the type of epithelium found in fallopian tubes.
   b. **Mucinous cystadenomas** represent 15% of all ovarian neoplasms. They are found bilaterally in 10% of patients. They can attain tremendous sizes, with tumors known to weigh 100 to 200 lb. There is some controversy as to whether these tumors are truly epithelial in origin or whether they represent a teratoma that has developed along a single cell line. If these gelatinous material filled tumors rupture, implantation of the benign tumor cells may occur over the peritoneal surfaces, leading to a condition known as pseudomyxoma peritonei. This condition may necessitate repeated laparotomies for the removal of gelatinous material. These tumors correspond to the type of epithelium found in the endocervix.

c. **Brenner tumors** represent 0.5% of all ovarian tumors and arise bilaterally in 10% of patients. Their peak incidence is in patients between 40 and 50 years of age. Most of these tumors are benign, but a malignant variety exists. Histologically, nests of epithelial cells with "coffee bean" nuclei are seen surrounded by strands of fibrous connective tissue. They correspond to Wathard cells found at several places in the Mullerian tract especially in the fallopian tube.

2. **Tumors of stromal cell origin.** Specialized stromal cells are present in the ovary to surround and "nurse" germ cells and to secrete hormones. Accounting for 5% to 10% of all ovarian tumors, stromal cell neoplasms may be associated with excessive hormonal release although most of these tumors are nonfunctioning. It should be remembered, however, that any ovarian neoplasm may exhibit excessive hormonal release.

   a. **Granulosa cell tumors** account for 1% to 2% of all ovarian tumors. They are unilateral in 90% of patients. Granulosa cell tumors present in various histologic patterns, but the constant characteristic is the presence of granulosa cells. Call–Exner bodies, which are small cavities containing eosinophilic fluid surrounded by granulosa cells, are often seen in the microfollicular histologic pattern of this tumor. These tumors usually occur late in the reproductive years and postmenopausally, but they are also seen in prepubertal children. Those tumors that produce estrogen cause a hyperplasia of the endometrium. Up to a 20% incidence of endometrial carcinoma has been reported in these patients. These tumors have low malignant potential, and if they do recur they do so several years after initial diagnosis. Although most functioning granulosa tumors are estrogenic, a small percentage may actually be androgen screening.

   b. **Thecoma** may occur alone or in conjunction with granulosa cell tumors or with fibromas. They are almost always benign and unilateral. Thecomas occur more often in older women than do granulosa tumors, and they are frequently estrogenic.

   c. **Sertoli-Leydig cell tumors** (often referred to as arrhenoblastomas or androblastomas) represent less than 0.5% of all ovarian neoplasms. They occur most frequently in young women (but can be seen at any age) and are unilateral in 95% of patients. Most are benign. These tumors have varying histologic appearances. Some are composed of only Sertoli cells arranged in tubules, others exhibit both Sertoli and Leydig cells, and still others are made up of pure Leydig cells containing Reinke crystals (hilus cell tumors) composed of remnant embryologic hilar Leydig cells. Some are undifferentiated and may resemble sarcomas or carcinomas. Although they are commonly associated with masculinization and androgen production, many of these tumors are endocrinologically inert and some may even be estrogen secreting.

d. **Gynandroblastoma** is an interesting rare tumor composed of well-differentiated sex chord stromal cells, both male and female. Although the cellular elements are well-differentiated, the vast majority of these tumors exhibit benign behavior. When they do recur, it is frequently after several years. These tumors may secrete estrogens or androgens.

3. **Tumors of germ cell origin** arise from progressive stages of differentiation of the toti-potential germ cells. They comprise 15% to 20% of all ovarian neoplasm and almost all varieties are malignant. However, the most common type, the mature cystic teratoma is almost always benign.

   a. **Teratomas** are the most differentiated germ cell tumors. Ninety-five percent of these are composed of the benign mature cystic forms also known as dermoid cysts. The rest are immature forms.

      (1) **Mature cystic teratomas** are the most common germ cell neoplasms, accounting for 10% of all ovarian neoplasms and 25% of all childhood tumors. Most commonly referred to as dermoid cysts, dermoids, or benign cystic teratomas, they occur most frequently during the early reproductive years (although they can be seen throughout life) and are bilateral 15% of the time. Mature elements from all three germ cell layers can be seen, though ectodermal elements, such as hair, sebaceous glands, and other dermal appendages predominate. Macroscopically, these are cystic tumors filled with sebaceous material. In 2% of patients, these tumors undergo malignant transformation. The malignant elements are usually squamous, and the condition is usually seen in postmenopausal patients.

      (2) **Solid mature teratoma.** A rare tumor, solid mature teratoma (also known as adult teratoma) occurs unilaterally and primarily in the first 2 decades of life. It should be classified as adult teratoma only if all elements are mature, in which case this tumor is benign.

      (3) **Monodermal teratomas** may be thought of as cystic teratomas where one germ cell line predominates over the others. The two most frequently mentioned are carcinoid and struma ovarii. Ovarian carcinoids are syndrome-pro-

ducing ovarian neoplasms in one-third of cases, without the requirement of liver metastasis. They are seen in slightly older age groups than are dermoid cysts. Struma ovarii appears microscopically exactly like mature thyroid tissue, producing thyroid hormones and in some cases causing a true thyrotoxicosis. Some of these tumors may be malignant and metastasize. Mucinous cystadenoma is thought by some to be a monodermal teratoma.

b. **Gonadoblastoma** is an uncommon tumor. It is usually seen in patients with gonadal dysgenesis, the majority of these patients being phenotypic females. Gonadoblastomas usually occur in the first three decades of life. They are composed of undifferentiated germ cells and sex chord stromal derivatives, such as granulosa cells or Sertoli cells. They are associated with dysgerminomas in 50% of patients.

4. **Stromal tumors** arise from supportive and vascular structures in the ovary. They are similar to tumors that may arise from these structures in any organ system of the body. Examples of stromal tumors include fibromas, leiomyomas, lipomas, lymphomas, and sarcomas.

## V. Differential diagnosis

### A. Common problems

1. The most important diagnosis that must be ruled out is **ovarian malignancy.** The way this is done is discussed in the diagnosis and management sections of this chapter (VI and VII).
2. **Functional ovarian cysts** are common in menstrual women.
3. **Leiomyomata** especially the pedunculated subserosal type, may mimic adnexal disease.
4. **Pelvic inflammatory disease** with either hydrosalpinx or tubo-ovarian complex or abscess can confound the diagnosis.

### B. Less common problems

1. **Bowel tumors (masses)** especially in older individuals, may represent benign or malignant tumors. However, in a population with an increasing number of older patients, retained feces, diverticular disease must be considered.
2. **Endometriosis**
3. **Torsion of an ovarian mass**
4. **Pelvic kidney**

## VI. Diagnosis

### A. Signs and symptoms

1. Most types of benign ovarian tumors do not cause symptoms and are consequently found serendipitously on palpation of a pelvic mass. Occasionally, these tumors are

functioning and systemic signs such as precocious puberty, irregular menses, or postmenopausal bleeding may be seen. Bladder and rectal pressure is seen in some cases, but it is more frequent when preexisting conditions have led to pelvic adhesions.

2. In premenarchal or postmenopausal women the ovaries are small and should not be palpable on bimanual pelvic examination. The palpation of a "normal sized ovary" (i.e., 3 cm × 2 cm × 1 cm) in a premenarchal or postmenopausal woman is abnormal and requires investigation as discussed below.

B. **Physical examination** should focus on the abdomen/pelvic areas. A thorough abdominal examination is followed by a complete pelvic examination with the collection of a Papanicolaou (PAP) smear. A rectovaginal exam is imperative to fully assess the physical characteristics of the mass. Determination of the size of an ovarian mass is important in deciding whether these masses will require surgical exploration at the outset, or whether observation and noninvasive management is appropriate.

C. **Laboratory and diagnostic procedures**

1. **Preoperative evaluation.** If the mass is suspicious for carcinoma and surgical exploration is appropriate, the standard preoperative laboratory studies should be made. These are discussed in Chapter 2, Care of the Hospitalized Patient.

2. **Tumor markers.** Certain tumors produce substances that may help identify them, called tumor markers. This association may also help determine if the mass is benign or malignant.

   a. **hCG and alpha-feto protein** are elevated in some germ cell malignancies.

   b. **CA-125** is elevated in nonmucinous epithelial ovarian malignancies.

   c. **Lactate dehydrogenase** (LDH) is frequently elevated in ovarian cancers.

3. **Imaging examinations**

   a. **Intravenous pyleograms** (IVP, or intravenous urogram) are useful when clinically indicated to evaluate for a pelvic kidney or ureteral obstruction or malposition. The plain abdominal anterior/posterior (AP) radiograph that initiates the IVP series will also show calcification or other distinguishing features (e.g., teeth leading to a diagnosis of dermoid cyst).

   b. **Barium enema** (BE, LGI, or lower gastrointestinal series) particularly in older women, to evaluate for intrinsic bowel pathology. Where there is clinical evidence of malignant disease, barium enemas are useful to evaluate for metastatic involvement of the bowel.

c. **Ultrasonography** is helpful in distinguishing between functional cyst and neoplastic ones, as the former are usually unilocular. When bimanual exam is difficult, such as in the obese woman, pelvic sonogram may be helpful. Precise measurement of the mass can also be obtained. The ultrasound may be confusing, because of its inability to distinguish between benign and malignant masses. Also, exophytic masses and pedunculated masses of the uterus, mesentery, omentum, and small bowel may all be misinterpreted by sonograph as an adnexal mass. Although transvaginal sonography can detect ovarian masses 1 cm or less in size, its use as a screening tool for ovarian cancer is currently not recommended.

d. **Computerized axial tomography** (CAT scan) is a newer technology, but often not worth the cost in terms of the additional information obtained. Each clinician will need to decide whether this expensive test will provide important information for the management of a specific patient.

4. **Invasive nonsurgical diagnostic procedures** that attempt to determine the histology of the lesions, such as transabdominal CAT scan aided aspiration or culdocentesis, should not be attempted. They may lead to spillage and spread of a localized malignancy, and in no way do they alter therapy. Even if the aspirate is benign, exploratory laparotomy is usually required in large lesions so that the risks of the invasive procedures are not justified.

## VII. Management

### A. Of the premenarchal female

1. Any adnexal mass discovered in a premenarchal female requires surgical evaluation by exploratory laparotomy.
2. The most likely cause would be a germ cell tumor. The possibility of malignancy, particularly dysgerminoma, is high, although the most common tumor is mature cystic teratoma (dermoid cyst).

### B. Of the reproductive-aged female (the menstrual-aged female)

1. **Probable functional ovarian cyst.** The most common cause of adnexal mass in this age group is a functional ovarian cyst. If the patient is having ovulatory cycles, the cyst should not persist through a normal cycle. If the patient is placed on oral contraceptives, the mass should resolve after 28 days. Functional cysts have been reported to occur in the measure of low dose triphasic oral contraceptives. This should be taken into account when selecting an oral contraceptive. These cysts usually arise from a

nonovulatory follicle or a corpus luteum and may be as large as 8 to 10 cm. This diagnosis is more likely if the adnexal mass is:

a. Cystic
b. 8 cm or less in diameter

2. **Probable nonfunctional ovarian cyst** If an adnexal mass is:
   a. Evaluated clinically as noted above and does not resolve in size.
   b. The adnexal mass is greater than 8 cm in diameter.
   c. The mass is solid or semisolid.
   d. The mass has other clinical characteristics suggestive that it is a nonfunctional cyst/mass (e.g., fixed to the pelvic side wall on physical examination).
   e. The mass is considered as a nonfunctional cyst and hence at a high potential for malignancy. An exploratory laparotomy is indicated.

C. **Postmenopausal female.** The ovary of the postmenopausal female is 1.5 × 0.75 × 0.5 cm after about the third year of menopausal life and therefore should not be palpable on pelvic examination. Any adnexal mass or palpable ovary in the postmenopausal female requires exploratory surgical evaluation. There is a 10% to 20% chance of finding malignancy in this situation, although the most common finding is benign ovarian or uterine neoplasia.

D. **Surgical management**

1. **Bowel preparation.** If the adnexal mass is immobile and fixed by what is suspected to be either a neoplastic, inflammatory, or endometriotic process, a bowel preparation should be taken prior to laparotomy. Then, if there is a bowel injury during a difficult resection, the bowel may be primarily repaired without sequela. Furthermore, if a neoplastic lesion is encountered and a bowel resection is required for optimal debulking, it can be carried out. A successful bowel preparation involves both a mechanical and an antibacterial regimen. A typical preparatory regimen follows.
   a. 4 L of polyethyline glycol/electrolyte solution (Go-Lytely solution) p.o. between 8:00 AM and noon the day before surgery.
   b. Erythromycin base 500 mg and neomycin 500 mg p.o. at 1:00 PM, 2:00 PM, and 8:00 PM the day before surgery.
   c. Clear liquids only for 24 hours prior to surgery.
   d. Fleets enema on the morning of surgery.
   e. Go-Lytely prep usually does not require fluid or electrolyte replacement, but these should nevertheless be checked after the bowel preparation is completed and prior to surgery.

2. **At laparotomy**
    a. The incision should be adequate so that the upper abdomen can be explored and appropriate surgical procedures performed in the event that the adnexal mass proves to be malignant. A midline incision accomplishes this readily and is recommended.
    b. Peritoneal fluid or washing should be done on entering the abdomen. This is accomplished by aspirating some of the peritoneal fluid from about the pelvis with a sterile syringe and sending the fluid for cytologic analysis. If no fluid is found, sterile saline is instilled and aspirated.
    c. The abdomen must be thoroughly explored manually and visually, starting at the diaphragm and working downward to the pelvis.
    d. The involved ovary must be handled carefully to avoid rupture. A difficult decision at the time of surgery in patients who want to retain fertility is whether to do a cystectomy or an oophorectomy. In dealing with ovarian neoplasia other than mature cystic teratoma, an oophorectomy should be done. Dermoids are best handled by cystectomy. One way to distinguish between the two is to lift the cyst out of the abdomen. Dermoids are filled with sebaceous material which hardens at room temperature; therefore the consistency of the mass will change. Frozen section pathological analysis of a part of a tumor may be of great help in determining the appropriate surgical procedure.
    e. Intraoperative and postprocedure measures should be taken to ensure fertility where applicable. Tissues should be handled carefully and gently so as not to damage them or to abrade their surfaces causing adhesion formation. Hemostasis should be meticulous for the same reasons. The contralateral ovary should be inspected, but if normal in size, and smooth in surface, it should be left alone. 100 cc of low molecular weight dextran instilled into the peritoneal cavity before closure of the abdomen decreases adhesion formation.

E. **Follow-up.** Most benign ovarian neoplasias are definitively treated with surgery and therefore the patient is at no greater risk of recurrence than the average woman. Therefore, no special follow-up procedures are necessary. The exceptions are specialized stromal tumors that may recur years after surgery. No specific diagnostic measures are practical other than to have the physician and patient be aware of the possibility of recurrence and thus have a high index of suspicion when physiologic abnormalities occur.

**III. Prognosis.** If careful histopathologic examination is carried out, and the ovarian neoplasia is truly benign, the prognosis is excellent. It is important to remove many sections of pathological material, particularly in large tumors. In some of these, small areas may be malignant.

## FALLOPIAN TUBES

The chapters on ectopic pregnancy, pelvic inflammatory disease, infertility, and endometriosis cover the management of tubal pathology in those areas. Some other benign fallopian tube diseases are:

**I. Granulomatous salpingitis** is rarely seen by most gynecologists in the United States. However, because the immigrant population has changed from a predominantly European to a mainly "Third World" mix, this disease may become more common.

- **A. Tuberculous salpingitis** is probably the most common variety of granulomatous salpingitis. The correct diagnosis necessitates a "team approach" by the pathologist and surgeon. Proper therapy involves anti-mycobacterial drugs (isoniazid 300 mg/d and ethambutol 1200 mg/d for several months). Less than 1% of infertile patients will have this disease.
- **B. Actinomycosis infection** is seen not infrequently in women with intrauterine devices, sometimes involving a unilateral mass. Proper therapy involves long-term treatment with oral penicillin (500 mg/d q.i.d. for 12 weeks).
- **C. Crohn's disease of the fallopian tube** can be seen in the presence of bowel involvement. The frequency of this diagnosis is increasing. Therapy involves oral steroids, often with the addition of metronidazole.
- **D. Other granulomas** may have foreign substances such as talc or mineral oil or infectious agents such as pinworm and schistosoma, as their causes. Infectious causes may be treated with the antibiotic or antiparasitic agent specific to the infecting organism, whereas granulomas from foreign substances are not treatable.

**II. Salpingitis isthmica nodosa.** This is a rare condition and pathologically looks like diverticula of the tubal epithelium into the muscularis of the tube, with surrounding hyperplasia of the smooth muscle. It can be thought of as "adenomyosis" of the fallopian tube. It is clinically significant because of its association with an increased incidence of infertility and ectopic pregnancy. There is no treatment for this anatomic abnormality.

**III. Benign cysts** frequently arise from Wolffian or Müllerian remnants. They are thin walled and fluid filled. Clinically they are important because they mimic ovarian neoplasia that necessitates laparotomy. On removal, careful attention should be paid to avoid injury to the mesosalpinx with consequent compromise of the ovarian blood supply. Occasionally these cysts may undergo torsion and present as an acute abdomen.

**IV.** **Benign tumors** of the fallopian tube are rare, and are clinically significant because of the necessity to exclude malignancy. They may also lead to infertility. Histologic varieties include epithelial, mesodermal, and mesothelial type as well as teratomas. Proper therapy is surgical excision.

## BIBLIOGRAPHY


Barber HRK, Graber EA. Gynecological tumors in childhood and adolescence. Obstet Gynecol Surv. 1973; 28:357.

Creasman WT. The adnexal mass; its diagnosis and management. Contemp Ob/Gyn. 1977; 9:45.

Goldstein SR, Subramanyam B, Snyder JR, Beller U, Raghavendra N, Beckman EM. The postmenopausal ovary: The potential role of ultrasound in conservative management. Obstet Gynecol. 1989; 73:8.

Saffos R, Benrubi G. Co-existing adenocarcinoma and cystadenofibroma of the ovary. South Med J. 1985; 78:478.

Scully RE. Ovarian tumors; a review. Am J Pathol. 1977; 87:686.

Spanos W. Preoperative hormonal therapy of cystic adnexal masses. Am J Obstet Gynecol. 1973; 116:551.

White KC. Ovarian tumors in pregnancy. Am J Obstet Gynecol. 1973; 116:544.

# CHAPTER 9

# Pelvic Relaxation

**Bertram H. Buxton**
**Robert L. Summitt, Jr.**

Pelvic relaxation is the loss of integrity of the structures that support the contents of the female pelvis. The result is a group of clinical symptoms, manifested by complaints of pelvic heaviness, discomfort and genital protrusion. These are accompanied by anatomic findings that are coincident with the weakened supportive structures (e.g., weakened cardinal ligaments associated with uterine prolapse). Understanding anatomic relations to clinical findings will lead to correct diagnoses and the application of appropriate therapeutic measures.

**I. Supportive anatomic structures of the female pelvis.** The following is a broad list of supporting structures that, when altered in basic integrity, lead to relaxation abnormalities.

- **A.** Bony pelvis.
- **B.** Pelvic diaphragm (levator ani muscle complex and its superior and inferior fascia) (Figs. 9.1, 9.2).
- **C.** Urogenital diaphragm (Fig. 9.3).
- **D.** Cardinal and uterosacral ligaments (supportive structures of cervix and upper vagina).
- **E.** Bulbocavernosus muscle and external sphincter ani muscle (supportive structures of lower vagina).
- **F.** Perineal body.

**II. Pelvic organs involved in pelvic relaxation and associated clinical manifestations**

- **A.** Bladder: cystocele, pelvic pressure, genital protrusion.
- **B.** Urethra: urethrocele (urethral detachment), stress urinary incontinence.
- **C.** Rectum: rectocele, defecatory dysfunction, genital protrusion.
- **D.** Uterus and cervix: uterine descensus (uterovaginal prolapse), pelvic pressure, genital protrusion.

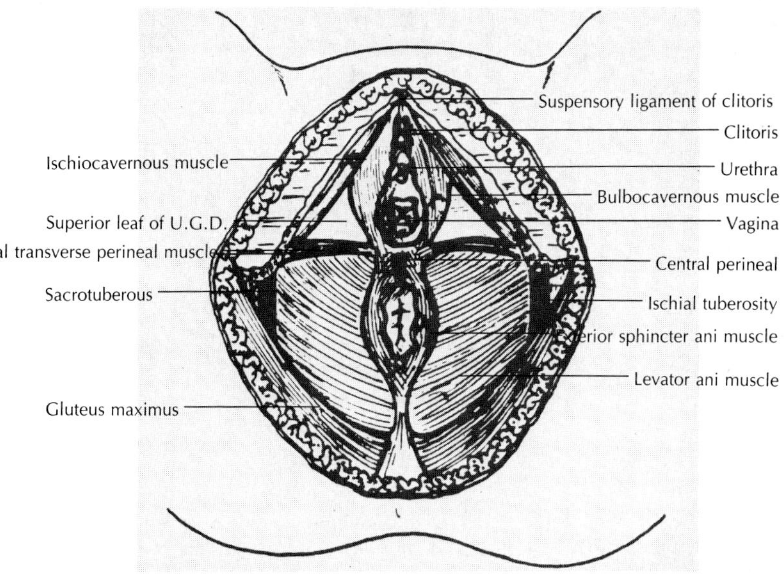


FIGURE 9.1. The pelvic diaphragm (viewed from above). The most critical element of the pelvic diaphragm is the pubococcygeus (or puborectalis) that surrounds the rectum, vagina, and uretha and that is connected to the peripheral tissues of the urogenital diaphragm (U.G.D.), the vagina, and the rectum stabilizing support of these structures. The lowest point of the pelvic floor is just anterior to the coccyx and the muscle mass inclines upward as it proceeds anteriorly to the symphysis pubis. Thus, the lower segment of the uterine corpus, the cervix, and the vaginal fornices normally rest on the levator plate (the posteriorly fused portion of the pubococcygeus muscle).

**E.** Vagina: anterior wall prolapse (cystocele, urethrocele, cystourethrocele); posterior wall prolapse (rectocele, enterocele); vault prolapse.

**F.** Omentum and bowel: enterocele, vault prolapse.

**III.** **Incidence.** The exact incidence of pelvic relaxation is unknown because of under reporting by patients and the lack of morbidity and mortality caused by its relatively benign manifestations. Institutions with an active gynecologic surgical service report that 10% to 15% of their major surgical procedures are associated with pelvic relaxation, the incidence varying with both the population served as well as the gynecologic surgeon's aggressiveness in surgically restoring normal pelvic support. Since 1950 the total numbers of cases of pelvic relaxation, as well as the numbers of severe cases of prolapse, have decreased. This is in part related to less frequent and less traumatic childbirth, more attentive management of the menopause, and closer health care monitoring of the aging patient.

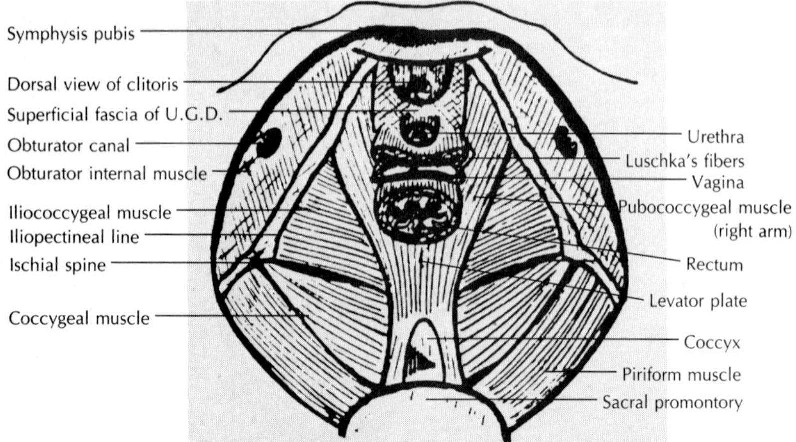


FIGURE 9.2. The pelvic diaphragm (viewed from below). Note the encircling pattern of the pubococcygeus (puborectalis) behind the rectum and the connecting fibers (Luschka's fibers) from this muscle to the vagina that reinforce the support function of this important portion of the levator ani. U.G.D. = urogenital diaphragm.

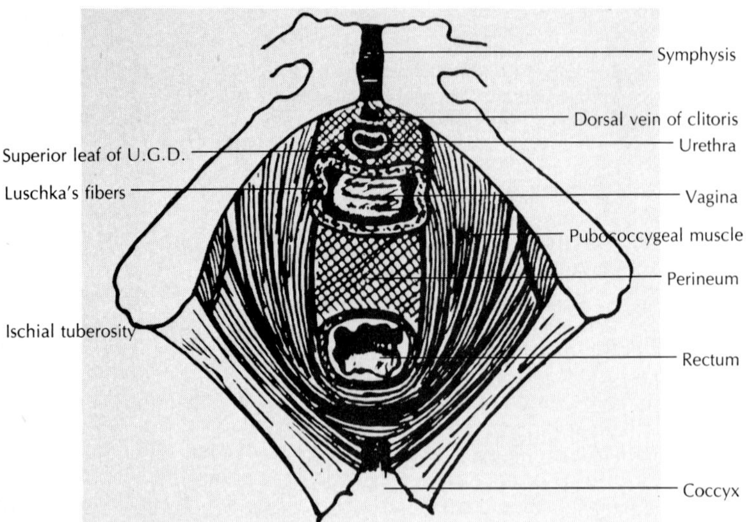


FIGURE 9.3. The perineum. Note the central anchoring role of the perineal body to which all important supporting structures of the pelvis from the level of the pubococcygeal muscle down are fixed (like the hub of a wheel). U.G.D.=urogenital diaphragm.

**IV. Morbidity** associated with pelvic relaxation consists of vague discomfort, diminished ability to carry out vigorous physical activity, and occasionally social embarrassment. Hypothetically, the recent reduction of individual parity and the increased use of cesarean section over midforcep delivery should reduce the incidence of pelvic relaxation. However, the effects on the incidence of pelvic relaxation by the current popularity of "natural childbirth" without episiotomy or elective low forceps to shorten the second stage of labor have yet to be determined.

## V. Etiology and pathophysiology of pelvic relaxation: Contributing factors

A. **Pregnancy and childbirth.** Although the exact mechanisms are debated, pregnancy and childbirth are considered the chief factors responsible for the development of pelvic relaxation, owing to:
   1. **A hormonally induced relaxing effect** on the pelvic supporting structures during pregnancy.
   2. **Progressive increase in intra-abdominal pressure** secondary to the enlarging uterus. In most cases, these forces may be counteracted to a degree by striated muscle exercise (Kegel's exercises).
   3. **Congenital weakness** in certain women, making them more likely to experience attenuation of critical supporting structures such as the cardinal and pubourethral ligaments.
   4. **Overdistention of the vaginal walls** by the birth process in some women, with resultant sagging of the vaginal walls.
   5. **Other birth trauma** resulting in laceration or avulsion of the pelvic and urogenital diaphragms, the vesicourethral supports, or the lateral vaginal connective tissue supports, thus contributing to the initiation of pelvic relaxation and eventual prolapse.
      a. Women with a wide forepelvis (gynecoid or flat) are more prone to anterior segment pelvic trauma causing cystocele development or downward displacement of the urethrovesical junction leading to the development of anatomic stress urinary incontinence.
      b. Women with a narrow forepelvis (anthropoid or android) tend to direct the focus of labor and childbearing forces into the wider posterior section of the pelvis in which case enterocele and/or rectocele are more likely to result. The repetitive effects of multiple pregnancies and births predispose the patient to greater damage. Therefore the trend toward fewer births among females in the industrialized nations will lessen exposure to such repetitive soft tissue trauma.

B. **Menopause and the aging process.** Birth-related pelvic support injuries are often not immediately recognized because of the integrity of striated muscle and connective tissue support. This support, however, may diminish postmenopausally abetted by aging. Menopause and the inevitable cellular changes secondary to aging are the second most common aggravating factors leading to loss of pelvic support.

1. Because of the estrogen receptors in the area of the bladder neck and urethra, estrogen loss results in decreased vascularity, leading to loss of urethral tone. This compromises the urethra's capacity for luminal compression resulting in urinary incontinence.
2. This progressive loss of vascularity also decreases support normally supplied by the cardinal ligaments and other endopelvic connective tissue components.
3. Age itself reduces both pliability and elasticity of collagenous tissues. In addition, cell populations are decreased resulting in less muscle and connective tissue mass needed for support.

C. **Race.** Although the exact reason for racial differences in the development of pelvic relaxation is not understood, it is well-known that black and Oriental women have a significantly lower incidence of pelvic relaxation than white females.

D. **Trauma** from accidental or sexual injury are rare causes of genital relaxation.

E. **Congenital defects.** Although congenital absence of supporting tissues or congenital weakness of such tissues are known to occur, this is an unusual etiology. Less than 2% of all cases of pelvic relaxation develop in nulliparous females, and most of these unfortunate women usually have lived a rigorous life of arduous labor contributing to their genital prolapse. However, acquired collagen deficiency disease may occasionally contribute to pelvic relaxation.

F. **Medical disorders.** Any condition that is associated with a chronic or repetitive increase in intra-abdominal pressure may be a factor in causing pelvic relaxation. Chronic obstructive pulmonary disease, chronic constipation, large pelvoabdominal tumors such as fibroids, ascites, and obesity have been implicated as contributing to the progressive loss of pelvic support.

## VI. Diagnosis of pelvic relaxation.

Symptoms of pelvic relaxation are divided into general symptoms and those that are specific for the particular type of pelvic relaxation. If all the various symptoms of pelvic relaxation coexist in the same patient, the condition is not only aggravating but may be incapacitating to an otherwise normal female with the capability of full physical and sexual function.

A. **General symptoms.** When general symptoms are present, more specific symptoms and relevant physical findings should be sought in order that appropriate corrective measures may be taken.

General symptoms are:

1. Pelvic heaviness.
2. Sacral backache.
3. Problems with intercourse such as looseness, obstruction, and/or pain.
4. "Bearing down" sensation, accompanied by a protrusion of a bulging mass beyond the introitus (if pelvic relaxation is severe).

B. **General physical examination.** The general procedure for examination in cases of pelvic relaxation rests on the following. These examination techniques are referred to as "strain, hold, and elevate" (S.H.E.).

1. After separation of the labia and replacing the vaginal contents (if necessary), the perineum is gently depressed with a Sims' speculum.
2. The patient is then asked to strain, and the sequence in which descent of the organs occurs is observed.
3. The patient is then asked to attempt to hold her vagina tightly closed, and the tone and strength of the pubococcygeal muscles laterally are assessed. (With normal support, the urethra, bladder and rectum retract from the vaginal axis during this.)
4. Then the vaginal vault is elevated using the vaginal examining fingers and the patient is asked to strain.
   a. If previous descent is corrected by this, lateral cervical vaginal defects are present.
   b. If the uterus and upper vagina descend together, uterovaginal prolapse is present. In the case of cervical prolapse, the cervix elongates and appears to prolapse while the uterine fundus remains stationary.
   c. If there is a bulging anteriorly, cystocele is present.
   d. A posterior upper vaginal bulge indicates an enterocele, or if lower down in the vagina, a rectocele is indicated.

C. **Specific symptoms and physical findings**

1. **Stress incontinence.** The symptom and condition of stress urinary incontinence are usually associated with descent of the bladder neck and proximal urethra. In addition to this descent, a downward and backward rotational movement of the urethrovesical junction away from its normal retropubic location also occurs. This anatomic alteration prevents equal transmission of the transiently increased intra-abdominal pressure to both the bladder neck and proximal urethra as well as to the bladder itself, thus forcing urine into the proximal urethra, and contributing to urinary incontinence.
   a. **History.** Anatomic stress urinary incontinence is present only during increased intra-abdominal pressure such as that caused by cough, sneeze, laugh, or

heel bounce. The patient may often notice this only in the sitting or standing position unless the urethrovesical neck dislocation is severe.

b. **Physical examination**

(1) **Demonstration of urine loss.** A Sims' speculum or finger separation of the introitus may be used to observe the bladder neck while the patient is straining downward or coughing. Posterior and downward rotation of the bladder neck is usually demonstrated. Objective loss of urine with this maneuver will make the diagnosis. If no urine loss is demonstrated supine, this maneuver should be repeated standing. It is important for the bladder to contain at least 300 mL of either urine, water, or saline prior to testing for urine loss.

(2) **Demonstration of urethrovesical junction hypermobility.** A catheter or cotton swab at the urethrovesical junction will angle sharply upwards by 30° or more when the patient strains if substantial disruption of the urethrovesical supports has occurred.

c. **Other tests.** Cystometry should be performed in all patients being evaluated for stress urinary incontinence. It is the only objective tool to confirm or rule out an unstable bladder as the cause of urinary incontinence. Multichannel urodynamic testing and/or urethroscopy, are indicated if there is a history of urgency, bed wetting, difficulty in stopping the urinary stream, nonstress-related incontinence, neurologic disease, or previous incontinence surgery (see Chapter 10, Gynecologic Urology).

**2. Cystocele**

a. **History and symptoms.** A cystocele may cause vague discomfort, pelvic pressure on standing, or may be associated with vaginal irritation and bleeding from ulceration of the exposed vaginal mucosa. Occasionally patients report that they have to replace the cystocele to urinate. Although stress urinary incontinence may be associated with a cystocele, it is not caused by the cystocele per se.

b. **Physical examination.** A cystocele is diagnosed by the demonstration of ballooning of the anterior vaginal wall behind the region of the bladder neck using the S.H.E. technique (see diagnosis of pelvic relaxation section, VI-B).

(1) **Mild,** asymptomatic (first-degree) cystocele is diagnosed if the vaginal wall does not protrude beyond the vaginal orifice on straining.

(2) **Moderate,** (second-degree) cystocele is diag-

nosed if the bladder bulge protrudes beyond the introitus on straining.

(3) **Severe,** (third-degree) cystocele is diagnosed if, even without straining, the cystocele lies outside the vaginal orifice.

c. **Residual urine** (urine left in the bladder after voiding) of large volume is usually not present in patients with a cystocele. If significant residual urine (100 mL or greater) accompanies a cystocele, chronic cystitis may be present and the possibility of a hypotonic bladder should be investigated by urodynamic evaluation. Voiding studies (uroflowmetry) should also be performed to evaluate the mechanism of micturition. By having the patient void and measuring the flow rate, abnormalities of detrusor contractibility (e.g., hypotonia) may be revealed.

3. **Uterine prolapse.** Prolapse of the cervical/vaginal midpelvic supports leads to inversion of the vagina and its vaults and descent of the cervix. If prolapse is mild, it is usually asymptomatic.

a. **History and symptoms.** Varying degrees of pelvic heaviness, pressure, and the perception of protrusion are common symptoms of moderate-to-severe prolapse. Sometimes prolapse and elongation of the cervix may occur without accompanying uterine descent. This is seen in cases of endometriosis, fibroids, or pelvic adhesive disease, which restrict downward migration of the uterine corpus but allow the cervix to elongate.

b. **Physical examination.** Uterine prolapse is present if the uterus and upper vagina descend together upon S.H.E. maneuver (see diagnosis of pelvic relaxation section, VI-B). The degree of uterocervical prolapse is assessed like other vaginal relaxations:

(1) **Mild (first-degree) prolapse** is characterized by descent of the cervix without protrusion beyond the introitus even with straining.

(2) **Moderate (second-degree) prolapse** is present when the cervix extends beyond the introitus upon straining.

(3) **Severe (third-degree) prolapse, or procedentia,** is present when, without straining, the cervix extends beyond the introitus. As in cystocele, ulceration with inflammation, bleeding, and thickening of the exposed cervical and vagina epithelium occur with procedentia. Complete procedentia is generally accompanied by the eversion of the vaginal walls, with associated cystocele and rectocele and a traction type of enterocele.

4. **Enterocele**
   a. **Types of enterocele**
      (1) **Traction enterocele** is a hernial sac led by the pouch of Douglas that descends with the uterus. The anterior wall of a traction enterocele is formed by the posterior wall of the uterus covered by its posterior visceral peritoneum. The lower portion of the posterior wall of the sac is covered by the enlongated cul-de-sac parietal peritoneum, and the contents may be omentum or ileum.
      (2) **Pulsion enterocele.** The congenital or pulsion type of enterocele results from a congenital weakness of the fascia of Denonvilliers, which ordinarily seals the superior margin of the rectovaginal septum. This type of enterocele is a peritoneal herniation of the pouch of Douglas separating the anterior wall of the rectum from the posterior wall of the vagina and occupies the rectovaginal space. It too may have ileum or omentum as contents.
   b. **History and symptoms.** Unless the enterocele is small and without intraperitoneal contents, the patient experiences pain on sitting, standing, or straining. Small enteroceles are often asymptomatic.
   c. **Physical examination.** A posterior upper vaginal bulge on S.H.E. indicates enterocele. An enterocele is differentiated from a rectocele by the absence of the examining finger in a posterior bulge on rectal examination.
5. **Rectocele**
   a. **History and symptoms.** Often there is a feeling of vaginal pressure or protrusion. If the rectocele is large, the patient may have to replace the rectal hernia to defecate.
   b. **Physical examination.** Rectocele is diagnosed by the observation, using the S.H.E. techniques (see diagnosis of pelvic relaxation section, VI-B) of a protrusion of the rectum into the posterior wall of the vagina, causing a ballooning out of the weakened posterior vaginal wall. A finger in the rectum falls into this sacculation of the anterior rectal wall and distends the weak posterior vaginal wall.
      (1) **Mild (first-degree) rectocele** is diagnosed if, with straining, it does not protrude beyond the introitus.
      (2) **Moderate (second-degree) rectocele** is diagnosed if the sacculation protrudes beyond the introitus on straining.

(3) **Severe (third-degree) rectocele** is diagnosed if protrusion occurs without straining.

6. **Loss of perineal support.** A relaxed lacerated perineum results in a perineal body that has lost some or all of its coordinated structural integrity, allowing less support for those structures that insert into it. These include the external sphincter ani muscles, bulbocavernosus muscles, the superficial transverse perineal muscles, and the pubococcygeus muscles as well as the lower anterior rectum and posterior vagina.
   a. **History and symptoms.** This condition is often asymptomatic but occasionally the patient will complain of introital looseness at the time of intercourse.
   b. **Physical examination.** Loss of perineal support is clinically evident prior to performing the speculum examination by observing a gaping introitus through which the anterior vaginal wall is easily visible and invites and aggravates the progress of a cystocele and/or urethrocele.

**VII. Treatment.** Surgery is not indicated in the asymptomatic patient. For the symptomatic patient, nonsurgical therapy should be discussed and offered prior to surgical intervention. Surgery should not, however, be withheld should the patient refuse initial nonsurgical therapy.

**A. Nonsurgical management of pelvic relaxation**

1. **Estrogen replacement therapy.** In estrogen deficient females, estrogen therapy increases vascularity and tone in the vagina, sometimes alleviating the need for surgery. Conjugated estrogen (Premarin) 0.625 mg p.o. q.d. or conjugated estrogen vaginal cream one-half applicator two to three times weekly is also useful as adjunctive therapy to both nonsurgical and surgical treatments. For patients unable to tolerate oral or vaginal estrogen, Estraderm-patches, 0.05 twice weekly can be used. With the uterus present, medroxyprogesterone acetate (Provera) 2.5 to 10 mg p.o. q.d. for 15 days every month should be added to avoid unopposed estrogen effect on the endometrium. Current practice suggests giving conjugated estrogen at 0.3 to 0.625 mg and 2.5 to 5 mg medroxy progesterone acetate every day.
2. **Kegel's exercises** are repetitive contractions of the pubococcygeus and can improve striated muscle tone and thus strengthen the pubococcygeus muscle significantly. This contributes to more effective lower vaginal and urethral function and structural support. They are primarily helpful for women in the reproductive-age group but are minimally useful in older women, especially when there is anatomic displacement of the urethrovesical neck or begin-

ning prolapse. Kegel's exercises are best taught by instructing the patient to simulate voluntarily stopping her urinary stream. Twenty-five repetitions at least four times a day are prescribed to increase tone. At the beginning, five to ten repetitions should be used; and repetitions should gradually increase each week.

3. **Pessary.** In symptomatic patients, pessary use has given way to the increased use of surgery even in the aged or infirm patient because of the increased safety of modern anesthesia, better preoperative and postoperative preparation and management and perhaps by the better health status of the older female today. However, some clinical situations justify use of a pessary.
   a. **Indications**
      (1) To support a prolapse in the early months of pregnancy. Because the enlarging uterus usually supplies sufficient support by its size, pessary support of the uterus after 14 to 16 weeks may not be necessary.
      (2) In women who wish to avoid surgery to preserve their childbearing potential.
      (3) In patients who are considered inoperable due to their medical status.
      (4) In other patients, usually aged and sexually inactive who steadfastly refuse surgical relief, who may obtain symptomatic relief without the risk of surgery.
      (5) In patients whose symptoms may or may not be attributable to pelvic relaxation, a "trial" of pessary to obtain relief with a return of symptoms when the pessary is removed verifies the appropriateness of surgery.
   b. **Types of pessaries** (Fig. 9.4)
      (1) **The Smith-Hodge pessary** or one of its newer variants is used for pregnant patients.
      (2) **Gelhorn, ring, donut, and inflatable pessaries** are effective in the type of patient listed in Sections VII-A-3-a- (3) and (4).
   c. **Adjunctive estrogen therapy.** Local or systemic estrogen is helpful in maintaining vaginal tissue tolerance to the pessary.
   d. **Follow-up.** Initially, patients should be seen and reexamined 1 week after the fitting of a pessary to ensure maintenance of position and assess tolerance. Afterwards, visits can extend to 3 to 6 months, with particular attention to examining the condition of the vaginal mucosa. Some patients can be instructed to remove, wash, and replace their own pessaries every 30 days.

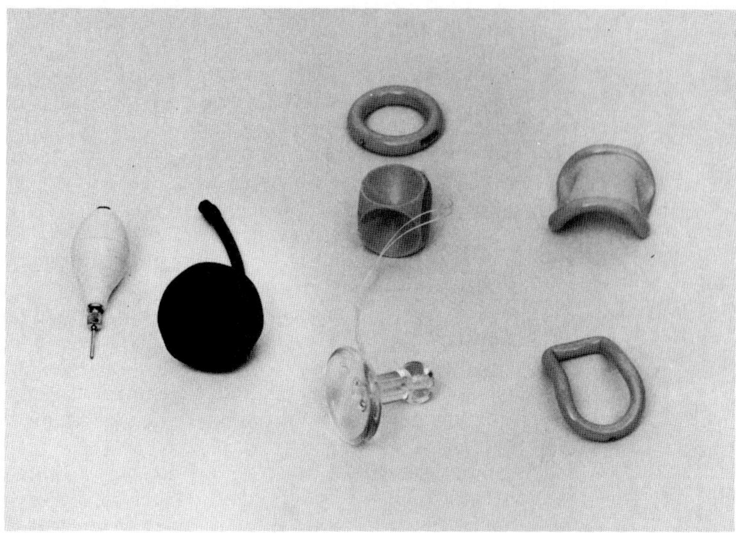

FIGURE 9.4. Types of pessaries. Beginning from the top and proceeding clockwise around the central pessary, the types are: ring pessary, Gehrung pessary, Hodge pessary, Gelhorn pessary, inflatable pessary with bulb. Center: cube pessary.

**B. Surgical management of pelvic relaxation**

1. **Indications.** Surgery should be undertaken only in the patient who is either still symptomatic after nonsurgical approaches have been attempted or desires surgical intervention in lieu of nonsurgical therapy.
2. **General principles.** Surgical treatment is designed to address the patient's specific deficits of pelvic support, and it is important to choose procedures that attempt to correct all the existing deficits. Also, it is important to use techniques that will protect the patient against recurrences and, if perceived as desirable by the patient, preserve a functional vagina for sexual intercourse. General guidelines for surgery are:
   a. Choose an appropriate procedure based on accurate preoperative evaluation and precise anatomic knowledge.
   b. Use estrogen replacement when indicated, both preoperatively and postoperatively (see treatment section, VII-A-1).
   c. Always obtain adequate exposure by adequate dissection.
   d. Avoid shortening the vagina to preserve sexual function and look for the opportunity of anchoring the vag-

inal apex posteriorly to the uterosacral ligaments, if feasible, or to the sacrospinous ligaments.

e. Plicate the uterosacral ligaments, closing the posterior peritoneum as close to the rectal reflection as possible to obliterate any potential enterocele.

f. Correct all pelvic support deficiencies, present and potential.

g. Avoid excising too much anterior or posterior vaginal wall so that the vagina is not too narrow.

h. Avoid overcorrection of a cystocele, thus causing anatomic stress urinary incontinence postoperatively.

3. **Surgery for uterine prolapse.** In North America prolapse of the uterus is usually managed by vaginal hysterectomy, although the British still use the Manchester-Fothergill procedure, in which the cervix is amputated and the cardinal ligaments are shortened and sewn to the cervical stump to provide uterine support.

4. **Surgery for cystocele.** Cystocele is corrected by an anterior colporrhaphy, which plicates the endopelvic fascia over the reduced bladder hernia and excises the excess stretched vaginal epithelium before repairing the vaginal incision.

5. **Surgery for rectocele (posterior colporrhaphy).** Rectocele is surgically managed in the same manner as the cystocele except that the perirectal fascia is used to maintain the reduced herniated rectal sac. Excess posterior vaginal epithelium is excised before the posterior vaginal wall is approximated.

6. **Surgery for loss of perineal support.** Perineorrhaphy is usually combined with the anterior-posterior or posterior vaginal repair. This consists of attaching all lower vaginal supporting tissues to the reconstructed perineal body. These supporting tissues are (from deep to superficial): the lower portion of the pubococcygeus muscles, the superficial transverse perineal muscles and fibers of the external sphincter ani. It is often necessary to excise scarred perineal skin and vaginal tissues. The vagina and the perineal skin edges are then reapproximated as in episiotomy repair.

7. **Surgery for enterocele**

   a. **Vaginal approach.** An enterocele must be identified before the posterior wall repair is initiated. It is necessary to carry the original posterior vaginal wall incision high enough to identify and repair this often latent defect. In a patient who has previously undergone hysterectomy, it may be detected by dissection up to the vaginal vault. The sac must be mobilized as with any hernia and the neck located and then tied off as high as possible being careful not to include the ureters. The sac is then usually excised.

b. **Abdominal approach.** If an enterocele or excessively deep cul-de-sac is found during an abdominal procedure, the Moschcowitz procedure may be used. This obliterates the cul-de-sac by a series of permanent sutures placed in ascending rows starting at the bottom of the sac and ending at the level of the uterosacral ligaments.

8. **Surgery for vaginal vault prolapse.** The surgical approach for correction of posthysterectomy vaginal vault prolapse may be either vaginal or abdominal. Either approach has distinct advantages and disadvantages. The selection is based on the presence of accompanying anatomic abnormalities and the degree of operator skill. The goal of correction is to re-establish normal vaginal position and function.

   a. **Vaginal approach.** The transvaginal sacrospinous fixation is performed through the same vaginal incision required for posterior colporrhaphy. In two-thirds of cases enterocele is present and should be repaired initially, as described above. The operator then dissects to the right sacrospinous ligament with his right hand, perforating the rectal pillar, and entering the pararectal space. The vaginal apex is attached to the sacrospinous ligament with permanent suture (O-Prolene®).

      (1) **Advantages**

         (a) Restoration of a functional vagina with normal upper horizontal axis.

         (b) In contrast to the abdominal approach, it allows simultaneous correction of cystocele, rectocele and enterocele.

         (c) Shorter operating time.

         (d) Extraperitoneal.

      (2) **Disadvantages**

         (a) May not be applicable to extremely short vaginal length.

         (b) Limited visual exposure.

   b. **Abdominal approach.** The transabdominal sacropexy is used to support an extremely short vagina or is used when the abdomen is entered for other reasons. The vaginal apex is attached to the sacral promontony with either a synthetic mesh (e.g., Mersiline®, Marlex®) or fascia lata.

      (1) **Advantage**

         (a) Allows support of the vagina when it is too short to reach the sacrospinous ligament.

      (2) **Disadvantages**

         (a) Does not allow simultaneous repair of cystocele. Combining a vaginal repair with transabdominal sacropexy would predispose to infection at the site of permanent sutures and mesh.

(b) Longer operating time.

(c) Greater risk of bleeding.

(d) Technically more difficult.

**9. Surgery for stress incontinence**

**a. Vaginal approach.** The correction of a displaced urethrovesical neck may be approached vaginally, particularly if there are coexistent correctable defects such as a large cystocele, uterine prolapse, enterocele, rectocele, or relaxed perineum.

(1) **Anterior colporrhaphy.** It is important to carry the anterior vaginal wall incision vertically up to the posterior lip of the urethra. The subvaginal connective tissue with the fused inferior surface of the urogenital diaphragm is dissected away from the vaginal skin. The urethra is freed by blunt dissection up to the vesical neck and if possible the remnants of the pubourethral ligaments, which usually have retained some degree of integrity, are used to restore the urethrovesical junction to its retropubic location. Buttressing these sutures with an additional layer of the subvaginal tissue should be performed. The use of polyglycolic sutures has improved the results of bladder neck reposition.

(2) The **modified Pereyra procedure** is a vaginoabdominal operation utilizing the periurethral fascia and endopelvic fascia. The primary dissection is made vaginally, similar to the anterior colporrhaphy, allowing identification of the fascial elements. Periuretheral and endopelvic fascia are bluntly dissected from the posterior pubic rami. A helical suture is then run through this band of tissue on each side of the urethra, leaving the ends long. A special needle is passed down from a small transverse abdominal skin incision, through the rectus fascia, rectus muscle, and guided subpubically into the vaginal incision. The needle is threaded with the two long ends of the sutures on each side of the urethra and brought back up and tied to each other across the midline of the anterior rectus fascia.

b. **Abdominal approach.** Transabdominal suspension of the urethrovesical junction may be done by a number of so-called "pin-up" procedures. The most popular of these are the Marshall-Marchetti-Krantz operation and the Burch procedure.

(1) **The Marshall-Marchetti-Krantz procedure** attaches the periurethral subvaginal connective tis-

sue by polyglycolic sutures to the fibrocartilage or periosteum of the symphysis.

(2) **The Burch procedure** uses the more lateral Cooper's ligament to suspend the bladder neck.

(3) **Other procedures.** Occasionally in patients with excessive scar tissue from previous failed operations or in those where only poor tissue is available, a sling of fascia lata, synthetic mesh, anterior rectus abdominus fascia, or even the round ligaments may be used to support the mobilized bladder neck and proximal urethra. The fascia lata, synthetic mesh, and rectus abdominus slings are sewn to the anterior rectus fascia.

## VIII. Prognosis

**A. Operative success.** The choice of the appropriate procedure and the use of good technique the first time around in the patient with tissue of reasonable integrity should produce 5-year success rates of 85% to 90%. Results are often excellent in cases where little functional or anatomic abnormality is present preoperatively.

**B. Operative failures.** The postoperative results to correct pelvic relaxation are unfortunately not 100%. The primary causes for operative failure include:

1. **Scarred or weak pelvic tissue.** Operations on patients who have scarred or weak tissue are prone to failure. Those with excessive scar tissue or thin, devascularized, weak tissues may need synthetic or extrapelvic tissue sling support. Meticulous attention must also be paid to principles such as hemostasis and delicate tissue handling.
2. **Poor choice of operation.** Although transabdominal bladder neck suspension has become the most popular route for the correction of anatomic stress urinary incontinence, the vaginal approach may, in the right hands, be equally successful, especially in patients with other deficits in vaginal and pelvic support. Individual patient needs and physician experience must weigh heavily in the proper selection of the optimal procedure.

## BIBLIOGRAPHY

Inmon WB. Pelvic relaxation and repair including prolapse of vagina following hysterectomy. South Med J. 1963; 56:577.

Netter FH. The Ciba collection of medical illustrations vol. 2, 1962. Reproductive system 1954, section 4, 5, and 7. New York: Curtis Publishing; 1962.

Nichols DH, Randall CL. Vaginal Surgery. Baltimore, Md: Williams and Wilkins; 1976.

Sciarra ED: Gynecology and Obstetrics. 51st ed. Philadelphia, Pa: Harper and Row; Vol. 1, Ch. 1, 61, 62, 63, and 85; 1988.

Tovel HMM, Dank V. Gynecologic Operations. Hagerstown, Md: Harper and Row; 1978.

# CHAPTER 10

# Gynecologic Urology

**Robert L. Summit, Jr.**
**John O.L. DeLancey**
**Thomas E. Elkins**

Because of the close embryologic and anatomic development of the lower urinary tract and genital tract, urinary complaints are some of the most common reasons that the female patient presents to the gynecologist. The close relationship of these systems makes them subject to similar anatomic, physiologic, and pathologic disorders. A disease process in one system will often adversely affect the normal function in the other. Therefore, symptoms tend to overlap and make accurate diagnosis difficult. The gynecologist must be aware of these pathophysiologic relationships, have a systematic approach for their evaluation, and be knowledgeable of specific lower urinary tract disorders.

Although urinary tract infection (UTI) is the most common lower urinary tract disorder, incontinence can be one of the most disabling conditions seen by the gynecologist. To evaluate and treat specific disorders of incontinence, the mechanism of urinary control should be understood. Continence is a learned mechanism of control over the micturition process. It is a complete neuropharmacologic and anatomic task.

## I. Components of urinary continence

The components that maintain continence and prevent uncontrolled urine loss include:

A. **Anatomic support** of the urethrovesical junction maintaining it in an intra-abdominal position.

B. **An internal urethral sphincteric mechanism** is composed of the following:

1. Urethral mucosal infolding providing a water-tight seal. It is estrogen dependent.
2. Elastic and connective tissue of the urethral wall.
3. Smooth muscle fibers in the urethral wall enhancing involuntary control over micturition.
4. Vascular content of the submucosal cavernous plexus.

C. **An extrinsic urethral sphincter** consisting of skeletal muscle has the following components:

1. Periurethral striated muscle fibers.

2. Muscles of the urogenital diaphragm (perineal membrane).

**D. Intact innervation** to all of these components providing modulation of their function.

Of the factors listed, those central to the problem of stress incontinence are: support of the proximal urethra and normal closure of the vesical neck.

## II. Evaluation of the patient with lower urinary tract complaints.

When the patient presents with specific lower urinary tract complaints, an organized and systematic evaluation process must be instituted. A specific history and clinical examination should be used. The history provides guidance for the evaluation. The clinical examination, in this field more than others, provides the definitive diagnosis. The clinical examination consists of neurological and physical examinations, later followed by specific urologic testing if necessary.

**A. History.** The history is composed of two parts; routine questioning and a 24-hour voiding diary.

1. **Routine questioning.** Disorders of the lower urinary tract share a pool of common symptoms. For simplicity, these symptoms can be grouped into two categories. The first category, irritative symptoms, includes complaints of urgency, frequency, dysuria, postvoid fullness, and suprapubic pain. The second category, incontinence, shares some symptoms with the previous category. However, stress incontinence and urge continence tend to be the primary complaints. The battery of questions addressed to the patient should review the following areas.
   a. Frequency of voiding
      (1) How often?
      (2) Nocturia?
      (3) Amount voided?
   b. Urgency (the inability to delay urination)
      (1) How severe?
      (2) Associated with urine loss?
   c. Urine leakage
      (1) If yes, when?
      (2) If yes, how does it affect the patient?
      (3) If yes, what preventive measures are taken?
   d. Voiding difficulties
      (1) Difficulty initiating voiding?
      (2) Discomfort or pain before, during, or after voiding?
      (3) Incomplete voiding?
      (4) Intermittent voiding?
2. **24-hour voiding diary.** This is valuable in obtaining a record of voiding habits, voiding frequency, voiding volumes, urgency, leakage, and intake. The patient keeps this journal during a day of normal activity. It may reveal disorders in

which the symptoms are obscured through direct questioning bias (Fig. 10.1)

**B. Clinical examination**

1. **Neurologic examination.** Uninhibited detrusor contractions can be the result of neurologic lesions. In patients with this condition, and others, a careful neurologic examination should be performed. The following neurological screening examination tests for intact motor and sensory response of nerve roots $L_1$–$S_4$ (those supplying the bladder). If neurologic deficit is noted, consultation is advised. It consists of:
   a. Testing sensation in lower extremity dermatomes by stroking over the thigh and leg.
   b. Assessing muscle strength through flexion and extension at the hip, knee, and ankle.

| TIME | AMT VOIDED | ACTIVITY | LEAK VOLUME | URGE PRESENT | AMOUNT/TYPE OF INTAKE |
|---|---|---|---|---|---|
| | | | | | |
| | | | | | |
| | | | | | |
| | | | | | |
| | | | | | |
| | | | | | |
| | | | | | |
| | | | | | |
| | | | | | |
| | | | | | |
| | | | | | |
| | | | | | |
| | | | | | |
| | | | | | |
| | | | | | |
| | | | | | |
| | | | | | |
| | | | | | |
| | | | | | |
| | | | | | |
| | | | | | |
| | | | | | |

FIGURE 10.1. The voiding diary. From Ostergard DR, ed. Gynecologic Urology and Urodynamics, 2nd ed. Copyright © Williams & Wilkins, Baltimore, 1985. Reprinted with permission.

c. Checking deep tendon reflexes.
d. Assess the presence of a Babinski sign.
e. Bulbocavernosis reflex test (stroke the perianal skin and observe contraction of the anal sphincter).

2. **Pelvic examination** is performed to assess conditions that may predispose to irritative symptoms or incontinence. Estrogen status of the vaginal mucosa, along with the presence of cystocele, rectocele, or prolapse are evaluated. The pelvic and anal muscle tones are also checked. Pelvic muscle tone is assessed during vaginal examination by having the patient contract her pelvic floor. This may be elicited by asking the patient to contract the muscles necessary to stop her urine stream. Anal muscle tone is assessed on rectovaginal examination by asking the patient to again contract her pelvic floor. Last of all, the anterior vaginal wall is assessed for the presence of a urinary fistula or diverticulum.

3. **Urine for culture and sensitivity** to rule out the presence of a UTI. A catheterized specimen is preferred, but a clean catch specimen may be considered acceptable if it is negative. A lower UTI can cause symptoms of incontinence as well as interstitial cystitis and urethral syndrome. Continuing evaluation in the presence of a UTI could either lead to an incorrect diagnosis or worsening of the patient's symptoms.

   If the urine culture reveals $10^5$ organisms/mL of urine, antibiotic treatment is instituted based on the sensitivities. Evaluation should not continue until the urine is recultured. If the repeat culture reveals bacteria, it must be determined whether bacteriuria is unresolved or recurrent, either because of persistence or reinfection. Unresolved bacteriuria implies the presence of bacteria despite therapy (e.g., resistant bacteria). Bacteriuria must have resolved before it can be classified as recurrent. Bacterial persistence refers to recurrence of the same organism, often secondary to an anatomic abnormality (e.g., infected renal calculus). These patients require an intravenous pyelogram (IVP). Reinfection refers to the presence of a different organism or serotype. The organisms usually arise from the vaginal or rectal reservoir. An IVP is not required. Instead, suppressive antibiotic therapy with either nitrofurantoin or trimethopri-sulfamethoxazole is administered. If bacteria are still present, an IVP is obtained. Once the urine culture is clear, the evaluation can continue.

4. **The Q-tip test** is performed to assess mobility and descent of the urethrovesical junction. Although not diagnostic for incontinence, this test aids in the evaluation of incontinence and may provide prognostic information as to treatment. The test is performed in the lithotomy position. A sterile, lubricated, cotton swab is inserted transurethrally into the

bladder, then withdrawn until resistance is felt. The angle of the cotton swab is measured from the horizontal at rest and again on maximum straining (Fig. 10.2). If the maximum straining angle from the horizontal is greater than 30 to 35°, this is felt to represent hypermobility of the urethrovesical junction and loss of anatomic support.

5. **Urethral calibration** may be of value in patients with voiding disorders, assessing urethral stenosis. It also provides information in patients with hypoestrogenism
6. **Cystometry** is used to test for the presence of detrusor instability and provides a pressure/volume study of bladder filling. This test may be performed in the office using a simple set-up consisting of a foley catheter, IV tubing, a central venous pressure manometer, and IV fluid. Bladder pressure is measured every 25 to 50 cc during filling and bladder capacity is assessed. Moderately priced cystometry systems are also available, allowing a more accurate and continuous measure of detrusor pressure. The most accurate means of cystometry uses multichannel urodynamic testing, allowing

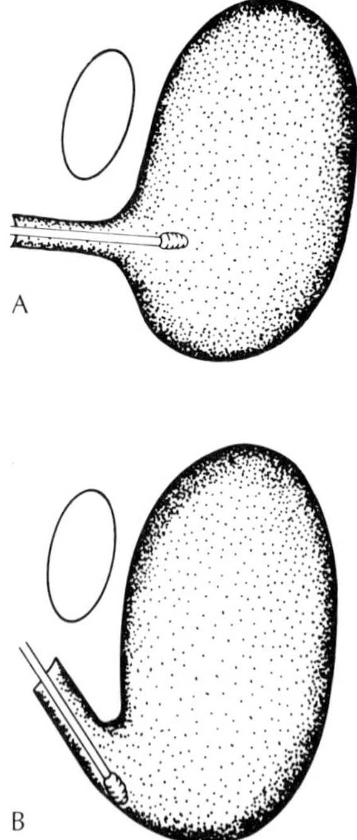


FIGURE 10.2. The Q-tip test. (A) Vesical neck position at rest. (B) Maximal angle changes from the horizontal with straining.

separation of true detrusor pressure from intra-abdominal pressure.

7. **Demonstration of urine loss.** To establish a diagnosis of incontinence, urine loss must be objectively demonstrated. Several tests may be used, including cystometry as noted above.
   a. **Cough stress test.** This is performed in the standing position with the patient having a full bladder. One leg is elevated on a stool and the patient is asked to cough vigorously while the urethra is observed for leakage.
   b. **1-hour pad test.** This test is performed by placing a preweighed pad into the patient's underwear and then having her perform a standard routine of exercises. After one hour, the pad is reweighed to determine leakage.
   c. Although each of these two tests is an excellent means for objectively demonstrating urine loss, neither test can always differentiate various types of incontinence. However, when combined with cystometry, accurate assessment can be made.
8. **Urethrocystoscopy** allows evaluation of the integrity and condition of the urethra, ureteral orifices, and bladder mucosa. The urethra can be assessed for evidence of chronic urethritis, mucosal atrophy, stenosis, and diverticulae. Dynamic evaluation for the vesical neck can be performed, visualizing opening of the urethrovesical junction during stress maneuvers, as might be seen in patients with stress incontinence. Although this technique is helpful in assessment of mobility and closure, it is highly subjective and subject to artifact because of the presence of the rigid tube within the urethra, and should not be considered a definitive procedure for the evaluation of vesical neck closure.

## III. Lower urinary tract conditions.

**III. Lower urinary tract conditions.** Below is a thorough, concise, list of the more common lower urinary tract conditions seen in the female patient. These conditions are rarely seen in their pure form, but more commonly present a diagnostic challenge to the clinician who must systematically differentiate several potential diagnoses using a careful history, thorough physical examination, and appropriate laboratory tests.

### A. Types of urinary incontinence

1. **Stress urinary incontinence**
   a. **Definition.** As defined by the International Continence Society, stress incontinence is a symptom, a sign, and a condition. The **symptom** indicates the patient's statement of involuntary urine loss with physical exertion. The **sign** denotes the observation of urine loss from the urethra immediately upon increasing intra-abdominal pressure. The **condition** is the socially unacceptable involuntary loss of urine that occurs when intravesical

pressure exceeds the maximum urethral pressure in the absence of detrusor activity.

Stress incontinence is usually caused by poor anatomic support of the proximal urethra. A few patients have stress incontinence with normal support because the intrinsic ability of the vesical neck to remain closed has been lost. In patients with stress incontinence, despite normal support, the usual treatments for stress incontinence secondary to hypermobility fail. Therefore a distinction between these two causes is essential. A procedure that increases closure pressure and creates some degree of obstruction should be used. The discussion here will be limited to stress incontinence related to poor support.

b. **Incidence.** Stress urinary incontinence is a common complaint in multiparous patients. Most normal women have occasional episodes of stress incontinence. Probably fewer than 5% of women will have symptoms severe enough to complain to a physician. This problem does, however, represent between one-third to one-half of female patients with urinary incontinence.

c. **History.** The history of stress urinary incontinence is fairly distinctive. A sudden increase in intra-abdominal pressure (e.g., laughing, sneezing, coughing, lifting) results in a simultaneous spurting of urine from the urethra. Although the actual amount of urine lost may be small, the condition may be so socially debilitating that a person must wear a perineal pad constantly or may actually confine herself to the house because of the fear of public embarrassment.

d. **Physical examination.** To make the diagnosis of stress incontinence, a physician must observe urinary leakage simultaneous with a cough and the patient must confirm that this is the type of urinary loss which is a problem for her. This examination should be elicited in the standing position with a symptomatically full bladder (e.g., cough stress test). The physical findings associated with stress urinary incontinence may vary markedly. Stress urinary incontinence may be present when minimal anatomic changes are noted. Extremely large cystoceles are rarely associated with stress incontinence. This is due to a kinking effect created in the urethra. On the other hand, a patient with a small or nonexistent cystocele may have marked urethral mobility with Valsalva and, as a result, have notable stress urinary incontinence. Uterine prolapse and generalized pelvic relaxation are common findings in patients with stress urinary incontinence, but it is unclear whether there is a direct causal relationship.

e. **Urodynamic assessment and findings**

(1) **Cystometric evaluation** shows the patient with stress urinary incontinence to have a normal residual urine volume of < 25 to 50 mL, and a bladder capacity that is within normal limits as well (350–500 mL). If uninhibited detrusor contractions are present, this may be the cause of the patient's incontinence. The frequent coexistence of stress incontinence along with uninhibited contractions is important to consider in establishing a diagnosis.

(2) **Urethrocystoscopy** may sometimes be a helpful diagnostic measure in the evaluation of a patient with stress urinary incontinence. In a patient with uncomplicated stress urinary incontinence, normal bladder mucosa and trigone are routinely encountered. The flaring of the vesical neck with Valsalva, or forceful coughing, can sometimes be seen, but artificial changes due to movement of the urethra over urethroscope can occur. In the patient with stress urinary incontinence, voluntary control of the urethra closure is usually intact. This may be visualized directly with the urethroscope, using either water or carbon dioxide as a study medium.

(3) **The Q-tip test** assesses urethral mobility but does not diagnose stress incontinence. Between 80% and 90% of women with genuine stress incontinence will demonstrate urethral hypermobility during Q-tip testing. However, 35% to 50% of continent women will also demonstrate hypermobility. Thus, this test is sensitive but not specific in the diagnosis of urinary incontinence. Urethral hypermobility in the patient with stress incontinence may represent a good prognostic sign with reference to cure when using standard incontinence surgery. The absence of urethral hypermobility should suggest reassessment of treatment options by the clinician.

(4) **Multichannel urodynamic testing** is one of the most accurate means to diagnose stress incontinence and allows differentiation from other causes of urine loss. By using microtransducer pressure catheters to measure intra-abdominal, urethral, and bladder pressures, computer subtraction allows the measurement of pressure created solely by the urethral musculature (urethral closure pressure) and detrusor muscle (true detrusor pressure). The following diagnostic studies are commonly performed during multichannel testing.

**Table 10.1. Drug Therapy for Urinary Incontinence**

| GENERIC DRUG (TRADE) | ACTION OR USE | SIDE EFFECTS | DOSE |
|---|---|---|---|
| DRUGS FOR UNINHIBITED DETRUSOR CONTRACTIONS | | | |
| Oxybutynin (Ditropan) | Anti-cholinergic (detrusor relaxation and antispasmotic) | Atropine-like | 5 mg p.o. t.i.d. |
| Imipramine (Tofranif) | Anti-cholinergic (detrusor relaxation)<br>Alpha-adrenergic stimulation (urethral tone increase) | Same as oxybutynin | 50–150 mg q.d.<br>25–75 mg q.d. (the elderly) |
| Dicyclomine (Bentyl) | Anti-cholinergic | Same as oxybutynin | 10–20 mg p.o. t.i.d. |
| DRUGS FOR GENUINE STRESS INCONTINENCE | | | |
| Phenylpropanolamine | Alpha-adrenergic | Somnolence<br>Hypertension | 75–150 mg q.d. |
| Ephedrine | Alpha-adrenergic | Same as phenylpropanolamine | 15–60 mg q.d. |
| Imipramine | Alpha-adrenergic<br>Anticholinergic | Same as oxybutynin | 50–150 mg q.d. |

(a) **The stress urethral pressure profile** is a measurement of urethral closure pressure throughout the urethra performed while the patient coughs repeatedly. Continent patients will maintain positive urethral closure pressure during coughs. Patients with stress incontinence typically demonstrate pressure equalization (the urethral closure pressure falls to zero or below). This is due to incomplete pressure transmission to the urethra. A relatively higher pressure is transmitted to the bladder, thus overcoming the ability of the urethra to maintain continence.

(b) **Cystometry** may be performed with great accuracy. The use of multiple channels allows the subtraction of abdominal pressure from bladder pressure, thus reflecting only the detrusor pressure and the possible presence of uninhibited detrusor contractions.

(5) **Pelvic ultrasound and flouroscopy,** with or without the assistance of bead chain or pressure catheter insertion, have also been shown to delineate the mobility of the proximal urethra that is so prominent in patients with pure stress urinary incontinence. Flouroscopics are also useful in depicting the amount of vesical neck distention, or funneling, that is often associated with significant urethral dysfunction and an open vesical neck. These tests are recommended especially for those cases that present an unusually difficult diagnostic challenge.

f. **Treatment of stress urinary incontinence**

(1) **Medical treatment** of stress urinary incontinence is usually reserved for those patients who are poor operative candidates or who have a mild degree of stress urinary incontinence that does not warrant surgery. Commonly used medications include those that produce sufficient alpha-adrenergic stimulation to increase urethral tone (Table 10.1).

(2) **Surgical treatment.** Eliminating abnormal mobility of the bladder neck and supporting the urethrovesical junction are the desired effects of surgical correction for stress urinary incontinence. A multitude of procedures have been used, with varying degrees of success. Vaginal approaches were first used in an effect to create an elevating shelf of tissue beneath the proximal urethra. These have been replaced by abdominal or abdominal-vaginal procedures, except in instances of significant pro-

lapse associated with only minimal incontinence. In such cases, a vaginal approach is optimal to manage both prolapse and incontinence. Abdominal procedures all attempt to elevate the urethra by upward fixation of periurethral and perivaginal tissues to either Cooper's ligament, the periosteum of the symphysis pubis, or the abdominal wall. Several of the more common procedures are described below:

(a) **Vaginal approach.** The anterior colporrhaphy, or Kelly plication, was formerly the mainstay of urinary stress incontinence surgery in gynecology. It is often performed in conjunction with a vaginal hysterectomy and/ or posterior colporrhaphy. In this operation, the periurethral-vaginal (fascial) tissues are plicated beneath the urethrovesical junction, elevating this structure to a position near the pubic symphysis. This is not a usual treatment for stress incontinence at present.

(b) **Abdominovaginal approach.** The procedures listed below may be used alone or in conjuction with a vaginal repair.

  (i) In the **Pereyra procedure,** as well as its modifications, the free ends of a suture that have been placed vaginally in the periurethral tissues, are passed through the space of Retzius and tied to the anterior rectus sheath, elevating the vesical neck. These sutures are passed using a long specialized needle, placed through a small suprapubic incision that eliminates the need for a large abdominal incision and a wide dissection of the space of Retzius.

  (ii) The **Stamey procedure** is a modification of the Pereyra procedure that includes endoscopic visualization of the bladder and bladder neck while the needles are being placed. Inclusion of a graft material to buttress sutures against the vaginal fascia is used.

(c) **Abdominal approach.** The procedures listed are useful when genital prolapse, which could warrant a vaginal approach, is not the primary problem, or when abdominal surgery is planned for coexistent considerations.

  (i) Suprapubic or abdominal procedures have been patterned after the **Marshall-Marchetti-Krantz procedure.** In this procedure, the periurethral vaginal tissue is identified through the space of Retzius and sutured directly to the periosteum of the pubic bone. A modification of this, the **Burch procedure,** elevates the vaginal tissue more laterally to the fibers of Cooper's ligament. Lee has described a further modification of the Marshall-Marchetti-Krantz procedure that includes an open-bladder technique to assist in dissection of the bladder neck and suture placement into the pubic symphysis.

(ii) A variety of **sling procedures** have been described, especially for the treatment of stress incontinence associated with an open vesical neck (type III stress incontinence). Fascia lata, rectus fascia, marlex strips, and other synthetic materials have been passed beneath the urethra and transfixed to more anterior, stationary structures to elevate the urethrovesical angle. Future challenges in gynecologic urology include the need to define the most appropriate procedure for individual patient situations.

**2. Uninhibited detrusor contractions (detrusor instability)**

a. **Definition.** Detrusor instability is usually defined as the cystometric presence of uninhibited detrusor contractions measuring 15 cm $H_20$ or greater while the patient inhibits voiding. Many patients can have this problem and yet have a normal cystometrogram because of the infrequency of their unstable contractions. Synonyms for this condition include: uninhibited contractions, irritable bladder, unstable bladder, urgency incontinence, and the outdated term, detrusor dyssynergia.

b. **Incidence.** Uninhibited detrusor contractions can occur in normal individuals when the bladder is greatly distented. When they occur in the presence of normal bladder capacity or when they cause incontinence, they are considered to be abnormal. Among women presenting for care with lower urinary tract symptoms (excluding bladder infections), approximately one-third will have demonstrable uninhibited detrusor contractions.

c. **Etiology and pathogenesis.** In early life, the bladder reflexively contracts when a certain volume of urine is contained within its lumen. When an individual learns to control urination, the detrusor muscle remains relaxed while the bladder fills, prevented from contracting by a constant inhibition from the cerebral cortex. These inhibitory impulses travel in the reticulospinal tracts of the spinal cord to the sacral micturition area. Removal of this inhibition allows the micturition reflex to begin. Uninhibited detrusor contractions occur either because the normal path of cortical suppression is disrupted or because the bladder muscle is so irritable that the normal inhibitory impulses are insufficient to keep the detrusor relaxed as the bladder fills. Normal cortical suppression may be impaired by damage to the cerebral cortex which can result from cerebral atherosclerosis, stroke, or trauma. The transmission of normally generated cortical impulses may be defective if the pontine mesencephalic reticular formation or spinal cord fibers carrying these impulses to the sacral micturition area are damaged. This can happen in conditions such as spinal cord injury and multiple sclerosis.

Damage to the lower motor neurons that run from the sacral micturition area to the detrusor and back abolishes the detrusor reflex and results in flaccid, acontractile bladder, and not in uninhibited detrusor contractions which follow upper motor neuron lesions. If the bladder muscle is irritable, it may contract despite normal inhibitory impulses. This can result from bladder or urethral infection, urethral diverticula, postoperative stricture or scarring of the urethra, foreign bodies (e.g., sutures, calculi), or interstitial cystitis.

It is possible that true stress urinary incontinence may cause uninhibited detrusor contractions. This hypothesis is inferred from the observation that in some patients who have both uninhibited contractions and stress urinary incontinence, the abnormal contractions resolve following successful incontinence surgery.

In the absence of overt neurological disease, uninhibited detrusor contractions are often idiopathic and a specific cause is not always found (although it should always be sought diligently).

d. **History.** When an uninhibited detrusor contraction occurs, it may give the patient a sense of urinary urgency or, if strong enough, may cause incontinence. One or both of these two problems may bring the patient to a physician for evaluation. Frequency, urgency, and urinary incontinence can all be caused by these contractions. Uninhibited detrusor contractions are either spontaneous or result from some provocative stimulus. Those that are provoked may result from the sound of running water, the touch of warm fluids, or may be set off by something physically stimulating to the bladder. Some patients may have uninhibited detrusor contractions in response to a cough or a sneeze. These patients may complain of urinary incontinence in response to these stimuli, thereby sounding like true anatomic stress incontinence. Cystometric demonstration that coughing elicits a detrusor contraction several seconds after the stimulus avoids the misdiagnosis of these patients as having stress urinary incontinence.

e. **Physical examination.** Unlike stress urinary incontinence, which is due to anatomic changes and in which physical examination plays an important diagnostic role, uninhibited contractions are a functional derangement and are not always associated with a specific anatomic change. Physical examination should be directed toward identifying the cause of the contractions. A careful neurologic examination is mandatory as are expression of the urethra looking for pus or urine from a diverticulum, and a search for findings of anatomic stress incontinence.

f. **Laboratory evaluations.** The diagnosis of uninhibited detrusor contractions may be confirmed by a detrusor contraction during bladder filling in the presence of the patient's attempt to inhibit urination. Laboratory investigation is therefore aimed at studying the detrusor activity and discovering the cause of uninhibited contractions.

   (1) **Cystometry** involves filling the bladder with fluid or gas while monitoring the pressure within the cavity. If the detrusor muscle contracts while the bladder is being filled, the pressure will usually rise by more than 15 cm $H_20$. This may occur spontaneously or be elicited by a provocative stimulus such as coughing or jarring the bladder. Because intra-abdominal pressure is transmitted to the bladder, a single channel measurement of bladder pressure represents the sum of intra-abdominal pressure and detrusor pressure. Measuring the pressure high in the rectum or vagina (that reflects intra-abdominal pressure) allows the differentiation of pressure increases caused by detrusor contraction from those caused by elevations in the intra-abdominal pressure. This is referred to as **multichannel cystometry.**

   (2) Other laboratory evaluation should include:
      (a) Search for bladder or urethral infection.
      (b) Determination of residual urine.
      (c) **Urethrocystoscopy** to look for visible lesions of the lower urinary tract.

g. **Treatment**

   (1) **Treatment of the underlying cause** of the uninhibited detrusor contractions should be initiated when

one is known. Infection should be treated with antibiotics (see Table 10.2), diverticula by excision or marsupialization, and urethral strictures and scarring by dilation.

(2) Pharmacologic relaxation of the detrusor muscle has proven to be effective treatment in the absence of a specific causative factor or as an adjunct to other therapy. Because the detrusor muscle is stimulated primarily by cholinergic nerves, anticholinergic medications have been the mainstay of therapy (Table 10.1). These medications all cause the usual side effects of atropine, but tolerance to these effects usually develops over time.

(3) **Bladder retraining drills** can be used to increase the patient's ability to suppress uninhibited detrusor contractions. This involves having the patient urinate on a predetermined schedule. The interval between voidings is short in the beginning, and lengthened progressively to teach the patient to suppress detrusor contractions for longer and longer periods of time. Beginning at 30 minute intervals, this can eventually be worked up to 3 to 4 hours between trips to the bathroom.

(4) **Biofeedback** techniques have also been helpful in treatment of uninhibited detrusor contraction.

3. **Other causes of urinary incontinence**

a. **Overflow incontinence** may be found in patients with a neurogenic or acontractile bladder. This can result from

**Table 10.2. Common Antimicrobial Medications Used for Lower Urinary Tract Infection**

| GENERIC DRUG (TRADE) | INDICATION | SIDE EFFECTS | DOSE |
|---|---|---|---|
| Nitrofurantoin (Macrodantin) | Cystitis | Gastrointestinal, dermatologic symptoms | 50 mg p.o. q.i.d. × 10–14 days |
| Trimethoprim-sulfamethoxazole | Cystitis | Gastrointestinal, dermatologic symptoms | 1 tablet p.o. 12 h |
| Ampicillin | Cystitis | Gastrointestinal, dermatologic symptoms | 500 mg p.o. q.i.d. × 10–14 days |
| Erythromycin | Urethritis | Gastrointestinal, dermatologic symptoms | 500 mg p.o. q.i.d. × 10–14 days |
| Tetracycline | Urethritis | Gastrointestinal, dermatologic symptoms | 500 mg p.o. q.i.d. × 10–14 days |

diabetes mellitus, extensive pelvic surgery (e.g., radical hysterectomy), or pelvic radiation therapy.

b. **Uninhibited urethral relaxation** can cause urinary incontinence in the absence of Valsalva or detrusor contraction.

c. **Extraurethral incontinence**
   (1) Ectopic ureter
   (2) Urogenital fistula (e.g., vesico-vaginal, urethrovaginal)

**B. Sensory urgency**

1. **Definition.** The sudden urge to urinate in the absence of a full bladder is called urgency. When this occurs in association with an uninhibited detrusor contraction, it is referred to as motor urgency. When it is not, it is termed sensory urgency.
2. **Incidence.** This problem acounts for approximately one-third of the patients seen with urinary complaints by gynecologists specializing in urologic investigations. If the urgency associated with acute UTI is included, sensory urgency becomes the single most common urologic symptom encountered by the gynecologist.
3. **Etiology and pathogenesis.** Sensory urgency is a symptom of irritation of the lower urinary tract, especially the urethra. Infection of the bladder or urethra, trauma to the urethra, hypoestrogenism, urethral syndrome secondary to chronic urethritis, interstitial cystitis, carcinoma in situ, strictures, functional spasm, chemical irritation, or allergy can all lead to sensory urgency. In addition, there are a number of patients who seem to have this symptom in the absence of any demonstrable lesion or irritant, and are felt to have it on an idiopathic basis. The possibility of organic disease should always be ruled out in these patients before the diagnosis is made. When there is no identifiable pathology, this problem is considered to be a condition in itself and not just a symptom of another disease process. It is commonly referred to as urethral syndrome.
4. **History.** The usual history is one of frequent, sudden urges to urinate. Often minimal amounts of urine are passed. Dyspareunia can be associated with this symptom. It is important to determine whether urinary tract infections have occurred in the past and whether the patient has had surgery on the bladder or urethra. Particular attention should be paid to patients who have hematuria, postvoid dribbling, or pyuria.
5. **Physical examination.** The urethra should be examined carefully to identify any evidence of infection as manifested by erythema of the meatus, tenderness to palpation, or the presence of pus with urethral expression. Evidence of vaginal infection or atrophy should be sought.

6. **Laboratory evaluation**
   a. **Urine culture and urinalysis** are mandatory.
   b. **Urethral culture** is indicated if urine culture and urinalysis are negative, and if the urethra manifests tenderness. Specifically, cultures should be obtained for chlamydia and gonorrhea.
   c. **Urethroscopy** is valuable as a tool to inspect the mucosa of the urethra directly and to evaluate its canal for diverticula, erythema, exudate, and strictures. Evidence of chronic urethritis in the absence of bacterial infection can lead to a diagnosis of urethral syndrome.
   d. **Cystoscopy** is an essential part of the evaluation when other tests fail to reveal an etiology and should be performed to evaluate the bladder for infection, interstitial cystitis, or neoplastic changes.
   e. **Urine cytology** should be performed in patients without an identifiable cause to rule out carcinoma in situ of the bladder.
7. **Treatment**
   a. **Antimicrobial therapy.** The treatment for urgency when it is a manifestation of UTI is antimicrobial therapy (see Table 10.2).
      (1) **Infection of the urethra** should be treated with erythromycin or tetracycline for 2 weeks in recognition of the role of chlamydia in infections of the urethra.
      (2) **Bladder infection** should be managed with medications that cover coliform bacteria, which typically cause these infections. Ampicillin or nitrofurantoin would be the first choice for outpatient therapy.
   b. **Urethral dilation and massage** has been used for the treatment of chronic urethritis, in the absence of bacterial infection. Performed every 2 weeks for two to three sessions, dilation is thought to provide improvement through expulsion of inflammatory exudate from periurethral glands, stretching submucosal fibrosis, relieving smooth muscle spasm, and correcting meatal stenosis. The treatment remains controversial, with little scientific data to support its efficiency.
   c. **Supportive counseling, psychotherapy and desensitization therapy** may prove useful if no pathology can be found. Sensory urgency may have a psychosomatic basis related to previous traumatic experiences such as sexual abuse or incest. These possibilities should be kept in mind and should be sympathetically explored.
   d. **Bladder retraining** (see pp. 158)

C. **Urethral diverticula**
   1. **Definition.** Diverticula of the urethra are saccular outpouchings of the urethral canal that are usually formed by cystic

dilation of one of the periurethral glands found in the submucosa of the urethra on its vaginal side.

2. **Incidence.** Diverticula of the female urethra are present in 4% to 5% of women and may cause symptoms of urethral irritation and postvoid dribbling. In certain cases, they may also be responsible for recurrent urinary tract infection. Although diverticula are demonstrable in a relatively large number of women as noted above, the fact that they cause clinical problems in less than 1% of the female population implies that many are asymptomatic and need no treatment.
3. **Etiology and pathogenesis.** Diverticula usually begin within the submucosa for the posterior urethral wall where a series of periurethral glands open into the mid and distal urethra. All of the periurethral glands are subject to infection with a number of organisms (e.g., gonorrhea, chlamydia, and others). These infections sometime lead to abscess formation or stricture of the gland orifice. Following the resolution of the infection, when the duct of the gland is blocked, a cyst forms, and when communication with the urethral lumen persists, a diverticulum results. Although it is usual to find a single diverticulum in a given patient, multiple diverticula are common and should be sought.
4. **History.** The symptoms of a diverticulum are related to its ability to cause irritation of the urethra and to discharge its contents into the urethral canal. Irritation may lead to dysuria and dyspareunia as well as frequency and urgency. When the contents of the diverticulum discharge into the distal urethra, it is noted by the patient as a dribbling of urine or purulent material after normal micturition has ended (postmicturition dribbling). Because stagnant urine retained in the diverticular sac favors the multiplication of bacteria, when this material is extruded into the urethra, it may reflux into the bladder and lead to treatable, but recurrent, cystitis.
5. **Physical examination.** Upon physical examination, a large diverticulum may be visible as a suburethral bulge seen within the vagina. They are confined to the posterolateral aspects of the urethra in the distribution of the periurethral glands and are most common in the middle third of the urethra. When urine or purulent material can be expressed from the bulge during physical examination, with subsequent disappearance of the bulge, the diagnosis is evident.
6. **Laboratory evaluation.** To confirm the clinical diagnosis, or to look for diverticula when classic physical findings are not demonstrable, a number of investigative techniques have been proven useful. Most depend on pressure which must be established in the urethra to open the lumen of the diverticulum and force fluid into it.
   a. **Urethroscopy,** with occlusion of the internal urethral

meatus (compressing it with a finger), can be used to visualize the orifice of the diverticulum.

b. **Positive pressure urethrography** performed by instilling contrast into the urethra with a special catheter (which occludes both proximal and distal urethra) is useful in forcing contrast into these lesions, thereby making them visible on radiographic images. Catheter types include the Tratner catheter and the Davis catheter.

c. **Urethral pressure profile.** A static urethral pressure profile, with a microtransducer pressure catheter, may reveal a depression in the profile curve, representing the position of the diverticular orifice.

d. Another technique that does not involve a special catheter involve placing contrast material in the bladder and having a patient begin to urinate with her finger over the external urinary meatus, thereby forcing the contrast into the diverticulum under pressure.

7. **Treatment.** Asymptomatic urethral diverticula require no treatment. When symptomatic, the treatment of urethral diverticula is usually surgical, although long-term antibiotic therapy and urethral dilatations may be helpful in some smaller lesions. If the diverticulum is acutely infected at the time of presentation, cultures should be taken and antibiotics used to treat the acute infection before surgical therapy is undertaken.

   a. **Excision of the diverticulum** can be accomplished transvaginally through a longitudinal incision over the mass. This may be easier if a small catheter is inserted into the diverticulum transurethrally before the procedure to make it easier to identify the sac during the operation. Careful dissection of the entire sac, with its excision at the neck, followed by repair of the urethra, suburethral tissues, and vaginal mucosa using fine suture, will give satisfactory results in most situations. Urethrovaginal fistula formation may occur, however, following this repair.

   b. **Marsupialization of the wall of the urethra and diverticulum to the anterior vaginal wall (Spence procedure)** is an alternative approach that requires less meticulous dissection. This technique is most suitable for diverticula in the distal one-third of the urethra because creating a permanent communication in this area, between urethra and vagina, is less likely to cause incontinence than it is in the upper two-thirds of the urethra. This procedure avoids the possibility of stricture or fistula formation which can occur after excision. It may lead to "spraying" during urination in a number of women, and occasionally to urinary incontinence, even when performed in the distal urethra.

## BIBLIOGRAPHY

Bates P, Bradley WE, Glen E. The standardization of terminology of the lower urinary tract. J Urol. 1979; 121:551.

Buchsbaum HG, Schmidt JR. eds. Gynecologic and Obstetric Urology. Philadelphia, Pa: WB Saunders; 1978.

DeLancey JOL. Structural aspects of the extrinsic continence mechanism. Obstet Gynecol. 1988; 72:296.

Karram MM, Bhatia N. The Q-tip Test: Standardization of the technique and its interpretation in women with urinary incontinence. Obstet Gynecol. 1988; 71:807.

Ostergard DR. Gynecologic Urology and Urodynamics. Baltimore Md, Williams and Wilkins; 1985.

Slate WG. ed. Disorders of the Female Urethra and Urinary Incontinence. Baltimore Md; Williams and Wilkins; 1982.

Staton SL. ed. Clinical Gynecologic Urology. St Louis, Mo: CV Mosby; 1984.

# CHAPTER 11

# Abortion

**Stephen R. Carr**
**Thomas G. Stovall**
**Charles R. B. Beckmann**

Abortion is the loss or termination of pregnancy before 20 weeks gestation calculated from the date of onset of the last menses. An alternative definition is delivery of a fetus with a weight of less than 500 g. The Committee on Terminology of the American College of Obstetricians and Gynecologists has proposed defining abortion as "expulsion or extraction of all or part of the placenta or membranes, without an identifiable fetus, or with a liveborn infant or a stillborn infant weighing less than 500 g. In the absence of known weight, an estimated length of gestation of less than 20 completed weeks (139 days) calculated from the first day of the last normal menstrual period may be used."

I. **Classification of abortion.** It is useful clinically to classify abortion by the gestational age at the time of abortion, by the cause of or indication for abortion, and by the clinical presentation.
   A. **Gestational age** is usually calculated from the first day of the last normal menstrual period.
      1. **First trimester abortion.** Conception to 12 completed weeks; often subdivided into early (conception to 6 weeks) and late (7 to 12 weeks).
      2. **Second trimester abortion.** Thirteen to 20 weeks of gestation.
   B. **Indication or cause**
      1. **Spontaneous abortion.** Abortion that begins without human intervention, a miscarriage in lay terms.
      2. **Elective (induced) abortion.** Abortion initiated by human intervention at maternal request.
      3. **Therapeutic (induced) abortion.** The guidelines of the American College of Obstetricians and Gynecologists for therapeutic abortion define the criteria for a therapeutic abortion as follows:
         a. When continuation of the pregnancy may threaten the life of the woman or seriously impair her health. In deter-

mining whether or not there is such risk to health, account should be taken of the woman's total environment, actual, or reasonably foreseeable.

b. When pregnancy has resulted from rape or incest. In this case the same medical criteria should be used in the evaluation of the patient.

c. When continuation of the pregnancy is likely to result in the birth of a child with grave physical deformities or mental retardation.

4. **Criminal abortion.** Termination initiated by human intervention outside an approved health-care facility.

C. **Clinical presentation** (Table 11.1)

1. **Threatened abortion.** Any vaginal bleeding, with or without pain, in a pregnancy before the 20th completed week of gestation where clinical judgement suggests that the pregnancy may continue. No cervical dilation or effacement is present.

2. **Inevitable abortion.** Uterine bleeding from a gestation of less than 20 weeks accompanied by cervical dilation but without expulsion of placental or fetal tissue through the cervix.

3. **Incomplete abortion.** Expulsion of some but not all of the products of conception before the 20th completed week of gestation.

4. **Complete abortion.** Spontaneous expulsion of all fetal and placental tissue from the uterine cavity before 20 weeks' gestation.

5. **Missed abortion.** The traditional definition is fetal death in utero before the 20th completed week of gestation but is retained in utero for 8 or more weeks. With the advent and widespread use of ultrasound, this term is not descriptive of early pregnancy loss. A new classification system has been proposed.

a. Anembryonic gestation (empty sac)—no fetus is present at a gestational age ≥ 7.5 weeks.

b. First trimester fetal death—death of the fetus in the first 12 weeks of gestation.

c. Second trimester fetal death—death of the fetus between 13 and 24 weeks gestational age.

6. **Septic abortion.** Abortion complicated by maternal infection of the genital tract (e.g., endomyometritis).

7. **Recurrent spontaneous abortion.** The loss of three or more pregnancies before 20 weeks gestation.

## II. Morbidity and mortality

### A. Morbidity

1. **Maternal morbidity.** The risk of morbidity in all abortions is decreased by medical attention at an early gestational age by competent experienced staff in an approved facility. Present data suggest an incidence of abdominal surgical procedures

**Table 11.1. Diagnosis and Treatment of Abortions**

| DIAGNOSIS | THREATENED ABORTION | INEVITABLE ABORTION | INCOMPLETE ABORTION | MISSED ABORTION |
|---|---|---|---|---|
| Symptoms | | | | |
| Crampy, bilateral lower quadrant pain | +/− | ++ | +++ | +/− |
| Symptoms of pregnancy | + | + | +/− | Usually |
| Amenorrhea | + | + | + | + |
| Vaginal bleeding | Spotting | Heavy | Heavy with clots | +/− and/or tissue |
| Physical exam | | | | |
| Cervix open | Usually not | Usually | Yes | +/− |
| Blood from cervix | Yes (min.) | Yes | Yes | +/− |
| Tissue from os | No | No | Yes | +/− |
| Uterus soft | Yes | Yes | +/− | +/− |
| Uterus tender | Often | Yes | Yes | Usually not |
| Abdomen tender | +/− | Usually | Usually | Usually not |

| | | | | |
|---|---|---|---|---|
| Laboratory tests | | | | |
| Urinary pregnancy test | +/− | +/− | +/− | Usually negative, often positive previously |
| β-hCG (RIA) | + | + | + | +/− |
| Ultrasound | Gestational sac if 6 weeks or more | Gestational sac if 6 weeks or more; +/− fetal movement; +/− halo sign | Unnecessary unless ectopic gestation or uterine anomally suspected | Disorganized cystic or collapsed intrauterine sac; +/− fetus or placenta |
| Treatment | Observation of patient, bed rest, treatment of infection, counseling, and support | Evacuation of uterine contents, counseling, and support | Evacuation of uterine contents, counseling, and support | Evacuation of uterine contents, counseling, and support |

hCG = human chorionic gonadotropin; RIA = radioimmunoassay.
From Beckmann RB, Thomason, JL, Abortion: Spontaneous and induced abortion in the first and second trimester. In: Ellis JW, Beckmann RB, eds. A Clinical Manual of Gynecology. East Norwalk, Conn: Appleton-Century-Crofts; 1983: 258-259. Courtesy of Berkeley Bio-Engineering, Inc., Langhorne, PA. Reprinted with permission.

coincident to abortion of about 3.9/1000 cases, including all causes, both related and unrelated to the abortion itself.

2. **Effects on future pregnancies.** Possible adverse effects on future pregnancies after elective abortion include midtrimester spontaneous abortion, preterm delivery, infertility, and low birth weight infants. Controversy exists over these associations and their interpretation.

B. **Mortality.** The risk of mortality from elective abortion is about 0.6 to 1.0 per 100 000 up to 8 weeks of gestation, doubling for each additional 2 weeks of gestation thereafter, as compared to the current maternal mortality of 8 to 10 per 100 000 live births. Thus, abortion and maternal mortality rates are probably equal at about 14 to 16 weeks of completed gestational age, with the value for abortion exceeding that for continued pregnancy thereafter. Dilation with suction and curettage carries the lowest risk, followed by intra-amniotic injection of (prostaglandin) $PGF_2\ \alpha$ or intravaginal $PGE_2$, and then hysterotomy/hysterectomy. Both the procedures and the gestational age of the pregnancy determine the individual risk.

## FIRST TRIMESTER ABORTION

I. **Prevalence.** About 15% to 20% of known pregnancies terminate in spontaneous abortion. Using more sensitive pregnancy tests (e.g., radioimmunoassay for the beta subunit of human chorionic gonadotropin), it is clear that pregnancy and spontaneous loss (often subclinical) occur far more frequently (40%). Thus, the true spontaneous abortion rate may be two or three times that previously suggested. About 80% of spontaneous abortions occur in the first trimester, with the incidence decreasing with increasing gestational age. If the woman has had one prior abortion, the rate of spontaneous abortion in a subsequent pregnancy is about 20%. If she has experienced three consecutive losses, her chance of having a subsequent loss is nearly 50%.

In addition, in the United States as many as one-quarter to one-third of all pregnancies are terminated electively.

II. **Etiology.** In early gestation, in utero demise usually precedes abortion, whereas later in pregnancy this may not be the case. A specific etiology for a pregnancy loss is often never ascertained; however, phenomena associated with spontaneous pregnancy loss include:

A. Pathologic ("blighted") ovum–anembryonic gestation.

B. Embryonic anomalies.

C. Chromosomal anomalies–50% to 60% of first trimester spontaneous abortions are chromosomally abnormal; the majority are numerical abnormalities.

D. Increased maternal age.

E. Incompatible intrauterine environment, for example, uterine anomalies such as septate uterus and bicornuate uterus, incompetent cervical os, and myomas.

F. Intrauterine device in place at the time of conception.
G. Teratogens and mutagens.
H. Severe maternal disease.
I. Maternal smoking.
J. Placental anomalies.
K. Maternal laparotomy—especially if performed before 16 to 20 weeks of gestational age.
L. Maternal trauma—often implicated, but unless it is extensive, maternal trauma probably plays a small part in the etiology of abortion.

III. **Threatened abortion** is common in the first trimester, occurring in an estimated 30% to 40% of pregnancies (Table 11.1).

A. **Symptoms**

1. **Vaginal bleeding** associated with threatened abortion is usually limited to light spotting. Other causes or such bleeding must be considered before the diagnosis is made, including cervical polyps, severe vaginal infection (especially trichomonas vaginitis), cervical cancer, gestational trophoblastic disease, ectopic pregnancy, trauma of the vagina or cervix, or irritation by a foreign body.
2. **Pain.** Crampy lower quadrant pain may or may not be present in patients with threatened abortion. The prognosis for carrying the pregnancy is worse when pain accompanies the bleeding.
3. In many cases it is impossible to distinguish between threatened abortion, completed abortion, and ectopic pregnancy. Thus, other diagnostic methods must be used.

B. **Physical examination**

1. The abdomen is usually not tender and the cervix is closed, although blood will be identified coming from the os.
2. No signs of labor (effacement or dilation), loss of tissue or fluid through the cervical os.
3. Cervical motion tenderness or adnexal tenderness on bimanual examination is usually not present.
4. After about 7 weeks gestation, the uterus feels soft on bimanual examination.

C. **Laboratory evaluation**

1. **Pregnancy test**
   a. A **urinary pregnancy test for human chorionic gonadotropin,** (hCG) is almost always positive especially if the pregnancy test being used has a sensitivity to 50 mIU/mL hCG. If the pregnancy test is negative an alternative diagnosis should be sought.
   b. **Serum assay for β-hCG by radioimmunoassay** is positive.
2. **Ultrasonography.** An intrauterine pregnancy will be routinely discovered on transabdominal ultrasound at 6 to 7 weeks gestational age or when the β-hCG is greater than

6500 mIU/mL. The gestational sac should have smooth contours. Transvaginal scanning has allowed the visualization of a gestational sac at an hCG titer of 1500 to 2000 mIU/mL. A fetal pole with demonstrable fetal heart action should be seen after 7 weeks gestation or if the gestational sac volume is calculated to be > 2.5 mL. A snowstorm pattern on ultrasound is characteristic of gestational trophoblastic disease.

3. **Evaluation of vaginal infection.** Vaginal examination for evidence of vaginal infection (culture for gonorrhea, saline, and potassium hydroxide [KOH] preparations) and a Papanicolaou (PAP) smear should be performed.
4. **Urinalysis and urine culture.** A clean voided urine specimen should be obtained for urinalysis. A urine culture and sensitivity should be obtained if indicated by urinalysis.
5. **Serum progesterone** can help differentiate a viable intrauterine pregnancy from a nonviable pregnancy (ectopic, completed abortion, intrauterine fetal demise). If the serum progesterone is < 5.0 ng/mL, the patient can undergo endometrial curettage without fear of interrupting a viable pregnancy. If the serum progesterone from a reliable laboratory facility is ≥ 25 ng/mL, the likelihood of an ectopic pregnancy is only 1.0% to 2.5%. Those patients with a progesterone level between 5.0 and 25 ng/mL should be further evaluated with serial hCG titers and ultrasound.
6. **Serial quantitative hCG titers.** A minimum increase of 29% and 66% should be seen in patients with a viable intrauterine pregnancy at 24 and 48 hours, respectively. (Note: Variation in hCG assay may be as high as 15% between titers.) Patients with a subnormal rise, plateaued, or falling level can safely undergo uterine evacuation without fear of interrupting a viable pregnancy. If chorionic villi are not recovered at the time of curettage, further evaluation for a possible ectopic pregnancy is warranted. This evaluation must be individualized and may include repeat hCG, ultrasound, and/or diagnostic laparoscopy.

D. **Treatment.** There is debate about the effectiveness of any measures in the treatment of threatened abortion, the argument being that these patients will eventually abort or not abort regardless of treatment. Nevertheless, therapy as indicated is appropriate.

1. **Bed rest or significant restriction in activity** is generally accepted as the most common and useful therapy. Hospitalization is rarely indicated, but may be if rest cannot be assured in the home.
2. **Counseling and reassurance** are important parts of the therapy for threatened abortion. The clinician should take the time to talk with the patient, fully explaining the situation, and answering all questions.

3. **Treatment of infection.** Any maternal infection that is discovered should be treated with appropriate therapy.
4. **Progesterone.** Supplementation with progesterone is ineffective in treating threatened abortion and may be teratogenic; it should not be used.
5. **Sedation.** In general, sedation should be avoided in favor of counseling and reassurance.

## IV. Inevitable abortion (Table 11.1)

A. **Symptoms.** The clinical signs of inevitable abortion are the same as those for threatened abortion, except that there is a judgement by the clinician that the bleeding is "so excessive" that the pregnancy is not salvageable. It is judgement based on clinical experience without definable diagnostic parameters.

B. **Physical examination**
1. The abdomen is sometimes tender.
2. The cervix may be effaced and dilated with blood but not tissue, coming from the cervical os.
3. Cervical tenderness on bimanual examination will usually be present.
4. After about 7 weeks gestation, the uterus will feel soft on bimanual examination.

C. **Laboratory evaluation** for inevitable abortion is the same as for threatened abortion, with the addition of maternal blood type and Rh determination.

D. **Treatment**
1. **Dilation, suction, and curettage.** Once the clinical judgement has been made that the pregnancy is nonviable, evacuation of the uterine contents is indicated, by dilation (if needed), suction, and curettage.
2. If the patient is Rh negative, $Rh_0$ (D) immune globulin (RhoGAM) should be given.

## V. Incomplete abortion.

**Incomplete abortion.** With incomplete abortion the loss of the gestation has begun and must be completed with medical assistance. All patients with incomplete abortion need surgical evacuation of the uterus to assure that there are no retained products of conception that may cause infection and/or hemorrhage (Table 11.1).

A. **Symptoms**
1. **Vaginal bleeding.** Vaginal bleeding, with the passage of blood and tissue and/or amniotic fluid is noted.
2. **Pelvic pain.** Central or slightly bilateral lower-quadrant pain, often described as labor-like, is noted. A sensation of fullness or pressure, with a desire to "bear down" as the process progresses may be described. Unilateral pain should alert the clinician to the possibility of ectopic gestation.

**B. Physical examination**

1. **Cervix.** The cervix is dilated and effaced and is usually tender on palpation. Blood is coming from the os, often with clots as well as products of conception, which may be found either in the vaginal canal or protruding from the os. The conceptus and placenta are often expelled simultaneously before the 10th week and separately thereafter. Myometrial contraction, which normally constricts the placental vascular bed and facilitates hemostasis may be impeded by retained tissues, especially placental tissue. The resulting hemorrhage may be profound. Therefore, appropriate precautions should be taken for such an eventuality, including the placement of a large bore intravenous catheter to allow rapid infusion of fluids and/or blood as required. Immediate removal of large pieces of protruding tissue at initial examination (by traction with a ring forceps) may reduce the bleeding significantly. The patient with tissue in the cervical os may also experience a vasovagal like bradycardia that responds promptly to removal of tissue from the cervix.
2. **Uterus.** The uterus may be more firm and smaller than expected for the stated gestational age because of loss of part of the products of conception. The uterus may also be tender upon palpation.

**C. Laboratory evaluation**

1. Pregnancy test, as for patients with threatened abortion.
2. Ultrasonography if there is clinical suspicion of ectopic gestation or uterine anomaly.
3. Maternal blood type and Rh.
4. Complete blood count (CBC).

**D. Treatment**

1. Dilation, suction, and curettage. Surgical evacuation of the remaining products of conception by dilation, suction, and curettage is required (see dilation, suction, and curettage, section X, for an outline of the procedure). This may be done on an inpatient or outpatient basis, depending on facilities. More advanced pregnancies, and those in which there is excessive hemorrhage (especially with anemia or hypovolemia) require hospitalization for transfusion and monitoring of maternal status. All tissues should be sent for pathologic examination, to identify the gestation and to screen for trophoblastic changes. Gross fetal or placental identification is often difficult due to maceration of the tissues by evacuation procedures or delay from the time of in utero demise.
2. **Observation (the completed abortion).** In some cases, all of the products of conception have been spontaneously expelled from the uterus. The patient may or may not be aware that the products of conception were passed. Physical examination reveals a relatively small, firm uterus with

a closed cervix and minimal bleeding. These findings are similar to the patient with an unruptured ectopic pregnancy. Ultrasound will show minimal or no intrauterine tissue or findings consistent with a small intrauterine blood clot. Serial measurements of the quantitative β-hCG will show a steady fall. Serum progesterone in the patient usually falls to < 1.0 ng/mL within 24 to 48 hours. With appropriate counseling, these patients may be followed at home without surgery. They should be instructed to call if they develop fever or chills, excessive pain, or copious vaginal bleeding.

3. **Antibiotic therapy**
   a. **Therapy for the febrile patient.** If the patient is febrile, broad-spectrum antibiotic therapy should be started, before the dilation and curettage (D & C) procedure if possible, but after appropriate cultures (aerobic and anaerobic) are taken. Appropriate antibiotic regimens are those used for the treatment of pelvic inflammatory disease (see Chapter 19).
   b. **Prophylactic therapy** with tetracycline (250 mg p.o. b.i.d. for 7 days, or doxycycline 100 mg p.o. b.i.d. for 7 days) is controversial but recommended by the authors. In many facilities, prophylactic tetracycline is given at the time of elective first trimester termination. The goal is to reduce the incidence of postabortal endometritis and pelvic inflammatory disease and their possible deleterious effects on fertility. We also recommend the use of methylergonovine acetate 0.2 mg every 4 hours for 24 hours to decrease the incidence of uterine atony.
4. **Counseling and reassurance** are of the utmost importance. It should be emphasized to the patient that most spontaneous first trimester abortions are nonrecurring. This is a key part of complete therapy.
5. **Rh isoimmunization prophylaxis.** If the patient is Rh negative, Rho (D) immune globulin (RhoGAM) should be given.
6. **Hysterotomy** may rarely be indicated in failed suction and curretage, but not as a routine method for abortion.
7. **Hysterectomy** may be indicated if there is concomitant uterine or other disease (e.g., uterine leiomyomata or chronic pelvic inflammatory disease with adhesions and chronic pain) that, of itself, would warrant hysterectomy. It is not an appropriate primary method of abortion, and is the rare case that requires hysterectomy.

VI. **Missed abortion/intrauterine fetal demise.** The concepts surrounding missed abortion have become somewhat obsolete with the almost routine use of ultrasound, and thus the newer classification.

A. **Symptoms.** Initially the patient may demonstrate the subjective symptoms of pregnancy followed by an episode diagnosed as threatened abortion. Thereafter, amenorrhea may persist, but the subjective signs of pregnancy may wane. Some patients have minimal vaginal spotting. Some patients may have no symptoms and/or persist in "feeling" pregnant.

B. **Physical examination.** Failure of the fetus to grow in accordance with length of amenorrhea and often regression in uterine size as the process of absorption of amniotic fluid and fetal maceration continue are consistent findings on serial antepartum examinations. Rarely, vaginal bleeding is noted.

C. **Laboratory evaluation.** A serial decline in the β-hCG titer and/or ultrasound examination showing intrauterine fetal demise and progressive disorganization of the intrauterine contents is diagnostic. Care must be taken not to miss the snowflake-like ultrasonographic pattern consistent with hydatidiform changes.

D. **Treatment.** An intrauterine fetal demise may be reabsorbed completely with resumption of menstrual cycles or it may proceed to an incomplete abortion. The treatment of intrauterine fetal demise (observation or surgical evacuation of the uterus) depends on which clinical path ensues as well as the wishes of the patient.

   1. **Observation.** With a diagnosis of intrauterine fetal demise in the first trimester, the patient may be followed as long as there is no evidence of infection or incomplete abortion on pelvic examination. The intrauterine fetal demise may be allowed to reabsorb without intervention.
   2. **Surgical evacuation of the uterus.** If clinical evidence suggests infection or incomplete abortion, or if the patient wishes surgical evacuation of the products of conception that remain in her uterus, a dilation, suction, and curettage may be performed. Generally, the patient wishes to evacuate the uterus as soon as possible.
   3. **RhoGAM.** If the patient is Rh negative, RhoGAM should be administered.
   4. **Counseling.** As with incomplete abortion, counseling is of the utmost importance for the psychological well-being of the patient.

VII. **Recurrent spontaneous abortion.** Although by definition, recurrent abortion does not occur until after three losses, many physicians begin work-up of the patient after two pregnancy losses. With recurrent loss, the emotional trauma is increased, and thus the counseling and diagnostic process must be outlined in detail for the patient. If the patient has a second trimester loss, she is more likely to have a uterine etiology for the loss, and the diagnostic evaluation should be begun after one mid-trimester loss.

A. **Etiology.** The etiologies for recurrent pregnancy loss are similar to those for a spontaneous abortion that is not recurrent. Karyotypic evaluation of the couple is abnormal in about 2% to 3% of fathers and 6% to 7% of mothers. Other possible etiologies include medical illness, immunologic factors, and structural abnormalities of the genital tract.

B. **Evaluation.** Diagnostic evaluation in this group of patients should include history and physical examination, evaluation for cervical incompetence, a CBC, thyrotropin assay, luteal phase endometrial biopsy, hysterosalpingogram, and karyotype. Other tests as indicated might include human leukocyte antigen typing and lupus anticoagulant antibody. No specific etiology for the recurrent loss is found in 35% to 45% of couples evaluated.

## VIII. Elective first trimester abortion.

Elective first trimester abortion follows the same treatment described for incomplete abortion. Simultaneous sterilization by tubal ligation may be performed without increased risk beyond that associated with the sterilization procedure itself.

## IX. Criminal abortion

A. **History.** The diagnosis of criminal abortion is entertained based on an index of suspicion raised by discrepancies in the patient's coherence and believability, her emotional status, the time and circumstances of her presentation for care, as well as her appearance and that of those who accompany her. For example, the woman who arrives at 3:00 AM complaining of the onset of bleeding while exercising, yet is calm and fully dressed with make-up, raises suspicion of criminal abortion.

(**Note:** Whether to report a suspected criminal abortion depends on the philosophy of the individual physician, the rules of the health-care facility, and the local and state legal statutes governing criminal abortion.)

B. **Physical and laboratory examination** is the same as for incomplete abortion, with the following additions:

1. Careful examination for trauma of any kind.
2. Gonorrhea, aerobic and anaerobic cultures, and a Gram stain should be taken from the endocervix.
3. Supine anterior–posterior and lateral and standing anterior–posterior radiographs of the abdomen and pelvis should be made to search for foreign objects or bowel perforation with a gas bubble under the diaphragm.

C. **Treatment**

1. **Dilation, suction, and curettage.** Removal of the remaining products of conception as in incomplete abortion is indicated.
2. **Broad-spectrum antibiotic therapy** should be begun as for pelvic inflammatory disease (see Chapter 19).
3. **Consultation** with a gynecologist and additional radiologic, and, if necessary, surgical evaluation of any suspected trauma.

4. **RhoGAM.** If the patient is Rh negative, RhoGAM should be administered.
5. **Tetanus toxoid.**

## X. Dilation, suction, and curettage.

**X. Dilation, suction, and curettage.** D & C is used in the first trimester in both induced and spontaneous abortions. In either case, morbidity caused by uterine perforation, cervical laceration, hemorrhage, and incomplete abortion increases after the 12th week of completed gestation. Suction, instead of sharp curettage, reduces the complication rate, lowers operative blood loss, and shortens operative time. The need for extensive sharp curettage (with the possibility of denuding the decidua basalis and causing hemorrhage or Asherman's syndrome) is lessened. There is little advantage, however, to a blunt rather than sharp curette, because it is the surgical technique rather than the instrument that causes most problems. An outline of the procedure follows, although the procedure should not be undertaken without appropriate supervised surgical training.

A. **Patient presentation/preoperative presentation.** A routine preoperative history, physical examination, and laboratory evaluation should precede the procedure.
   1. The patient's bladder should be empty, with catheterization if necessary to ensure that the bladder is empty.
   2. Perineal shaving is unnecessary, as no decrease in infectious or surgical morbidity in shaved patients has been demonstrated.

B. **Procedure**
   1. An anesthetic technique appropriate to the patient should be selected. If general or regional anesthesia is chosen, it is administered at the start of the procedure. If local anesthesia is chosen, for example, paracervical block, it is administered at the appropriate time in the procedure. Consultation with an anesthesiologist is appropriate.
   2. A careful bimanual examination under anesthesia is performed. A weighted vaginal speculum or a Graves bivalve speculum is placed. The cervix and the vagina are identified and cleaned with an antiseptic solution such as providone-iodine (Betadine®). If the patient is awake, the Graves speculum may be more comfortable and hence preferable.
   3. The anterior lip of the cervix is then grasped with a tenaculum, ring forceps, or Allis clamp and pulled outward gently to lengthen and straighten the endocervical canal and, to some extent, the uterine cavity. Care must be taken not to place the tenaculum too high so as to impinge on the bladder or to pull too hard so as to pull the tenaculum through the cervical tissue, lacerating it. Placing the tenaculum vertically rather than horizontally will decrease the likelihood of pull-through lacerations. A

second tenaculum may be used if significant traction is anticipated.

4. Uterine depth and direction is then carefully ascertained with a uterine sound, first within the endocervical canal, and then part way into the uterine cavity (Fig. 11.1). This helps determine the need for dilation, as well as further estimating the size and direction of the uterine cavity, which will aid in the subsequent instrumentation. Pratt or Hegar dilators are then slowly used as needed to dilate the cervix sufficiently to allow instrumentation and removal of the products of conception (Fig. 11.2). Laceration of the cervix may be avoided by the slow and gentle use of these instruments. There is no rush to complete dilation.
5. Dilation may be difficult, especially in nulliparous patients. This is also true in elective and some missed abortions compared with the treatment of the inevitable or incomplete abortion. The use of laminaria tents may help with difficult dilation, as well as reducing the incidence of cervical trauma or laceration. Made from the stems of a seaweed *(Laminaria japonica),* laminaria are small sterile

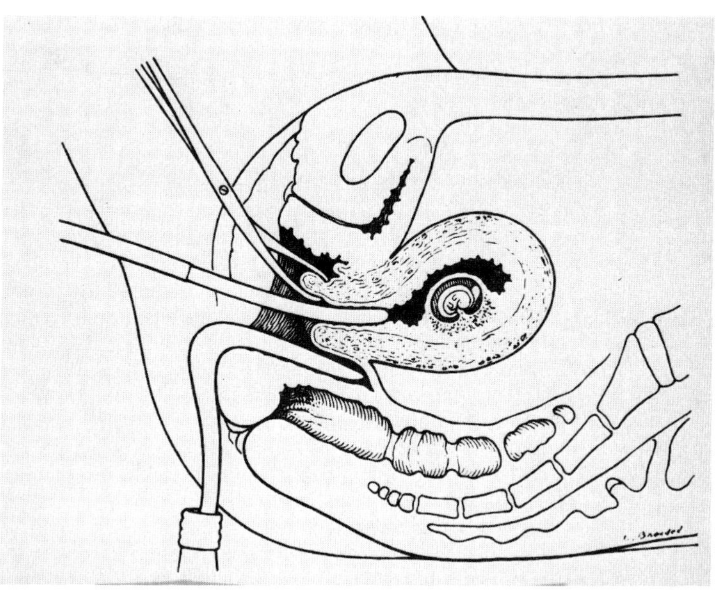

FIGURE 11.1. Sounding of the uterus with weighted vaginal speculum in place and anterior lip of the cervix grasped with a tenaculum. From Quilligan EJ, Zuspan F. Douglas-Stromme Operative Obstetrics. 4th ed. New York: Appleton; 1982:184. Reprinted with permission.

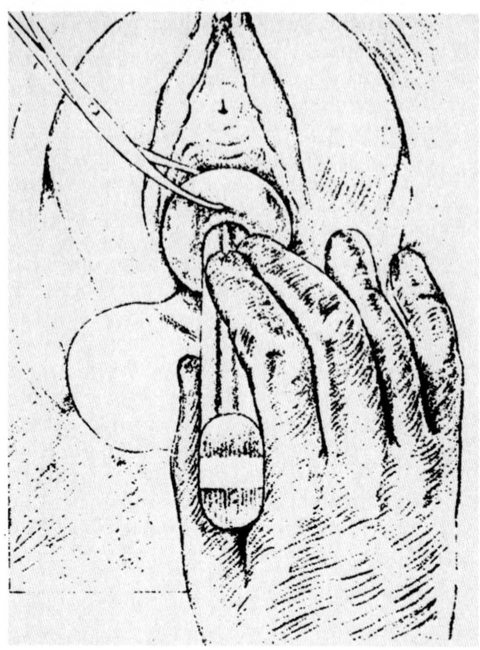

FIGURE 11.2. Dilation of the cervix. From Quilligan EJ, Zuspan F. Douglas-Stromme Operative Obstetrics. 4th ed. New York: Appleton; 1982:185. Reprinted with permission.

"sticks" of material that are carefully placed into the endocervical canal and then beyond so that their tips just pass the internal os but without rupturing the membranes. They come in three sizes, small (3 to 5 mm in diameter), medium (6 to 8 mm), and large (8 to 10 mm). The size that may be tightly fit, but not forced, through the os is chosen. Over the next 8 to 12 hours the hygroscopic "water-seeking" seaweed slowly expands (often three to five times its original diameter) facilitating a slow and minimally traumatic dilation. Often sufficient dilation is left to be done. Concerns about an increased incidence of infection with the use of laminaria has proven unjustified.

6. If a vacuum suction is to be used, it is inserted, without the suction being engaged. Thus suction machine has previously been set up and tested to show that it maintains an appropriate amount of suction (usually 50 to 60 mm Hg).
7. An intravenous infusion of oxytocin is begun "piggyback" into the main intravenous line as the suction procedure is begun (20 to 40 U of oxytocin in 1 L of solution

is usually sufficient). This oxytocin infusion is maintained during the procedure and for 1 hour afterward. Blood loss is thereby significantly reduced and uterine tone increased, the latter decreasing the chances of uterine perforation of the pregnancy-softened uterine wall.

8. Suction is then applied, and the suction tip is gently rotated in the uterine cavity to remove the products of conception (Fig. 11.3). This may need to be done several times to remove all of the tissue. Sufficient repetition is indicated by the absence of retrieval of tissue, a frothy bloody return, and a "rough, scratchy" and/or "gritty" feeling on the tip of the suction catheter against the uterine wall. Rotation rather than "in out" suction minimizes the risk of perforation. Sometimes, tissue pieces too large to pass the cannula are encountered. These are easily removed with an ovum or other forceps, whereupon the suction procedure may be completed. Such pieces should be checked routinely at the end of these procedures. The size of the suction tip chosen will vary with the gestational age, the estimated size of the uterus, and

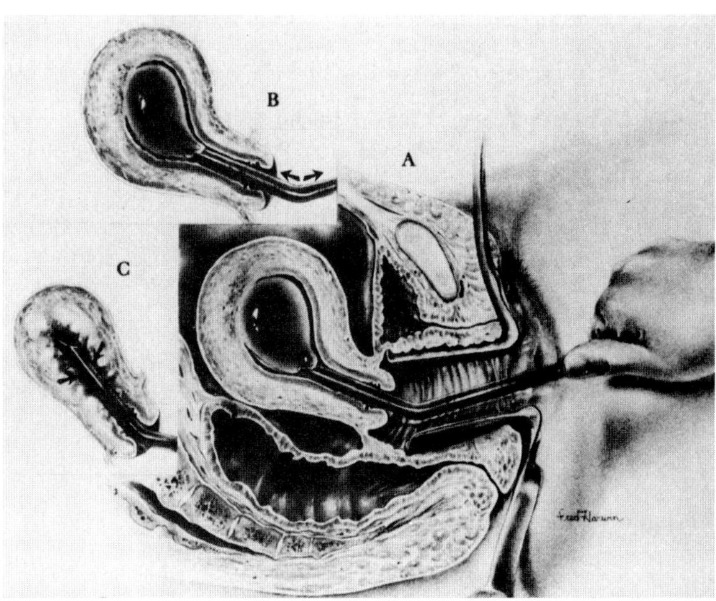


FIGURE 11.3. Suction curettage. (A) Suction tip inserted through cervical canal. (B) Suction applied, with uterine contraction due to the suction process as well as intravenous oxytocin infusion. (C) Empty uterus contracted about the suction tip. From Quilligan EJ, Zuspan F. Douglas-Stromme Operative Obstetrics. 4th ed. New York: Appleton; 1982:186. Reprinted with permission; also courtesy of Berkeley Bio-Engineering, Langhorne, Pa.

the amount of dilation accomplished. Tips vary from 7 to 12 mm in diameter and in general the number of the tip size should correspond to the estimated weeks of gestation.

9. Sharp curettage may be used to check for retained products, or as a primary method of uterine evacuation. In the latter case, blood loss is increased somewhat. In either case, the sharp curette is gently introduced into the uterine cavity and pulled out under mild pressure in smooth, even strokes. Excessive pressure may lead to perforation or denuding of the basalis. To help avoid this, the curette should be held in thumb and forefinger only, so that excessive pressure cannot be exerted.
10. After the products of conception are removed, all implementation is removed, and the sites of the traction or tenaculum insertion on the cervix are checked to ensure that there are no lacerations and that any bleeding is ceasing.

C. **Examination following procedure.** A second careful bimanual examination at the end of the procedure is essential, to help check for completeness of procedure (feel for a firm not boggy uterus), trauma, for example, developing hematoma, and for adnexal abnormality, for example, a combined gestation.

## XI. Complications of abortion

A. **Hemorrhage** is usually associated with retained products of conception and/or uterine atony. Other causes include uterine tumors, uterine perforation, or other trauma and infection.

B. **Incomplete abortion.**

C. **Uterine perforation** is estimated to occur in 0.8 to 1.5/1000 abortions. Physician inexperience and marked anteflexion or retroflexion of the uterus are the most common causes of uterine perforation. When perforation is suspected, prompt cessation of the procedure (if in progress) and evaluation of the possible perforation (site, maternal status) and gestation (abortion not begun, complete, incomplete) is made. Table 11.2 suggests a clinical classification of such perforations and their therapy. The use of diagnostic laparoscopy has reduced the need for laparotomy by more than one half.

D. **Pelvic infection.**

E. **Failure to recognize simultaneous ectopic pregnancy.**

F. **Uterine synechiae (Asherman's syndrome).**

G. **Cervical incompetence.**

H. **Cervical scarring and stenosis.**

I. **Cervical laceration.**

J. **Postabortal syndrome.** Other terms synonymous with postabortal syndrome are postabortal hematometra, postabortal uterine atony, and "redo" syndrome. In this syndrome, although the cervix remains open, blood clots collect within the uterine cavity (sometimes quickly, sometimes after several days) causing a swollen, tender uterus associated with fever and crampy pain. Oxytocics may help by stimulating uterine contractions, but reevacuation of the uterine contents by suction curettage is the treatment of choice. Antibiotics should be administered as if the patient were infected and hospitalization should be considered, especially if the patient has a hematocrit less than 30 or is febrile.

**Table 11.2. Clinical Classification and Treatment of Uterine Perforation During Abortion**

| CLINICAL CLASSIFICATION | TREATMENT |
|---|---|
| A. Immediate recognition with cessation of the procedure (suspected or actual perforation by any instrument including suction cannula with no suction applied). | |
| 1. Complete abortion. Perforation after contents of uterus completely evacuated. | In hospital observation of clinical status, serial CBCs, for at least 48 hours. |
| 2. Intact sac. Gestation undisturbed. | As above then readmit in about 2 weeks for repeat surgical evacuation. |
| 3. Incomplete abortion. Perforation occurs during evacuation; uterus partially emptied. | Immediate diagnostic laparoscopy. Laparotomy and repair if needed. Completion of abortion, either transcervically under laparoscopic observation or, if laparotomy, via uterine rent if transcervical approach inappropriate. |
| B. Delayed recognition after operative manipulation (suction or curettage). No abdominal contents identified.<br>Uterine evacuation may have been attempted before possible perforation was recognized.<br>1. Complete abortion.<br>2. Intact sac.<br>3. Incomplete abortion. | All require immediate diagnostic laparoscopy with laparotomy if indicated (bowel trauma, uncontrolled bleeding, etc.). For B.2 and B.3: Abortion may be completed as in case A.3 above. |
| C. Perforation with identification of abdominal contents (bowel, omentum, fat, etc.).<br>1. Complete abortion.<br>2. Intact sac.<br>3. Incomplete abortion. | All require immediate laparotomy and surgical repair as needed. For C.2 and C.3: Abortion may be completed as in case A.3 above. |

Adapted from Walden W, Birnbaum S. Classifying perforations that occur during abortion. Contemp Obstet Gynecol, Medical Economics Company, 1980; 15:47.

K. **Failed abortion with continuation of pregnancy** is uncommon, estimated to occur at an incidence of 0.07/100 cases (46 cases in a series of 65 045 elective first trimester terminations).

## ABORTION IN THE SECOND TRIMESTER

There are many problems associated with both elective and therapeutic second trimester termination of pregnancy, including medico–legal and psychosocial, as well as purely medical problems. Such procedures are best done in facilities where they are performed routinely by an experienced staff exposed to these procedures on a regular basis. If second trimester termination is considered, documentation of gestational age by ultrasound if necessary is imperative prior to starting the procedure.

I. **Techniques.** There are several techniques for second trimester abortion. The choice depends on gestational age, the medical status of the patient, and the skills of the physician. In many cases it is the latter factor that is appropriately most important.

A. **Dilation and evacuation.** In the United States there are two opinions about transcervical uterine evacuation beyond 12 completed weeks of gestation. One view is that the morbidity and mortality are much decreased with dilation and evacuation as compared to other second trimester techniques until 16 weeks of completed gestational age. The technique is similar to the technique used in first trimester dilation and suction or curettage except that surgical forceps are usually needed to remove fetal parts, especially the calvarium.

B. **Prostaglandin induction.** Prostaglandin administration results in labor and abortion. Two administration methods are commonly used; intra-amniotic injection and placement of vaginal preparations.

1. Intra-amniotic injection of $PGF_2\ \alpha$ is often used for second trimester termination after 16 weeks gestational age. This route of administration for $PGF_2\ \alpha$ is successful in most cases within 48 hours, with a mean time to abortion of 20 to 31 hours. About 10% will abort incompletely and about 2% will fail to abort. About 15% to 20% of patients require a second prostaglandin injection without augmentation with intravenous oxytocin administration. Oxytocin administration, especially after membranes are ruptured, reduces evacuation time significantly. Great care must be taken, however, in the administration of this combination to avoid uterine hyperstimulation, water intoxication, or other metabolic complications. To avoid transient fetal survival, combinations of $PGF_2\ \alpha$ and saline have been used to good effect. However, they do have the disadvantage of exposing the patient to some degree of the risks of hypertonic saline that are not inherent in the use of prostaglandins alone. In the event of the failure, uterine malformation may be the cause, and evaluation for it should be

made so that appropriate therapy may be begun if indicated. Ultrasonography plays a key role in this evaluation.

2. $PGE_2$ vaginal suppositories are especially useful in missed abortions of advanced gestational age and in intrauterine fetal demise in advanced pregnancy. $PGE_2$ is available in 10-mg suppositories, placed every 2 to 4 hours. Augmentation with oxytocin, especially after membrane rupture, is helpful in many cases. If used, careful monitoring of the severity of contractile activity is important.
3. Adverse reactions to prostaglandin use include:
   a. Cervical or vaginal laceration and fistulae formation
   b. Infection
   c. Delayed or incomplete abortion (especially retained placenta)
   d. Uterine rupture
   e. Nausea, emesis, and diarrhea
   f. Hypotension
   g. Tachycardia
   h. Disseminated intravascular coagulation
   i. Exacerbation of asthma, which is a contraindication to the use of prostaglandins for abortion

C. **Laminaria** may be used in conjunction with other methods to speed the cervical dilation process in a manner that is less damaging to the cervix.

D. **Hysterotomy** is occasionally indicated when maternal status prohibits the use of other methods of abortion, but is outdated as a primary method of abortion. Because of the vertical uterine scar made during the procedure, further pregnancies must be delivered by cesarean section. A desire for permanent sterilization is not an indication to use hysterotomy as a primary method of abortion. This procedure has the highest morbidity and mortality rate of all abortion procedures, and should be used only when all other methods have been exhausted.

E. **Hysterectomy**
1. Indications
   a. Uterine or other gynecologic pathology that by itself would have warranted the procedure.
   b. Serious irreparable damage to the uterus.
   c. Hemorrhage control following abortion by another method.
2. **The technique is the same as for cesarean hysterectomy.** In the event that the operation is done for uterine trauma, careful attention to anatomy is imperative, especially the bladder and ureters. The complications are those of hysterectomy, with increased risk of involvement of the bladder and ureters.

F. Maternal blood type and Rh should be determined and Rh immunoglobulin administered if indicated.

G. All tissues retrieved should be sent to the pathology lab for dating and for screening of trophoblastic changes.

## BIBLIOGRAPHY

Akhter A, Flock M, Rubin G. Safety of abortion and tubal sterilization performed separately versus concurrently. Am J Obstet Gynecol. 1985; 152:619.

Cowchock S, Dehoratius R, Wapner R, Jackson LG. Subclinical autoimmune disease and unexplained abortion. Am J Obstet Gynecol. 1984; 150:367.

Hemminki K, Mutannen P, Saloneimi I. Smoking and the occurrence of congenital malformations and spontaneous abortions: Multivariate analysis. Am J Obstet Gynecol. 1983; 145:61.

Hern W. Abortion Practice. Philadelphia, Pa: JB Lippincott; 1984.

Hertz J. Diagnostic procedures in threatened abortions. Obstet Gynecol. 1984; 64:223.

Kaunitz AM, Hughes JM, Grimes DA, Smith JC, Rochat AW, Kafrissen ME. Causes of maternal mortality in the United States. Obstet Gynecol. 1985; 65:605.

Kaunitz AM, Rovira E, Grimes DA, Schulz KF: Abortions that fail. Obstet Gynecol. 1985; 66:533.

Lubbe W, Liggins G. Lupus anticoagulant and pregnancy. Am J Obstet Gynecol. 1985; 152:322.

McDonough P. Repeated first-trimester pregnancy loss. Am J Obstet Gynecol. 1985; 153:1.

Miodovnik M, Lavin JP, Knowles HG, Holroyde J, Stys SJ. Spontaneous abortion among insulin-dependent diabetic women. Am J Obstet Gynecol. 1984; 150:372.

Park T, Flock M, Schulz K, Grimes DA. Preventing febrile complications of suction curettage abortion. Am J Obstet Gynecol. 1985; 152:252.

Peterson WF, Berry FN, Grace MR, Gulbranson CL. Second-trimester abortion by dilatation and evacuation: An analysis of 11,747 cases. Obstet Gynecol. 1983; 62:185.

Sachs ES, Jahoda GJ, VanHemel JO, Hoogeboom AJM, Sandbuyl LA. Chromosome studies of 500 couples with two or more abortions. Obstet Gynecol. 1985; 65:375.

Stovall TG, Ling FW, Cope BJ, Buster JE. Decreasing the incidence of ruptured ectopic pregnancy utilizing serum progesterone. Am J Obstet Gynecol. 1989; 160:1425–1431.

Stray-Pederson B, Stray-Pederson S. Etiologic factors and subsequent reproductive performance in 195 couples with a prior history of habitual abortion. Am J Obstet Gynecol. 1984; 148:140.

Stubblefield PG, Monson RR, Schoebaum SC, Wolfson CE, Cookson DJ, Ryan KJ. Fertility after induced abortion: A prospective follow-up study. Obstet Gynecol. 1984; 63:186.

Verp MS, Rzeszotarski MS, Martin AO, Sipson J. Relationship between Y-chromosome length and first trimester spontaneous abortion. Am J Obstet Gynecol. 1983; 145:433.

# CHAPTER 12

# Ectopic Pregnancy

**Thomas G. Stovall**
**Charles R. B. Beckmann**

An ectopic pregnancy occurs when the blastocyst implants on any tissue other than the endometrium that lines the uterus.

**I. Incidence.** One in every 40 to 100 pregnancies is an ectopic gestation. The incidence has tripled since 1970, but is dependent on the population studied.

**II. Sites of occurrence**

A. **Fallopian tube.** Ninety-seven percent of ectopics occur in the tube (ampullary most common followed by the isthmic and interstitial portions).

B. **Abdominal pregnancy** (1.0%)

1. **Primary.** A primary abdominal pregnancy occurs when fertilization and implantation take place in the peritoneal cavity.
2. **Secondary.** A secondary abdominal pregnancy is more common and occurs when implantation follows tubal abortion or rupture.

C. **Uterine** (1.5%)

1. **Cornual** - ectopics are usually difficult to diagnose. Profuse bleeding may occur if rupture occurs.
2. **Cervical.** Implantation occurs in and around the internal cervical os. Although rare, these patients present with profuse bleeding early in pregnancy.

D. **Ovarian pregnancy** is rare (0.5%).

E. **Heterotopic pregnancy.** One in every 30 000 ectopics is a combined intrauterine and ectopic pregnancy.

**III. Morbidity and mortality**

A. **Morbidity and mortality.** Despite a reduction in mortality for ectopic pregnancy, it remains a major cause of maternal morbidity and mortality, comprising 5% to 6% of all maternal deaths in the United States. It is the leading cause of maternal mortality in the first trimester and the single leading cause of maternal deaths for black women. Because of early diagnosis and better treatment methods, morbidity is also significantly reduced although still substantial.

B. **Subsequent fertility.** Overall, the subsequent pregnancy rate following an ectopic pregnancy is only 60%, with about 40% of these being recurrent ectopics. The chance of a subsequent live birth following surgical treatment of an ectopic pregnancy is approximately 40%.

C. **Recurrent ectopic pregnancy.** The recurrence rate of ectopic pregnancy for patients with a previous tubal ectopic pregnancy is 15% to 20%. This recurrence rate is dependent on the treatment modality, status of the contralateral tube, and other associated infertility factors as well as the underlying etiology of the ectopic itself.

## IV. Etiology. Common etiologies include:

A. **Pelvic inflammatory disease** (PID) is the most common cause of ectopic pregnancy because of tubal mucosal damage. The patient who has had PID is at high risk for ectopic pregnancy, with an estimated incidence as high as one in four pregnancies.

B. **Intrauterine device (IUD).** The concurrent use of an IUD is associated with an increased rate of ectopic pregnancy, in part because of the association of IUD use with pelvic infection. The past use of an IUD is associated with an increased ectopic rate. 9% to 13% of all pregnancies that occur with an IUD in place are extrauterine. Also, an increased incidence of ovarian pregnancy has been observed, such that 12% to 20% of ectopics are ovarian in the presence of an IUD and without an IUD only 0.48% are ovarian. The risk increases with the duration of IUD use. The overall relative risk has been eliminated at two to three times.

C. **Tubal ligation or tubal reconstructive surgery.**

D. **Previous pelvic surgery** including appendectomy, especially if there was appendicial rupture, abscess formation, or postoperative surgical infection is also an associated risk factor.

## V. Pathogenesis

A. Following implantation, the duration of viability for the ectopic pregnancy, the degree of invasion of maternal tissues, and risk to the patient is dependent on implantation site. In cases of ectopic pregnancy of the distal fallopian tube, early rupture and/or tubal abortion are more likely compared to interstitial tubal pregnancy where the potential for growth is greater. Great variation exists, however, as demonstrated by reports of advanced ectopic pregnancies in all possible sites, occasionally progressing to fetal viability. Initially, there is implantation of the fertilized ovum into the tubal mucosa, followed by rapid invasion of trophoblast, with extension from the tubal lumen into the connective tissue between the serosa and endosalpinx. A hematoma in this space grows as the pregnancy advances leading to bleeding from the distal aspect of the tube.

**B. The decidual cast.** The uterine lining proliferates in response to the presence of human chorionic gonadotropin (hCG), undergoing irregular shedding as hCG production wanes in association with demise of the ectopic pregnancy. This causes the irregular, sometimes profuse vaginal bleeding often seen with ectopic pregnancies.

**C. Arias-Stella.** This pathologic endometrial change is not unique to or diagnostic of ectopic pregnancy. As originally described, it consists of hypertrophy, hyperchromatism, pleomorphism, and an increase in mitosis in the secretory cells of the endometrium.

## VI. Differential diagnosis

**A.** Abortion (threatened, incomplete, complete)
**B.** Corpus luteum cyst
**C.** Appendicitis
**D.** PID
**E.** Endometriosis
**F.** Cystic ovarian masses, with or without torsion
**G.** Heterotopic pregnancy

**VII. Natural history.** The natural history of ectopic pregnancy is varied. At one extreme there is acute pain, hemorrhage, shock, and even death. At the other extreme, there may be no symptoms with the implantation undergoing resorption or tubal abortion at an early stage. Spontaneous resolution of tubal pregnancies without symptoms and without surgical intervention has been reported. To date, there are no laboratory tests, clinical signs, symptoms, ultrasound, or laparoscopy characteristics which will predict spontaneous resolution with a high degree of certainty.

**VIII. Diagnosis.** When an ectopic pregnancy is ruptured, an acute abdomen and shock are often encountered. The patient complains of generalized crampy lower quadrant pain, often accompanied by referred pain in the shoulder caused by diaphragmatic irritation by intraperitoneal blood. Other signs and symptoms may be obscured by pain and shock. The abdomen may be rigid, with guarding, rebound, and decreased or absent bowel sounds. This condition requires swift diagnostic confirmation, initial emergency measures, and immediate surgery. One should not, however, be misled by the patient who appears to be in no distress, as there is great variation in the presentation of patients with significant intra-abdominal bleeding. When an ectopic pregnancy is unruptured, diagnosis is based upon careful history with risk factor assessment, physical examination, pregnancy testing, serum progesterone screening, ultrasonography, dilation and curettage, and laparoscopy.

**A. Signs and symptoms**

1. A **classic triad of symptoms** is consistently described for the patient who presents with a ruptured ectopic pregnancy.
   a. **Abdominal and/or pelvic pain** is seen in 90% to 100% of patients with a ruptured ectopic. It is often described as colicky, characteristically unilateral but sometimes bilateral, and sometimes on the opposite side from the ectopic pregnancy, in which case it is usually associated with a symptomatic corpus luteum cyst.
   b. **Amenorrhea** is present in 78% to 85% of patients.
   c. **Vaginal bleeding,** from minimal spotting to bleeding comparable to a menstrual period, occurs in 75% to 85% of patients. Scant bleeding or vaginal spotting is encountered most often.
2. **Other signs and symptoms**
   a. **Subjective symptoms of pregnancy** such as breast tenderness, nausea, and urinary frequency are seen in 50% to 75% of patients.
   b. **Referred shoulder pain,** if present, results from diaphragmatic irritation by hemoperitoneum. The severity of such pain does not correlate with the amount of intra-abdominal bleeding.
   c. Listlessness, syncope, and fainting while straining at bowel movement are less commonly seen.
   d. When an unruptured ectopic pregnancy is present, the patient is most often asymptomatic, or has only minor symptoms that could be attributed to an intrauterine pregnancy.

**B. Physical examination.** When the ectopic pregnancy is ruptured, the physical examination is often limited by time constraints resulting from the need to treat shock and hypovolemia as well as physical limitations caused by the pain and abdominopelvic rigidity of the acute abdomen. Extensive examination is often possible in the patient with an unruptured ectopic pregnancy, but the great variation in findings that are encountered makes diagnosis a considerable challenge.

1. **Vital signs.** A slight elevation in temperature may be found, especially with a hemoperitoneum, but rarely above 101°F (38°C) if uncomplicated by concurrent infection. Blood pressure and pulse rate are usually normal, although a slight tachycardia associated with pain or anxiety is not uncommon. Tachycardia and hypotension are seen with ruptured ectopic pregnancy, although young healthy women have considerable cardiovascular reserve so that blood loss may be quite extensive before any noteworthy changes in heart rate and blood pressure are manifest.

2. **Abdominal examination** often reveals a surgical acute abdomen in the patient with ruptured ectopic pregnancy, characterized by rigidity, rebound, diminished or absent bowel sounds, and occasionally distention. When the ectopic pregnancy is unruptured, the abdomen may be soft with active bowel sounds, or may demonstrate some guarding, tenderness, or rebound in one or both lower quadrants. Only rarely are there decreased bowel sounds or abdominal distention.
3. **Pelvic examination**
   a. **Tenderness.** With ruptured ectopic pregnancies, pelvic examination is typically characterized by pain on cervical motion and tenderness of the uterus and adnexae with palpation.
   b. **Cul-de-sac.** In ruptured ectopics, the cul-de-sac may be distended with blood causing a bulging of the septum into the posterior vaginal fornix.
   c. **Cervix and decidual cast.** The cervix may be normal in appearance, or it may be discolored (bluish) and soft. Some degree of cervical motion tenderness is common. The cervix may also be open, with passage of blood and occasionally tissue, the latter often confused with incomplete abortion. The tissue passed is a decidual cast. It is passed, whole or in fragments, as the viability of the gestation wanes.
   d. **Uterus.** The uterus may be soft, tender, and enlarged, or may seem normal. Deviation of the uterus to one side may indicate the presence of an adnexal mass, but this may represent a large corpus luteum as well as an ectopic gestation. A cornual pregnancy may palpably simulate an enlarged uterus.
   e. **Adnexa and adnexal mass.** A discrete adnexal mass or fullness is found in less than one-half of patients with an ectopic pregnancy so that the absence of an adnexal mass does not rule out ectopic pregnancy. Conversely, a palpable mass may represent a corpus luteum of early pregnancy or other ovarian neoplasm, so that a palpable adnexal mass does not equate with the presence of an ectopic pregnancy.
4. **History and physical examination** with assessment of risk factors is correct in less than 50% of cases. In unruptured ectopics, the majority of correct diagnoses cannot be made without further testing.

**C.** Laboratory examination and diagnostic procedures

1. **A complete blood count** (CBC) to determine the patient's hematologic status as a potential surgical candidate is mandatory.
2. **Blood type** and antibody determination are essential.
3. **Pregnancy testing.** Current urinary pregnancy tests using

monoclonal antibody technology are sensitive (often to 50 mIU/mL β-hCG); if positive, a pregnancy, but not its location, is established; if negative, pregnancy of any location is unlikely. If the physician wishes to use quantitative β-hCG titers in the analysis of the pregnancy, a more sensitive serum pregnancy test should be done. Radioimmunoassay (RIA) for hCG using β-hCG antibodies (RIA for β-hCG) is sensitive, detecting gestation as early as 8 to 10 days postfertilization as the result of a test sensitivity of 0.5 to 10 mIU/mL of serum. Radioimmunoassay for β-hCG is pregnancy specific, as the antibody is raised against the β-subunit of hCG that is dissimilar to the β-subunit of luteinizing hormone. With a negative serum β-hCG ectopic pregnancy can be effectively discounted. Each physician must learn which tests are available in his or her hospital as well as the sensitivities and characteristics of each. Human chorionic gonadotropin, produced by the syncytiotrophoblast, indicates a pregnancy but does not identify location. Because hCG levels may be low in ectopic pregnancy, the more sensitive the test, the higher the frequency of positive results. Human chorionic gonadotropin concentrations plotted individually or in a serial comparative manner against the duration of amenorrhea, has little diagnostic value, as the actual time of ovulation and conception are not known for most patients. Also, 10% of women with normal gestation with have a single hCG level lower than the 90% confidence limits set for a particular gestational age (Fig. 12.1). Combined pregnancy, multiple ectopic pregnancies, or a viable ectopic pregnancy may not fit this pattern and may demonstrate relatively high hCG titers. Rarely, nonpregnancy-associated ectopic production of hCG by carcinoma of the bronchus, stomach, liver, pancreas, and breast, and multiple myeloma and melanoma, may confuse the clinical situation.

4. **Serum progesterone** concentrations in ectopic pregnancy are generally lower than in normal pregnancy controls. Only 2% of ectopics have a progesterone of >25 ng/mL, 80% are <15 ng/mL, and 40% to 45% of patients have a serum progesterone level of <5.0 ng/mL. There have been no viable pregnancies associated with a serum progesterone of <5.0 ng/mL. A serum progesterone should be obtained in all patients at risk for ectopic pregnancy, and in all patients with first trimester bleeding. Patients with a progesterone <5.0 ng/mL can safely undergo dilation and curettage without fear of interrupting a viable intrauterine pregnancy. Serum progesterone has a wide application as a screening test for ectopic pregnancy and appears to be a useful tool to further direct the evaluation in the patient thought to have an ectopic.

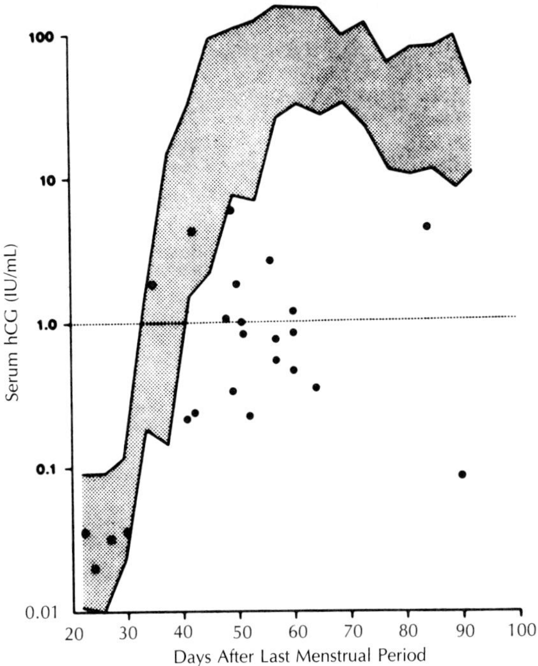


FIGURE 12.1 Serum beta-human chorionic gonadotropin (β-hCG) levels determined by radioimmunoassay (RIA) techniques in 24 women with ectopic pregnancies. The normal pattern on hCG secretion seen during the first trimester of uncomplicated pregnancy is indicated by the hatched area. Each point represents a single sample from a woman with an ectopic pregnancy. The dotted line represents the level of detection of most commercial pregnancy tests. From Rasor JL, Brunstein DG. The rapid modification of the beta-hCG radioimmunoassay: Use as an aid in the diagnosis of ectopic pregnancy. Obstet Gynecol. 1977; 50:557. Copyright 1977 by the American College of Obstetricians and Gynecologists. Reprinted with permission.

5. **Ultrasonography.** In the patient who is not acutely ill with a positive pregnancy test and findings suggestive of ectopic pregnancy, ultrasonography is indicated. At defined hCG titers, ultrasound is excellent for identifying an intrauterine pregnancy because the gestational sac is clearly seen against the homogenous uterine shadow.
   a. **Interpretation of sonograms in ectopic pregnancy**
      (1) **Pregnancy identification.** The prominent ring of echoes against the uniform density of the uterus of an intrauterine pregnancy (Fig. 12.2) is recognized by transabdominal ultrasound at 5 to 6 weeks of gestation measured from the first day of

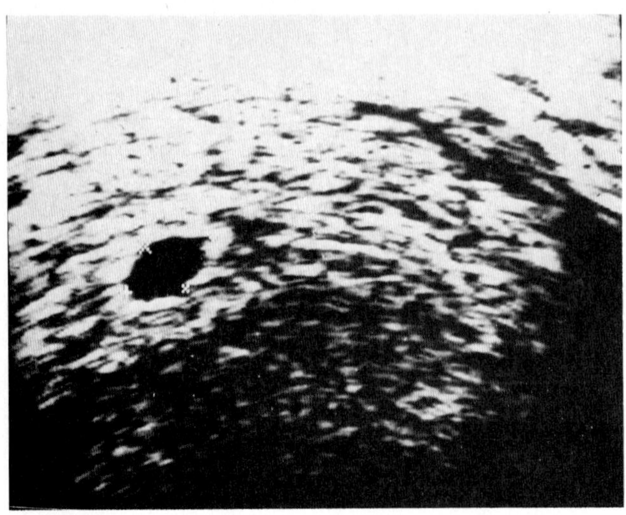

FIGURE 12.2. Sonography of early intrauterine pregnancy.

the last menstrual period, when the chorionic sac is 10 mm in diameter. Fetal heart activity is seen by 7 weeks. Transvaginal ultrasound is able to identify an intrauterine pregnancy 1 to 2 weeks earlier. When an intrauterine pregnancy is demonstrated, extrauterine pregnancy is effectively excluded (except for the rare combined pregnancy). Quantitative values for β-hCG may aid in evaluation of the sonographic images. It has been suggested that a range of 6000 to 6500 mIU/mL of β-hCG may be used as a "discriminatory hCG zone" for transabdominal ultrasound and hCG levels for transvaginal ultrasound are in the range of 1500 to 2000 mIU/mL hCG. The pregnancy may be assumed to be an ectopic if not identified in the intrauterine position. Below these values the sonographic diagnosis of intrauterine pregnancy may not be possible. In this case, serial evaluation or combination testing with other diagnostic modalities may be indicated.

(2) **Blighted ovum.** Care must be taken not to confuse the early normal intrauterine pregnancy with a nonviable blighted ovum, characterized by an intrauterine echo with an irregular internal wall shadow, a volume of less than 2.5 cc, and the absence of a fetal pole.

(3) **Decidual cast.** Blighted ovum, and to a lesser extent early intrauterine pregnancy, may in turn be confused with a decidual cast.

(4) **Other sonographic findings.** With all the sophistication of analysis and technique presently available, it is important to keep in mind the scope of disorders that may confuse the ultrasonographic evaluation of the pelvis for ectopic pregnancy. A differential list of the common ultrasonographic findings is presented in Table 12.1. Rarely, an ectopic pregnancy may be sonographically identified in the adnexae or other extrauterine position thus fulfilling Kobayashi's ultrasound criteria for ectopic pregnancy:

(a) Diffuse, amorphous uterine echoes.
(b) Uterine enlargement.
(c) Absence of intrauterine sac.
(d) An extrauterine irregular mass or poorly defined extrauterine mass, containing some echoes.
(e) At times, an extrauterine ectopic fetus is seen.

(5) **Ultrasonographic procedures.** When using transabdominal scanning, it is important to provide adequate bladder distention. The distended bladder pushes bowel and other structures from the top of the uterus so that their shadows do not confuse the ultrasound picture coming from within the uterus, and in addition provides an anatomic reference point for the many structures found in the pelvis. Such distention may be provided by giving the patient fluids (either oral or intravenous) or by placing a Foley catheter and distending the bladder with sterile saline solution. Care must be taken to neither overdistend or underdistend the bladder. Overdistention is a common error, flattening and deforming the uterus and any structures that may be contained therein. An exception is found in the case of the retroverted uterus, however, in which overdistention may help in resolution of the intrauterine details by straightening the uterus. With transvaginal scanning, bladder distension is neither required nor desirable.

**6. Culdocentesis** may be indicated when the diagnosis of intraperitoneal bleeding is uncertain. Note that hemoperitoneum is not always symptomatic. Culdocentesis is not a test for ectopic pregnancy, but rather for hemoperitoneum. In light of laparoscopy and potential nonsurgical management and since 50% to 60% of patients with unruptured

**Table 12.1. Differential Diagnostic Criteria for the Ultrasound Evaluation of Ectopic Pregnancy**

| ULTRASOUND FINDINGS | DIFFERENTIAL CONSIDERATIONS |
|---|---|
| Uterus | |
| Central linear band | Decidual band<br>Abnormal intrauterine gestation (abortion, blighted ovum)<br>Intrauterine pregnancy less than 5 to 6 weeks |
| Enlargement | Normal variant<br>Myomas<br>Adenomyosis<br>Intrauterine pregnancy |
| Sac | Intrauterine pregnancy greater than 5 to 6 weeks<br>Abnormal intrauterine gestation<br>Intrauterine blood clot<br>Gestational sac in a fallopian tube that has undergone muscular hypertrophy<br>Fluid accumulation with endometritis |
| Adnexa mass | Differential for solid adnexal masses<br>Corpus luteum (± bleeding) |
| Ring, dense shell echo | Tubo-ovarian abscess<br>Appendiceal abscess<br>Diverticulosis<br>Ovarian cyst<br>Bicornuate uterus with intrauterine pregnancy in one horn<br>Endometriosis (endometroma)<br>Hydrosalpinx<br>Gestational sac in hypertrophied fallopian tube<br>Cornual pregnancy<br>Intrauterine pregnancy in fundal leiomyoma<br>Fluid-filled loop of small bowel<br>Pedunculated uterine myoma |
| Fetal pole | Pregnancy, probably abnormal/ectopic<br>Combined pregnancy |
| Pelvis | |
| Cul-de-sac echo | Blood (ruptured ectopic, tubal abortion, ruptured cyst, ruptured leiomyosarcoma, bleeding ulcer, etc.)<br>Ascites<br>Ovarian cyst |

From Hallatt JG. Ectopic pregnancy associated with the intrauterine device. A study of several cases. Am J Obstet Gynecol. 1976; 125:755. Reprinted with permission from Mosby-Year Book Inc.

ectopics have a small amount of blood in the cul-de-sacs, the role of culdocentesis has been lessened. Please see Chapter 34; the section on culdocentesis expands fully on the procedure.

7. **Dilation and curettage (D&C).** Examination of endometrial tissue is indicated in the presence of an intrauterine fetal demise (progesterone <5.0 ng/mL and/or abnormal rise or plateau or fall in hCG titer). Such tissue examination has not been useful in the diagnosis of ectopic pregnancy if the Arias-Stella reaction is formed because it is absent in about one-half to three-fourths of patients and, like the decidual reaction, may be associated with other disorders. The absence of chorionic villi, however, is highly suggestive of either ectopic pregnancy, or completed abortion and further investigation, involving laparoscopy, laparotomy, or other diagnostic testing, may be indicated. In some circumstances, intrauterine pregnancy may be possible in a patient whose clinical presentation suggests ectopic pregnancy: The possibility of a viable intrauterine pregnancy in light of the available evidence should be discussed with the patient, and D&C avoided when possibility of intrauterine pregnancy is strong.
8. **Diagnostic laparoscopy**
   a. **Indications.** Diagnostic laparoscopy is the standard by which other diagnostic methods are measured and should be used for:
      (1) **Uncertain diagnosis.**
      (2) **Hemodynamic stability.** When the patient is hemodynamically stable and without significant hemoperitoneum, diagnostic laparoscopy allows direct evaluation of the pelvis. This procedure allows a timely, early diagnosis of unruptured ectopic pregnancy. When an unruptured ectopic gestation is discovered, conservative treatments are more likely to be feasible.
   b. **Contraindications**
      (1) Unstable patient.
      (2) Abdominal hernia or repair is a relative contraindication to laparoscopy.
      (3) Evidence of ileus.
9. **Combination testing.** Because no single noninvasive modality can diagnose an ectopic pregnancy in all situations, algorithms combining several of the above-mentioned diagnostic modalities are useful (Fig. 12.3).

## IX. Surgical treatment

In most areas, laparotomy is performed routinely, and is the preferred method for treating this ectopic pregnancy. This requires hospitalization for 3 to 5 days, with loss of 3 to 6 weeks of occupational

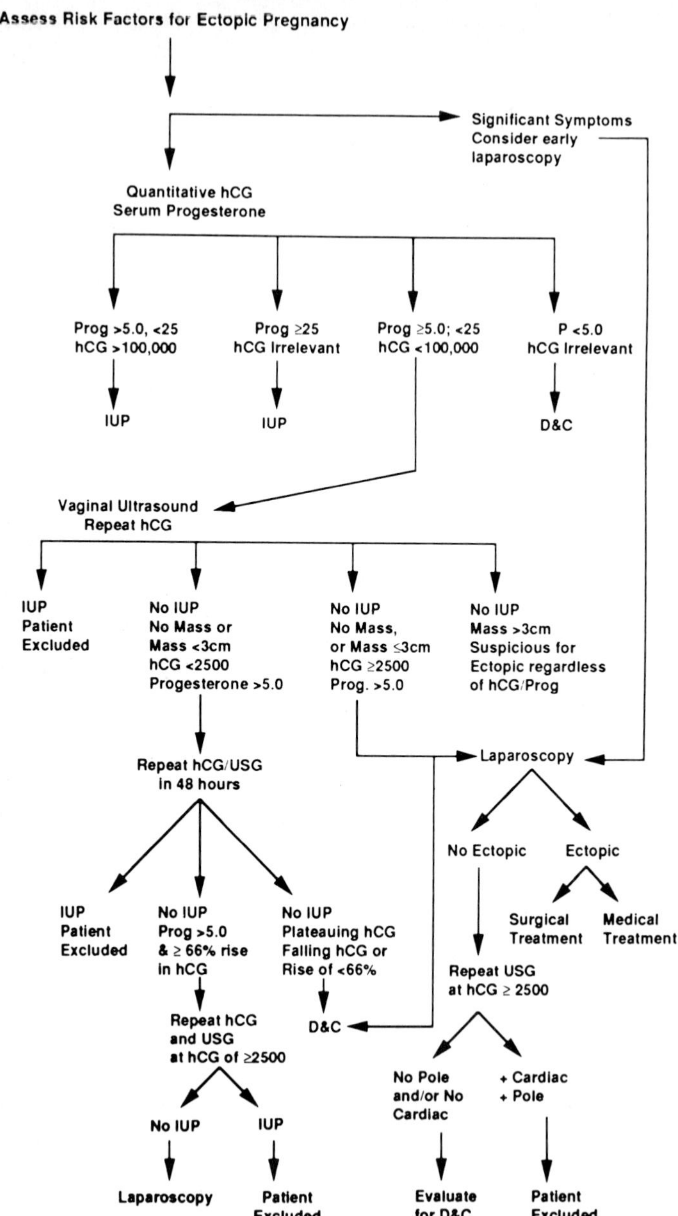


FIGURE 12.3. Diagnostic algorithm for suspected abnormal pregnancy. IUP = intrauterine pregnancy; hCG = human chorionic gonadotropin; D&C = dilation and curettage; USG = ultrasonogram; Prog = progesterone.

productivity. Laparoscopic removal has greatly decreased the trauma of surgery and shortened hospital stay, but must be performed by a skilled operative laparoscopist. Most procedures traditionally done as a laparotomy case now may be done as a laparoscopic procedure.

A. **Surgical considerations.** Once the diagnosis of ectopic pregnancy is entertained, the surgical decisions depend on:
   1. **Surgeon.** As a rule, only a surgeon cognizant of techniques to minimize damage to the reproductive tract should undertake the surgical care of ectopic pregnancy.
   2. **Clinical status of the patient.** Two general rules apply:
      a. The primary objective is the arrest or prevention hemorrhage.
      b. When a patient presents in shock, the minimal surgery necessary should be chosen to reduce the operative risk in an already hemodynamically unstable patient.
   3. **Future fertility.** The patient's desire for potential further reproductive capability is paramount. Any procedure that could render the patient sterile should be avoided.
   4. **Timing of surgery.** Immediate therapy is indicated once the decision has been made to treat the ectopic pregnancy surgically.
   5. **Laparoscopic surgery.** Laparoscopic management has been prospectively compared to laparotomy management. Both methods appear to be equal with respect to future reproductive outcomes. Laparoscopic treatment requires a greater degree of surgical skills, but decreases costs, decreases hospital stay, and avoids the risk of laparotomy. Laparotomy is generally indicated if:
      a. The patient is hemodynamically unstable.
      b. The skills of the surgeon favor laparotomy.
      c. The patient has a contraindication to laparoscopy.
      d. The ectopic is cornual or abdominal.
   6. **General principles of surgical management**
      a. Minimize adhesion formation by:
         (1) Minimize handling of tissue.
         (2) Use of gentle irrigation with heparinized Ringer's lactate (5000 U/L).
         (3) Intra-abdominal installation of dextran solution. The usual amount placed in the abdomen is 50 to 100 cc.
         (4) Meticulous hemostasis. Methods include ligation of small bleeders with fine, nonreactive suture (polyglactin or nylon), bipolar electrocautery damage, and the injection of small amounts of dilute pitressin solution into the bleeding tissue.

(5) Washing of all talc from gloves before surgery to prevent talc granuloma.

(6) Use of minimally reactive suture materials (polyglactin or nylon) to decrease the likelihood of adhesion formation.

b. Various perioptive medications (steroids, antihistamines, antibiotics) have been suggested, singly or in combinations. No regimen has been of proven value. Antibiotic therapy is indicated if there is evidence of active infection. Commonly used regimens include cefoxitin, 2 g intravenous piggyback q6 h or pipericillin, 2 g intravenous piggyback q8 h for 48 hours. Doxycycline (100 mg p.o. b.i.d.) has also been recommended because of the association of ectopic pregnancy with chlamydia infection.

7. **Management of the contralateral fallopian tube.** Although the contralateral fallopian tube often appears normal on gross inspection, as many as one-half have significant microscopic abnormalities. Careful inspection of the tube is important (with discussion of findings in the operative note) but microsurgical intervention is not advisable at initial surgery.

8. **Choice of ablative or nonablative surgical management.** Ablative surgery (salpingectomy, salpingo-oophorectomy, hysterectomy) may be necessary if irreparable damage has been done to the reproductive structures. When possible, however, conservative surgical procedures (salpingostomy, partial salpingectomy) should be performed, especially when the patient desires to maintain her maximal reproductive capability. In general, the initial surgery should be restricted to removal of the ectopic pregnancy and preservation of as much of the reproductive tract as possible. Reconstructive surgery should be done at a second operation after tissue edema and hyperemia have resolved and a complete reproductive evaluation of the patient has been completed.

9. **Specific surgical management.** The choice of surgical procedure depends on the specific implantation site of the ectopic pregnancy, the amount of anatomic damage done by the ectopic pregnancy (whether ruptured or unruptured), and the patient's desire for future fertility. In each case the operating surgeon must weigh these factors to decide upon the appropriate surgical approach.

a. **Ablative surgery**

(1) **Ipsilateral salpingectomy** is the most commonly performed procedure, primarily because it is rapid, simple, and efficient. The procedure is indicated if the fallopian tube is damaged beyond repair or if the extra time needed for a

nonablative procedure is not justified based on the patient's desires for future fertility. When a salpingectomy is performed, care must be taken to preserve the vascular supply of the ipsilateral ovary.

(2) **Oophorectomy** is indicated only if the ovary is damaged beyond salvage, or if the ovary contains pathology for which oophorectomy is indicated. Ipsilateral oophorectomy was formerly common management. This is thought to reduce recurrent ectopics caused by ovum transmigration and associated delay in ovum pickup. There is no evidence to support this concept. Thus, all viable ovarian tissue should be retained.

(3) **Hysterectomy** may be indicated if there is extensive damage to the reproductive tract or, if there is concomitant disease of the uterus which under other circumstances would warrant hysterectomy. Hysterectomy as a routine matter is not indicated even if both fallopian tubes are damaged because in vitro fertilization and other techniques are available for the couple who desires pregnancy. (**Note:** Cornual resection has been advocated in the past to decrease the incidence of repeat ectopic pregnancy, especially the isthmic type. However, no data support its effectiveness, and it may actually lead to an increased incidence of interstitial ectopic pregnancy and uterine rupture. In addition, intrauterine pregnancy following cornual resection may have to be delivered by cesarean section because of the risk of uterine rupture at the site of the cornual resection.)

b. **Nonablative surgery**

(1) **Linear salpingostomy (with and without closure)** is performed if possible on the antimesenteric border of the tube to minimize disruption of the fallopian tubes blood supply. Whether to close the incision is controversial and a decision left to the surgeon.

(2) **Segmental resection and subsequent midtube reanastomosis** is used in isthmic tubal pregnancy when linear salpingostomy is not feasible because of the extent of damage to the fallopian tube. Whether to proceed with anastomosis at the first operation is an individualized surgical decision. It does provide a nidus for infection. To remove this tissue a D & C is a wise precau-

tion, provided preservation of a possible viable intrauterine pregnancy is not desired by the patient.

10. **Rh immunoglobulin (RhoGAM) therapy** should be administered to all Rh negative, unsensitized women within 72 hours of surgery for ectopic pregnancy.

## X. Nonsurgical (medical) management

As a result of the generally poor reproductive outcome, costs, risk, and morbidity of surgical treatment, nonsurgical treatment methods are now being used in some medical centers.

### A. Methotrexate (MTX)

1. **Treatment approach.** One possible treatment protocol (Table 12.2) summarizes the use of MTX. Contraindication to MTX treatment includes:
   a. Ectopic pregnancy rupture
   b. Cardiac activity in the ectopic
   c. Size >3.5 cm

**Table 12.2. Methotrexate Treatment Protocol for Unruptured Ectopic Pregnancy**

| DAY | TIME | THERAPY |
|---|---|---|
| 1 | Variable | CBC*, SGOT†, MTX‡, β-hCG‖ |
| 2 | 8:00 AM | CBC, SGOT, CF§, β-hCG |
| 3 | 8:00 AM | MTX, β-hCG |
| 4 | 8:00 AM | SGOT, CF, β-hCG |
| 5 | 8:00 AM | MTX, β-hCG |
| 6 | 8:00 AM | CBC, SGOT, CF, β-hCG |
| 7 | 8:00 AM | MTX, β-hCG |
| 8 | 8:00 AM | CF, β-hCG |

*CBC = complete blood count with differential and platelet count.
†SGOT = serum glutamic-oxaloacetic transaminase.
‡MTX = intramuscular methotrexate, 1.0 mg/kg.
§CF = intramuscular citrovorum 0.1 mg/kg.
‖β-hCG = quantitative beta-human chorionic gonadotropin.

**NOTE:**
1. MTX stopped when there is a 15% decrease in two consecutive hCG titers.
2. Once MTX is given, CF is always given.
3. No vitamin containing folic acid and no alcohol should be used during treatment; abstaining from intercourse is also necessary.
4. Contraception is prescribed for 2 months following treatment completion.
5. Incidence of side effects is 2% to 5%.
6. Incidence of failure (nonresponders or tubal rupture) is 3% to 5%.
7. Protocol is outpatient.

Successful treatment occurs in 96% of patients meeting these criteria.

2. **Reproductive function following MTX treatment.** Treatment of unruptured ectopic pregnancy by MTX-CF (methotrexate-IM citrovorum) assists in restoration of tubal anatomy and does not impair return of menses. The pregnancy rates following this form of therapy appear to be better than those achieved by traditional surgical methods.

B. **Antiprogesterone drugs.** RU-486 is a progesterone receptor blocker that works at the site of implantation to compete for available progesterone binding sites. RU-486 has been demonstrated effective in terminating intrauterine pregnancy in the first trimester with about 80% efficacy. Preliminary data on treatment of ectopic pregnancy with RU-486 has been disappointing, but in the cases reported to date, the ectopic gestation was probably too advanced. As treatment of ectopic pregnancy occurs earlier, this drug will need to be reassessed.

C. **Nonintervention.** Observation without treatment has been shown effective. The following criteria may be used to determine eligibility for this form of treatment:

1. Falling hCG titer
2. Implantation in an extrauterine part of the oviduct
3. No active bleeding
4. Tubal serosa intact
5. Implantation fully visualized laparoscopically
6. Transverse diameter not >3 cm

Potential problems include tubal rupture, the formation of a persistent or chronic ectopic, and tubal damage. Before this form of treatment gains wide popularity, a "marker" is needed to determine which ectopics will respond without treatment. As a general rule, the vast majority of patients should be treated either medically or surgically.

D. **Future treatment methods**

1. **MTX KCl (potassium chloride) injection by ultrasound.** Injection of MTX or KCl into the ectopic gestation by ultrasonographic needle guidance has been described with successful outcome. The experience with this method is limited.
2. **Prostaglandin injection.** Prostaglandin $F_2$ can be injected directly into the ectopic site using ultrasound, or at the time of laparoscopy. Clinical trials in this area are also limited.

XI. **Prognosis for tubal ectopic pregnancy.** In less than 50% of women who undergo conservative surgery or have one undamaged tube, subsequent intrauterine pregnancy occurs. The chance of intrauterine pregnancy following ectopic pregnancy is approximately four times greater than a repeat ectopic pregnancy. The great variation noted is the result of many factors, including not only the ectopic pregnancy and the surgery involved in its care, but also the fertility status of the patient and her partner, the underlying causes of her ectopic pregnancy, and her general health. Each case therefore requires individual evaluation before comment may be made to the patient about her reproductive future.

**XII. Interstitial ectopic pregnancy.** Interstitial ectopic pregnancy occurs in one per 2500 to one per 5000 live births. Compared to tubal ectopic pregnancy, interstitial implantation provides a larger mass of uterine tissues into which the gestation may grow and a larger vascular supply to nourish the process. Interstitial ectopic pregnancies therefore develop further and become symptomatic later than ampullary ectopic pregnancies. When they rupture, they are more likely than ampullary tubal ectopic pregnancies to bleed profusely, causing severe shock. Levels of hCG are often higher than in tubal ectopic pregnancy because of this tendency toward delayed diagnosis.

- **A. Diagnosis.** The duration of amenorrhea may be longer and the onset of pain and/or vaginal bleeding may be delayed compared to similar tubal ectopic pregnancies. Physical examination is similar to tubal ectopic pregnancy except that interstitial ectopic pregnancy often demonstrates uterine asymmetry with marked tenderness on palpation in the area of irregularity. The laboratory evaluation is similar to that for tubal ectopic pregnancy.
- **B. Management.** Cornual resection is indicated when the procedure will leave a functional uterus and the patient desires to preserve her reproductive capability. The fallopian tube is usually damaged so as to make its removal (salpingectomy) desirable. Hysterectomy is indicated if the uterus is damaged beyond repair. Ovarian tissue should be preserved whenever possible. Pregnancy following cornual resection is associated with an increased risk of uterine rupture, especially if the cornual resection is deep enough that the uterine cavity was entered. In the latter case, cesarean section is recommended for future pregnancies.

**XIII. Rare types of ectopic pregnancy**

- **A. Combined pregnancy.** Because the diagnosis of combined pregnancy is usually missed at the time of first treatment, the morbidity is increased. How much it is increased over that of simple tubal ectopic pregnancy or simple spontaneous abortion is unknown because of the rarity of combined pregnancy. Once the correct diagnosis of combined pregnancy is made, a management appropriate for each pregnancy of the set must be formulated. The fetal salvage rate for the intrauterine component of a combined pregnancy is about one in three, the most likely event being spontaneous abortion in the first trimester. Diagnostic dilation, suction, and curettage should be made available to the patient if required.

B. **Abdominal pregnancy**

1. **Morbidity and mortality.** Maternal mortality is rare, although maternal morbidity is high because the diagnosis is made preoperatively in less than one-half of cases and because of the extent of damage to abdominopelvic organs associated with hemorrhage. A 10% to 20% overall fetal salvage rate is described for abdominal pregnancy. Of surviving infants, one-third to one-half will have some degree of deformity.
2. **Diagnostic signs and symptoms**
   a. Studdiford's criteria for diagnosis of primary abdominal pregnancies.
      (1) Presence of normal tubes and ovaries with no evidence of recent or past pregnancy.
      (2) No evidence of uteroplacental fistula.
      (3) The presence of a pregnancy related exclusively to the peritoneal surface and early enough to eliminate the possibility of secondary implantation following primary tubal nidation.
   b. Secondary abdominal pregnancy results from early tubal abortion or most commonly as a result of tubal rupture.
   c. In addition to the classic triad of amenorrhea, pain, and abnormal uterine bleeding, signs and symptoms of abdominal pregnancy may include persistent nausea and emesis, unusually painful fetal movements, severe abdominal cramping not characteristic of round ligament pain.
   d. **Physical examination** characteristic findings include abnormal fetal presentation, palpation of the uterus separate from the fetal parts, or cervical displacement from its expected position.
   e. **Laboratory examination and diagnostic procedures.** After 16 weeks' gestation, fetal ossification allows direct visualization of the fetus and the fetal parts are often posterior to the lumbar spine in a true lateral x-ray of the pelvis. Demonstration of the fetus outside of the uterus on ultrasound is diagnostic.
3. **Management.** The management of abdominal pregnancy is to remove the fetus surgically. The placenta is also removed if it can be removed in an en bloc dissection. Otherwise, it is left in situ to avoid the hemorrhage that will ensue if it is disturbed from its abnormal implantation site.

C. **Ovarian pregnancy**

1. **Diagnosis.** Diagnostic criteria of Spiegelberg include:
   a. The tube, including the fimbria ovarica is intact.
   b. The gestational sac definitely occupies the normal position of the ovary.

c. The sac is connected to the uterus by the ovarian ligament.

d. Ovarian tissue is demonstrable in the walls of the sac. The history and physical examination for ovarian pregnancy is similar to that for tubal ectopic pregnancy with two exceptions:

(1) Continued menses, which may appear normal, seem to be relatively common in patients with ovarian pregnancy.

(2) An adnexal mass is felt more often in patients with ovarian pregnancy (80% to 90% of cases) than in patients with tubal ectopic pregnancy.

2. **Management.** Surgical removal of the ectopic pregnancy is indicated, although preservation of as much ovarian tissue as possible is appropriate.

D. **Cervical pregnancy.** The morbidity and potential for mortality is high because of the associated profuse hemorrhage and the surgical treatment often required, which is hysterectomy.

1. **Diagnosis.** Cervical pregnancy demonstrates amenorrhea, but the vaginal bleeding is painless rather than painful. Upon examination the cervix is soft, thin-walled, round rather than conical, and disproportionally large. The examination is often confusing, with the cervical–uterine complex referred to as an hour-glass shaped uterus.

2. **Management.** If there is a strong desire for pregnancy in the future, an attempt may be made at sharp curettage. Vaginal packing is sometimes helpful to control the profuse bleeding that may ensue. Cervical cerclage type procedures that ligate the cervical branch of the uterine artery have been reported to help in the control or bleeding in this situation, and may be tried. If the bleeding cannot be controlled, abdominal hysterectomy will be required. When diagnosis is made early, usually by ultrasound, MTX has been reported to be successful.

## XIV. Future directions

The future holds much promise in the treatment of this disease state. Earlier diagnosis is making more conservative treatment possible. Nonlaparoscopic medical management is proving to be more feasible in many cases. The development of a single test, or set of tests that will predict resolution without any form of intervention will further reduce the morbidity associated with treatment, and will hopefully improve future reproductive potential.

## BIBLIOGRAPHY

Beckmann CRB, Sampson, M. Ultrasonographic diagnosis of interstitial ectopic pregnancy. J Clin Ultrasound. 1984; 12:304.

Beral V. An epidemiological study of recent trends in ectopic pregnancy. Br J Obstet Gynaecol. 1975; 82:775.

Bernstein, D, Holzinger M, Ovadia J. Conservative management of cervical pregnancy. Obstet Gynecol. 1981; 58:741.

Boronow RG, McElin TW, West RH, Buckingham JC. Ovarian pregnancy. Am J Obstet Gynecol. 1965; 91:1095.

Clark C. Cervical pregnancy. A review of the literature and report of a case. Obstet Gynecol. 1960; 16:454.

Conrad M, Johnson J, James A. Sonography in ectopic pregnancy. In: Sanders R, James A. eds. Ultrasound in Obstetrics and Gynecology. New York: Appleton–Century–Crofts; 1977: 114–121.

DeCherney A, Kase N. The conservative surgical management of unruptured ectopic pregnancy. Obstet Gynecol. 1979; 54:451.

Grimes D, Geary F, Hatcher R. Rh immunoglobulin after ectopic pregnancy. Am J Obstet Gynecol. 1981; 140:246.

Hallatt J. Repeat ectopic pregnancy: A review of 123 consecutive cases. Am J Obstet Gynecol. 1975; 122:520.

Kadar N, Caldwell B, Romero R. A method of screening for ectopic pregnancy and its indications. Am J Obstet Gynecol. 1981; 138:253.

Kadar N, DeVoe G, Romero R. Discriminatory hCG Zone: Its use in the sonographic evaluation for ectopic pregnancy. Obstet Gynecol. 1981; 58:156.

Lund J. Early ectopic pregnancy: Comments on conservative treatment. J Obstet Gynaecol Br Commonw. 1955; 62:1.

Lundstrom V, Bremme K, Eneroth P, Nygard I, Sundvall M. Serum beta-human chorionic gonadotropin levels in the early diagnosis of ectopic pregnancy. Obstet Gynecol Surv. 1980; 35:261.

Pauerstein CJ, Croxatto HB, Eddy CA, Ramzy I, Walters MD. Anatomy and pathology of tubal pregnancy. Obstet Gynecol. 1986; 67:301.

Schneider J, Berger C, Cattell C. Maternal mortality due to ectopic pregnancy: A review of 102 deaths. Obstet Gynecol. 1977; 49:557.

Schoen JA, Nowak RJ. Repeat ectopic pregnancy. Obstet Gynecol. 1975; 45:542.

Stangel J, Gomel V. Techniques in conservative surgery for tubal gestation. Clin Obstet Gynecol. 1980; 23:1221.

Steadman G. Combined intrauterine and extrauterine pregnancy. Obstet Gynecol. 1953; 2:277.

Stovall TG, Kellerman AL, Ling FW, Buster JE. Emergency department diagnosis of ectopic pregnancy. Annals of Emerg Med. 1990; 19:1098–1103.

Stovall TG, Ling FW, Buster JE. Outpatient chemotherapy for unruptured ectopic pregnancy. Fertil Steril. 1989; 51:435–438.

Stovall TG, Ling FW, Buster JE. Reproductive performance after methotrexate treatment of ectopic pregnancy. Am J. Obstet Gynecol. 1990; 162: 1620–1624.

Stovall TG, Ling FW, Cope BJ, Buster JE. Preventing ruptured ectopic utilizing a single serum progesterone. Am J Obstet Gynecol. 1989; 160:1425–1431.

Stovall TG, Ling FW, Smith WC, Felker R, Rasco BJ, Buster JE. Successful nonsurgical treatment of cervical pregnancy with methotrexate. Fertil Steril. 1985; 50:672–674.

Timor-Tritsch I, Rottem S, Thaler I. Review of transvaginal ultrasonography: A description with clinical application. Ultrasound Quarterly. 1987; 6:1–3.

# CHAPTER 13

# Gynecologic Problems in Children

**David Muram**

The reproductive tract in the premenarchal girl is different in structure and function from the genital tract of the adult female. These anatomic differences require that for premenarchal patients the examining physician use specially designed equipment (e.g., vaginoscope, Huffman's virginal vaginal speculum) to avoid undue discomfort and consequent anxiety about future examinations.

Not only are there differences in anatomy requiring special instrumentation, there are also disease processes and conditions that are either specific to or more common during childhood. It is important for the gynecologist to be familiar with this aspect of gynecology so that he or she can provide for the comprehensive care of patients, and at the same time provide expert consultation services for other physicians.

## I. Anatomic considerations

**A. Newborn.** During the first few weeks of life, the newborn female is affected by estrogens transferred across the placenta. The vagina at birth is about 4 cm long. The uterus is enlarged, measuring 4 cm in length, has no axial flexion, and a ratio between cervix and corpus of 3:1. The external genitalia are affected as well: The labia majora are bulbous; the labia minora are thick and protruding. The clitoris in the child is relatively large. The ovaries, which arise from the $T_{10}$ level are abdominal organs in early childhood, and are not palpable on pelvic or rectal examination. A vaginal discharge admixed with blood is common secondary to endometrial shedding that results from the falling serum estrogen levels derived from the maternal circulation.

**B. Early childhood** (14 days to 8 years). The genital tract receives little estrogen stimulation during early childhood. The vagina is slightly longer than in the newborn female (5 cm in length). The mucosa is thin and atrophic and therefore has little resistance to trauma and infections. The vagina has neutral or slightly alkaline secretions and is colonized with mixed bacterial flora. Following birth, the uterus regresses in size. By age 5,it regains the same size as it was at birth. The cervix in childhood is flush with the vaginal vault. It is not palpable, and the external genitalia shows lack of estrogenic stimulation as well. The labia majora are flat, the labia minora and hymen are extremely thin. The clitoris is relatively small.

C. **Late childhood.** Between the ages of 8 and 10 years, the vagina elongates to 8 cm in length, the mucosa becomes thicker, the corpus uteri grows, and the ratio of cervix to corpus is 1:1. The cervix is still flush with the vaginal vault. The vaginal maturation index shows mainly parabasal cells but also intermediate cells and occasional superficial cells. The external genitalia show some signs of estrogen stimulation: The mons pubis thickens; the labia majora fill out; the labia minora are rounded; and the hymen becomes thicker.

D. **Puberty.** In the premenarchal years (ages 10–13), the vagina reaches its adult length (10–12 cm). It is more distendable and the mucosa becomes thick and moist. The vaginal secretions are acidic, and lactobacilli are present. The differential growth of the uterine corpus and cervix is pronounced. The corpus is twice as large as the cervix. The cervix is clearly separated from the vaginal vault by the appearance of vaginal fornices. The ovaries descend into the true pelvis and the external genitalia achieve adult appearance.

## II. Examination of the young child

A. **General procedure.** In examining small children it is often helpful to have the mother hold the child on her lap. This maneuver gives the child a sense of security. The child should be asked to help with the examination. When the child separates her own labia, she is distracted and is less tense. Often the examiner places the child's hand over his or her own. It gives the child the impression that she has complete control over the examination.

1. **Indications for sedation.** When the child is apprehensive, sedation may be helpful. This can be achieved by using a standard pediatric cocktail such as a combination of demerol 50 mg/cc, thorazine 12.5 mg/0.5 cc, and phenergan 12.5 mg/0.5cc. The usual dose is 1 cc for every 20 lb (9 kg) of body weight with a maximum 2 cc dose. Sedation, however, is not sufficient even for minor procedures (e.g., biopsy).
2. **Indications for general anesthesia.** When the child is extremely apprehensive or if the child has been hurt previously, it is advisable to examine her under general anesthesia. Forceful examination is not justified. Not only is it psychologically traumatic, but the child may be injured by the instruments as she struggles to free herself. Most children, however, can be examined without resorting to general anesthesia.

B. **Gynecologic examination** of young girls is composed of four parts:

1. **Inspection and palpation of vulvar structures.** The examiner must identify each vulvar structure and answer the three following questions:
   a. Does it appear normal?
   b. Is it in its proper location?
   c. Would it function normally later in life?
2. **Inspection and palpation of other sex areas** (i.e., breast, axillary hair, skin). The physician must record the patient's height, weight, and general body contours. The presence or absence of breast tissue needs to be noted. In addition, one must also note the presence or absence of sexual hair, facial hirsutism, and general body hair. The skin is inspected for the presence of acne as well as abnormal pigmentation and fibromatous lesions.
3. **Visualization of the vagina and cervix.** Visualization of the lower vagina can be achieved in most patients simply by separating the labia and depressing the perineum. By positioning the child in a knee-chest position and asking her to bear down (Valsalva maneuver) a great deal of vaginal mucosa can then be inspected. However, the upper vagina and the cervix in many prepubertal children can be seen only by using a small vaginoscope. In the older child, following pubertal development, the Huffman-Graves vaginal speculum is an ideal instrument.
4. **Bimanual abdominal-pelvic examination** (performed rectally in the prepubertal child) is always a part of the gynecologic examination. Palpation of the uterus is most easily accomplished at birth or after puberty. During childhood only a small central mass of tissue, which probably represents the cervix and not the corpus, can be felt. The rectal examination reveals no other palpable mass. Pelvic masses in this age group require careful evaluation to rule out neoplasms. Patency of the anal canal is established at the same time.

## III. Congenital malformation of the genital tract

A. Most congenital malformations of the external genitalia are evident at birth. Some disorders result in ambiguity of the external genitalia and thus the child's sex may be in doubt (see Chapter 24). Conditions that affect the upper genital tract (e.g., absent uterus, absent vagina), are diagnosed at puberty or shortly after.

B. An imperforate hymen may give rise to the condition of hydrocolpos. This is the result of accumulation of vaginal secretions behind the obstructing membrane. The affected newborn child may be fretful and have difficulties urinating. On examination, one finds a lower abdominal cystic swelling, a palpable cystic mass on rectal examination, and a tense, bulging membrane at the introitus. Occasionally, when endometrial shedding occurs, the vaginal fluid is tinged with blood; this condition is called hematocolpos. The treatment is incision of the occluding membrane. If undiagnosed during childhood, when menses begin the blood accumulates in the vagina and uterus. The result is retrograde menstruation and an increased incidence of endometriosis and infertility. The diagnosis can be confirmed by sonographic evaluation of the pelvis. At the same time, the kidneys need to be visualized because there is a 10% incidence of renal tract abnormalities in association with Müllerian duct malformations.

## IV. Vulvovaginitis

A. **Incidence.** Vulvovaginitis accounts for over 70% of all pediatric gynecology referrals.

B. **Pathophysiology.** A young child is more susceptible to infections of the vulva and vagina for the following reasons:

1. Lack of estrogen, which makes the vaginal mucosa thin and atrophic.
2. Contamination by stool and other debris in young girls in whom perineal hygiene is often less than adequate.
3. There is some evidence to suggest that the immune mechanisms of the vagina are impaired in children.

C. **Symptoms** of vulvovaginitis vary from minor discomfort to relatively intense perineal pruritus accompanied by a minimal to copious foul-smelling discharge. Inspection of the genitalia reveals an area of redness and soreness, which may be minimal, or may extend laterally to the thighs and backward to the anus.

D. **Causative organisms.** In general, vaginal infections can be divided into three groups:

1. **Nonspecific infections.** These represent contamination of the vagina with multiple organisms, usually of enteric origin, due to poor perineal hygiene.
2. **Secondary innoculation.** These are infections with a specific organism that causes a primary infection elsewhere (i.e., pharyngitis, strep throat). Infection of the vagina occurs following bacteremia or innoculation with the patient's hands.
3. **Specific infections.** These are infections secondary to specific organisms, for example, sexually transmitted disease (e.g., gonorrhea, herpes).

E. **Evaluation**

1. **Collection and examination of vaginal secretions** may be done directly from the vagina using a saline-moistened cotton tip swab. Alternatively, warm saline can be instilled into the vagina using a small syringe and catheter and then collected for examination. The vaginal fluid obtained should be evaluated for:
   a. Smears for bacteriology and Gram stain.

b. Bacterial and mycotic cultures.
c. Wet prep for:
   (1) Micotic organisms potassium hydroxide (KOH).
   (2) Red blood cells.
   (3) Vaginal epithelium (estrogen effect).
   (4) Trichomonads.
   (5) Parasitic ova.

2. **Vaginoscopy.** In children in whom an infection is documented for the first time, vaginoscopy can be delayed. However, in children with a recurrent vaginal infection, an infection refractory to treatment, or when a foul-smelling, or bloody discharge is present, a thorough vaginal inspection is necessary. Examination is necessary not only to determine the extent of infection but to exclude the presence of foreign bodies or neoplasms.

**F. Treatment**

1. **Vulvar hygiene.** In all instances close attention is given to vulvar hygiene, and both parents and child need to be properly instructed. In patients with nonspecific vaginitis, this is the treatment of choice, and is curable in the majority of patients. These instructions must include the use of sitz baths and anal wiping from front to back. The child is instructed to sit in the tub, open her thighs and wash the vulvar area with warm water and soap. There is no need to put soap in the vagina. Following the bath, the child is told to pat dry the vulvar area. On occasion, the parents may wish to apply a small quantity of baby powder or corn starch to the vulva to assure that the area is kept dry.
2. **Discontinuation of topical irritant.** In rare instances, allergic reactions to creams or chemical agents are the cause of irritation. Discontinuation of contact with these chemicals alleviates the symptoms and prevents recurrences.
3. **Antibiotic therapy.** The treatment of vulvovaginitis requires determination of the exact etiology. If a specific organism is found, it should be treated with an appropriate antibiotic agent to which the organism is sensitive. If a specific organism cannot be identified, a course of broad-spectrum antibiotics may be prescribed, although this treatment is less likely to be effective than when the specific infectious organism is known. In all cases where acute infection is seen, a sample of the vaginal discharge should be sent for culture and sensitivity. However, therapy may be started with ampicillin or a similar preparation, and change the medication if indicated by the culture results.
4. **Topical hydrocortisone.** When pruritus is intense hydrocortisone cream may be necessary to alleviate the itch. This may be given as triamcinolone 0.1%, applied as a thin film to the affected area twice daily for 5 to 7 days.

5. **Estrogen therapy.** When the infection is severe, and a significant denudation of the vaginal mucosa is noted, a short course of estrogen treatment can be given to promote healing of vulvar and vaginal tissues. A small quantity of conjugated estrogen vaginal cream is applied as a thin film to the vulva and with a finger just inside the vagina twice daily for 5 to 7 days.

V. **Foreign bodies.** If insertion of a foreign body into the vagina is the cause of vulvovaginitis, usually the child does not recall inserting the object. Even if she does, she rarely admits to it. Recurrences are quite frequent when an object was inserted intentionally into the vagina. In most instances, foreign bodies are lodged accidentally in the vagina. The most commonly found objects are small pieces of toilet paper. These appear as amorphous conglomerates of grayish material, in which white and red blood cells are embedded. The presence of foreign bodies in the vagina induces intense inflammatory reaction that produces a bloody, foul-smelling discharge. When these foreign bodies are located in the lower third of the vagina, they can be seen when the labia are separated and the perineum is depressed. Most can be irrigated and removed with warm saline. Vaginoscopy is indicated for removal of large foreign bodies and to confirm that no other foreign bodies are present in the upper vagina.

VI. **Pinworms**

A. **Incidence.** Severe or chronic nocturnal perianal pruritus suggests the presence of pinworms *(Enterobius vermicularis).* The pinworm is the most common helminth in the United States. Humans are the only susceptible host and there are no intermediate hosts. When ingested, the ova hatch in the duodenum. The adult female migrates during the night from the cecum to the perianal and vulvar region to deposit up to 12,000 eggs per worm. Occasionally the worm can be found on the perineum or even in the vagina.

B. **Symptoms.** In addition to perianal pruritus, occasionally vulvovaginitis exists with variable symptoms and signs. Note, that not every child with pinworms has vulvovaginitis. However, when recurrent infections particularly when associated with nocturnal pruritis are present, an effort should be made to rule out the presence of pinworms.

C. **Diagnosis.** Using sticky Scotch® tape, the perineum is dabbed early in the morning prior to bathing, and the tape is then examined under a microscope. When characteristic ova are seen, the diagnosis is made. When vulvovaginitis is present, it is due to a nonspecific infection with enteric coliforms, which are carried into the vagina from the anus by the adult worm.

D. **Treatment.** Medication is given to the patient and every member of the family using mebendazole (Vermox) 1 tablet per person as a single dose. Clothes and linens should be washed to prevent reinfestation.

## VII. Lichen sclerosus

A. **Incidence.** Lichen sclerosus of the vulva is an hypotrophic dystrophy that usually affects women in the postmenopausal age group. Occasionally it is seen prior to puberty, usually affecting young children.

B. **Clinical features.** Histologically, the findings in the postmenopausal age group and young children are similar, including a flattening of the rete pegs, hyalinization of the subdermis tissues, and keratinization.

The lesion has no known malignant potential, provided only hypoplastic dystrophy is present. The classic clinical presentation is flat, ivory papules that may coalesce into plaques. In extreme cases, the whole vulva may be involved, but usually the lesion does not extend beyond the middle of the labia majora nor encroach into the vagina. The clitoris is frequently involved as well as the fourchette and the posterior anorectal area. Sometimes there are skin lesions affecting extragenital areas. Although most lesions appear predominantly white, some of them do have pronounced vascular markings, tend to bruise easily forming bloody blisters, and are susceptible to secondary infections.

C. **Symptoms** include vulvar irritation, dysuria, and pruritis. Scratching is quite common and occasionally may provoke bleeding or lead to secondary infection.

D. **Treatment**

1. Many treatment regimens have been proposed using various creams such as hydrocortisone, estrogen, progesterone, and testosterone. In the postmenopausal age group, testosterone is most commonly used and alleviates most symptoms.
2. In young girls, the use of testosterone is not recommended. Treatment would consist mainly of improved local hygiene, reduction of trauma and the use of hydrocortisone creams (triamcinolone 0.1% applied to the affected area twice daily) to alleviate the itch. Such treatment should be short in duration and may be repeated when exacerbation occurs.

E. **Prognosis.** Marked improvement in the symptoms and the appearance of the skin lesions occur following puberty. Over 50% of the children improve significantly during puberty. Although histologic confirmation of the hypoplastic nature of these lesions is necessary in the postmenopausal age group, it is usually not indicated in children. The lesion has no malignant potential and if it appears to be lichen sclerosus to the experienced observer, histological confirmation is not necessary.

## VIII. Labial adhesions

A. **Incidence.** Labial adhesions are quite common in prepubertal children. The condition may exist to some extent in many children and remain asymptomatic and thus unrecorded. It is important to recognize this condition because it is often mistaken for congenital absence of the vagina by the unexperienced observer. Such diagnosis creates unnecessary parental anxiety.

B. **Etiology.** The etiology is not known, but the lesion is probably related to the low levels of estrogens in the prepubertal child. The skin covering the labia is extremely thin, and local irritation causes scratching, which may denude the labia. The labia then adhere in the midline, stick to each other and re-epithelialization occurs on both sides. The labia remain fused in the midline.

C. **Symptoms.** Most children with a small degree of labial fusion are completely asymptomatic. When symptoms occur, they usually relate to interference with urination or the accumulation of urine behind the membrane. Thus dysuria, pain with urination, and recurrent vulvar and vaginal infections are the cardinal symptoms. On rare occasions when complete occlusion is present, urinary retention may occur.

D. **Treatment.** If asymptomatic, minimal to moderate degrees of labial fusion can be left untreated. When treatment is necessary, a thin film of conjugated estrogen cream is applied twice daily for 7 to 10 days and may separate the labia. When medical treatment fails or when severe urinary symptoms or retention exist, surgical division of the fused labia is then indicated.

E. **Prognosis.** Recurrence of labial fusion is quite common. This is due to the estrogen deficiency state that exists until puberty. Following puberty the condition resolves spontaneously, not to recur until after the menopause. Improved perineal hygiene and removal of irritants from the vulva may prevent recurrences. Proper instructions to the mother and child should be given.

## IX. Urethral prolapse

A. **Pathophysiology.** The urethral mucosa is an estrogen dependent tissue. During childhood, it is thin and atrophic. Occasionally the urethral mucosa prolapses through the urethral meatus. Because of venus obstruction, the prolapsed tissue becomes swollen and occasionally undergoes necrosis.

B. **Diagnosis** of urethral prolapse is easy when a central orifice is seen and a protruding tumor is found superior to the vagina where the urethral meatus is located. Occasionally the tumor may be mistaken to be arising from the vagina. If that is the case, examination under anesthesia and identification of the urethral orifice in the center of the mass may be necessary to define the true nature of this lesion.

C. **Therapy.** When the lesion is small and urination is unimpaired, a short course of therapy using conjugated estrogen cream (Premarin cream, small amount applied twice daily for 5 to 7 days) is beneficial. If urinary retention is present, if the lesion is large and necrotic, or if the child is examined under anesthesia, resection of the prolapsed tissue and insertion of an indwelling Foley catheter for 24 hours is the treatment of choice.

## X. Vaginal bleeding

Vaginal bleeding in early childhood, regardless of duration and quantity, is always of clinical importance. When vaginal bleeding occurs in children, two groups of conditions should be considered. In the first, the bleeding is caused by a local vulvar or vaginal lesion. The more common vulvar and vaginal disorders causing bleeding in children are listed in Table 13.1, and are discussed in greater detail throughout this chapter. In the second, the bleeding arises from the endometrium itself, usually as a manifestation of precocious puberty. Obviously, diagnosis and treatment of vaginal bleeding requires a detailed examination. A medical history and careful inspection of the external genitalia will determine the cause of bleeding in many

**Table 13.1. Etiology of Vaginal Bleeding in Children Over 7 Days of Age**

I. Caused by vulvar and vaginal disorders
   - A. Vulvovaginitis
   - B. Foreign bodies
   - C. Trauma
   - D. Urethral prolapse
   - E. Vulvar skin disorders
   - F. Botryoid sarcoma
   - G. Adenocarcinoma of the cervix or vagina

II. Caused by endometrial shedding
   - A. Physiologic
     - 1. Newborn withdrawal bleeding
   - B. Early sexual development (incomplete form)
     - 1. Premature menarche
   - C. Early sexual development (complete forms)
     - 1. Immature hypothalamic-pituitary-ovarian axis
       - a. Exposure to estrogens
         - (1) In the food chain
         - (2) Medications
       - b. Endogenous estrogen production
         - (1) Functional ovarian cysts
         - (2) Ovarian neoplasms
         - (3) Other hormone-producing neoplasms
     - 2. Mature hypothalamic-pituitary-ovarian axis
       - a. Costitutional precocious puberty
       - b. Central nervous system lesions
       - c. McCune-Albright syndrome

children with vulvar lesions. Vaginoscopy and examination under anesthesia are the mainstays of evaluation to exclude the presence of local vaginal lesions (i.e., tumors, foreign bodies, etc.). Vaginoscopy is required to visualize the upper third of the vagina, to remove foreign bodies, or to exclude penetrating injuries. In infancy and childhood, the hymenal orifice normally will admit a 0.5 cm vaginoscope. An instrument of 0.8 cm diameter can be used to examine most older premenarchal girls. Although some patients cooperate well in the office, many young patients are apprehensive and vaginoscopy is best performed under general anesthesia. If the aperture is too small for an instrument to be passed without discomfort, vaginoscopy should not be further attempted without general anesthesia. Indeed, persistent manipulation of the sensitive tissues without anesthesia will be traumatic and counterproductive.

Bleeding that arises from the endometrium itself usually represents endometrial shedding, often as the result of sexual precocity. Sexual precocity is the onset of sexual maturation at any age that is 2.5 standard deviations earlier than the norm. The appearance of any of the secondary sexual characteristics before 8 years of age or onset of menarche prior to age 10 is considered precocious. Occasionally, for reasons that remain unclear, only one sign of pubertal development will be present (e.g., breast development, menstruation). It may be caused by transient elevation in the levels of circulating estrogens, or alternatively, may be due to extreme sensitivity of the target tissues to the very low, prepubertal level of sex hormones. However, endometrial bleeding may be the result of estrogen stimulation from exogenous sources (e.g., medications) or endogenous sources (e.g., granulosa cell tumor). When endometrial shedding occurs, the following evaluation is recommended to determine the etiology.

**A.** Determination of blood estradiol or, alternatively, by the cytologic evaluation of a vaginal smear (maturation index) to determine estrogen stimulation.

**B.** Gonadotropin-releasing hormone stimulation test to assess pubertal development.

**C.** Pelvic ultrasound and sometimes computed tomography (CT) of the abdomen and pelvis to exclude gonadal or adrenal neoplasms.

**D.** CT of the head to rule out central nervous system lesions.

## XI. Embryonic carcinoma of the vagina (botryoid sarcoma)

**A. Incidence.** These rare tumors are most commonly seen in the very young age group — 3 years of age or less — although they may be present at birth. These tumors arise in the submucosal tissue and spread rapidly beneath an intact vaginal epithelium. The vaginal mucosa then bulges into a series of polypoid growths, which gives the lesions the name botryoid sarcoma. Occasionally masses of tumors are bulging through the vaginal orifice. The lesions usually involve the vagina but the cervix may be affected as well, particularly in an older child.

**B. Diagnosis.** The diagnosis is made by histologic evaluation of a biopsy specimen. Note that a routine microscopic evaluation may erroneously diagnose these lesions as benign. Striated muscle fibers are not always seen under light microscopy and most of the tumor demonstrates myxomatous changes. Under those circumstances electron microscopy may be required to confirm the diagnosis of embryonal rhabdomyosarcoma.

**C. Treatment.** In recent years, the treatment of these lesions has improved significantly. Combination chemotherapy using vincristine, actinomycin-D, and cyclophosphamide has been used with great success. The chemotherapy should be continued for at least 6 months, at which time the tumor is re-examined and re-biopsied. If the tumor is then amenable to surgical removal, radical hysterectomy, and vaginectomy are then performed. The ovaries are preserved and exenteration is not recommended. Following surgery, chemotherapy should be continued for another 6 to 12 months. If the tumor is unresectable, radiotherapy is used to reduce tumor size and control tumor growth. Electron microscopy may determine whether or not the tumor has responded to chemotherapy by demonstrating only nonviable tumor cells in a biopsy specimen. This information may be valuable in deciding further treatment.

**D. Prognosis.** The prognosis for children with embryonal carcinoma of the vagina in children is favorable, provided the diagnosis is established immediately when symptoms appear. Overall cure rates in excess of 50%, and as high as 80%, have been reported.

## BIBLIOGRAPHY

Cowell CA. The gynecologic examination of infants, children, and young adolescents. Pediatr Clin North Am 1981; 28:247–266.

Dewhurst CJ. Practical Pediatrics and Other Gynecology. New York, NY: Marcel Decker; 1981.

Dewhurst Sir J. Botryoid sarcoma of the cervix and vagina in children. In: Progress in Obstetrics and Gynecology. Studd J, ed. Edinburgh: Churchill Livingstone; 1983; 3:151–157.

Dewhurst, Sir John. Female puberty and its abnormalities. Edinburgh: Churchill Livingstone; 1984.

Emans SJH, Goldstein DP. Pediatric and Adolescent Gynecology. Boston, Mass: Little, Brown; 1977.

Grant DB. Vaginal bleeding in childhood. Pediatr Adolesc Gynecol 1983; 1:173.

Heller ME, Savage MO, Dewhurst J. Vaginal bleeding in childhood: A review of 51 patients. Br J Obstet Gyneacol 1978; 85:721.

Huffman JW, Dewhurst CJ; Capraro VJ. The Gynecology of Childhood and Adolescence. 2nd ed. Philadelphia, PA: WB Saunders Co; 1981.

Lavery JP, Sanfilippo JS. eds. Pediatrics and Adolescence in Gynecology. New York: Springer–Verlag; 1985.

Mercer LJ, Mueller CM, Hajj SN. Medical treatment of urethral prolapse. Adolesc Pediatr Gynecol 1988; 1:182–184.

Muram D. Genital tract trauma in pre-pubertal children. Pediatr Ann 1986; 15:616–620.

Muram D. Pediatric and adolescent gynecology. In: Pernol ML, Benson RC, eds. Current Gynecologic and Obstetric Diagnosis and Treatment. Norwalk, Conn: Appleton-Century-Crofts; 1987: 563–585.

Muram D, Massouda D. Vaginal bleeding in children. Contemp Obstet Gynecol 1985; 27:41–52.

Stovall TG, Muram D. Labial adhesion as a cause of acute urinary retention. Adolesc Pediatr Gynecol 1988; 1:203–204.

## CHAPTER 14

# Pelvic Pain and Dysmenorrhea

**Roger P. Smith**

## ACUTE PELVIC PAIN

Acute abdominal and pelvic pain account for a large number of emergency room and short notice office visits. Although most acute abdominal pain is of nongynecologic origin, pelvic organs are often involved.

Acute pelvic pain is almost always associated with morbidity of some degree. Sometimes including intense short-term pain and other times involving collapse. Acute pelvic and abdominal pain frequently are harbingers of significant physiologic disturbances that can carry life-threatening significance.

### I. Pathophysiology

The perception of acute pelvic pain can be produced by five common mechanisms: perforation, distention, ischemia, inflammation, and hemorrhage. Pain from the pelvic organs occurs through small afferent fibers that accompany sympathetic nerves. These enter the spinal cord at T10, T11, T12, and the L1 levels. Their course carries them through the uterine, cervical and pelvic plexuses, the hypogastric nerve, the superior hypogastric plexus (the presacral nerve), as well as the lumbar and lower lumbar sympathetic chain. Exact pathways are difficult to trace with certainty, making therapeutic approach to blocking pain sensation difficult. Once afferent fibers pass through the dorsal roots and enter the spinal cord, the signal they carry is subject to modulation at the local, segmental, and supraspinal levels. Because visceral structures do not have cortical representations, the sensation of pain is generally referred to superficial areas of the body. These areas are usually those with similar innervation as that of the viscus. Hence, the complaint of pain may be similar for widely different etiologies.

### II. Etiology

Table 14.1 presents the various causes of acute pelvic pain, which include gynecologic, urologic, and gastrointestinal disorders, as well as a few other rarer conditions.

**Table 14.1. Differential Diagnosis of Acute Pelvic Pain**

- I. Gynecologic causes
  - A. Adnexal
    1. Infection
    2. Ectopic pregnancy
    3. Torsion of pelvic mass or organ
    4. Ovarian cyst (bleeding)
    5. Ovulatory pain
  - B. Uterine
    1. Abortion
    2. Fibroid tumors
    3. Infection
- II. Urologic causes
  - A. Infection
  - B. Calculi
  - C. Tumors
- III. Gastrointestinal causes
  - A. Inflammatory
    Appendicitis, gastroenteritis, ulcerative colitis, ulcer disease, irritable bowel syndrome, diverticulitis, mesenteric adenitis, biliary disease
  - B. Mechanical
    Constipation, herniation, obstruction, torsion, intussusception
  - C. Other
    Embolism, infarct, parasites
- IV. Other
  - A. Aneurysm
  - B. Muscular
    Strains, rectus hematoma
  - C. Biochemical
    Sickle cell crisis, acute intermittent porphyria, heavy metal poisoning, black widow spider bites
  - D. Neurologic
    Tabes, herpes (shingles)

## III. Differential diagnosis

### A. Gynecologic causes

#### 1. Adnexal

a. **Infection.** Pelvic inflammatory disease (PID) accounts for almost 7% of nontraumatic emergency room visits for abdominal pain, second only to gastroenteritis as a specific diagnosis. Severity can range from an acute diffusely tender salpingitis, to a smoldering tubo-ovarian abscess. The hallmark of PID is low abdominal pain even though this symptom may be absent in as many as 6% of cases. In over 80% of patients symptoms will have been present for less than 15 days and frequently can be counted in hours. When the history reveals menstruation and tampon use, toxic shock syndrome must be included in the differential diagnosis.

b. **Ectopic pregnancy.** The pain of an ectopic pregnancy is usually lateralized at first and may become diffuse if there is intraperitoneal bleeding. If rupture occurs, the intraperitoneal bleeding that sometimes occurs can be life threatening. Irritation of the posterior cul-de-sac by leaking blood can cause a bearing down sensation reminiscent of constipation. With improved pregnancy tests, a positive result is generally found. Some elevation of the white blood count is common and a low grade fever may be present if leakage has occurred over an extended period. Vaginal bleeding need not be present.

c. **Torsion of a pelvic mass.** An adnexal or pedunculated pelvic mass, such as a fibroid, may twist on its mesentery leading to compromise of blood supply and ischemia. The resultant pain is generally strong, abrupt, and made worse by movement. Its onset is occasionally related to a change of body position, although this history is generally unreliable. The pain is generally lateralized and directly associated with a tender, painful pelvic mass. With time, peritoneal irritation will lead to more diffuse pain, rebound tenderness and tenderness on motion of the cervix.

d. **Cystic masses** do not generally cause pelvic pain. When a cystic mass is suddenly distended, however, pain may be acute in onset, especially when bleeding occurs within the mass. These masses may also cause discomfort with rupture or with torsion. Bleeding into a cyst and torsion both will produce similar symptoms and are frequently reported as being iliac or inguinal in location. Bleeding that is self-limited may cause intermittent symptoms with period of improvement or even complete resolution. Examination will generally reveal the mass.

e. **Ovulatory pain** (Mittelschmerz). Although not generally painful, ovulation can, on occasion, cause discomfort. The pain is frequently described as sharp, with an element of dull aching. It is usually well-localized and should occur only at approximately 14 days prior to the next menstrual flow. It should not be present in women taking oral contraceptives, premenarchal or postmenopausal women. A careful history may well elicit similar past episodes.

**2. Uterine causes**

a. **Spontaneous abortion.** Although variable in intensity and duration, crampy, lower abdominal pain is an almost constant finding in spontaneous abortion. Vaginal bleeding, a menstrual history commensurate with pregnancy, and pregnancy test should be helpful. Because abdominal tenderness is generally not present, any tenderness suggests a re-evaluation of the possibility of ectopic pregnancy.

b. **Fibroid tumors.** Uterine fibroids only rarely present with the symptoms of abdominal pain. Pain is only created in the presence of distention or ischemia due to bleeding or necrosis in rapidly growing myomas, or because of ischemia should a pedunculated fibroid undergo torsion. History and physical examination will generally make the diagnosis apparent.

c. **Infection** limited to the uterus will generally only occur after delivery, abortion (spontaneous or induced), or instrumentation. Cervical discharge and signs of ascending infection and salpingitis will often be present.

**B. Urologic causes**

1. **Infection.** Urinary tract infections (UTIs) account for slightly more than 5% of cases of nontraumatic abdominal pain seen in emergency rooms. The discomfort of lower UTIs is generally pelvic, suprapubic, and lower abdominal. A history of frequency and dysuria is commonly present and fever (when present) is generally mild. Upper UTIs (pyelitis, nephritis) will present with more generalized signs of infection and tenderness in the costovertebral area. Pain in these cases may radiate toward the pelvis, but seldom originate there. Urinalysis will separate these causes from others in the differential.
2. **Urinary calculi.** The pain of urinary calculi is among the worst encountered from any cause. Classically originating in the flank and radiating to the groin on the affected side, the pain will be intense and unrelieved by the patient's position. Palpation of the abdomen and pelvis does not usually elicit tenderness. Palpation over the kidney on the involved side often causes pain. A urinalysis revealing hematuria, combined with an acute course and lateralized signs and symptoms, will help to differentiate this problem from urinary tract infection.
3. **Tumors.** Like gynecologic tumors, tumors in the urinary tract are generally painless unless torsion, bleeding, infarct, or infection occur. Physical examination may reveal a mass, directing the course of further investigation.

**C. Gastrointestinal causes**

1. **Gastrointestinal inflammatory problems** (e.g., gastroenteritis, colitis, etc.) account for the most common causes of acute abdominal pain. Most of the processes involved will give a similar picture of diffuse abdominal pain or colic, and fever. Early nausea and vomiting are frequent. The history, progression of symptoms, and physical findings, combined with blood counts and selected serum chemistry studies, will generally separate the various etiologies (Table 14.1).
2. **Mechanical distention** of any hollow abdominal organ can

cause acute pain. In the gastrointestinal tract, this can happen gradually, as with constipation, or abruptly, as with herniation and obstruction. History will generally be helpful in establishing a differential diagnosis but, in extreme cases, a diagnosis may not be established without exploratory surgery.

3. **Other causes.** The organs of the gastrointestinal tract are not immune to accidents such as embolism, infarct, or parasitic infection. As with mechanical causes, history and other physical findings may be helpful, but therapy may have to be directed toward stabilization before a specific diagnosis is made.

D. **Other miscellaneous causes**

1. **Aortic aneurysm.** Abdominal or pelvic pain can accompany dissection, leakage, or rupture of an abdominal aortic aneurysm.The presence of a pulsatile mass suggests the diagnosis. If the patient's condition permits, ultrasound may be useful in confirming the diagnosis.
2. **Muscular disorders.** Abdominal pain can originate from the structure of the abdominal wall itself. Strains and hematomas are the most likely causes and the patient's history will often direct the diagnostic process. The pain reported is usually well-localized and involves point tenderness.
3. **Biochemical disorders** of both an inborn and acquired nature are unusual causes of abdominal pain. Some to be considered are: sickle cell crisis, acute intermittent porphyria, heavy metal poisoning, and toxins (e.g., black widow spider bite).
4. **Neurologic disorders.** Neuralgia due to tabes dorsalis and herpetic radiculopathy (shingles) may cause abdominal pain.

## IV. Diagnosis

A. **Signs and symptoms** associated with abdominal and pelvic pain can be many and varied. Rapid and thorough evaluation of each sign and symptom must be carried out. Many potentially life-threatening conditions present as abdominal or pelvic pain. In general, the more acute and catastrophic the symptoms, the greater the risk to the patient. Signs of diffuse peritonitis (rigidity, rebound, depressed or absent bowel sounds, fever) are also indications of significant pathological disturbance and risk. A bluish discoloration of the peri-umbilical area (Cullen's sign) may be present in patients with intra-abdominal bleeding, but is rarely found.

B. **Physical examination**

1. **Basic assessment.** Measurement of blood pressure (in two positions if blood loss is suspected), pulse rate, and body temperature is imperative. Evaluation of heart and lungs

should also be included, with its priority determined by the patient's history and general condition.

2. **Abdominal examination.** When performing the abdominal examination, it is often useful to begin by asking the patient to indicate "where it hurts." The area involved, as well as the way in which the patient points, will be helpful in evaluating the degree of localization. Gentle palpation to evaluate for masses and tenderness should be carried out. Where possible, every effort to avoid discomfort will be rewarded by a more cooperative patient and ultimately more valuable information. With gentle palpation, true rigidity as opposed to voluntary guarding can be elicited. Finding a mass will help to direct further evaluations. A diffuse, dough-like consistency to the abdomen is suggestive of intraperitoneal bleeding and may suggest additional testing. Deeper palpation and an evaluation of rebound tenderness are next carried out. When significant peritonitis is present, bowel sounds will generally be absent. Gentle palpation with the stethoscope provides an opportunity to confirm earlier findings, freed from the patient's expectation of discomfort associated with manual palpation.
3. **Pelvic and rectal examination.** No evaluation of the patient with abdominal or pelvic pain is complete without a pelvic and rectal examination. This should include a speculum examination of the cervix for blood or discharge. Palpation of the uterus and adnexa for masses and tenderness will do much to add or subtract from the list of possible causes. Peritoneal irritation may be indicated by discomfort when the cervix and uterus are moved by the examining hand. Rectal examination may be confirmatory and may also reveal signs of masses and bleeding that can change the direction of further investigation. Motion of the peritoneum by way of rectal examination will again cause discomfort when inflammation exists.

C. **Laboratory, x-ray, ultrasonography**

1. **Complete blood count (CBC).** A CBC represents the corner stone of the laboratory evaluation. This will help to identify inflammatory processes by virtue of elevations in the white blood count as well as alterations in the differential count. The hemoglobin or hematocrit will be helpful in the evaluation of possible blood loss. It should be remembered that these parameters will not accurately reflect acute, uncompensated blood loss.
2. **Urinalysis** is a quick and inexpensive way to evaluate the role of the urinary tract in the development of the patient's pain. It also provides information as to the patient's metabolic status.
3. **Cervical culture and Gram stain.** When a purulent cervical discharge is present, a Gram stain and culture of the dis-

charge for gonorrhea and chlamydia are helpful. Empiric antibiotic therapy should be based on the clinical picture and the Gram stain, rather than the results of the culture that can take 48 hours or more to return.

4. **Pregnancy testing.** The use of a sensitive pregnancy test such as the newer urinary pregnancy test for presence of human chorionic gonadotropin is also an important part of the evaluation when a pregnancy associated problem is suspected.
5. **Imaging by x-ray and ultrasonography.** Imaging by x-ray and ultrasonography have only limited value as screening tools. X-ray examination may confirm air–fluid levels or the presence of free air in the peritoneal cavity (suggestive of bowel perforation). Ultrasonography can help identify pelvic masses when present. When ectopic pregnancy is suspected, it may be useful if it demonstrates an intrauterine pregnancy.
6. **Serum chemistries.** An evaluation of serum chemistries may be useful in evaluating gastrointestinal, or biliary causes, as well as general status. These tests should be used based on specific possible diagnoses and are generally not of value as "screening tools."

D. **Culdocentesis** can be useful in the evaluation of the patient with pain. When nonclotting blood, purulent fluid, or fecal material are revealed, they can contribute significantly to the diagnostic process. It should be remembered that culdocentesis is an invasive procedure and the information gained has limitations. The use of this adjunct to the physical examination must be reserved for only those patients where the information gained will outweigh the discomfort and risk involved (see Chapter 34—Common Office Gynecologic Procedures).

## V. Management

The management of the patient with abdominal or pelvic pain is directed towards stabilization, pain relief, and specific therapy directed at correcting the cause. Because many types of acute abdominal and pelvic pain may be caused by processes that can be life threatening, it is important to never ignore the possibility that diagnostic evaluations may have to be limited in favor of supportive measures. Blood replacement and fluid therapy for external or intraperitoneal bleeding may be required. Support and antibiotics in aggressive doses may be indicated. Exploratory surgery to both diagnose and correct a significant intraperitoneal process is often required.

## VI. Prognosis

The prognosis for the patient experiencing acute abdominal or pelvic pain should generally be good. A good outcome is predicated upon a correct and timely diagnosis of the underlying cause of discomfort, combined with prompt and appropriate therapy.

# SECONDARY DYSMENORRHEA AND CHRONIC PELVIC PAIN

## I. Incidence

A. In general, the incidence of **dysmenorrhea** is difficult to estimate with any accuracy. It is safe to say that between 10% and 15% of women suffer sufficient disability such that they lose time from work, school, or home on a monthly basis. Between 50% and 90% of women will suffer this degree of disability at least once during their reproductive years. The magnitude of this problem can be appreciated because there are approximately 40 million women of reproductive age in the United States. Dysmenorrhea is most common in younger women, but it may extend throughout the reproductive years.

B. The incidence of **chronic pelvic pain** is much lower than that of secondary dysmenorrhea, but chronic pelvic pain represents a source of significant disability. It often requires a great deal of time and resources, from both physician and patient, to make a diagnosis and establish treatment.

C. Because the same processes that cause secondary dysmenorrhea may also be a source for chronic pelvic pain between menstrual periods, these two subjects will be treated together.

## II. Morbidity and mortality

Menstrual pain may vary from a mild inconvenience, to a severe disability. It may be as mild as lower abdominal cramping or pressure, or it may be as severe as extreme pain, nausea, vomiting, diarrhea, and collapse. Although not directly life threatening, it can be a source of significant morbidity. In 1940, it was estimated that over 140 million hours were lost from the work force because of dysmenorrhea.

## III. Etiology

Secondary dysmenorrhea is caused by, or is "secondary to," identifiable pathological or iatrogenic conditions acting on the uterus, tubes, ovaries, or pelvic peritoneum. Pain generally results when these processes alter pressure in or around the pelvic structures, change or restrict blood flow, or cause irritation of the pelvic peritoneum. These processes may act in combination with the normal physiology of menstruation to create discomfort, or they may act independently with their symptoms becoming noticeable during menstruation. When symptoms occur between menstrual periods, these processes may be the source of chronic pelvic pain.

## IV. Differential diagnosis

The possible etiologies of secondary dysmenorrhea may be broadly classified as being intrauterine and extrauterine (Table 14.2). Almost any process that can affect the pelvic viscera and cause acute pain can be a source for chronic pain or secondary dysmenorrhea.

**Table 14.2. Differential Diagnosis of Secondary Dysmenorrhea**

I. Intrauterine causes
  A. Adenomyosis
  B. Myomas
  C. Polyps
  D. Intrauterine contraceptive device (IUD)
  E. Infection
  F. Cervical stenosis and cervical lesions
II. Extrauterine causes
  A. Endometriosis
  B. Tumors (fibroids, malignant)
  C. Inflammation
  D. Adhesions
  E. Psychogenic
  F. Pelvic congestive syndrome
  G. Nongynecologic causes
III. Idiopathic

Because the treatment of these pain syndromes is based on treating the underlying cause, the importance of the differential diagnosis should be apparent.

A. **Intrauterine causes**

1. **Adenomyosis** is a condition characterized by a benign invasion of the endometrium into the uterine musculature, often accompanied by a diffuse overgrowth of the musculature as well. This condition is reported in 25% to 40% of hysterectomy specimens. Grossly, the uterus will be slightly enlarged and generally symmetrical. A colicky dysmenorrhea and menorrhagia are the most frequent presenting complaints for a patient with adenomyosis. The pain seen in adenomyosis is often referred to the rectum or the sacrum. Endometriosis is thought to be coexistent in about 15% of cases. The final diagnosis of adenomyosis is histologic (see Chapter 7—Benign Diseases of the Uterus).
2. **Leiomyomata uteri** are the most frequently occurring human tumor and are reported to occur in 20% of women over 30, and 30% of women over 40 years of age. These tumors may range in size from very small to over 100 lb in weight. They can occur in any part of the uterus, cervix, or the broad ligament. Those most likely to be a cause of secondary dysmenorrhea create distortion of the uterus and uterine cavity. Pain is thought to arise from disruption of the normal uterine muscle activity or from altered intrauterine pressures. The diagnosis of fibroids will generally be made based on the physical examination findings of an enlarged and distorted uterus (see Chapter 7—Benign Tumors of the Uterus).
3. **Polyps**. Although an infrequent cause for dysmenorrhea, pedunculated masses within the uterine cavity can be a source of menstrual pain. When large enough to be symp-

tomatic, these growths are detectable by virtue of uterine enlargement or herniation through the cervix.

4. **Intrauterine contraceptive devices.** A common iatrogenic cause for secondary dysmenorrhea is the intrauterine contraceptive device (IUD). The presence of this foreign body causes an increase in uterine activity that may be painful. This is especially common for women who have not had children. History and the presence of the IUD string on physical examination should provide an adequate clue (see Chapter 17—Contraception and Sterilization).
5. **Pelvic infection.** It is the consequences of infection, rather than the infection itself, that are generally responsible for secondary dysmenorrhea or chronic pelvic pain. Scarring and intraperitoneal adhesions lead to restricted motion of the pelvic viscera, and thus pain. This pain may only be apparent during menstruation, intercourse, bowel movements, or physical activity, or it may be constant and chronic in character. A history of pelvic infection, especially of repeat episodes, combined with a painful pelvic examination, thickening of the adnexa, and restricted motion, should all add to the suspicion (see Chapter 19—Sexually Transmitted Diseases and Pelvic Inflammatory Disease).
6. **Cervical stenosis.** Often blamed in the past as a source of dysmenorrhea, cervical stenosis and cervical lesions are only rarely the source of menstrual or other pelvic pain. Inspection of the cervix on speculum examination will reveal the presence of a lesion, but cervical stenosis can only be assessed by the use of a probe. Because this is a generally uncomfortable procedure, it is not advised unless all other causes have been investigated. (see Chapter 6—Benign Diseases of the Cervix and Vagina).

**B. Extrauterine causes**

1. **Endometriosis** is a condition in which tissue resembling normal uterine mucous membrane occurs aberrantly in various locations outside the uterus. The chief locations where endometrial implants are found are: the ovaries; uterosacral ligaments; rectovaginal septum; the pelvic peritoneum of the uterus, fallopian tubes, rectum, sigmoid colon, and bladder; and more distant locations such as the umbilicus and vagina. The implants of endometrial tissue may vary from the size of a pin head, to large pelvic masses of several centimeters. Endometriosis is most common in white women between 30 and 40 years of age. Whereas about 8% to 10% of patients will present with acute symptoms, most patients present complaining of severe dysmenorrhea with symptoms referred to the back and rectum. In a patient demonstrating symptoms and signs consistent with chronic pelvic inflammatory disease, the presence of nodules in the uterosacral area should point toward the possibility of endometriosis (see Chapter 26—Endometriosis).

2. **Tumors** that are either benign or malignant, arising in, or spreading to, the uterus or adnexal structures, may be a cause of dysmenorrhea or pelvic pain. Although an unusual cause of pain alone, the presence of a mass on pelvic examination should prompt the physician to consider all possible types of tumors, not just "fibroids" (see Chapters 30, 31, 32 on Gynecologic Oncology).
3. **Inflammation.** Chronic inflammation can be a source for chronic pelvic pain and dysmenorrhea. This may occur because of the active effects of inflammation, or by virtue of the scarring and damage done by past episodes. In the past, chronic inflammatory processes such as tuberculosis were occasionally found, although this is an uncommon diagnosis today (see Chapter 19—Sexually Transmitted Diseases and Pelvic Inflammatory Disease).
4. **Adhesions** arising from old inflammatory processes or surgical intervention can be a source for chronic pelvic pain, and less frequently, dysmenorrhea. Although generally not apparent on physical examination, the patient's history should be helpful in evaluating this possible cause.
5. **Psychogenic** dysmenorrhea was once thought to be relatively common. As frequently occurs, when we do not have an explanation for the patient's complaint of pain, it is very easy to dismiss it as "all in their head." Much has been written about the various personality types believed to be associated with dysmenorrhea and chronic pelvic pain. As we have learned more about both secondary and primary dysmenorrhea, it appears that few patients truly have "psychogenic" dysmenorrhea. Although there is no doubt that dysmenorrhea affects different patients to different degrees and in different ways, and that any attempt to substantiate complaint such as pain can be used as a way to gain attention or other psychological ends, this is not a common reason for the complaint of dysmenorrhea. In cases of chronic pain, there is often a strong overlay of psychological symptoms as the pain itself becomes the disease. In approximately 5% to 10% of patients with chronic pelvic pain, no definite cause can be identified. This adds to the confusion about the true role of psychological factors in the complaint of pelvic pain. In general, listening to the patient will often give clues as to the likelihood of this etiology. Worsening of symptoms during times of stress, "inconvenient" recurrences that remove the patient from unpleasant situations, and other signs of emotional components should all make the physician suspicious. Only after other physical causes have been eliminated should this diagnosis be made.
6. **Pelvic congestive syndrome.** The term pelvic congestive syndrome is generally applied to patients who complain of either chronic pelvic pain or recurrent dysmenorrhea although few or no clinical findings exist. Some authors have

reported that some of these patients demonstrate enlarged or engorged pelvic veins when examined by laparoscopy. This has prompted the hypothesis that the engorgement leads to the complaints of pelvic heaviness and pain. This has not been adequately explored as a clinical entity, and would be a tenuous diagnosis to make.

7. **Musculoskeletal** pain may result from disorders of the lumbosacral spine, abdominal wall, and pelvic floor muscles. Examination directed toward these specific areas, possibly with the assistance of a physical therapist, will occasionally lead to the diagnosis.
8. **Nongynecological disorders.** The bladder, rectum, sigmoid, and diseases thereof can all be a potential source for chronic pelvic pain. Each of these areas should be included in both the history and physical evaluation of the patient with the complaint of pain. The same processes that can cause acute pain, can also be responsible for a more chronic process (see acute pelvic pain, section III–B, C, D).

## V. Diagnosis

A. **Signs and symptoms.** The signs and symptoms involved in secondary dysmenorrhea and chronic pelvic pain can be many and varied. In general they will be referable to the underlying etiology. The complaint of gastrointestinal symptoms, urinary difficulties, back problems, or the like should alert the physician to the possibility of nongynecological causes. The complaints of heavy menstrual flow combined with pain suggest uterine changes such as adenomyosis, myomas, or polyps. The complaint of pelvic heaviness, or change in abdominal contour, should raise the possibility of intra-abdominal neoplasia. Fever, chills, and malaise should suggest an inflammatory process. The coexisting complaint of infertility may suggest that endometriosis is a possibility. When the patient notes that her symptoms started only after placement of an IUD, the probable cause is evident.

B. **Physical examination.** The physical examination will generally provide clues to the diagnosis, if not the diagnosis itself. Pelvic examination should initially be performed with one hand only, to avoid confusion of pain originating from the abdominal wall, as opposed to the pelvic organs. The presence of asymmetrical, or irregular enlargement of the uterus should suggest myomas, or other tumors. Symmetrical enlargement of the uterus is often present in cases of adenomyosis and occasionally when intrauterine polyps are present. The presence of painful nodules in the posterior cul-de-sac and restricted motion of the uterus is suggestive of endometriosis. Restricted motion of the uterus is also found in cases of pelvic scarring from adhesions, or inflammation. Inflammatory processes often cause thickening of the adnexal structures. This thickening may be palpable on physical examination.

C. **Laparoscopic examination.** In many cases of pelvic pain, laparoscopic examination of the pelvic organs may be necessary to complete the diagnostic process. This valuable tool is usually reserved for a later portion of the evaluation, once more conservative investigative measures have been used.

D. **Laboratory.** The laboratory evaluation of the patient with secondary dysmenorrhea or chronic pelvic pain is limited. Blood counts may help to evaluate the presence of ongoing or excessive blood loss. Sedimentation rates may help to identify the presence of chronic inflammatory processes, but are, of necessity, nonspecific.

E. **Radiological evaluation** of the patient is generally restricted to the evaluation of nongynecological etiologies, such as those of the gastrointestinal or urinary tract. Ultrasound examinations of the pelvis may be useful. Ultrasound can demonstrate the presence and extent of myomas, adnexal and other tumors, or locate an intrauterine IUD.

## VI. Management

Whenever possible, the treatment of both secondary dysmenorrhea and chronic pelvic pain is directed toward correcting or removing the underlying causative factors. Whereas analgesics, antispasmodics, and birth control pills may have some temporary benefit, only specific therapy aimed at correcting the cause will ultimately be successful. This may range from removing an offending IUD to antiestrogen therapy for endometriosis, from removal of a polyp to hysterectomy. Physical therapy, directed toward postural abnormalities and key muscular weaknesses, may either totally relieve pain or at least provide enough improvement to allow adequate daily functioning. In those few patients in whom no specific diagnosis may be established, and intractable, debilitating pain is present, presacral neurectomy or laser ablation of the uterosacral ligaments may be useful. These are generally reserved for those patients in whom no other therapy has been useful. Whereas some reports claim up to 85% relief from pain, these procedures are far from innocuous and their use should be limited.

## VII. Prognosis

When the proper diagnosis is made, and appropriate therapy is instituted, the majority of patients will obtain relief of their pain and return to normal function. Unfortunately however, there are those patients who will receive little or no improvement in their pain. These patients can be difficult to deal with and may become clinically depressed. Continued attempts at relieving physical complaints, accompanied by proper psychological counseling and emotional support are basic requirements of the physician and support staff.

## PRIMARY DYSMENORRHEA

### I. Incidence

The incidence of primary dysmenorrhea is similar to that of secondary dysmenorrhea. It is uncommon for true primary dysmenorrhea to occur during the first three to six menstrual cycles of a young woman. The incidence of primary dysmenorrhea is greatest in women in their late teens to early 20s. The incidence then declines with age, but even women in their 40s may be affected. It appears that the incidence is not affected by childbearing.

### II. Morbidity

The pain of primary dysmenorrhea is often greater than that experienced with secondary dysmenorrhea. In addition to pain, these patients often experience debilitating nausea, vomiting, diarrhea, and symptomatic vasoconstriction. These symptoms are often a source of significant disruption in the lives of patients with primary dysmenorrhea.

### III. Etiology

Primary dysmenorrhea occurs because of either an increase in uterine prostaglandin (PG)$F_2$-alpha, an increased sensitivity to prostaglandins, or both. $PGF_2$-alpha is a potent uterine muscle stimulator. Increased levels of $PGF_2$-alpha leads to an increase in uterine contractile activity, ischemia, and pain. $PGF_2$-alpha is also a potent stimulator of the smooth muscle of the gastrointestinal tract, leading to the symptoms of nausea, vomiting, and diarrhea.

### IV. Pathogenesis and pathophysiology

A. **Prostaglandins** are derivatives of fatty acids commonly found in the cell wall. The production of various prostaglandins is shown in Figure 14.1. Prostaglandin production in the uterus increases under the influence of progesterone, reaching a peak at, or soon after, the start of menstruation. Once menstruation begins, formed prostaglandins are released from the shedding endometrium. In addition, the necrosis of endometrial cells provides increased substrate for the synthesis process. Two main prostaglandins are made in the uterus; $PGF_2$-alpha and $PGE_2$. $PGF_2$-alpha is a potent smooth muscle stimulator and vasoconstrictor. $PGE_2$ is a potent vasodilator and platelet disaggregator. $PGE_2$ has been implicated as a cause of primary menorrhagia.

B. **The uterine activity** found in patients with primary dysmenorrhea can be striking. During normal menstruation, contractions of 50 to 80 mm Hg, lasting 15 to 30 seconds are not uncommon. These generally occur with a frequency of from one to four contractions in 10 minutes. Resting pressure in the uterus is generally 5 to 15 mm Hg. In women with dysmenorrhea, contractions may have peak pressure in excess of 400 mm Hg, last longer than 90 seconds, and have less than 15 seconds of

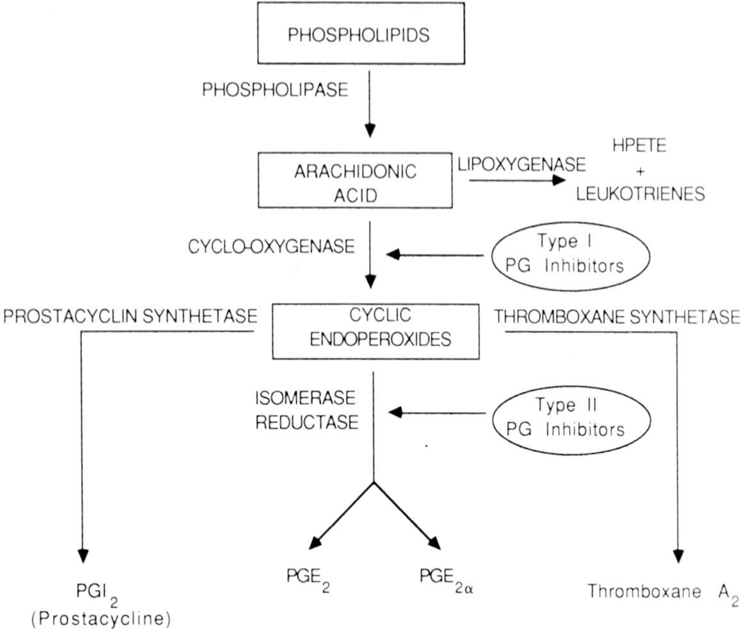


FIGURE 14.1. Biosynthesis of prostaglandins. Adapted from Smith, RP. Drug therapy for dysmenorrhea. Ill Med J 1986; 169:22–25. Reprinted with permission.

rest at a baseline pressure sometimes as high as 80 to 100 mm Hg. Pressures of this magnitude and duration cause significant ischemia.

C. **Pain mechanism.** The exact mechanism that creates the sensation of pain is unknown. Recent studies show a strong correlation between pain and pain relief, and the parameters of uterine work, maximal pressures, frequency and quality of contractions, rate of pressure change, and the quality of "rest" between uterine contractions. With the exception of rate of change, these parameters all have intuitive bearing on perfusion and ischemia. Further research into uterine blood flow and a better understanding of the phenomenon of pain itself, may help to resolve these questions.

## V. Differential diagnosis

The most important differential diagnosis to consider is that of secondary dysmenorrhea. Although the history and the patient's description of symptoms is often characteristic, the diagnosis of primary dysmenorrhea should not be made without thoroughly evaluating and eliminating other possible causes.

## VI. Diagnosis

A. **Signs and symptoms.** Patients with primary dysmenorrhea generally present with the complaint of recurrent, month-after-month, spasmodic lower abdominal pain occurring on the first 1 to 3 days of menstruation. The pain is diffusely located in the suprapubic area with radiation around and through to the back. The labor-like pain is described as "coming and going," and the patient will often use a fist opening and closing to illustrate their description. This pain is often accompanied by moderate to severe nausea. Vomiting and/or diarrhea are not infrequent. Patients often double up into a fetal position in an effort to gain relief. Many patients will report having tried a heating pad or hot water bottle in an effort to decrease their discomfort.

B. **Physical examination** of a patient with primary dysmenorrhea should be normal. There should be no palpable abnormalities of the uterus or adnexa. Speculum and abdominal examinations should similarly be normal. Patients examined during the time of actual symptoms often appear pale and "shocky." The abdomen will be soft and nontender, and the uterus normal.

C. **Laboratory, x-ray, ultrasonography.** The use of these modalities is limited to evaluating possible causes of secondary dysmenorrhea only (see secondary dysmenorrhea and chronic pelvic pain, section V-D,E).

## VII. Management

A. **Analgesics**

1. **For mild pain,** minor analgesics such as aspirin, acetaminophen, propoxyphene, or their compounds have found wide use.
2. **For severe pain,** or pain that is not responsive to minor analgesics, potent major analgesics are often required. Whereas these agents provide good pain relief, their potential side effects may render the patient unable to function normally. Useful agents and their compounds are:
   a. Butalbital (Fiorinal), 1 or 2 tablets p.o. q4 h.
   b. Oxycodone (Percodan), 1 tablet p. o. q6 h.
   c. Pentazocine (Talwin), 1 tablet p. o. q3–4 h.
   d. Promethazine (Synalgos), 2 tablets p.o. q4 h.
   e. Codeine, 30 to 60 mg tablets p.o. q4 h.
   f. Meperidine (Demerol), 50 to 100 mg q4–6 h.

B. **Oral contraceptives**

Because anovulatory cycles are less likely to have symptoms of primary dysmenorrhea, one approach has been to modify the menstrual cycle itself. Suppression of ovulation with oral contraceptive agents does provide many patients with complete or partial improvement. The use of oral contraceptives yields a thinner, more atrophic, endometrium, with much less prostaglandin. This, in turn, causes the menstruation to be shorter, lighter, and have less cramping. Relief is not always complete, and many patients do not want, or cannot take, these medications. In patients who desire contraception, and have no contraindications, they may be a reasonable choice. Any of the standard oral contraceptives are satisfactory for this purpose (see Chapter 17—Contraception and Sterilization).

C. **Pain prevention**

1. **Nonsteroidal anti-inflammatory (NSAI) drugs** (Table 14.3). The most practical method of suppressing uterine activity has been by reducing the level of prostaglandin through prostaglandin synthetase inhibitors and/or reducing the sensitivity of the myometrial receptors using NSAI drugs.

   a. **Classes of NSAI drugs.** There are two broad classes of NSAI compounds (enolic acids, carboxylates), each with sub-groups (Fig. 14.2).

**Table 14.3 Clinical Drug Usage in Dysmenorrhea and Pelvic Pain***

| DRUG (TRADE NAME) | INITIAL DOSE | FOLLOWING DOSE |
|---|---|---|
| Acetic/salicylic acids | | |
| Indomethacin (Indocin®) | 25 mg | 25 mg t.i.d. |
| Tolmetin (Tolectin®) | 400 mg | 400 mg t.i.d. |
| Sulindac (Clinoril®) | 200 mg | 200 mg b.i.d. |
| Diflunisal (Dolobid®) | 1000 mg | 500 mg q12 h |
| Diclofenac (Voltaren®) | 75–150 mg | 75 mg b.i.d. |
| Propionic acids | | |
| Ibuprofen (Motrin®, Rufen®)† | 400 mg | 400 mg q4 h |
| Naproxen (Naprosyn®)† | 500 mg | 250 mg q6 8h |
| Naproxen sodium (Anaprox®)† | 550 mg | 275 mg q6 8h |
| Fenoprofen calcium (Nalfon®) | 200 mg | 200 mg q4 6h |
| Ketoprofen (Orudis®) | 75 mg | 75 mg t.i.d. |
| Fenamates | | |
| Mefenamic acid (Ponstel®)† | 500 mg | 250 mg q4 6h |
| Meclofenamate (Meclomen®) | 100 mg | 50–100 mg q6 h |
| Pyrazolones | | |
| Phenylbutazone (Azolid®, Butazolidin®) | 100 mg | 100 mg t.i.d. |
| Oxicams | | |
| Piroxicam (Feldene®) | 20 mg | 20 mg qd |

*Consult full prescribing information before using any of these drugs.
†FDA approved for primary dysmenorrhea.

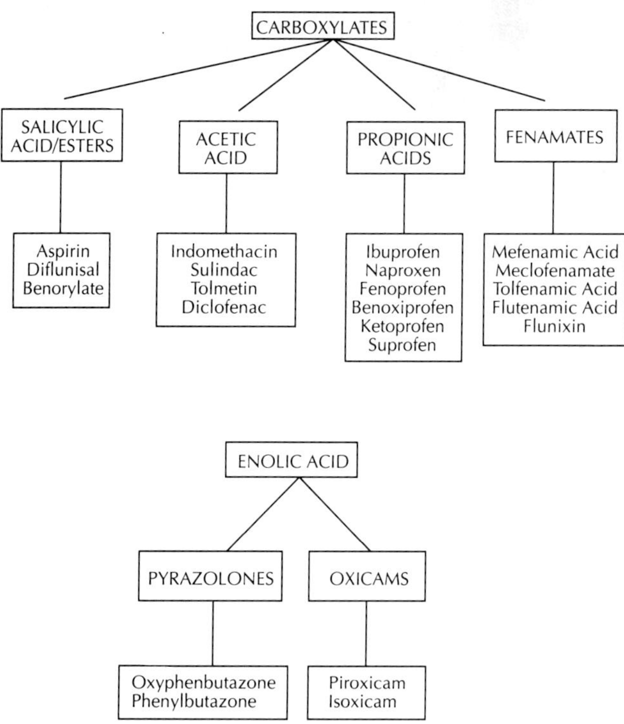


FIGURE 14.2. Nonsteroidal anti-inflammatory drugs. Adapted from Smith, RP. Drug therapy for dysmenorrhea. Ill Med J 1986; 169:22–25. Reprinted with permission.

(1) **Enolic acids.** Drugs of the enolic acid type appear to be primarily Type II inhibitors of prostaglandin synthesis. These agents act through the inhibition of the isomerase/reductase step in the formation of $PGE_2$ and $PGF_2$-alpha. The most frequently used agent in the enolic acid groups are phenylbutazone and piroxicam. Whereas phenylbutazone (Azolid, Butazolidin) is an effective short-term analgesic for musculoskeletal pain (through anti-prostaglandin activity), its relative toxicity has limited its use. Piroxicam (Feldene) has a long half-life (50 hours) that allows once a day dosage. Its action as an anti-inflammatory drug is well-established, but its use as an analgesic or for the indication of dysmenorrhea has not been fully evaluated.

(2) **Carboxylates.** It is the carboxylates that have the most day-to-day use for pain relief and dysmen-

orrhea. Within this major group there are four families of compounds that have individual characteristics. The salicylic acids and esters appear to inhibit cyclo-oxygenase by the donation of their acetyl group to the enzyme. The most recognized agent in this group, aspirin, has a low potency for reducing prostaglandin synthesis and, hence, has had little clinical utility in the treatment of moderate or severe dysmenorrhea. Increased potency is seen in the acetic acid groups. Although sulindac (Clinoril) must undergo reduction to a sulfide form before becoming active, most of the drugs in this group are effective as anti-inflammatory and analgesic agents. In several studies, indomethacin has shown usefulness in treating dysmenorrhea, but a moderate incidence of side effects has also limited the use of this and most other drugs in this class for treating dysmenorrhea.

The most commonly used drugs for dysmenorrhea come from two carboxylate classes: arylalkanoic acids (propionic acid derivatives) and anthranilic acids (fenamates).

Of the propionic acid derivatives currently available, only ibuprofen (Motrin, Rufen) and naproxen (Naprosyn, Anaprox) are approved and commonly used for this indication. Other drugs of this class (benoxiprofen, ketoprofen, fenoprofen) have been used for pain relief or arthritis therapy.

The fenamates are potent prostaglandin synthetase inhibitors, but in addition have been shown to antagonize the actions of already formed prostaglandins. In the United States, mefenamic acid (Ponstel) is approved for dysmenorrhea and clinical studies supporting the use of meclofenamate (Meclomen) are well under way. The dual action of synthesis inhibition and direct antagonism should give these agents an edge in efficacy.

b. **Drug choice.** In the majority of clinical settings, the agents most commonly employed will be mefenamic acid (Ponstel), naproxen sodium (Anaprox), and ibuprofen (Motrin, Rufen). Clinical dosages for these drugs and the other NSAI agents are shown in Table 14.3. Once an agent is selected it should be tried over the course of two to four cycles before success or failure is assessed. If therapy is unsuccessful, some patients may still have favorable responses to another NSAI drug. This second choice should be chosen from a different chemical class for the best chance of success. Patients should be reminded to take their medication at the onset of menstruation or symptoms, and maintain consistent medication for as long as symptoms would normally last if medication had not been taken.

c. **Side effects.** The physician should always be aware of the potential for side effects with any medication. Although side effects for these three medications are infrequent and generally mild, serious side effects are possible. The short duration of use in dysmenorrhea limits the risk of serious side effect. If pain relief is not complete, patients should be warned not to add additional analgesics, especially other NSAI agents, because of possible potentiation of gastrointestinal and other side effects.

2. **Drugs that suppress uterine activity.** By suppressing uterine activity, it is possible to interrupt the process by which dysmenorrhea pain is created. Drugs such as calcium antagonists (nifedipine), or spasmolytic agents (isoxsuprine, papaverine, ritodrine) may suppress uterine activity in the laboratory, but their side effects have limited clinical usefulness.

## VIII. Prognosis

Through careful evaluation of the individual patient's symptoms and physical findings, it should be possible to make the diagnosis of primary dysmenorrhea and select the most appropriate mode of therapy. When at least partial relief of the symptoms of dysmenorrhea is not achieved, serious reappraisal of the original diagnosis of primary dysmenorrhea is indicated.

## BIBLIOGRAPHY

Smith RP. The use of nonsteroidal anti-inflammatory drugs in primary dysmenorrhea. Ill Med J 1986; 169:22-25.

Stenchever MA. Dysmenorrhea and premenstrual syndrome. In: Droegemueller, Herbst, Mishell, Stenchever, eds. Comprehensive gynecology. St Louis: CV Mosby Co.; 1987; pp. 941–952.

Ylikorkala O, Dawood MY. New concepts in dysmenorrhea. Amer J Obstet Gynecol 1978; 130:833-847.

# CHAPTER 15

# Premenstrual Syndrome

**Joyce M. Vargyas**
**Frank W. Ling**

The premenstrual syndrome (PMS) is a cyclical symptom complex that begins from 5 to 11 days prior to the onset of menses, is unique to each patient in type and degree of symptoms, and disappears with the onset of menses or shortly thereafter. Another description of PMS, which resulted from a workshop at the National Institute of Mental Health in 1983, describes the syndrome as a constellation of mood, behavior, and/or physical changes that have a regular cyclical relationship to the luteal phase of the menstrual cycle, are present in most, if not all cycles, and are remitted by the end of the menstrual flow with a symptom-free interval of at least 1 week each cycle. An important aspect of all descriptions of the premenstrual syndrome is the timing of symptoms and an emphasis on a symptom-free follicular phase.

## I. Incidence and classification of PMS

A. **Incidence.** Because of the great variation in signs and symptoms, the range of reported incidences for PMS is large. The incidence of PMS is reported to vary between 20% and 90% of women. It appears that approximately 70% of women will have some physical or emotional premenstrual symptomatology that is clearly cyclic in nature. However, only approximately 20% of all women will have symptoms severe enough to interfere with daily functioning. The disease seems to be most prevalent in women from 30 to 40 years of age and is more frequently encountered in women who have a history of postpartum depression or affective illness. It also appears to be more prevalent in women who have first-degree relatives with a major depressive disorder. Women with at least one child have a higher incidence of PMS when compared to nulliparous women.

B. **Classification.** The various subgroups of PMS as described by Guy Abraham are seen in Table 15.1. There is considerable overlap between subgroups, and most women complain of more than one set of symptoms. The most commonly reported

**Table 15.1. Premenstrual Syndrome Divided into Categories According to Major Symptoms**

| PMT-A | PMT-C |
|---|---|
| Tension | Hypoglycemic episodes |
| Anxiety | Increased appetite |
| Mood swings | Headaches |
| Nervousness | Sweet cravings |
| Irritability | |
| **PMT-D** | **PMT-H** |
| Depression | Weight gain |
| Confusion | Abdominal tenderness |
| Crying | Breast tenderness |
| Forgetfulness | Swelling of extremities |

From Vargyas JM. Premenstrual syndrome in infertility. In: Mishell and Davejan, eds. Contraception and Reproductive Endocrinology. 2nd ed. Oradell, NJ: Medical Economics Books; 1986. Reprinted with permission.

symptoms are those of the PMT-A group: anxiety and irritability. Anywhere from 70% to 100% of PMS sufferers complain that this symptom complex is the most severe of those they experience. The second most common group of complaints are those of somatic origin (PMT-H). Approximately 60% of patients with PMS complain of breast tenderness, weight gain, and bloating. Symptoms associated with hypoglycemia are reported by approximately 45% to 50% of PMS sufferers and are the least frequent symptoms (PMT-D). The incidence of this is approximately 35%. The patients who do have the symptoms of severe depression are those who also have the most severe PMS in terms of incapacitation. These are the women who seem to have the highest degree of premenstrual absenteeism from work and suicidal ideation.

**II. Morbidity and mortality.** The impact of PMS is seen socially and economically both for the patient as well as work colleagues, family, and friends. There appears to be a greater absenteeism from work during the premenstrual period. Women report an inability to concentrate, a lack of interest, forgetfulness, and a lack of coordination, resulting in decreased efficiency and productivity even in those patients who do not miss any days from work. Likewise, because of irritability and emotional outbursts, working relationships become strained during the premenstrual period. The patient's spouse, significant others, and offspring will report noticeable differences in the PMS sufferer, depending on the phase of the cycle. There appears to be more frequent altercations between the patient and her spouse or significant other. Most women also report a loss of interest in sex as well as a decreased frequency of sexual intercourse during this time period. There is a loss of patience in dealing with children and likewise a decrease in nurturing. A large percentage of women with major affective illnesses report a premenstrual exacerbation of illness-related symptoms. This data is substantiated by the knowledge that there are more psychiatric hospital admissions and more suicide attempts during premenstrual phase when compared with the follicular phase. Also, women with a history of a major depressive illness are more likely to develop premenstrual symptoms even after the depressive episode has ended.

**III. Etiology and pathophysiology.** Because the symptoms of PMS are numerous and varied, and because no single etiology has been identified to explain the cause of the syndrome, several mechanisms for the pathogenesis of PMS have been described.

**A. Fluid imbalance** studies have shown that in normal women luteal phase levels of angiotensin, renin, and aldosterone are elevated when compared to the follicular phase. When patients with generalized premenstrual symptomatology are compared to controls, aldosterone levels have not been shown to be elevated. However, one study indicated that there were elevated levels of aldosterone in women with weight gain and bloating as the predominant symptomatology (PMT-H) when compared to a control population. Certainly it is possible that some of these luteal phase hormonal alterations account for a few of the symptoms of PMS, particularly those of weight gain, breast tenderness, edema, and abdominal bloating. Although studies indicate that women subjectively feel that they have gained weight, many have no measurable weight gain when evaluated on a daily basis.

**B. Elevated prostaglandin (PG) levels.** Luteal phase $PGF_2$ and $PGE_2$ have been demonstrated to be elevated in the luteal phase when compared to the follicular phase. In addition, peripheral serum metabolites of prostaglandins, prostaglandin levels in endometrium, and prostaglandin levels in menstrual fluid of dysmenorrheic patients are elevated when compared to those women with no dysmenorrhea. Nonetheless, no studies have been performed evaluating prostaglandin levels in premenstrual syndrome patients when compared to levels of prostaglandins in control patients. It is important not to confuse the diagnosis of dysmenorrhea with the diagnosis of premenstrual syndrome, although any one single patient can experience both of these problems.

**C. Nutritional imbalance.** Investigators have found that women with PMS have a higher intake of salt and refined carbohydrates and a lower intake of foods high in nutrition and vitamins than in asymptomatic women. Also, glucose tolerance tests given in the luteal phase of the cycle are flattened when compared to the follicular phase with glucose levels falling below 60 ng/mL. The symptom of sweet cravings combined with the aberrations in carbohydrate metabolism result in premenstrual hypoglycemic episodes. These episodes are thought to be correlated with crying outbursts and violent behavior.

D. **Neuroendocrine alterations.** Many of the central nervous system neurotransmitters that are altered in depression, such as serotonin, dopamine, and norepinephrine, are thought to be altered in the luteal phase of the menstrual cycle. It has been shown that progesterone has an effect on serotonin metabolism and that estradiol levels alter the turnover rate of dopamine and norepinephrine. Most of these findings have been demonstrated in the animal model and as yet have not been shown to be altered in PMS. However, the concept of varying levels of steroids affecting the neurotransmitters responsible for mood and behavior as an explanation for the cyclical emotional changes that occur throughout the menstrual cycle is promising as a model for the etiology of PMS. Central opioid activity is influenced by the fluctuating levels of gonadal steroids throughout the menstrual cycle. β-endorphin levels affect mood and behavior, and fluctuate under the influence of progesterone and estrogen. It has been reported that patients with PMS have lower-than-normal luteal phase endorphins (i.e., PMS patients have lost central opioid tonus). These complex interactions may be shown as important factors in the etiology of PMS.

E. **Unproven theories**

1. **Steroid imbalance.** The original hypothesis concerning abnormal luteal phase steroid levels as an etiological factor in PMS was based on empirically founded observations of clinical improvement in women receiving progesterone suppositories for treatment. From these findings stemmed the hypothesis that women with PMS have lower progesterone levels, higher estradiol levels, and therefore an altered $E_2$/P ratio when compared to controls. Studies of daily luteal phase steroid levels in PMS patients and controls did not substantiate this hypothesis. Two studies demonstrated a slightly lower progesterone and higher estradiol level in patients, but only on three of the premenstrual days. In one of the studies the alterations were found only in patients whose predominant symptomatology was anxiety. Symptomatology in most PMS patients has a duration of 7 to 14 days. Therefore the slight alterations on three isolated premenstrual days do not seem to serve as a pathophysiological explanation for PMS. Subsequent studies have demonstrated no alterations in luteal phase steroid levels in patients when compared to controls.
2. **Elevated prolactin level.** Many studies have been performed comparing luteal phase prolactin levels in PMS patients with those of controls. None of these studies demonstrated an elevated prolactin level in the subject group. All information thus far indicates that prolactin is not an etiological factor in any of the symptomatology of PMS.

**IV. Differential diagnosis.** Any process that results in anxiety, depression, premenstrual and menstrual discomfort, or disturbance of optimal functioning may be included in the differential diagnosis.

**A. Common differential diagnoses**

1. Situational diagnosis
2. Affective disorders
   a. Unipolar
   b. Bipolar
3. Dysmenorrhea (see Chapter 14—Pelvic Pain and Dysmenorrhea)
   a. Primary
   b. Secondary

**B. Less common differential diagnoses**

1. Psychosis
2. Eating disorders
3. Mastodynia

## V. Diagnosis

**A. Patient history**

1. **PMS.** Most important in making the diagnosis is a history of a symptom-free follicular phase in contrast to the luteal phase emotional and physical disturbances. Likewise, the following historical factors are important in diagnosing and characterizing the type and extent of the patient's premenstrual symptomatology.
   a. Age at onset of symptomatology.
   b. Number of days per cycle symptoms are experienced.
   c. Most significant symptoms.
   d. Degree of severity—social interactions, incapacitation.
   e. Variations from cycle to cycle.
   f. Symptomatology during use of oral contraceptives.
   g. Symptomatology during pregnancy.
   h. History of postpartum depression.
   i. Previous treatment for PMS.
2. **Situational depression.** Recognition of acute situational anxiety and depression related to external stress is important. Because of extensive publicity concerning PMS in the lay press, many women undergoing major life transitions relate emotional liability to PMS rather than facing the problems confronting them. Careful questioning concerning marital or relationship problems, occupational changes, or recent childbirth or child-rearing difficulties must be elicited in the history. If a positive response to any of the questions is obtained and the onset of symptoms coincides in time with the onset of the premenstrual symptomatology, the diagnosis of an adjustment disorder may be made. However, it must be noted that PMS may coexist with an adjustment disorder.

3. **Affective disorders** may be suspected based on thorough history taking. A past history of psychotherapy, use of psychotropic medications, psychiatric hospitalizations, or suicide attempts are important factors in making the diagnosis. A family history of any of the above problems is also critical because of the genetic basis for many of these disorders. Note that women with psychiatric disorders most often have premenstrual exacerbations of their symptomatology and therefore may have the concurrent diagnoses of PMS and an underlying affective disorder. An accurate determination of the extent of each of the problems is important for proper treatment to be initiated.
4. **Dysmenorrhea.** Many women misinterpret the term PMS for menstrual discomfort and cramping. Women who have dysmenorrhea and symptoms related to prostaglandin release such as low back pain, nausea, diarrhea, and anterior thigh pain a few days immediately prior to menses and during menses without the luteal phase emotional changes may simply have primary or secondary dysmenorrhea. This differential diagnosis can be made by routine questioning concerning the most predominant symptomatology experienced.
5. **Mastodynia.** Similar to the isolated diagnosis of dysmenorrhea, premenstrual breast tenderness and engorgement may be the predominant symptomatology experienced without the cyclic mood swings. This diagnosis may be elicited upon history taking.
6. **Eating disorders.** Approximately 15% of high school and college women have an eating disorder such as bulimia or anorexia nervosa. Often they request diuretics, complaining of premenstrual weight gain and bloating despite an actual weight that is significantly lower than average for their height. If there is a large discrepancy between perceived body image and actual weight coupled with a history of compulsive dieting, extensive use of diuretics and laxatives, or a history of food binging and vomiting, then this diagnosis must be considered. However, the diagnosis of an eating disorder may be separate or in conjunction with the diagnosis of PMS.

B. **Physical examination.** There is no specific physical finding to aid in the diagnosis of PMS. A complete routine physical examination is necessary for all new gynecological patients and may help in determining organic causes of secondary dysmenorrhea and chronic pelvic pain. Breast tenderness may be found if the examination is performed in the luteal phase.

C. **Testing**

1. **PMS symptomatology questionnaire.** The single most important step in assessment and evaluation of PMS is the use of a **self-rated prospective daily diary of symptoms.** Retrospective reporting has been shown to be inaccurate and

unreliable. The patient must complete on a daily basis a form that enables her to report symptoms throughout the entire cycle. An example of such a form is seen in Figure 15.1.

a. **Procedure.** The patient rates the severity of each symptom she experiences from 0 to 3 (none to severe), beginning with the first day of menses. Bleeding is charted to indicate the onset and duration of the menstrual flow. An initial morning temperature may be taken and graphed on a basal body temperature chart to determine when ovulation occurs. This enables the physician to tabulate a "luteal phase score" in comparison to a "follicular phase score." A daily weight is charted to determine if premenstrual weight gain does occur. Likewise the occurrence and severity of dysmenorrhea is recorded.

b. **Interpretation.** It may be necessary to have the patient complete two cycles prior to diagnosing or categorizing the nature and severity of the individual's problem because of cycle-to-cycle variations in symptomatology. The baseline forms may be used for both initial assessment of the disease process and the response to therapeutic measures.

   (1) **The suspected diagnosis of PMS is confirmed** if other previously mentioned disorders are ruled out and if the patient has a significant increase in symptomatology during the luteal phase. Most patients have essentially little or no symptomatology during the follicular phase. A "total luteal phase score" and a "total follicular phase score" may be obtained by adding total daily scores in each phase of the cycle, excluding the menstrual days that are usually high because of extensive physical symptomatology. Most often in PMS subjects, the total luteal phase score will be three to six times higher than the follicular phase score.

   (2) **If the patient reports a significant degree of symptomatology throughout the menstrual cycle,** it is necessary to look for etiological factors unrelated to PMS as previously described in the differential diagnosis. The predominant type of symptom complex can be evaluated from detailed examination of the diary. There is most often a significant degree of overlap between subgroups. Nevertheless many patients will have a tendency to score highest on those symptoms relating to anxiety such as irritability, tension, and irrational behavior. Others will tend to rate themselves higher on symptoms relating to depression such as decreased self-esteem, confusion, and fatigue.

Many patients will simply report those symptoms relating to water retention or others will have symptoms related to prostaglandin release such as headache and dysmenorrhea. Although somewhat simplistic and tedious, a clustering of symptom complexes is useful in determining the best treatment modality for the patient.

2. **Psychiatric evaluation.** If an underlying chronic emotional disorder is suspected from either the history or a high follicular phase score, psychological or psychiatric assessment is warranted. Optimally, the patient should be referred to a psychiatrist for an open-ended interview. Psychological testing may be used in conjunction with the interview and the type of test used is based on the individual preference of the examiner. Commonly used standardized tests include the Beck's Depression Scale, The Hamilton Anxiety Rating Scale, and the Structured Clinical Interview for the Diagnostic and Statistical Manual of Mental Disorders, 3rd ed., revised. The interpretation of the results is most meaningful if administered both in the follicular and luteal phase of the cycle.

VI. **Treatment.** Because the presentation of PMS is diverse and because no single treatment modality has been shown to work for all patients, the therapeutic approach must be individualized, depending on the type and severity of the patient's symptomatology and her response to therapy.

A. **Conservative measures.** The initial management of the PMS patient should consist of supportive and educational steps without the use of medications. Thirty percent of patients diagnosed as having PMS will respond well to this treatment. Those who do not may be treated with regimens supplemented with medication chosen to reduce the most disturbing symptoms not improved by conservative treatment.

1. **Support.** Reassurance from the physician has been found to be most helpful. It is imperative to let the patient know that her problems are not uncommon and that measures will be taken to try to improve her quality of life.

2. **Education.** Daily charting of symptomatology will help the patient identify more clearly the most troublesome symptomatology and the days of the cycle when symptoms are most severe. Monitoring daily symptoms also helps the patient obtain a degree of control in her life. Coping measures may be used by avoiding destructive or difficult social interactions and, if possible, avoiding major decision making.

3. **Diet**

a. **Salt.** The patient should be instructed to reduce her salt intake. This should decrease some of the water retention-related symptomatology. The discomfort from

Name ______________________ Age: _______ Height: _______ Weight: _______

Grading of Menses

0 - None
1 - Slight
2 - Moderate
3 - Heavy
4 - Heavy and clots

Grading of Symptoms (complaints)

0 - None
1 - Mild, present but does not interfere with activities
2 - Moderate, present and interferes with activities but not disabling
3 - Severe, disabling, unable to function

| DAY OF CYCLE | 1 | 2 | 3 | 4 | 5 | 6 | 7 | 8 | 9 | 10 | 11 | 12 | 13 | 14 | 15 | 16 | 17 | 18 | 19 | 20 | 21 | 22 | 23 | 24 | 25 | 26 | 27 | 28 | 29 | 30 | 31 | 32 | 33 | 34 | 35 | 36 |
|---|---|---|---|---|---|---|---|---|---|---|---|---|---|---|---|---|---|---|---|---|---|---|---|---|---|---|---|---|---|---|---|---|---|---|---|---|
| Date | | | | | | | | | | | | | | | | | | | | | | | | | | | | | | | | | | | | |
| Menses | | | | | | | | | | | | | | | | | | | | | | | | | | | | | | | | | | | | |

PMT-A

| | | | | | | | | | | | | | | | | | | | | | | | | | | | | | | | | | | | | |
|---|---|---|---|---|---|---|---|---|---|---|---|---|---|---|---|---|---|---|---|---|---|---|---|---|---|---|---|---|---|---|---|---|---|---|---|---|
| Nervous tension | | | | | | | | | | | | | | | | | | | | | | | | | | | | | | | | | | | | |
| Mood swings | | | | | | | | | | | | | | | | | | | | | | | | | | | | | | | | | | | | |
| Irritability | | | | | | | | | | | | | | | | | | | | | | | | | | | | | | | | | | | | |
| Anxiety | | | | | | | | | | | | | | | | | | | | | | | | | | | | | | | | | | | | |

PMT-H

| | | | | | | | | | | | | | | | | | | | | | | | | | | | | | | | | | | | | |
|---|---|---|---|---|---|---|---|---|---|---|---|---|---|---|---|---|---|---|---|---|---|---|---|---|---|---|---|---|---|---|---|---|---|---|---|---|
| Weight gain | | | | | | | | | | | | | | | | | | | | | | | | | | | | | | | | | | | | |
| Swelling of extremities | | | | | | | | | | | | | | | | | | | | | | | | | | | | | | | | | | | | |
| Breast tenderness | | | | | | | | | | | | | | | | | | | | | | | | | | | | | | | | | | | | |
| Abdominal bloating | | | | | | | | | | | | | | | | | | | | | | | | | | | | | | | | | | | | |

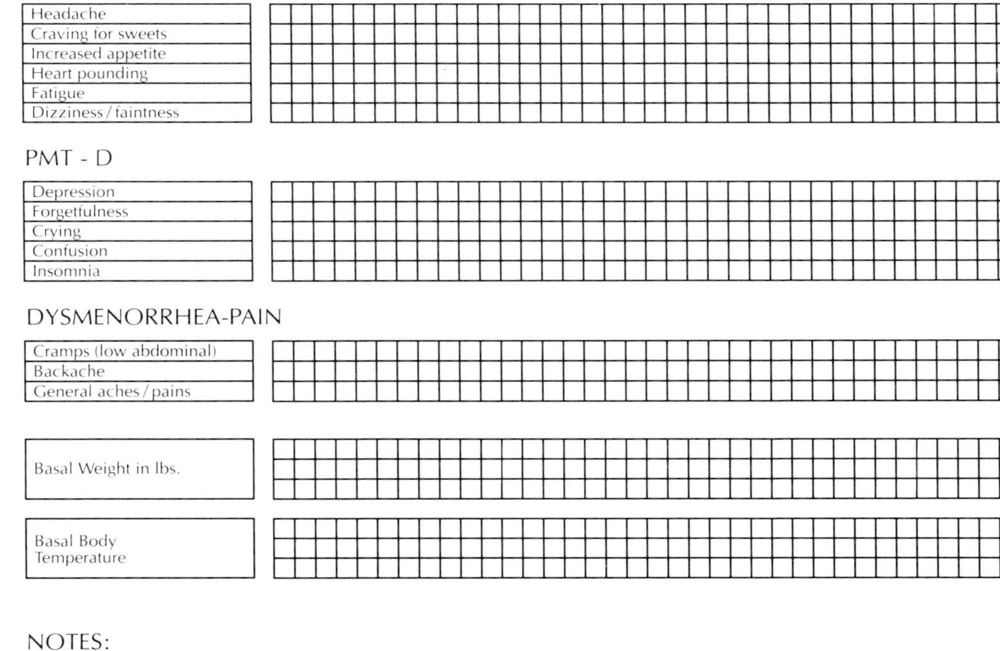

PMT - C

Headache
Craving for sweets
Increased appetite
Heart pounding
Fatigue
Dizziness / faintness

PMT - D

Depression
Forgetfulness
Crying
Confusion
Insomnia

DYSMENORRHEA-PAIN

Cramps (low abdominal)
Backache
General aches / pains

Basal Weight in lbs.

Basal Body Temperature

NOTES:

FIGURE 15.1. Premenstrual syndrome symptomatology questionnaire. Adapted from Vargyas JM. Premenstrual syndrome. In: Mishell DR, Jr., and Davajan V, eds. Infertility, Contraception and Reproductive Endocrinology, Second Edition, 1986, p. 354. Reprinted by permission of Blackwell Scientific Publications, Inc., Cambridge, Mass.

bloating and edema, and concerns about weight gain also affect her emotional liability.

b. **Refined sugar.** Foods containing refined sugar should likewise be reduced to attempt to decrease the reactive hypoglycemia secondary to altered carbohydrate metabolism. This restriction may likewise decrease mood swings.

c. **Caffeine** in the diet should also be minimized to avoid physical and emotional manifestations. Education as to foods with caffeine should be included (coffee, chocolate, soft drinks, and some medications).

4. **Exercise.** The patient should be instructed to follow a regular exercise routine with some aerobic activity included in the regimen. The type of activity chosen is based on personal preference. The advantages of exercise for the PMS patient are numerous. Stress reduction and increased self-esteem are apparent. The transient but significant increase in central β-endorphin levels may be helpful for mood elevation.

5. **Vitamin $B_6$** (pyridoxine) supplementation may be added to the diet. Three hundred to 500 mg daily in oral preparation is recommended based on the studies performed thus far. Peripheral neuropathy has been reported at levels over 1500 mg/d. Therefore the patient must be instructed that this is not a completely benign medication. The neuropathy is reversible upon discontinuation of the medication.

B. **Diuretics.** If the patient still has significant symptoms of water retention despite dietary salt restrictions, oral diuretics may be prescribed with instruction to be used only as needed.

1. Hydrochlorothiazide, 25 mg to 50 mg with potassium supplementation.
2. Dyazide (hydrochlorothiazide 25 mg/triamterene 50 mg), daily without the need for potassium supplementation.
3. Spironolactone, 25 mg twice to three times daily.

C. **Prostaglandin inhibitors** can be given to those patients with significant premenstrual and menstrual pain including headache, cramping, low back pain, breast tenderness, and generalized discomfort. Any one of the many available prostaglandin inhibitor products may be used for patients using adequate birth control measures (see Chapter 14—Primary Dysmenorrhea section, IV-A). The prostaglandin inhibitors are contraindicated in women who have a history of gastritis or peptic ulcer disease. The medication should be taken only as needed. Taking the medication with meals helps to avoid gastric irritation.

D. **Anxiolytics.** In patients who are unresponsive to conservative measures and who have a significant degree of premenstrual anxiety and irritability, newer short-acting antianxiety agents may be prescribed.

1. Buspirone is a nonsedating, nonaddictive serotonergic an-

xiolytic which, in higher doses, may have antidepressant effects. The initial dose is 5 mg t.i.d. with meals. Effects of the medication are not apparent for 10 to 14 days.

2. Alprazolam is efficacious in the treatment of anxiety. It has some antidepressant effects as well. The initial dose is 0.25 mg twice or three times daily. The medication should only be given on the days before menses when the patient is symptomatic according to previously recorded symptom records. The patient may take half the premenstrual dose during the first 2 days of menses if needed.

E. **Antidepressants.** Patients who are unresponsive to the above measures and have a significant degree of premenstrual depression may be **referred to a psychiatrist for antidepressant medication and supportive therapy.** Many of these patients have some degree of follicular phase symptomatology as well. The patients must take the medication on a daily basis and beneficial effects are usually realized 2 to 3 weeks after initiation of treatment. Continued contact and support with the primary referring physician is beneficial but because of a significant degree of side effects the administration of the antidepressant medication should be monitored by a psychiatrist.

F. **Progesterone.** All double-blind placebo-controlled crossover trials have shown progesterone suppositories to be no more effective than placebo in the treatment of PMS. Although this therapy has been popular based on published retrospective case reports, there are currently no scientific data to support this treatment. Vaginal or rectal suppositories of 50 to 200 g during the luteal phase have been reported useful in some patients. Studies using Provera (medroxyprogesterone acetate) have not demonstrated relief of symptoms with this form of therapy.

G. **Gonadotropin-releasing hormone agonists.** Newly available agonists that ablate hormonal fluctuations have been noted to be useful for both emotional and physical symptoms. Short-term side effects such as hot flashes have been successfully managed with estrogen replacement therapy without the return of PMS symptoms. Data on long-term therapy are not available and concerns of potential osteoporosis and other problems must be considered.

VII. **Prognosis.** Most patients referred for symptoms of premenstrual syndrome will show improvement if appropriate measures are taken. A thorough assessment process with careful attention to the differential diagnosis of those patients presenting with PMS will result in appropriate and successful treatment for many women who have been misdiagnosed. With the use of conservative measures and the addition of medication when necessary, most women with PMS will show a significant improvement in their symptoms and quality of life.

## BIBLIOGRAPHY


Abraham GE. Premenstrual tension. Current Problems in Obstet Gynecol 1980; 3:12.

Andersch B, Hahn L, Andersson M, Isaksson B. Body water and weight in patients with premenstrual tension. Br J Obstet Gynaecol 1978; 85:546.

Backstrom T, Carstensen H. Estrogen and progesterone in plasma in relation to premenstrual tension. J Ster Biochem 1974; 5:257.

Golub LJ, Menduhe H, Conly SS. Weight changes in college women during the menstrual cycle. Am J Obstet Gynecol 1965; 91:89.

Halbreich U, Endicott J. Possible involvement of endorphin withdrawal or imbalance in specific premenstrual syndromes and postpartum depression. Med Hypoth 1981; 7:1045.

Katz FH, Romjh P. Plasma aldosterone and renin activity during the menstrual cycle. J Clin Endocrinol Metab 1972; 34:819.

Maddocks S, Hahn P, Moller F, Reid RL. A double-blind placebo-controlled trial of progesterone vaginal suppositories in the treatment of premenstrual syndrome. Am J Obstet Gynecol 1986; 154:573.

Mechelahis AM, Yoshida H, Dormis JC. Plasma renin activity and plasma aldosterone during the normal menstrual cycle. Am J Obstet Gynecol 1975; 123:724.

O'Brien PM, Craven D, Selby C, Symonds EM. Treatment of premenstrual syndrome by spironolactone. Br J Obstet Gynaecol 1979; 86:142.

Reid RL, Yen SSC. Premenstrual syndrome. Am J Obstet Gynecol 1981; 139:85.

Sampson GA. Premenstrual syndrome: A double-blind controlled trial of progesterone and placebo. Brit J Psychiat 1979; 135:209.

Vargyas JM. The use of progesterone in the premenstrual syndrome. Abstract presented at the annual meeting of the American Fertility Society, Chicago, Ill, September, 1985.

Wardlow SL, Wehrenberg WB, Kerin N, Autunes JL, Franty AG. Effects of sex steroids on endorphin in hypophyseal portal blood. J Clin Endocrinol Metab 1982; 55:877.

Wood D. The treatment of premenstrual syndrome symptoms with mefenamic acid. Br J Obstet Gynaecol 1982; 87:306.

# CHAPTER 16

# Sexual Problems

**Domeena Renshaw**

Sexual dysfunctions are impaired, incomplete, or absent expressions of normally recurrent sexual desires and responses.

**I. Normal sexual physiology and sexual response.** At any age, from in utero to the senium, the definition of orgasm relates to a build-up of general and genital vasoneuromuscular tensions. In both men and women, temperature, heart rate, breathing, and blood pressure all increase to a peak with orgasm, then subside with pleasurable relaxation. In women the clitoris becomes erect and the vagina lubricates by transudation; in men, the penis becomes erect, pre-ejaculatory emission occurs, and then there is an ejaculation (5 cc) of semen (sperm, prostatic, and seminal vesicle fluids). During orgasm there is a sudden discharge of tensions, tonic-clonic muscle contractions of all large and small muscles of the body (including the pubococcygeus) followed by a return to the pre-excitement state. The stimulus may be oneself (masturbation or fantasy), another person (same or opposite sex), or another species (animal) the latter being rare. In their 1979 comparative study, Masters and Johnson found no consistent differences in the sexual responses of heterosexual and homosexual women and men. It must be emphasized that for the male and female, the phases of the sexual responses are similar, but the average timing of the cycle is fourfold longer for women (Fig. 16.1). This information allows the anorgasmic woman to be patient with herself as she learns her own responses and also the timing difference explains why only 20% to 30% of women attain a coital climax. The clitoris is the analog of the penis and has lateral crural roots attached to the pelvic arch where the periosteum has vibratory end organs that respond well to a pulsating shower or a vibrator. Unlike the penis, the clitoris has neither reproductive nor urinary function. It is purely for sexual arousal. A woman and her physician need to realize this basic information. A climax always involves both clitoris and vagina, whether the stimulus is directly on the clitoris or indirectly by a pulley action of the labial attachments stimulating the clitoris and crurae during coitus. The sen-

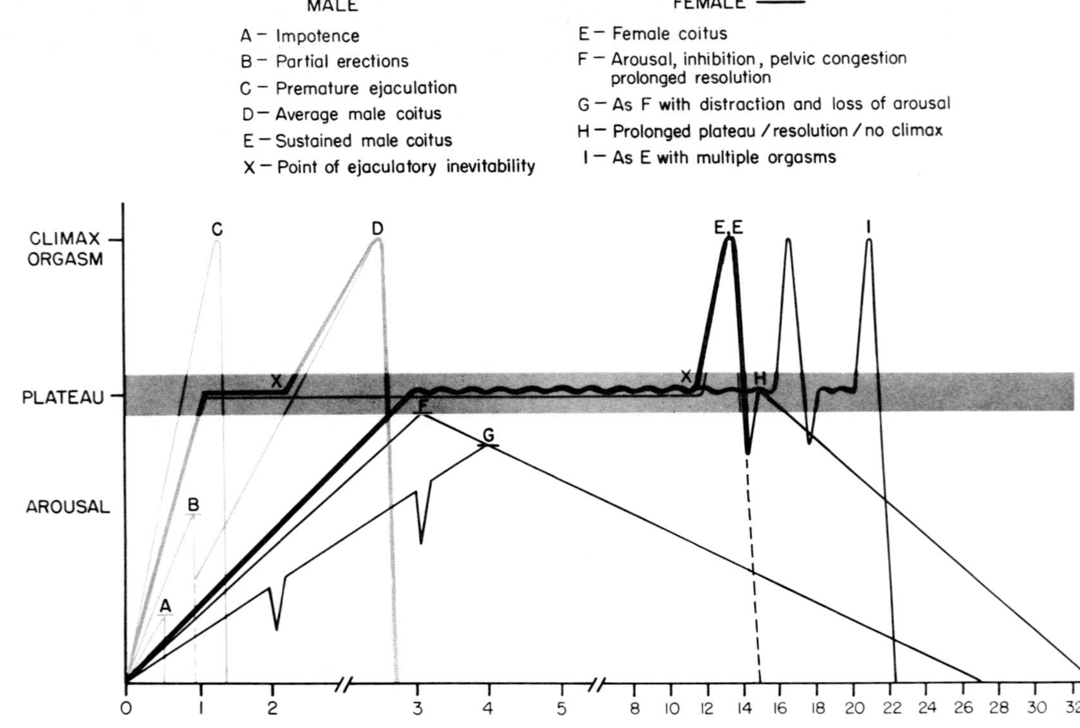


FIGURE 16.1. Comparison of the sexual response cycle in males and females.

sations will, of course, differ with coitus and partner closeness but the physiological end result of a climax is the final relaxation whatever the mode. One climax is not "better or worse" than another, they only differ. The sensationalized Grafenberg spot ("G-spot") is as yet histologically unsubstantiated as a separate organ or area of prostatic-like tissue. Grafenberg wrote that this area at the trigone of the bladder was erogenous and when stimulated digitally, caused copious vaginal secretions and orgasms. It is still controversial.

## II. Sexual dysfunction

A. **Incidence.** Sexual questions or problems perplex every developing boy, girl, teen, and adult. "Am I sexually normal?" is perhaps the most common concern about the sexual self, feelings, and behaviors. Few find answers to these questions at home. Only rarely do school programs and textbooks provide an accurate sex education beyond the menstrual cycle. Many sexual inaccuracies and myths are learned from peers, x-rated magazines, cable TV, and video cassettes. From these, a new set of concerns results: "What's wrong with me?" (that I am celibate or not an Olympic sexual athlete as portrayed on the screen). The gynecologist can play a valuable role as the medical authority to assist a patient to sort out fact and fantasy. Basic accurate sexual information and reassurance may be all that is required. A sexual dysfunction may exist (by estimate) in about 50% of marriages. When difficulties with pleasurable climactic resolution of appropriate sexual arousal occur, they may be accepted as transient or become problematic when there is subjective concern or discomfort. In some cases partner dissatisfaction may for the first time precipitate awareness of a dysfunction in a previously accepting individual (e.g., premature ejaculation, anorgasmia, or sexual apathy). Because of changing social attitudes, sexually active single women or men may as readily consult a physician for a sexual problem as their married peers. There are no statistics on the incidence of sexual dysfunction in single adults of either sex.

B. **Morbidity and mortality.** The personal and social morbidity of sexual problems and dysfunction is high. Mortality, however, is rare. Only when a woman feels desperate about attaining sexual release and/or satisfying her partner may she threaten, attempt, or succeed at suicide. Her suicidal statement should not be trivialized and will need psychiatric consultation.

C. **Etiology**

1. **Physical causes.** The physical problems that can cause sexual dysfunction are multiple. Important specific causes include:

    a. **Intact hymen.** Despite 2 decades of tampon advertising, there are women who do not use them. Some of these women present with dyspareunia or vaginismus and are unaware that they have an intact hymen. Both the woman and her husband/partner may on occasion not know this fact. Physical examination will quickly make the diagnosis. Use of a mirror during the physical examination is helpful to educate the patient and her partner by visualizing the hymen, and is an important part of their sex therapy. Hymenectomy is indicated, especially to allow an unconsummated marriage to come to coitus.

b. **Vaginitis**
   (1) Infectious vaginitis may cause itching, discomfort, or concern about hygiene and may present as transient dyspareunia or sexual avoidance. Medical therapy specific to the infection is indicated and may be concurrent with necessary sex education.
   (2) Atrophic vaginitis caused by estrogen deficiency may occur with natural or surgical menopause. Because of an absence of vaginal lubrication in these patients, there may be acute coital pain on entry and with the friction of intercourse, "it hurts like a knife" may be the woman's complaint. Pelvic examination will usually confirm the diagnosis. Estrogen replacement therapy is indicated in most cases along with sex education and the use of lubricants for coitus (for example, KY Jelly®, saline, or baby/mineral oil).

c. **Endometriosis** may present as dyspareunia, although some women may adapt to the cyclic discomfort. Upon diagnosis, based on physical examination and usually laparoscopy, medical treatment, danocrine (Danazol) or gonadotropin-releasing hormone agonist is often used, especially in childless patients. This treatment may result in atrophic vaginitis and dyspareunia. Patients should be warned and advised to use abundant lubrication for coitus, and/or change coital position.

d. **Congenital abnormalities.** Agenesis of the vagina may present as "vaginismus" as the patient confuses her sensations to be of vaginal origin when it is perineal pain. Other symptoms may cause special problems, such as the patient with a complaint of dyspareunia and found to have a double vagina.

e. **Endocrine abnormalities**
   (1) **Hypothyroidism** may present with loss of libido in addition to classic signs and symptoms such as weight gain, dry skin, and hair loss. Whether the restored libido upon thyroid replacement therapy may be related to weight loss and general energy return is uncertain, but it is notable in most patients.
   (2) **Hyperprolactinemia,** with or without associated hypothyroidism, may present with lowered libido,

galactorrhea, and infertility. With appropriate evaluation and therapy utilizing bromoergocriptine mesylate, galactorrhea is suppressed and libido is usually restored as the serum prolactin level is reduced.

f. **Side effects of medications.** Many medications may cause lowered libido and/or orgasmic difficulties so that the clinician who takes a careful sexual and medical history may be able to make the chronological connections even when such a connection is not evident to the patient. Specific medications have been known to have reversible, negative impact on sexuality: antihypertensive, psychotropic, antipsychotic, antidepressant, and antianxiety medications are especially prone to such effects. In some cases the patient's physician may alter the drug and/or dosages or time of administration to improve sexual function while maintaining the needed drug's therapeutic effects. Other approaches include brief sexual counseling such as advising "loveplay" before an evening or morning dosage of medication to take advantage of the time when the blood level of the drug is lowest. Most of all, discussing the medication associated sexual problem with a patient will give relief from self-blame. In addition, the patient can develop a good adaptation to and compliance with her required medical regimen.

2. **Psychologic and social causes.** There are many intrapsychic and interpersonal factors that may impede pleasureable sexual exchange: fear of pain or inflicting it; fear of pregnancy or impregnation; fear of contracting or transmitting infection, acquired immunodeficiency syndrome (AIDS), or cancer; and fear of performance failure or of being ridiculed or rejected. Most may be unfounded or overemphasized, but all require discussion to diffuse their negative effects. Early traumatic sexual experiences may also be troublesome, ranging from discovery of and punishment for normal masturbation to childhood sexual abuse and/or teen or adult rape (inside or outside of marriage). If the patient is a minor, sexual abuse or attempted abuse must be reported to child protection authority by Federal mandate (not required if the patient is of age).

   Three basic questions may greatly assist the clinician in evaluating such problems:

   a. Did you have any sexual experience that was upsetting to you at any age? If yes, discuss the details.
   b. How did you handle it at the time?
   c. How much does it affect you now?

**D. Pathogenesis.** All people may be born with similar genital apparatus, but capacities to be aroused and to respond differ. These capacities depend on intact central nervous system, peripheral and autonomic nerves, plus muscles, blood vessels, and end organs. Additional factors include each person's personality, early and current life experiences as well as the response to internal and external erotic stimuli: pleasurable, painful, or conflictual.

## III. Sexual problems or questions brought to physicians

A. **Anorgasmia.** Failure to achieve orgasm is a common complaint. Some women are unsure whether they are orgasmic, especially if a different or excessive body response is expected. The gynecologist's explicit questions can determine whether a woman is truly anorgasmic and simultaneously be educational for the patient: What happens to your breathing? Your heart rate? Your body muscles? Do you feel a change in the clitoris and the vagina? Do you feel small contractions involuntarily in the whole body and lower vagina and then total body relaxation? If she is uncertain, then suggest that she check herself, read one of the self-help books (see bibliography), and ask again on her next visit. This approach gives dignity to her question and accurate medical information. Proper charting of the problem of the anorgasmia complaint is important. In addition, suggested home masturbatory activities help the patient gain important insight, and self-help reading allows for the accurate collection of appropriate medical information.

B. **Orgasm during sleep.** Like men, women can have an orgasm during sleep. During Rapid Eye Movement (REM) sleep, women of all ages, like men, have normal sexual arousal, accompanied by rapid breathing, increased heart rate, clitoral engorgement, and vaginal lubrication (erections and occasional nocturnal emissions for men), raised blood pressure, an orgasm, and then relaxation. At times, there is a remembered sexual dream. Sleep is unconscious and uninhibited by daytime controls. The woman who is concerned by this phenomenon can be reassured she is quite normal. Also, the report is prognostically good in an anorgasmic woman because if she can have an orgasm in sleep, she will soon attain a conscious climax.

C. **Climax during vaginal delivery.** This is not common, but possible, and normal with pudendal nerve stimulation.

D. **Sexual arousal or climax during breast-feeding.** This is a normal undifferentiated nipple reflex orgasmic response that may occur even with a breast pump. With high levels of prolactin, some lactating women report a transient sexual apathy.

E. **Intercourse or orgasms during pregnancy.** Both intercourse and orgasms during pregnancy are fine unless there is vaginal bleeding or premature rupture of membranes that are contraindications to intercourse.

F. **Resuming intercourse after delivery.** This should be possible when the genital area has healed. A pelvic exam should be done before intercourse is resumed.

G. **Feeling depressed and apathetic sexually.** Clinical depression causes insomnia, crying, sadness, and decrease in appetite for food, sex, and life, lasting 3 to 6 weeks or more. It responds well to the use of a single bedtime dose of tricyclic antidepressants (doxepin hydrochloride [Sinequan], 25 to 125 mg p.o. daily in divided doses; amitriptyline hydrochloride [Elavil], 25 to 125 mg p.o. daily in divided doses) used for about 6 weeks or until the depression lifts. When antidepressants are used properly, hypnotics are unnecessary and are contraindicated because of their potential for creating dependency and chemically aggravating a depression.

H. **Posthysterectomy sexual changes.** If the ovaries are not removed at the time of hysterectomy, the presurgery sexual pattern should continue or even improve if, for example, there were pregnancy fears or dyspareunia. Because there are myths that women become fat and sexless after the uterus is removed, patients who undergo hysterectomy benefit from preoperative counseling and assurance that their femininity and desirability will not be altered, that the vagina will remain receptive and elastic, and that excessive weight gain will occur only if overeating and/or underactivity follow the surgery.

I. **Painful orgasms with an intrauterine device (IUD).** A minority of women with IUDs have complained of painful orgasm. This is the result of uterine contractions on the inserted IUD during a climax. Removal of the IUD relieves the symptom.

J. **Sexual apathy.** If no physical (endocrine—pituitary or thyroid) cause of sexual apathy can be found, then anorgasmia, which may produce the attitude of "there's nothing in sex for me," should be investigated. Questions about masturbatory frequency, marital or relationship conflict, medications, alcohol or drug abuse, and if there are other partners (selective apathy) should also be asked.

K. **Sexual expression** is the only instinct where deliberate, sustained control or even complete suppression does not result in a threat to the life of the individual, as would cutting off breathing, eating, sleeping, elimination, or circulation. Celibacy, for example, is a normal choice. When **"loss of desire" (HSD or hypoactive sexual desire)** is the presenting complaint, it is important to carefully differentiate preferred abstinence from selective nonfunction with a particular partner, while desire for sexual relations with another partner or alone (masturbation) continues.

## IV. Diagnosis

### A. Signs and symptoms (DSM-III-R diagnoses)

1. **Hypoactive sexual desire (302.71):** Taking into account age, health and context of the woman's life and whether she or her partner perceives the lack of desire as a source of distress.

2. **Female sexual arousal disorder (302.72):** Partial or complete failure despite adequate focus, intensity, and duration (in the absence of organic factors) to attain or maintain vaginal lubrication and clitoral dilation–response until completion of the sex act.
3. **Inhibited female orgasm (302.73):** Recurrent and persistent inhibition (not due to organic cause) manifested by a delay in or absence of orgasm following a normal sexual excitement phase of adequate focus, intensity, and duration.
4. **Functional dyspareunia (302.76):** Coitus associated with recurrent and persistent genital pain not caused exclusively by a physical disorder.
5. **Functional vaginismus (306.51):** Recurrent and persistent involuntary spasms of the pubococcygeus musculature of the outer third of the vagina (not caused by a physical disorder) that interfere with coitus.
6. **Sexual aversion disorder (302.79):** Persistent or recurrent extreme aversion to, and avoidance of almost all genital contact with a sexual partner. There is often high concomitant physiological anxiety.
7. **Atypical psychosexual dysfunction (302.70):** Sexual dysfunctions not included in other classifications, for example no erotic sensations or complete anesthesia despite physical evidence of sexual excitement or orgasm, extremely rapid achievement of orgasm, etc.

**B. Physical examination**

1. **Physical examination.** A complete general physical examination including a complete genital examination is an essential aspect of the evaluation of a woman complaining of a sexual dysfunction.
2. **Sexological examination.** In addition, an educational sexological examination is done, with the nurse chaperone present and her partner (if she consents to his being there). It is bonding to a couple to gain the body knowledge with the physician authority giving permission to look and understand. The woman's index finger is placed on her clitoris, then her husband's or partner's finger over hers, which she removes so he also can feel the clitoris. He stays for the pelvic and speculum examination, which the woman watches with the head of the table elevated while she holds a hand mirror so she may see each step. The perineal and genital sensations supplied by the pudendal nerves, the circular pubococcygeus muscles of the lower vagina (instruct her to contract tightly then relax), the mucosa, lubrication, cervix and so on are all explained. This is a highly professional medical examination with educational dialogue and documentation that it was done including the name of the nurse attendant. At no time is the sexological exam to be an exercise of sexual stimulation in the office. Therefore, the physician's request for her partner's presence, the use of a nurse chaperone, and the placement of the patient's own

finger, then the partner's, on the clitoris are all essentials for standard ethical practice. Arousal is only appropriate in the privacy of the patient's own home and is prescribed by the gynecologist as standard home sex therapy.

C. **Lab studies.** Those studies clinically indicated on the basis of the physical examination should be performed.

## V. Management

### A. Therapy

1. An explicit general health and sexual history face-to-face from each partner separately is optimal. However, a written history sheet can be completed by the woman and her sexual partner (if she has one), before the next visit if there is not sufficient time for an oral history during the patient's initial visit.
2. A thorough physical examination including a sexological examination (for sex education) should be conducted.
3. If the clinician perceives from the history or the physical examination, a possible cause or connection between the sexual symptoms and an earlier experience, this should be explained to the patient as part of her sexual counseling. For example, "Since your unplanned third pregnancy, there seems to be sexual avoidance; Is that correct?" Another example, "Childbirth, pain, and even death seemed to have been recurrent themes when you were little. Is it possible that this relates to your present fear of pregnancy and intercourse?"
4. Reassure the patient that the sexual problem is potentially reversible after the physical examination has been completed.
5. Direct the patient and her partner to self-help reading (see the Self-Help Reading List of this chapter). Sensate Focus exercises are a major part of standard sex therapy to be done at home, and allow partners to concentrate first on relaxed sensual closeness rather than sexual contact. Light or firm touch pleasuring explores the entire skin (with the exception of breasts and genitals) and directs attention away from performing sexually. This (paradoxically) is often highly sexually stimulating. The couple or the solo woman can often proceed at home to subsequent steps in Sensate Focus activities, namely genital massage.
6. Sexual fantasy is an essential part of normal arousal. The patient is encouraged to think of romantic/arousing books, movies, or courtship experiences while doing the home loveplay. This is a essential to sexual arousal.
7. Follow-up should occur every 1 or 2 weeks for five or six office visits to supervise and direct the couple or solo patient. Explain that about 80% of sexual dysfunctions improve when such techniques are used. If appropriate time and effort have not been taken to do the home exercises, discussion should be held with the patient or couple to

determine why the avoidance, and rectify the problem so that home exercises can continue.

8. Refer the patient to a reputable sex clinic for more intensive therapy, if her sex problem does not respond to the outlined therapy within six visits.
9. Refer the patient or couple for marital counseling if there are marked relationship frictions preventing cooperative sex therapy or if there are residual issues after the sex symptom is reversed.
10. Meet with a colleague as a male–female team for a complex case or talk it over with a colleague in consultation.

B. **Specific therapy for functional vaginismus.** Functional vaginismus (recurrent and persistent involuntary spasms of the musculature of the outer third of the vagina) not caused by a physical disorder that interferes with coitus may be the cause of a marriage or relationship being unconsummated. These are challenging cases and may be tenaciously resistant to therapy. Reassure and encourage the patient by telling her, "I will be patient, this may take five or six visits for you to relax to complete your pelvic examination. I cannot go further or faster than you can go, but I will stand by you all the way—." A preferred technique is to have the woman patient in stirrups and tell her first to tightly contract (paradoxical intention) the pubococcygeus muscle. "Tight, tighter—Is that the best you can do? Close your eyes tight; purse up your mouth; tighten the rectum; now the lower vagina tight. Great! Now relax. Take a long deep breath in—hold it in to the slow count of four. Now open your mouth and breathe out to the slow count of four. Relax—" (This is an anti-Valsalva maneuver). On the exhalation insert a single lubricated finger. "Now tighten again!!" There is usually surprise. On the next open mouth exhalation, one can insert two fingers, then a child-size speculum.

Sometimes the patient is anxious, clammy, sweating, hyperventilating, or crying. Reassure and instruct her, and sometimes her partner too, in deep slow breathing and relaxation because the partner may be more upset than the patient during the procedure. Whether to include the partner depends on a clinical assessment of his level of anxiety and thus degree of direct involvement in the problem. The onset of anxiety has probably happened to the patient a hundred times or more at home. Do not get into a power struggle or force the patient, but give her the option to stop: "When you're ready we'll try again." Meanwhile, instruct her to practice at home. Tell her to lie down and insert her own lubricated index finger (this is preferable to metal dilators because she attains double sensory contact—finger and vagina—plus the physician is thus giving not only permission but prescription to touch her genitals). Tell the couple that when they are at home, (relaxed, lying down with no outside distractions) the patient should spend 5 to 15 minutes twice daily, for 2 days doing relaxed, open-mouthed, slow exhalations (out breaths) with simultaneous vaginal insertion of her lubricated index finger; similarly for the following 2 days she should insert two of her fingers, then the next 2 days she should insert her partner's lubricated finger, guided by her. The partner should be asked to "Come back if this does not work." At that time the patient may be very anxious; if this is the case, suggest the use of a small amount of thiothixene (Navane) 2 mg daily for the next 4 weeks. During this time suggest that she repeat the above protocol of finger exercises. Once she successfully completes these exercises, suggest she wear a lubricated tampon all day to attain and accept sensations in the vagina. The next therapeutic step is for the couple to spend time (about 15 minutes) in foreplay, then, use lubrication (saliva, mineral or baby oil) on the penis and on the vaginal introitus. The patient is to mount and "stuff" the flaccid penis (although awkward) into the vagina from the woman-on-top position. These exercises allow her to be active and to control while the partner is instructed to be passive and receptive during these graded steps so the patient will not be fearful, thinking "you're going to hurt me." Once she has successfully inserted the flaccid penis she is told to relax and contract the pubococcygeus tight as she did during her office visit. In this voluntary way she may get in touch with herself in a more relaxed way, make peace with her sexual self, and overcome her panic. She will now be able to become an active participant in finding a comfortable relaxed coital position.

**VI. Prognosis.** For the first time in centuries the outlook is optimistic for the reversal of unpleasant sexual symptoms because of scientific sex education and the home application of sex therapy exercises of relaxed pleasuring. These are available in self-help books (see the Self-Help Reading List at the end of the chapter). Because there are only a few sex clinics and they are often overloaded, sex therapy merits a diagnostic trial by the primary physician (often a gynecologist) and is best provided for women patients—solo, in a group therapy instructional setting, or a couple by a sensitive gynecologist. There is no sexology subspecialty. The knowledge has been available for almost 2 decades and is waiting for wider application, especially by women's doctors and informed gynecologists.

## BIBLIOGRAPHY

Beck AT, Ward CH, Mendelson M, Mock J, Erbaugh, J. An inventory for measuring depression. Arch Gen Psychiatr 1961; 4:561–571.

Grafenberg E. The role of the urethra in female orgasm. Int J Sexol 1950; 3:145.

Lief H, ed. Sexual Problems in Medical Practice. Monroe, Wis: American Medical Association; 1981.

Hamilton M. The assessment of anxiety states by rating. Br J Med Psychol 1959: 32:50–55.

Masters W, Johnson V. Human Sexual Response. Boston, Mass: Little, Brown & Company; 1966.

Masters W, Johnson V. Human Sexual Inadequacy. Boston, Mass: Little, Brown & Company; 1970.

Masters W, Johnson V. Kolodony R. Sex and Human Loving. Boston, Mass: Little, Brown and Company; 1986.

Renshaw DC. Sexual problems in old age, illness, and disability, Psychosomatics 1981; 22:975–985.

Renshaw DC. Communication in marriage. MAH 1983; 17:199–220.

Renshaw DC. Relationship therapy for sex problems. Comp Ther, 1983; 9:32–36.

Rosensweig N, Pearsall FP. Sex Education for the Health Professional, New York: Grune & Stratton; 1978.

Spitzer RL, Williams BJ, Gibbon M, First MG: Instruction Manual for the Structured Clinical Interview for DSM-III-R. New York: Biometrics Research Dept, New York State Psychiatric Institute; 1987.

## SELF-HELP READING LIST

Barbach LG. For Yourself (women). New York: Doubleday; 1975.

Belliveau F, Richter L. Understanding Human Sexual Inadequacy. New York: Bantam Books; 1970.

Kitzinger, S. Women's Experience of Sex. New York: G P Putnam; 1983.

Masters W, Johnson V, Kolodny R. Sex and Human Loving. Boston, Mass: Little Brown Co.; 1986.

The Boston Women's Health Book Collective. Our Bodies, Ourselves: A Book by and for Women. New York: Simon and Schuster; 1975 and 1982.

Simon, Sidney. Touching, Caring, Feeling. Niles, Ill: Argus Communications; 1976.

CHAPTER 17

# Contraception and Sterilization

**John C. Jarrett**
**George M. Ryan, Jr.**

Requests for contraceptives and contraceptive counseling are the more frequent reasons women visit their obstetrician–gynecologist. This chapter outlines the various methods that are currently available, the effectiveness (Table 17.1), and the advantages and disadvantages of each method to provide the physician with an overview of contraception and a basic framework for deciding which method is most suitable for each individual patient. Whereas these issues are always of importance, they may be especially so during the puerperium when one considers the practical, financial, and family–planning aspects of contraception. Some methods of contraception may not be well-suited for postpartum use. To be safe and effective in the puerperium, consideration must be given to the woman's altered physiologic status as a result of pregnancy, and to issues such as breast feeding and infant well-being.

**Table 17.1. Effectiveness of Contraceptive Methods**

| METHOD | EFFECTIVENESS (IN PREGNANCIES PER 100 WOMAN YEARS OF USE) |
|---|---|
| Rhythm methods (natural family planning, e.g., calendar method, temperature method, cervical mucus method, symptothermal method) | 20–30 |
| Withdrawal (coitus interruptus) | 20–25 |
| Spermicides (creams and jellies, foams, foaming tablets, and suppositories) | 2–40 |
| Vaginal sponge | 15 |
| Condoms | 10–15 |
| Intrauterine devices | 3–5 |
| Combined oral contraceptive | 1–2 |
| Depomedroxyprogesterone acetate (Depo-Provera) | <1 |
| Hormonal postcoital preparations | <1 |

## "NATURAL" METHODS OF CONTRACEPTION

I. **Rhythm method (natural family planning techniques).** The rhythm method is the contraceptive choice of 4% of American couples. The basic principle of all rhythm methods is abstinence during the fertile period.

A. **Techniques**

1. **Calendar method.** The lengths of six to twelve consecutive menstrual cycles are recorded. The beginning of the fertile period is estimated by subtracting 18 days from the shortest cycle length. The end of the fertile period is estimated by subtracting 11 days from the length of the longest cycle.
2. **Temperature method.** Daily basal body temperatures are recorded using a basal body thermometer. Abstinence is practiced from the beginning of menses until 3 days after the rise in temperature associated with ovulation.
3. **Cervical mucus of ovulation method.** This method depends upon the ability of the woman to recognize the increased and clearer cervical mucus associated with rising estrogen levels and impending ovulation. The mucus is clear and increased in amount as compared to the secretory milky colored or opaque cervical mucus seen in the nonovulatory or "safe" intervals. Abstinence is practiced from the first awareness of increased, clearer mucus until 4 days after maximal mucus secretion. Abstinence from intercourse is required during menses, as mucus cannot be properly evaluated when mixed with blood. Intercourse should not occur on consecutive days in the early preovulatory period, as mucus cannot be properly evaluated for 24 hours after intercourse.
4. **Symptothermal method.** This method combines the cervical mucus method with either the calendar or temperature method. Abstinence is required from the earliest day indicated by either method to the latest day indicated by either method.
5. **Other methods.** There are biochemical changes (e.g., enzyme activity) and physical changes (e.g., electrical resistance) in vaginal, cervical, and salivary secretions as a result of cyclic hormonal fluctuations. Commercially marketed methods are available to monitor these changes and thereby predict the fertile period. The effectiveness of these methods in the general population is as yet undetermined. Hormonal assays for urinary estrogen, metabolites of progesterone, and gonadotropins are now available for home use. Some allow prediction of ovulation and some only confirm ovulation. Again, their usefulness in the general population is as yet undetermined.

B. **Effectiveness.** The effectiveness of natural methods varies widely, depending on the patient population and method used. The overall pregnancy rate with natural methods of contraception is about 20 to 30 pregnancies per 100 women years of use.

C. **Advantages and disadvantages**

1. **Advantages.** Natural methods of contraception may be used by couples who object to other forms of contraception; they are cost free (with the exception of the commercially available methods that monitor biochemical or physical changes), and they are universally available.
2. **Disadvantages.** Natural methods require long periods of abstinence from vaginal intercourse and extensive user education and motivation. There are concerns over the aging of gametes and the incidence of spontaneous abortion and congenital anomalies.

D. **Postpartum.** Natural contraceptive methods are all difficult to use effectively during the puerperium. Cyclic timing is invalidated by the preceding pregnancy, and many of the symptomatic changes can be difficult to reliably monitor. Resumption of cyclic menstrual function following delivery can occur at unpredictable intervals. In non-breast-feeding women, normal pituitary function is present by the fourth to sixth week postpartum. Resumption of ovulation may also occur as early as the fourth to sixth postpartum week. Furthermore, menses cannot be used as an indicator of the return of function as a significant proportion of woman ovulate prior to the first menses. Breast-feeding does delay pituitary and ovulatory function. Lactating women are unlikely to ovulate prior to the tenth week postpartum, although ovulation as early as 5 weeks postpartum in a breast-feeding woman has been reported.

II. **Withdrawal (coitus interruptus).** Coitus interruptus is withdrawal of the penis from the vagina prior to ejaculation, which must occur outside of the vagina and away from the immediate perivaginal area to be an effective contraceptive method. It is practiced frequently in Europe but is used regularly by only 2% of American couples.

A. **Effectiveness**

1. **Method.** The theoretical effectiveness based on perfect use and compliance is 9 to 15 pregnancies per 100 woman years of use.
2. **User.** The actual effectiveness in practice is 20 to 25 pregnancies per 100 woman years of use.

B. **Advantages.** Withdrawal requires no mechanical or chemical devices, may be practiced under any circumstances, and is free.

C. **Disadvantages.** Withdrawal demands a high level of self-control, may markedly decrease the enjoyment of intercourse, and is associated with a high failure rate, even if adhered to, due to the occasional unnoticed release of sperm into the vagina or onto the perineum.

D. **Postpartum.** There are no additional advantages or disadvantages to the use of this method postpartum, and there are no contraindications to this method during the postpartum interval.

## BARRIER METHODS OF CONTRACEPTION

I. **Spermicides** are the primary form of contraception of about 3% of American women.

A. **Effectiveness**

1. **Method.** The theoretical effectiveness based on perfect use and compliance is 9 to 15 pregnancies per 100 woman years of use.
2. **User.** While one recent review reported effectiveness as 78% (22 pregnancies per 100 women years of use) the actual effectiveness in practice is reported to vary from 2 to 40 pregnancies per 100 woman years of use. This is dependent on the degree of professional instruction, the population studied, and user motivation. There does not seem to be a significant difference among the various forms of spermicide.

B. **Types.** Spermicides are available as creams and jellies, foams, foaming tablets, and suppositories.

C. **Composition.** All spermicides contain an inert base or vehicle, and an active ingredient, most commonly a surfactant such as nonoxynol-9, which disrupts the integrity of the sperm membrane.

D. **Advantages.** Spermicides are associated with few side effects or user risks, are inexpensive, easily available, and are convenient when intercourse is infrequent. Some protective effect against the transmission of venereal diseases is also offered.

E. **Side effects.** Spermicides can cause local irritative responses on rare occasions. There is some concern about the potential systemic effects of transvaginal absorption of the active ingredients, but no significant studies have yet demonstrated any specific adverse effects.

F. **Postpartum.** Spermicide preparations are as safe in the puerperium as at other times.

II. **Vaginal sponge.** The vaginal sponge is a polyurethane device that is impregnanted with the spermicide nonoxynol-9, thereby combining features of the barrier and spermicides.

A. **Effectiveness.** The failure rate of vaginal sponges approaches that of the diaphragm and spermicides, approximately 15 per 100 woman years of use.

B. **Advantages.** Vaginal sponges are available over the counter and may be left in place, providing protection for 24 hours and through multiple acts of intercourse. A reduced risk for chlamydial and gonorrheal infections has been reported.

C. **Disadvantages.** Use of vaginal sponges has been associated with toxic shock syndrome. Therefore, vaginal sponges should not be used during menstruation, in women with a history of toxic shock syndrome (TSS), or left in place for more than 30 hours.

D. **Postpartum.** There are no additional advantages or disadvantages and no additional contraindications to the use of the vaginal sponge during the postpartum interval.

**III. Condoms** are thin sheaths, most commonly made of latex, which prevent the transmission of sperm from the penis to the vagina. Worldwide they are the most widely used form of contraception but are the primary form of contraception of only about 12% of American couples. The discovery of the acquired immune-deficiency syndrome (AIDS) has led to renewed recognition of the potential role of the condom as protection against sexually transmitted diseases (STDs).

A. **Effectiveness**

1. **Method.** The theoretical effectiveness based on perfect use and compliance is 2 to 3 pregnancies per 100 woman years of use.
2. **User.** The actual effectiveness in practice is 6 to 30 pregnancies per 100 woman years of use. Failures are due to nonuse, inadequate application, vaginal penetration prior to application, failure to withdraw the penis from the vagina while still erect, or tears or breaks in the condom sheath.

B. **Advantages**

1. Condoms are easy to use, inexpensive, available over the counter, and offer protection against venereal disease transmission.
2. Condoms are the only nonpermanent form of male contraception currently available.
3. Condoms can be used as an effective adjunct to other forms of contraception.

C. **Disadvantages.** The use of condoms necessitates interruption of lovemaking for application and may decrease tactile sensation.

D. **Side effects.** Rare allergic reactions have been reported. In cases of allergic reaction, natural skin condoms may be used.

E. **Postpartum.** Condoms alone, or in conjunction with a spermicidal agent, are considered by many to be a good form of "interval" contraception for the puerperium. Effectiveness is to a great extent dependent on how these contraceptive devices are used.

**IV. Diaphragms** are shallow rubber cups with flexible metal rims that are placed in the vagina to cover the cervix. They function both as mechanical barriers and as receptacles for spermicidal agents, which must accompany diaphragm use. They are the primary form of contraception of about 8% of American women.

A. **Effectiveness**

1. **Method.** The theoretical effectiveness based on perfect use and compliance is 2 to 3 pregnancies per 100 woman years of use.
2. **User.** The actual effectiveness in practice is 10 to 15 pregnancies per 100 woman years of use.

B. **Types**

1. **The arcing spring diaphragm** is the first choice of many physicians for routine use. The rim of the arcing spring diaphragm is a sturdy, double metal spring. Its firm construc-

tion allows use in cases of cystocele, rectocele, mild pelvic relaxation, and uterine retroversion. Furthermore, insertion may be easier because of the flexibility of the rim.

2. **Coil spring.** The rim of the coil spring diaphragm is spiral-coiled and sturdy, but it is best suited for women with good vaginal tone and no uterine displacement.
3. **Flat spring.** The rim of the flat spring diaphragm is flat and more rigid than the other types of diaphragms. It is best suited for women with good vaginal tone and a shallow symphyseal arch or long, posterior cervix.

C. **Fitting.** Most diaphragms are available in sizes ranging from 55 to 105 mm. Diaphragms should fit snugly between the posterior fornix, pubic symphysis, and lateral vaginal walls, yet cause no discomfort. If a diaphragm is too small, it may slip out during sexual excitation because of resultant vaginal elongation. If a diaphragm is too large, it may buckle, cause discomfort, or even vaginal ulceration.

D. **Advantages**

1. Diaphragms may be inserted up to 6 hours prior to intercourse.
2. Diaphragms offer some protective effect against transmission of certain STDs.
3. Diaphragms are an effective form of contraception for women who have infrequent intercourse.

E. **Disadvantages**

1. Diaphragm use may be associated with an increased incidence of urinary tract infections.
2. Some couples have difficulty with the physical presence of the diaphragm and/or problems with the insertion or removal of the diaphragm or with the timing of these activities.
3. Spermicide and/or latex sensitivity produces local reactions in 2% to 4% of patients.
4. TSS has been reported with both diaphragm and sponge use and has led to recommendations to avoid these methods during menses and to limit the time they are left in place to no more than 24 hours.

F. **Postpartum.** Diaphragms are acceptable and effective, but care must be taken to insure an adequate fit following childbirth, as alterations in vaginal dimensions may occur at delivery and during the puerperium.

V. **Intrauterine devices (IUDs).** Introduced in the early 1900s, IUDs are used today by 7% of American women. Unfortunately, in the 1980s IUDs were essentially withdrawn from the market by their manufacturers because of the escalating costs of product litigation (see complications of IUDs section, E). However, in 1988 a new copper IUD (ParaGard®) was introduced in the United States. Presently, both this IUD and the Progestasert® IUD, which was introduced in 1976, are available for the physician to meet the contraceptive needs of patients. None of the other IUDs described below are currently available, but they are still present in many patients and are therefore included here.

A. **Effectiveness.** IUDs have a failure rate of 3 to 5 pregnancies per 100 woman years of use.

B. **Types of IUDs and their mechanisms of action**

1. **Lippes Loop™** is a serpentine-shaped device composed of inert polypropylene plastic, available in sizes of A through D. It does not require replacement at regular intervals and is the most widely used type of IUD. IUDs made of inert substances evoke a sterile inflammatory response in the endometrium consisting of mononuclear cells, foreign body giant cells, plasma cells, and macrophages. These may engulf the sperm or ovum, or inhibit implantation of the blastocyst. Inert substance IUDs also increase prostaglandin and immunoglobulin production in the uterine environment and produce asynchronous development of the endometrium.
2. **Saf-T-Coil®** is an inert polypropylene device in a T configuration with helically shaped arms, available in two sizes. Like Lippes Loop™ it does not require replacement at regular intervals. Its mechanism of action is also like that of the inert substance Lippes Loop™.
3. **Copper-bearing devices** are polypropylene devices available in both "T" and "7" configurations with a small copper wire wrapped around the ascending arm which releases a systemically insignificant amount of copper a day. Copper-bearing devices produce an inflammatory response that is accentuated by the presence of the copper. Cupric ions may also interfere with several enzyme systems in the endometrium that are important in implantation and increase prostaglandin synthesis. Copper-bearing devices are smaller than other types of IUDs and may be more appropriately suited for nulliparous women. **These devices require replacement every 3 years,** as their effectiveness is markedly diminished upon complete dissolution of the copper. The Copper T380A (ParaGard®) is the currently available device of this type and is "T" shaped with copper on both the stem and the arms. It is marketed for 4 years of use prior to replacement.
4. **Progestasert®** is a "T"-shaped polypropylene device with progesterone impregnated in the ascending arm of the device, which releases 65 μg of progesterone per day. The response to the local levels of progesterone maintains the endometrium in a decidualized state. The device must be replaced yearly. It is smaller than other types of IUDs and may be more appropriately suited for nulliparous women.

C. **Insertion of IUDs** in today's climate of medico–legal risk requires that extensive informed consent efforts be made and a recommended format is included with the ParaGard® IUD. The patient must sign the document prior to insertion of the IUD.

1. **Contraindications to the IUD**
   a. **Absolute contraindications**
      (1) Pelvic infection
      (2) Pregnancy
      (3) Cervical or uterine malignancy or unresolved abnormal Papanicolaou (PAP) smear
      (4) Postpartum until uterine involution is complete
   b. **Relative contraindications**
      (1) History of pelvic infection or gonorrhea
      (2) History of ectopic pregnancy
      (3) Uterine anomalies or leiomyomata
      (4) Hypermenorrhea and dysmenorrhea (the Progestasert® may be therapeutic for these problems for some women)
      (5) Valvular heart disease
      (6) Impaired immunity either from disease or iatrogenic in nature (transplant patient, chemotherapy patient, chronic steroid use)
      (7) Concern for future fertility
2. **Timing of insertion.** This is usually recommended during menses to avoid pregnancy, but under appropriate circumstances an IUD may be inserted at any time. After pregnancy, IUDs are most commonly inserted only after complete uterine involution has occurred.
3. **Insertion technique.** Before an IUD is inserted, informed consent must be obtained from the patient. Negative results for a recent PAP smear and gonorrhea culture should be available.
   a. Bimanual examination should be done to exclude pelvic abnormalities and pregnancy and to determine uterine axis and position.
   b. Clean the ectocervix with an antiseptic solution.
   c. Place a tenaculum on the anterior lip of the cervix.
   d. Paracervical anesthesia may be administered if desired.
   e. Sound the uterus to ascertain the depth and direction of the uterine cavity.
   f. Using sterile technique, load the IUD into its applicator.
   g. Insert the applicator into the cervical canal using mild traction on the tenaculum.
      (1) **Plunger technique.** The inner plunger pushes the IUD into the uterine cavity once the outer sheath is past the internal os.
      (2) **Withdrawal technique.** The outer barrel is inserted into the fundus of the uterus and then withdrawn with the inner plunger in place.
   h. Leave the strings long (2–3 inches)–they may be cut shorter later if needed.
   i. Repeat the bimanual examination.

**D. Lost IUD.** A "lost IUD" is when the patient cannot find the string of an IUD she believes to be in place. Most commonly, a speculum examination will reveal the string and the patient may be reassured. If no string is found and the patient is unaware of having spontaneously lost her IUD, further evaluation for the presence and position of the IUD is required followed by removal if indicated by an abnormal location for the IUD.

1. **Lost IUD location**
    a. Pregnancy should be excluded by a urine pregnancy test before other evaluation is done.
    b. Gentle probing with a uterine sound or cotton swab may discover the IUD and even allow the relocation of its strings in the vagina without dislodging of the IUD. If the IUD is in the lower uterine segment, it should be removed by traction on the strings as this position is not efficacious for contraception.
    c. Ultrasonography may be used to ascertain IUD location. Posterior–anterior and lateral pelvic x-rays may be obtained after placing a different type of IUD, uterine sound, or radio-opaque catheter in the uterus for use as a reference point.
2. **Removal of a lost IUD.** The following guidelines should be followed for removal of an IUD:
    a. If the strings are visible, simple traction with forceps will usually suffice to remove the IUD.
    b. If the IUD is demonstrable in the uterine cavity, an IUD hook or Novak curette may be used. Occasionally dilation and curettage (D&C) or hysteroscopy will be necessary to manipulate and remove the IUD.
    c. If the IUD is outside the uterine cavity, it should be removed by laparoscopy or laparotomy, because it may induce the formation of significant adhesions.

**E. Complications of IUDs**

1. **Infectious disease.** Users of IUDs are twice as likely as noncontraceptive users to develop pelvic inflammatory disease (PID). They are 4.5 times more likely to develop inflammatory disease than users of oral contraceptives, and 3.3 times more likely than users of barrier methods. Women under age 25, those with multiple sexual partners, and those with a history of prior PID are at increased risk for all complications, especially PID. The risk of infectious complications is greatest during the first month after insertion.
2. **Ectopic pregnancy** occurs in 2.9% to 8.9% of women who conceive with an IUD in place. Although current or past IUD use does not increase a woman's risk of ectopic pregnancy overall, if pregnancy does occur the ratio of ectopic to intrauterine pregnancies is increased.
3. **Uterine perforation** occurs in about one of every 1000 patients, occurring most commonly at the time of insertion.

4. **Alterations in vaginal bleeding.** Menstrual blood loss may be increased by 20% to 50% for patients using copper IUDs, although it may actually be diminished with a Progestasert® IUD. Menstrual blood loss can be effectively reduced by the use of prostaglandin synthetase inhibitors. Intermenstrual bleeding is not uncommon in general as well as in women with IUDs. About 15% of women will request removal of their IUD because of bleeding problems.
5. **Expulsion of IUDs.** There is a 10% spontaneous expulsion rate during the first year of use.
6. **Intrauterine pregnancy**
   a. **Spontaneous abortion.** If the IUD is not removed, the incidence of spontaneous abortion is 55%. If the IUD is removed, the incidence of spontaneous abortion is reduced to 20% to 25%.
   b. **Second trimester loss.** If the IUD is left in place, the risk of miscarriage is ten times greater than that of a control population. If it is removed during the first trimester, there is no increased risk. The risk of septic second trimester fetal loss is increased 26fold if an IUD is left in place.
7. **Dysmenorrhea.** IUD use (except the Progestasert®) is commonly associated with dysmenorrhea, which may be relieved by prostaglandin synthetase inhibitors.

## HORMONAL METHODS OF CONTRACEPTION

I. **Combination oral contraceptives** are the most widely used form of reversible contraception in the United States.

A. **Effectiveness.** The failure rate is one to two pregnancies per 100 woman years of use. Oral contraceptives are the most effective of all nonpermanent forms of contraception. However, effectiveness is reduced if the estrogen content of a given pill is less than 30 μg.

B. **Steroid components and their mechanisms of action.** There are currently 31 different combination pills available in the United States. Many of these are available in both 21 and 28 day packets. The 28 day packets contain seven inert tablets and 21 tablets containing hormones so that the patient is instructed to take a pill a day so as to facilitate remembering to start the next cycle on time. They are formulated from synthetic estrogens and progestins and administered for 21 days with a seven-day hiatus to allow for withdrawal bleeding. Newer formulations, the so-called biphasic or triphasic pills combine a steady or slightly varied dose of estrogen with varying doses of progestins as outlined in T 17.2. These formulations allow for the administration of a lower progestin dose. The rates of pregnancy and clinical problems, such as breakthrough bleeding, remain similar to those of other oral contraceptive pills.

1. **Estrogens**
   a. **Ethinyl estradiol** and **mestranol** are the two estrogens used in oral contraceptives. The hepatic conversion of mestranol to ethinyl estradiol accounts for its metabolic activity. These two compounds may be considered clinically equipotent, although some evidence suggests ethinyl estradiol may be more potent by a factor of 1.6.
   b. **Mechanisms of action.** The estrogen component of oral contraceptives enhances the negative feedback of the progestin on luteinizing hormone, (LH), suppresses follicle-stimulating hormone secretion, and stabilizes the endometrium to prevent irregular bleeding.
2. **Progestins**
   a. The **five currently available progestins are all derivatives of 19-nortestosterone.** The removal of the 19-carbon from testosterone alters the major metabolic effect from androgenic to progestogenic. The addition of the ethinyl group at C-17 enhances this effect and allows for oral activity. The available progestins, their relative potencies, and their estrogenic and androgenic effects are listed in T 17.3. The difference in these may be useful to consider when managing some of the minor side effects of the pill.
   b. **Mechanisms of action.** The progestin components of oral contraceptives suppress the secretion of LH by a negative feedback effect on the hypothalamus and/or pituitary, produces a decidualized endometrium that is not receptive to implantation, produces thick cervical mucus that may impede sperm penetration, and may alter tubal motility.

C. **Indications and contraindications for oral contraceptive use**
1. **Indication.** Any woman who desires a nonpermanent contraceptive method, wishes to use an oral contraceptive, and has no medical or other contraindication to the use of oral contraceptives.
2. **Absolute contraindications**
   a. Thrombophlebitis, thromboembolic disorders, cerebrovascular disease, coronary artery disease, or a history of these conditions.
   b. Undiagnosed abnormal genital bleeding
   c. Impaired liver function
   d. Pregnancy
   e. Known or suspected malignancy of the breast or reproductive system
3. **Relative contraindications.** The following conditions dictate careful consideration of the risk–benefit ratio for the patient and the necessity to informed consent before prescription of combination oral contraceptives:

**Table 17.2. Combination Oral Contraceptives**

| TRADE NAME | ESTROGEN | μg/TABLET | PROGESTOGEN | mg/TABLET |
|---|---|---|---|---|
| Brevicon | Ethinyl estradiol | 35 | Norethindrone | 0.5 |
| Demulen | Ethinyl estradiol | 50 | Ethynodiol diacetate | 1.0 |
| Enovid-E | Mestranol | 100 | Norethynodrel | 2.5 |
| Enovid 5 mg | Mestranol | 75 | Norethynodrel | 5.0 |
| Levlen | Ethinyl estradiol | 30 | Levonorgestel | 0.15 |
| Loestrin 1.5/30 | Ethinyl estradiol | 30 | Norethindrone acetate | 1.5 |
| Loestrin 1/20 | Ethinyl estradiol | 20 | Norethindrone acetate | 1.0 |
| Lo/Ovral | Ethinyl estradiol | 30 | Norgestrel | 0.3 |
| Modicon | Ethinyl estradiol | 35 | Norethindrone | 0.5 |
| Norinyl 2 mg | Mestranol | 100 | Norethindrone | 2.0 |
| Norinyl 1+80 | Mestranol | 80 | Norethindrone | 1.0 |
| Norinyl 1+50 | Mestranol | 50 | Norethindrone | 1.0 |
| Norlestrin 2.5/50 | Ethinyl estradiol | 50 | Norethindrone acetate | 2.5 |
| Norlestrin 1/50 | Ethinyl estradiol | 50 | Norethindrone acetate | 1.0 |
| Ortho-Novum 2 mg | Mestranol | 100 | Norethindrone | 2.0 |
| Ortho-Novum 1/80 | Mestranol | 80 | Norethindrone | 1.0 |
| Ortho-Novum 1/50 | Mestranol | 50 | Norethindrone | 1.0 |
| Ortho-Novum 1/35 | Ethinyl estradiol | 35 | Norethindrone | 1.0 |
| Ortho-Novum 10/11 | Ethinyl estradiol | 35 | Norethindrone | 0.5 for 10 days |
| | Ethinyl estradiol | 35 | Norethindrone | 1.0 for 11 days |

| | | | | |
|---|---|---|---|---|
| Ortho-Novum 7/7/7 | Ethinyl estradiol | 35 | Norethindrone | 0.5 for 7 days |
| | Ethinyl estradiol | 35 | Norethindrone | 0.75 for 7 days |
| | Ethinyl estradiol | 35 | Norethindrone | 1.0 for 7 days |
| Ovcon 50 | Ethinyl estradiol | 50 | Norethindrone | 1.0 |
| Ovcon 35 | Ethinyl estradiol | 35 | Norethindrone | 0.4 |
| Ovral | Ethinyl estradiol | 50 | Norgestrel | 0.5 |
| Ovulen | Mestranol | 100 | Ethynodiol diacetate | 1.0 |
| Tri-Levlen | Ethinyl estradiol | 30 | Levonorgestel | 0.05 for 6 days |
| | Ethinyl estradiol | 40 | Levonorgestel | 0.075 for 5 days |
| | Ethinyl estradiol | 30 | Levonorgestel | 0.125 for 10 days |
| Tri-Norinyl | Ethinyl estradiol | 35 | Norethindrone | 0.5 for 7 days |
| | Ethinyl estradiol | 35 | Norethindrone | 1.0 for 7 days |
| | Ethinyl estradiol | 35 | Norethindrone | 0.5 for 7 days |
| Triphasil | Ethinyl estradiol | 30 | Levonorgestrel | 0.05 for 6 days |
| | Ethinyl estradiol | 40 | Levonorgestrel | 0.075 for 5 days |
| | Ethinyl estradiol | 30 | Levonorgestrel | 0.125 for 11 days |
| Zorane 1/50 | Ethinyl estradiol | 50 | Norethindrone acetate | 1.0 |
| Zorane 1.5/30 | Ethinyl estradiol | 30 | Norethindrone acetate | 1.5 |
| Zorane 1/20 | Ethinyl estradiol | 20 | Norethindrone acetate | 1.0 |

Adapted from Jarrett JC, II. Contraception. In: Ellis JW, Beckmann RB, eds. A Clinical Manual of Gynecology. East Norwalk, Conn: Appleton-Century-Crofts; 1983: 416–417.

**Table 17.3. Oral Contraceptive Progestogens***

| PROGESTOGEN | RATIO OF PROGESTATIONAL POTENCY* | RELATIVE ESTROGENIC POTENCY† | RELATIVE ANTIESTROGENIC EFFECT‡ | RELATIVE ANDROGENICITY§ |
|---|---|---|---|---|
| Norethindrone | 1 | 0.3 | 2.5 | 1.6 |
| Norethynodrel | 1 | 2.1 | 0.0 | 0.0 |
| Norethindrone acetate | 2 | 0.9 | 25.0 | 2.5 |
| Ethynodiol diacetate | 15 | 0.4 | 1.0 | 1.0 |
| Norgestrel | 30 | 0.0 | 18.5 | 7.6 |

*Different results may be obtained depending on the assay used. Some of these values are based on animal studies, and therefore should be used only as approximations.
*From Greenblatt RB. Med Sci May, 1967; 37–49.
†Relative to ethinyl estradiol-100. From Jones RC, Edgren RA. Fertil Steril 1973; 24: 284.
‡From Dickey RP. ACOG Sem Fam Plan 1974; 32.
§From Tausk M, de Visser J. International Encyclopedia of Pharmacology and Therapeutics. Elmsford, NY: Pergamon Press; 1973: section 28, chap 28.
Source: From Jarrett JC. Contraception. In Ellis JW, Beckmann RB, eds. A Clinical Manual of Gynecology. East Norwalk, Conn: Appleton-Century-Crofts; 1983: 419. Reprinted with permission.

a. Diabetes
b. Hypertension
c. Migraine headaches
d. Hemoglobinopathies, (e.g., sickle cell or sickle C disease)
e. Congenital hyperlipidemia
f. Cholestatic jaundice during pregnancy
g. Varicose veins
h. Epilepsy
i. Uterine leiomyomata
j. Cigarette smoking, especially in women over age 30
k. Women over age 35
l. Elective surgery (the pill should be discontinued 4 weeks prior to any elective surgery)
m. Women who are breast-feeding (the pill decreases the quantity and quality of lactation and some drug crosses the placental barrier to the fetus)

**D. Administration**

1. **Low-dose pills** (30 or 35 μg of estrogen) should be used for all women as the pill of initial therapy.
2. **When to take the pill (pill schedules).** If the pill is begun on the fifth day of the menstrual cycle, contraceptive protection is afforded during the first cycle. Some pills are packaged so as to encourage starting them on Sunday, which may cause the patient to start the pill other than on the fifth day of the menstrual cycle. This should be taken into account when counseling the patient about protection during the first pill cycle. Oral contraceptive pills should be taken at the same time every day. Developing this habit may reduce the risk of missing a pill. Taking the pill at bedtime will often decrease any nausea that may occur. There is no good rationale for recommending routine pill-free intervals.
3. **Missing pills.** If the patient misses one pill, she should take it as soon as possible and take the next pill on schedule. If two pills are missed, the pills should be discontinued for 7 days and another form of contraception used for the remainder of the cycle. Alternatively, two pills may be taken each of the following days, but another form of contraception should be used for the remainder of that cycle.
4. **When to start the pill after pregnancy**
   a. If an abortion or miscarriage has occurred at less than 12 weeks' gestation, the pill can be started immediately.
   b. If an abortion or miscarriage occurs after 12 weeks' gestation, the patient should wait 1 week before starting the pill.
   c. Following delivery after 28 weeks in a nonnursing patient, the patient should wait 2 weeks before starting the pill.

5. **Follow-up care for pill users**
   a. Patients should be seen 6 to 8 weeks after the initial visit when the pill is prescribed. Blood pressure should be checked for elevation, which if discovered will require re-evaluation of pill use. In addition, other evidence of side effects should be sought and managed as appropriate (see hormonal methods of contraception section, I-F). Proper use of the pill should also be confirmed. Yearly visits thereafter are appropriate in the absence of complicating factors.
   b. Regular laboratory evaluation of glucose or lipid levels may be indicated in patients at particular risk for diabetes or hyperlipidemia.

E. **Clinical problems associated with pill use**
1. **Breakthrough bleeding** occurs in up to 10% of patients using oral contraceptives as a result of insufficient estrogen to stabilize the endometrium, and is therefore more common with the low-dose pills. The bleeding will abate after two or three cycles in most patients, and reassurance may be the only treatment needed. If the bleeding persists after two or three cycles, switching to a pill with a higher estrogen–progestin ratio may be helpful. Alternatively, a 7-day course of conjugated estrogens or ethinyl estradiol may be administered around the time of bleeding in conjunction with the pill.
2. **Amenorrhea** occurs in about 1% of patients and is more common with the low-dose pills. It is a result of insufficient estrogen stimulation to endometrial growth resulting in inadequate endometrium for withdrawal bleeding to occur. There is no evidence that prolonged amenorrhea while on the pill has any adverse effects. This will often be adequate assurance for the patient who is taking the pill properly and in whom, therefore, there is virtually no chance of pregnancy. If the amenorrhea is of concern to the patient, a pill with a higher estrogen content may be prescribed (Table 17.2).
3. **Post-pill amenorrhea** is defined as amenorrhea of 6 months' or more duration following discontinuation of the pill. It occurs in less than 1% of patients and is more common in women with a prior history of menstrual irregularity. For this reason, the pill should be used with caution in young women who have not established regular menses. Post-pill amenorrhea is not related to the type of pill or the duration of pill use but is instead most likely related to the pill's suppression of the hypothalamus. The incidence of pituitary adenomas is increased in this group of patients.
4. **Weight gain.** Some minor weight gain is frequently reported but usually responds to dietary restriction.
5. **Chloasma,** a mask-like hyperpigmentation of the skin, is a rare problem with low-dose pills. It is often transient, but in some cases may be permanent.

6. **Androgenic effects.** Acne, oily skin, and mild hirsutism may occur. Use of a less androgenic pill may alleviate this problem.
7. **Depression** is usually a mild problem that may be alleviated by the administration of vitamin $B_6$. Discontinuation of the pill and use of another form of contraception may be necessary.

**F. Side effects and major complications of pill use**

1. **Vascular thrombosis** is the major risk factor associated with pill use, accounting for virtually all of the increased risk of mortality in pill users. Virtually all of the significant data were collected prior to the advent of the current low dosage pills. Smoking and aging are significant risk factors for the development of vascular complications. Virtually all of the increased risk is concentrated in patients who smoke, particularly after the age of 30, and in nonsmokers after the age of 35.
   a. **Deep venous thrombophlebitis and pulmonary embolism.** The risk of these problems is increased 5.7fold by pill use and is estrogen related. The incidence in one series was decreased from 25.9 to 7.2 cases per l00 000 by lowering the estrogen content from 75 μg to 50 μg or less.
   b. **Myocardial infarction.** The risk of myocardial infarction is proportionate to the estrogen dose. The dosage and type of progestin may also be a significant factor, thus suggesting that use of the lowest effective progestin dose may be advisable. The presence of other risk factors such as obesity, hypertension, and hyperlipidemia increase the risk and are therefore relative contraindications. The increased risk for these patients may persist even after discontinuation of the pill.
   c. **Cerebrovascular accidents.** This complication is usually heralded by headaches, which must therefore be carefully evaluated in pill users. The risk of thrombotic stroke is increased threefold to fourfold and that of hemorrhagic stroke, twofold. The incidence of cerebrovascular accident in pill users is 1/10 000 woman years.
2. **Lipid metabolism.** Plasma triglycerides and cholesterol are elevated with pill use, as are low-density lipoproteins. High-density lipoproteins are decreased. These effects may be related to the increased incidence of vascular phenomena in pill users. A decrease in the amount of progestin as in some of the low-dose or "phasic" pills may decrease the magnitude of these effects. The type and the amount of progestin may be the determining factors of the lipoprotein-cholesterol changes.
3. **Carbohydrate metabolism.** Estrogens and progestins produce an increased peripheral resistance to insulin. Fifteen percent to 50% of women on the pill will develop

impaired glucose tolerance. No impairment of glucose tolerance in a group of women taking a pill containing 35 μg of ethinyl estradiol and 0.4 mg of norethindrone has been demonstrated. The clinical significance of the elevated blood sugar in normal women is unclear but may be of importance in women with latent, subclinical, or gestational diabetes.

4. **Hypertension.** Five percent of pill users develop significant hypertension after 5 years of use. This is thought to involve alterations in the renin–angiotension system, because there is an eightfold increase in angiotensinogin in pill users. Sodium retention may also be a factor.
5. **Liver adenomas** are benign solitary or multiple tumors that are extremely vascular and prone to hemorrhage. They are a rare but recognized side effect of pill use and the occurrence is related to duration of pill use and dose. Fifty percent of patients with liver adenomas present with right upper quadrant or epigastric pain, and 40% have a palpable mass. The principal potential danger of liver adenoma is hemorrhage. An adenoma may regress upon discontinuation of the pill.
6. **Gallbladder disease.** The risk of gallstones and cholecystitis is increased twofold in pill users and is probably related to increased cholesterol saturation.
7. **Neoplasms**
   a. **Cervix.** An association between oral contraceptives and cervical neoplasia has not been established.
   b. **Uterus.** Oral contraceptives are associated with a decreased risk of endometrial carcinoma.
   c. **Breast.** There appears to be no association between breast cancer and pill usage. The pill affords some protection against the development of benign breast disease.
8. **Pregnancy complications.** Congenital anomalies of the VACTERL (vertebral, and, cardiac, tracheal, esophageal, renal, and limb) type are increased if the pill is taken through the first trimester. The incidence of spontaneous abortion or stillbirth after discontinuation of the pill is not increased. There is a twofold increase in twinning in patients who become pregnant soon after discontinuing the pill. Patients should be encouraged to wait two or three cycles after discontinuing oral contraceptives prior to attempting pregnancy.
9. **Postpartum.** Oral contraceptives should be started by nonlactating women between 2 and 3 weeks after delivery. This minimized the risk of postpartum thrombophlebitis and provides suppression prior to the initiation of ovulation. Oral contraceptives should probably not be used by breast-feeding women because of potential passage of exogenous hormones into the breast milk.

**G. Noncontraceptive benefits ascribed to oral contraceptive use**

1. Decreased incidence of breast carcinoma.
2. Decreased incidence of endometrial carcinoma.
3. Decreased incidence of ovarian carcinoma.
4. Decreased incidence of rheumatoid arthritis.
5. Decreased incidence of PID.
6. Decreased incidence and severity of iron-deficiency anemia associated with menorrhagia.
7. Decreased incidence of symptomatic ovarian cysts requiring invasive evaluation.

**II. Progestin-only pills (mini-pills).** Progestin-only pills contain 350 μg of norethindrone or 75 μg of norgestrel. The contraceptive effect depends on alterations in the endometrium and cervical mucus; suppression of LH is incomplete and a significant number of women who take mini-pills will ovulate. Irregular bleeding is common and frequently results in discontinuation of this method of contraception. The failure rate of progestin-only pills is 2.5%. Progestin-only pills may be used in patients for whom estrogens are contraindicated, although the effect of the progestin must be considered. Progestin-only pills must be taken continuously. The incidence of ectopic gestations is increased if pregnancy does occur in a patient using progestin-only pills. When used in the puerperium, they should be started between the second and fourth postpartum weeks. It is controversial whether they are safe for use in lactating women.

**III. Depomedroxyprogesterone acetate (DMPA; Depo-Provera)** is not FDA approved for use in the United States as a contraceptive method, although it is widely used throughout the world. The recommended does is 150 mg IM every 3 months; the contraceptive effect of 150 mg is maintained for 4 months, so some margin of error is provided. The failure rate is less than one pregnancy per 100 woman years. The mechanism of action is to block the LH surge and alter the endometrium and cervical mucus so that they are less receptive.

**A. Advantages**

1. Infrequent administration.
2. Provides an extremely effective means of contraception for women in whom other methods are contraindicated.
3. Estrogen levels are maintained at an early follicular phase level. There are no hypoestrogenic side effects.
4. Produces amenorrhea which may be desirable in patients who have problems with menstrual hygiene, such as the mentally handicapped.

**B. Concerns and disadvantages**

1. Unpredictable vaginal bleeding may occur, especially during the first treatment cycle. Short courses of supplemental estrogen are therapeutic.
2. Because of the long-acting nature of the preparation, there may be some delay in return of menses and fertility upon

discontinuation. However, these effects do not appear to persist beyond 8, or at most, 12 months.

3. Weight gain of 5 to 10 lbs is not uncommon.
4. There is no evidence linking breast carcinoma and oral contraceptive use in humans. A link was noted in one study using beagle dogs, but this relationship has not been reproduced in other animal studies or in data from human use.

C. **Postpartum.** When used in the puerperium, the initial dose of DMPA should be administered at 2 to 3 weeks after delivery in non-breast-feeding women; the method is not recommended in lactating women.

IV. **Postcoital contraception.** Postcoital contraception entails the use of agents to prevent pregnancy following an episode of unprotected intercourse during the fertile phase of the cycle.

A. **Indications for postcoital contraception** include sexual assault or abuse, condom breakage or diaphragm displacement during intercourse or failure to use adequate protection (especially common in young women during their first sexual experience). **Pre-existent pregnancy must be excluded prior to therapy.**

B. **Available methods**

1. **Hormonal** methods must be initiated as soon as possible after coitus, preferably within 24 hours but no later than 72 hours. Mechanisms of action of hormonal methods include asynchronous development of endometrium, alteration of tubal motility, and direct or indirect luteolysis.
   a. Diethylstilbestrol (DES) 25 mg p.o. b.i.d. for 5 days (FDA approved).
   b. Ethinyl estradiol 2.5 mg p.o. b.i.d. for 5 days.
   c. Conjugated estrogens 10 mg t.i.d. p.o. for one menstrual cycle. (**Note:** An antiemetic should be given with these agents because of the nausea that they elicit (e.g., prochlorperazine [Compazine], 10 mg. p.o. or p.r.n. as suppository, q8 h in a non-p.r.n. regimen starting at the start of postcoital therapy.)
   d. Norgestrel and ethinyl estradiol (Ovral) two tablets b.i.d. for 1 day—should produce withdrawal bleeding.
2. **Mechanical.** The insertion of copper-bearing IUD within 5 days of intercourse has been reported to be an effective method of postcoital contraception. However, the cautions about IUD insertion may limit the usefulness of this method. The insertion of an IUD into a victim of sexual assault–abuse should be discouraged.

C. **Effectiveness of postcoital therapy.** Most studies report failure rates of postcoital therapy as less than 1%. Most failures are due to delay in treatment, poor patient compliance, or repeated unprotected intercourse.

D. **Side effects and cautions.** Patients must have adequate short-term follow-up to exclude complications and failures. This also provides the opportunity for contraceptive counseling.

1. Nausea and vomiting are frequent with hormonal methods of postcoital contraception. An anti-emetic should be prescribed.
2. If pregnancy does occur, the incidence of ectopic gestation is increased for all methods of postcoital contraception.
3. Because of concerns over possible teratogenic effects of the high doses of estrogen, abortion should be considered if pregnancy occurs despite hormonal postcoital therapy.

## SURGICAL METHODS OF CONTRACEPTION

I. **Female sterilization.** In 1982, 22% of all married women had undergone sterilization. There are estimated to be over 15 000 000 sterilized adults in the United States, and sterilization (tubal ligation and vasectomy) is currently the most commonly used form of contraception.

A. **Approaches and techniques**

1. **Laparotomy** is most commonly used for puerperal sterilization. The use of the mini-laparotomy as a means of achieving interval sterilization is gaining increasing favor, primarily because a specimen may be sent for pathologic confirmation of successful surgery. Various techniques that are commonly used include:
   a. **Madlener.** A loop of tube is elevated and the base is crushed with a clamp. The crushed area is then ligated using nonabsorbable suture.
   b. **Pomeroy.** A loop of tube from the middle third of the tube is elevated, ligated with plain gut, and excised.
   c. **Irving.** The tube is divided and the proximal stump is buried in the wall of the uterus. The distal stump is buried in the leaves of the broad ligament.
   d. **Cook.** Similar to the Irving technique but the proximal stump is buried in the round ligament.
   e. **Kroener.** The fimbriated portion of the tube is excised.
   f. **Aldridge.** The fimbriated end of the tube is buried in the broad ligament.
   g. **Uchida.** The mesosalpinx is injected with a saline-epinephrine solution. It is then incised to expose the tube itself. The serosa of the proximal end is then stripped off and the majority of the proximal segment is removed and the stump ligated with nonabsorbable suture and placed back in the broad ligament. The distal end is ligated and the broad ligament closed with the distal stump left outside the broad ligament.
   h. **Partial or total salpingectomy.** A part or all of the tube is removed.
   i. **Cornual resection.** The tube is ligated 1 cm from the cornua and excised from the cornua. The distal end can be buried in the broad ligament, and the proximal

wound may be covered with the round and broad ligaments.

2. **Laparoscopy.** In 1976, 38% of all female sterilizations were performed by laparoscopy.
   a. **Bipolar electrical methods.** The current passes from one jaw of the instrument to the other jaw. This method is used for "coagulation only" techniques and carries less risk of accidental burns than unipolar cautery. Coagulation techniques include:
      (1) **Coagulation, transection, and recoagulation.** The addition of transection, recoagulation, or even biopsy does not decrease the failure rate, and may lead to an increased rate of complications.
      (2) **Coagulation and transection.**
      (3) **Coagulation only** may be performed at one or several sites on the tube. Multiple sites are preferred, creating a coagulated segment of at least 3 cm in length.
   b. **Silastic bands.** With the use of a special applicator, a knuckle of fallopian tube, in the isthmic portion, is elevated and a small silastic band is placed around the base of the knuckle. Tears in the mesosalpinx may occur in up to 3% of patients, especially if the tubes are thickened or scarred. Greater immediate and late postoperative pelvic pain may occur with this technique.
   c. **Spring-loaded clips.** The clip is placed across the isthmic portion of the tube and occludes the lumen with minimal tissue destruction.
3. **Uncommonly used techniques.** Some techniques of surgical sterilization are now uncommonly used. These include:
   a. **Unipolar electrical cautery by laparoscopy.** A low-voltage high-frequency current is passed from the laparoscopic instrument through the patient to a "ground plate," from which it returns to the generator. This carries the serious risk of inadvertent burns to bowel, bladder, or skin. For this reason, unipolar cautery has been largely replaced by other techniques and its use should no longer be encouraged.
   b. **Thermocoagulation by laparoscopy.** Low-voltage electricity heats the instrument which then actually sears the fallopian tubes.
   c. **Colpotomy.** An incision is made in the posterior fornix, the tube is "delivered," and then ligated by one of the above techniques, often fimbriectomy. This technique carries a higher morbidity rate than other techniques and is used infrequently.
   d. **Culdoscopy.** A special instrument is inserted into the posterior cul-de-sac, the tube visualized, grasped, and delivered into the vagina and ligated. This is a technically difficult procedure and is rarely used.

e. **Hysteroscopy.** The techniques of thermocoagulation and electrocoagulation as well as mechanical occlusion with sclerosing agents or tubal plugs have been attempted through the hysteroscope. Unacceptable failure and complication rates have been encountered. At the present these techniques must be considered experimental.

B. **Timing of sterilization procedure**

1. **At the time of cesarean section,** the techniques most commonly used are the Pomeroy or Irving sterilization techniques.
2. **Postpartum** tubal ligation can be performed through a minilaparotomy. If performed within 48 hours, there is no increase in infectious morbidity. The procedure adds little time to the hospital stay and avoids the need for a second hospitalization.
3. **Interval sterilization.** With respect to timing of interval sterilization, it is wise to wait at least 8 weeks postpartum for an abdominal approach and 6 months for a vaginal surgical procedure. Interval sterilization is best done during the proliferative phase to avoid luteal phase pregnancies, although a concomitant D&C obviates this requirement.

C. **Sequelae of sterilization.**

1. There is some evidence of altered pituitary-ovarian function after tubal ligation. The incidence of menstrual irregularity may be due to an alteration in ovarian blood supply.
2. Some reports suggest that the incidence of dysmenorrhea may be increased. However, when controlled for age, previous gynecologic problems and previous contraceptive methods, no increase has been demonstrated.
3. Subjective complaints of decreased sexual enjoyment, a worsening of general health status, and depression are not uncommon. These symptoms may represent ambivalence or negative feelings about the decision to be sterilized.

D. **Reversal of surgical sterilization.** Approximately 3% to 4% of sterilized women regret their decision to be sterilized and 1% of sterilized women request reversal of the sterilization procedure. Of those requesting reversal, 89% were younger than 30 years of age at the time of sterilization. Unstable marital relationships are present at the time of sterilization in 50% of those requesting reversal. Reasons for requesting reversal of sterilization include change in marital status (63%), crib death (17%), desire for more children (10%), personal tragedy (4%), and various psychological problems (6%).

E. **Failure rates.** Pregnancy occurring after tubal ligation may be ectopic in 10% to 60% of cases. Any poststerilization pregnancy should be considered an ectopic until proven otherwise. The published failure rates for the various methods are

1. Madlener 14/1000
2. Pomeroy 4/1000

| | | |
|---|---|---|
| **3.** | Cornual resection | 29/1000 |
| **4.** | Irving | <1/1000 |
| **5.** | Kroener | 18/1000 |
| **6.** | Uchida | 0/1000 |
| **7.** | Cautery | 1 to 4/1000 |
| **8.** | Silastic band | 3.3/1000 |
| **9.** | Spring clip | 2 to 25/1000 |

**F. Informed consent.** Providing proper informed consent is one of the most important aspects of preparing the patient for sterilization. The level of satisfaction with being sterilized is directly related to the degree of satisfaction with presterilization counseling. In addition to an explanation of the operative technique to be used, alternative methods should be presented. The permanence of the procedure should be emphasized but not guaranteed. Failure rates for the tubal ligation procedure should be reviewed. Complications and side effects, during and after the procedure, should be discussed.

**II. Male sterilization.** Vasectomy is the surgical interruption of the vas deferens in the scrotum. Male sterilization accounts for about 11% of all contraceptive methods. Approximately 250,000 vasectomies are performed each year in the United States.

**A. Effectiveness.** The failure rate is less than one per 100. Azoospermia does not occur immediately and must be documented prior to resumption of unprotected intercourse.

**B. Complications**

1. **Minor postoperative pain and swelling of the scrotum** are common, but serious complications are rare. Sperm granulomas may occur in as many as 20% of patients.
2. **Sperm immobilizing and agglutinating antibodies** have been demonstrated in a significant percentage of males after vasectomy.
3. **The relationship between vasectomy and possible long-term sequelae** such as altered immune status, changes in coagulation status, and atherosclerosis are currently under investigation.

**C. Reversibility.** Reports have indicated the presence of sperm in the ejaculate of 90% of men who have undergone vasectomy reversal and pregnancy in 70% of the partners of patients undergoing reversal.

**III. Abortion** is discussed in Chapter 18. In any event, abortion should not be viewed as a contraceptive method but rather one possible alternative to contraceptive failure.

## INVESTIGATIONAL METHODS OF CONTRACEPTION

The perfect contraceptive has not yet been developed, but it would be one that could be used for long periods of time without significant side effects. It should be 100% effective and 100% reversible. Investigations are under way.

I. **Barrier methods.** More effective and less displeasurable methods are being developed. Long-acting spermicides and spermicidal-impregnated condoms, diaphragms and sponges hold promise.

II. **IUDs** that are impregnated with antifibrinolytic substances or prostaglandin synthetase inhibitors, as well as ones that can be inserted immediately postpartum, are being tested. However, the future of IUD use is clouded by medico-legal considerations.

III. **Hormonal methods.** Much of the work in the investigation of improved hormonal methods of contraception is being directed toward the use of agonists and antagonists of LH releasing hormone. Hormone-impregnated vaginal rings may soon be available. Agents are also being sought that will specifically block hormonal action at a given level (e.g., endometrium, ovum, or blastocyst). Injectable long-acting silastic implants of several progestin compounds are also currently under investigation.

IV. **Vaccines** that would produce immunity to implantation hormones (e.g., human chorionic gonadotropin or to sperm are under investigation).

V. **Sterilization.** Many sterilization techniques, which would allow easier and more effective reversibility, are being developed for both males and females.

## BIBLIOGRAPHY

Bacharach CA. Contraceptive practice among American women: 1973–1982. Fam Plann Perspect 1984; 16:253.

Bottiger LE, Boman G, Westerhelm B. Oral contraceptives and thromboembolic disease: Effects of lowering oestrogen content. Lancet 1980; 1:1097.

Corson SL, Derman RJ, Tyrer LB. Fertility Control. Boston, Mass: Little, Brown and Company; 1985.

Cramer DW, Schiff I, Schoenbaum SC, Gibson M, Bellisle S, Albrecht B, Stillman RJ, Berger MJ, Wilson E, Stadel BV, Seibel M. Tubal infertility and the intrauterine device. N Engl J Med 1985; 312:941.

Edelman DA. Vaginal contraception: An overview. Int J Gynaecol Obstet 1984; 22:11.

Foreman H, Stadel BV, Schlesslman S. Intrauterine device usage and fetal loss. Obstet Gynecol 1981; 58:669.

Grady W, Hayward M, Yogi J. Contraceptive failure in the United States: Estimates from the 1982 National Survey of Family Growth. Fam Plann Perspect 1986; 18:200.

Grimes DA. Reversible contraception for the 1980's. JAMA 1986; 255:69.

Hatcher RA, Guess F, Stewart F. Contraceptive Technology 1984–1985. New York: Irvington Publishers Inc.; 1984.

Meade TW, Greenberg G, Thompson SG. Progestogens and cardiovascular reactions associated with oral contraceptives and a comparison of the safety of 50 mcg and 30 mcg estrogen preparations; Br Med J, 1980; 280:1157.

Mishell DR, Rosenfield A, Spellacy WN, Andrews WC, Grimes DA. Dialogues in Contraception. Lyndhurst, NJ: Health Learning Systems; 1985.

Nash HA. Depo-Provera: A review. Contraception 1975; 12:377.

Ory HW. Mortality associated with fertility and fertility control: 1983. Fam Plann Perspect 1983; 15:57.

Rosenberg MJ, Rojanapithayakorn W, Feldblum PJ, Higgins JE. Effect of the contraceptive sponge on chlamydial infection, gonorrhea, and candidiasis. JAMA 1987; 257:2308.

Royal College of General Practitioners. Oral Contraceptives and Health: An Interim Report. London, England: Pitman; 1974.

Royal College of General Practitioners. Further analysis of mortality in oral contraceptive users. Lancet 1981; 1:541.

Silber SJ. Vasectomy and vasectomy reversal. Fertil Steril 1978; 29:125.

# CHAPTER 18

# Sexual Assault

**Charles R. B. Beckmann**
**Linda L. Groetzinger**
**Sylvia Lessman**
**Michael L. Bolos**

Sexual assault and abuse of adults and children is a physically and emotionally traumatic experience shared by many people. Evidence suggests that at least one in four female children under 18 years of age and probably an equal number of male children, one in four adult women, and an unknown number of adult men are victims. Worse yet, because of the stigmas placed on victims by society in general, and within the medical and legal systems in particular, only one-tenth of these victims of violence seek help from anyone. Instead, most victims suffer in silent aloneness, internalizing their feelings rather than sharing them with others. Victims who do seek help often find themselves as traumatized by caregivers as they were from those who assaulted them. This chapter identifies the problem of sexual assault and child sexual abuse. It teaches caregivers to overcome their own discomfort and misconceptions so that they are able to assist victims, and to suggest care plans that will facilitate the actual care of victims. A cautionary note: Caring for sexual assault and abuse victims requires specific knowledge and skills as well as good intentions and common sense. Such care is best done using a multidisciplinary team approach, as individual caregivers (physicians, nurses, social workers) rarely have all the knowledge and skills needed to provide for all of the victim's needs.

Whereas much of this chapter addresses the care of female victims, some sections are written in a gender neutral format and also provide information about the responses of male victims. This approach is consistent with the nature of the problem and provides additional illumination about the tragedy of sexual assault and abuse. For example, when a woman is assaulted, her sense of control and sense of safety is attacked, but not her sense of herself as a feminine person; conversely, male victims often feel their masculinity is attacked in addition to issues of safety and control.

## I. Sexual assault

### A. Definition

1. **Physical contact.** Sexual assault involves the unlawful and nonconsensual physical contact of one person by another person or people. The classic case is forced sexual inter-

course of a female victim by a male rapist. The more general definition includes any action involving acts that in a consensual setting would be sexual, or that involve genital structures in such a manner that the victim perceives a sexual intrusion, performed upon a person against his or her will by one or more male or female perpetrators, or where the victim is forced to perform sexual acts upon the perpetrator(s).

2. **Violence and nonconsent.** All sexual assaults are acts of violence performed against the victim's will. The most important common element is nonconsent, always associated with threatened or actual physical and/or emotional force. The lack of control (especially over his or her own body) that the victim experiences is the most serious immediate emotional problem faced by the victim of sexual assault.
3. **Trauma.** While all sexual assaults are traumatic, significant physical trauma (e.g., knife wounds, severe beating) is uncommon, occurring in perhaps 5% of cases although in one series the incidence is reported as 12%. Murder seems less common than severe trauma. Twenty-five percent to 50% of victims do have some minor physical trauma, usually bruising or minor cuts or abrasions. Threats of violence, often with the brandishing of weapons, are common.
4. **Pregnancy.** There is no evidence that pregnancy results any more or less frequently in unprotected fertile female victims of sexual assault than in a similar group of unprotected fertile females engaging in consensual sexual activity. The latter group have a pregnancy rate of 5%.

B. **Prevalence.** Sexual assault is an underreported event because many victims choose to remain silent. Based on the F.B.I.'s estimate that 90% of sexual assaults are not reported, extrapolation of studies concerning general and specific populations suggests that one in every four women, one in every four children, and an unknown number of men are victims of sexual assault.

II. **Emotional impact of sexual assault.** The rape trauma syndrome is the term used to describe a specific form of acute stress reaction to a life-threatening situation: rape. The reaction begins during the assault at the moment when the victim feels that he or she has lost control and has no way out of the situation. The response is described in three phases.

A. **Acute phase.** The acute phase of rape trauma syndrome is seen in the first hours to the first days after the assault.

1. **Early acute stage.** The early acute phase of rape trauma syndrome occurs in the time immediately after the disclosure of sexual assault and/or of the sexual assault itself.
   a. **Psychological symptoms.** The psychological symptoms of acute phase rape trauma syndrome are common to any acute stress reaction to a life-threatening situation. This psychological trauma is often masked by individu-

alized coping mechanisms and/or initial reaction of shock. The physical and emotional responses to any physical trauma suffered during the assault are admixed with these responses. The victim may experience dismay, disbelief, acute and generalized fear, and/or may appear to be subdued, stunned, numb, quiet, and resistant to talking about the event. This is a volatile state when the patient may go from tears to casual-seeming social conversation and back again without warning or seeming reason. The patient may exhibit varying degrees of anxiety when discussing potential consequences of the assault. These include family reactions, the acquisition of sexually transmitted diseases (STDs), the possibility of pregnancy, the police interview, and the possibility of pressing charges and entering into the legal system process. The patient may experience flashbacks and "relive" parts of the attack. Reassurance that he or she is safe at the time, and giving the victim as much control over what is happening as reasonable for the clinical situation is the best method of dealing with this distressing anxiety.

b. **Retreat to routine activities.** A retreat to routine activities is a common reaction of the sexual assault victim, often before seeking police or medical care. Activities such as cleaning the house or going to the bank are the victim's attempt to regain a sense of self and of control. These actions should not be construed as an indication of less severity of physical and/or emotional trauma reported by the patient, nor be taken as reason to doubt the veracity of the patient's report of assault.

c. **Cognitive dysfunction.** Victims may appear preoccupied or distracted. In defense against the pain of realization of what has happened, the victim may defocus discussion from actual events and may have difficulty in giving a history of the attack or of other recent or even past events. The patient may focus on apparent irrelevancies or unrelated aspects of her normal life. The patient may have considerable difficulty concentrating, in giving her medical history, or in describing her usual life. The apparent inconsistencies in the patient's history are distressing to the patient and are often of concern to health professionals and law enforcement officials. Sensitive, nonjudgemental persistence can assist in reestablishing cognitive control. These inconsistencies and the minimization of the severity of the event are a reflection of the crisis of self-esteem that all patients undergo and the fears the patient has about the reactions of others.

d. **Communicating and coping with pragmatic issues.** A relief in the generalized anxiety and an improved emotional and cognitive state is usually seen when the victim discusses the events of the sexual assault with supportive health care providers, family, and/or friends. Because victims often have less opportunity than they would like, or is needed, to share the flood of anxiety, fear, anger, and self-reproach that they experience, health-care providers can serve a vital function as facilitative listeners. The patient may use such defenses against anxiety and stress as minimizing the event, blaming herself, becoming silent, and declining to tell family or friends. While being sensitive to the patient's discomfort, and the needs that such defenses serve, the health-care professional can convey patience, let the victim set the pace for care, and facilitate some discharge of anxiety through whatever the patient's means of release may be. In addition, the victim needs particular help with pragmatic concerns such as how to get home (or where to go if home is not an appropriate place). Issues of pregnancy, STDs, whom and how much to tell about the experience, and preparation for feelings that may arise during the subsequent days and weeks are matters that are important to discuss before the patient leaves the care area.

2. **Late acute stage.** After hours or days, as the initial numbness or shock begins to diminish, the patient may notice minor or previously overlooked physical symptoms. These may include vague abdominal pain, gastrointestinal irritability, genitourinary pain or burning, and bruises or lacerations to other parts of the body. These must be medically evaluated and treated, and the symptoms or injury discussed with the victim. Similarly, as the emotional numbness of the early acute stage diminishes, many victims experience tension headaches, loss of appetite, sleeplessness, fear, embarrassment, anger, revenge, self-blame, and especially fears of further violence and death.

**B. Middle phase**

1. **Reorganization or adjustment.** The middle or second phase of the rape trauma syndrome has been called the outward adjustment phase. During this time the victim seems to resolve issues about the assault and come to deal with his or her life in a controlled manner. These solutions are often disruptive of the victim's life. Such unworkable plans include never going out at night, never answering the phone when the patient is alone, and so forth. Eventually these plans fail the crisis state, leading to the reorganization phase. It is important for the health-care team to realize that this is a transition phase and that more difficult times will follow for the victim. Recognition of the transient but difficult nature of this time is important.

2. **"Poor judgement is not a rapable offense!"** During this middle phase victims may ignore aspects of the personal impact of the assault, both actual and potential. This is exemplified by return to usual activity at an intensified level, or in failing to return to the hospital for follow-up medical and/or emotional care. Intellectual rationalization of how the event occurred, and attempts to define just how to prevent a recurrence are common. The victim often expresses a sense of responsibility for his or her victimization or for having "failed" to prevent it. Such thoughts are an effort to re-establish a sense of control and in that sense are appropriate. Unfortunately, they also may often include conclusions ("I was responsible because I was out at night") or plans ("I'll never go out at night again") that are not only inappropriate but often detrimental. A good phrase to share with victims about these issues is that "Poor judgement is not a rapable offense!" Understanding this concept is important for victims, their friends and family, and others including health-care providers and law enforcement officials.

C. **Late phase.** The late, or reorganization, phase is the final stage of the rape trauma syndrome, beginning at the end of the middle phase when the victim begins a re-examination of himself or herself and/or his or her life. During this re-examination, most victims experience some feelings of disorganization. This phase determines the long-term resolution of the assault and may last for a considerable time, depending to a great extent on the quality of support the victim has received in the first two phases of her recovery.

1. **Readjustment.** During this phase, the victim needs to talk about the readjustment process, feelings of self-blame, vulnerability, rage, and change. Feelings of generalized and specific vulnerability and safety concerns will persist but their intensity will diminish over time. Sometimes long-standing issues are triggered by the reactions to the assault; sometimes reactions to the assault are hidden until triggered by some other event such as a new relationship, pregnancy, or legal action involving the prosecution of the assailant(s). There may be specific life-style changes, such as moves to a new residence or to a new city, employment changes, and changes in sexual partners and friends.
2. **Dreams.** Many victims experience a marked change in their dreams during the late phase. They may experience dreams that range from fearful re-enactment of the assault to dreams involving mastery of the experience, often in ways that may be disturbingly violent. Victims need to discuss these changes openly to keep their perspective.
3. **Reactions requiring specific intensive intervention.** Some victims exhibit severe emotional reactions, on occasion compounded by the use of drugs and alcohol, or exacerba-

tion of pre-existing emotional problems including acute psychosis. Others may become totally silent. Both extremes are warning signs requiring intervention by a social worker, psychologist, or psychiatrist depending on the specific problems.

D. **Special issues for the male victim.** Based on the limited experience with male victims of sexual assault (relatively little as compared to that with female victims), males seem to have an additional emotional burden. Male victims often seem to feel that their male identity—their masculinity—has been attacked, and that their masculinity is questionable in both their own eyes and in those around them. This view may be because many male victims are assaulted by males, but it may also represent a society view that men are the attackers, and that a male victim is somehow less male for having become the victim of attack. Health-care professionals should be alert for this additional burden male victims may carry.

III. **Initial evaluation and management of sexual assault victims** usually occurs in an emergency service department. More frequently, however, disclosure of sexual assault is occurring in clinics and doctors' offices as well as in nonmedical settings such as schools, churches, and women's centers. After arriving in the health-care setting, a protocol for care is important so that the victim is surrounded by professionals who are clearly caring as well as knowledgeable about the problem. This controlled and confident care environment helps the victim and health professionals deal effectively with the difficult tasks at hand. These tasks include responding to the emotional needs of the patient, medical evaluation and treatment, collection of forensic specimens, and helping the patient to handle interaction with police officials. A set of forms that will guide the health-care team through these tasks, providing a structured format for recording information and detailing plans, is helpful. The forms on pp 303 to 312 present the outline for the contents of such a set.

A. **First activities**

1. **Initial emotional support**

a. Immediately upon disclosure the victim should be taken to a quiet private area, thus minimizing exposure to interruption and embarrassment. It must be remembered that the victim has had an assault on his or her sense of privacy and control and has a great need to regain some sense of composure and control. **It is best that a supportive member of the health-care team remain with the victim at all times.** By encouraging the patient to talk while demonstrating a positive, supportive, nonjudgemental demeanor, this member of the health-care team begins the care process and sets the tone for the tasks that are to come.

b. Child victims of sexual assault and/or abuse provide special problems in evaluation and management. Child is defined differently in different locales and for different purposes, but in general a victim is a child from the medical standpoint until puberty. Most state statutes regarding child abuse and neglect follow the recommendations of the National Center for Child Abuse and Neglect in defining a child as anyone under 18 years of age. For other legal matters, child may be defined as under fourteen or sixteen, upon the individual state statutes and the matter at hand. In some states a pregnant child may be considered an adult with the right to sign consents for care but still be covered in the other provisions of child abuse statutes.

Although some child victims are assaulted by strangers, over 90% are long-term (years) victims of abuse by persons known to the family, most often parents and relatives. These children are in a difficult position, often sensing that what happened is wrong, yet loving and being dependent upon the abuser and wishing him or her no harm. Further, the abuser usually has offered the child a combination of enticements ("It feels good, doesn't it?") and threats ("Mommy will leave Daddy if you tell, and she will hate you.") which make the situation difficult for the child. **Child victims must be interviewed alone.** By the end of the evaluation a decision must be made as to the safety of returning the child to the home environment.

This initial interview and those that follow are best done by professionals trained in this specialized aspect of pediatric interviewing. These professionals must be aware and follow the local and state statutes about child sexual abuse reporting and take them into consideration as they care for the patient and his or her family.

**2. Triage.** As soon as possible after arrival in the health-care setting, a nurse or physician skilled in trauma triage should determine if the victim has sustained significant trauma (e.g., broken bones, knife wound). This task rarely requires more than a brief history and cursory physical examination (including vital signs) that does not require that the patient disrobe.

a. **Significant trauma.** If the victim has suffered significant trauma, the care appropriate to the trauma should be initiated. As much attention as possible to the other physical and emotional traumas of sexual assault should be given, with a clear communication to the patient that rapid attention to his or her injuries is being done to prevent permanent damage or death.

b. **No significant trauma.** If no significant trauma has been sustained, the victim may be cared for according to an established sexual assault care protocol similar to that offered in this chapter.

3. **Consents for care.** As in all health-care situations, a written consent for care should be obtained from the patient, from his or her guardian if the patient is a minor or unable to give consent for other reasons, or from the senior physician or health care administrator if the patient is unable to consent because of injury. This consent has special importance in the care of sexual assault victims, as it is especially important to start the process of continued reinforcement of the patient's sense of control. In the case of a minor, or if the victim is not able to offer consent, care may be provided on an emergency basis without formal consent. In addition, most states provide that care may be given to a child without the consent of the parents or guardian if the medical or social conditions warrant, usually with a court order. Indeed, in many states, care in a child abuse situation may be given without a specific court order. In many states, an age is specified at which a minor may consent or withhold consent.
4. **Initial contact with police.** In accord with local reporting requirements for a crime, a report of sexual assault and abuse cases for children should always be made and for adults made at the victim's request or if required by law. The victim is not required to cooperate with the police, and the health-care team should support him or her in making a decision on this matter. Nevertheless, cooperation with police and other legal authorities is clearly associated with improved emotional outcomes for victims; therefore, the health-care team should encourage victims to work with the police.

   During this initial period, police will need to interview the victim about the immediate circumstances of the sexual assault: where it happened, how it happened, information about the assailant(s), and any help that can be offered toward apprehension of the assailants. In most circumstances this initial contact should be limited to discussion of this information, with a more detailed discussion with police after the victim has completed his or her initial medical care.
5. **Child welfare authorities.** Most states require that a report be made to child welfare authorities of all suspected cases of child sexual assault or abuse in which parent, guardian, child-care provider, a person known to the victim or residing in the home of the child, is suspected; or in which parental neglect is viewed as a contributing factor to the child's victimization. In any event, this is good practice because the experienced professionals who will respond to this call will provide a depth of evaluation not possible in the health-care setting.

B. **History.** Figures 18.1 (Patient Information), 18.2 (Sexual Assault/Sexual Abuse History), and 18.3 (Patient History) present the historical information that should be obtained. More than one member of the team will obtain information and all should use such forms for the recording of this information. It is important that all team members sign and date all the pages of these forms upon which they have made contributions, and that the physician in charge sign and date all materials.

1. **Talking about the assault**
   a. Talking about the events of the sexual assault in the setting of a warm, supportive health-care program is painful but is not an additional trauma (i.e., it is not "being raped again").
   b. Child victims may have neither the vocabulary nor sense of safety to talk about their experience. The experienced pediatric interviewer will use language appropriate to the child's age and background and may rely on techniques such as drawing pictures of what happened and the use of anatomically correct dolls so that the child can show what happened in the relatively safe environment of play. Care must be taken not to ask leading questions of the child so that the interview is deemed unusable in a court of law.
2. **The medical record.** Clarity and brevity are of value in the medical records of sexual assault victims. However, in the case of the presentation of the victim's memory and reactions to a sexual assault there is considerable controversy as to whether to present the information as a summary of the victims statements and an evaluation of the victim's feelings or as a series of direct quotations from the patient. The argument for the former is that, as a professional's summary, it is not only valid but also effective for health care and legal needs. In this way, the risk of later questions being raised in court about apparent inconsistencies may be reduced. The argument for the latter is the opposite, that such summary "colors" the information with the professional's views and feelings. There is insufficient information to make a clear recommendation as to which approach to follow, although it is the opinion of the authors that in most cases the accurate and well-stated professional's summary is sufficient and indeed preferable.

C. **Physical examination and laboratory evaluation,** including the collection of forensic specimens. Figures 18.4 (Physical Examination) and 18.5 (Laboratory Evaluation) present the physical examination and laboratory evaluation for sexual assault and abuse victims, including the collection of forensic specimens.

1. **Examining the victim of sexual assault**
   a. A thorough physical examination with the collection of medical and forensic specimens is important for medical and legal reasons. The sex of the examining physi-

cian is not as important as the development of a warm caring health-care environment. Indeed, an empathetic physician of the same sex as the assailant may be of benefit to help the patient regain control of his or her interpersonal skills. Also, allowing the patient throughout the examination to consent for specific parts of the examination will assist the patient in regaining control. This is especially true for invasive maneuvers such as speculum examination of the vagina or examination of the rectum.

   b. Child victims may not be able to permit all of the components of the physical examination, especially genital and rectal examinations. If the child cannot permit the examination but the history, circumstances, and that portion of the physical examinations that can be done suggests the need for a full physical examination (specifically a genital and rectal examination), examination under anesthesia is the safest and most humane procedure. Sedation in the outpatient setting is dangerous medical practice, is rarely effective, and should be avoided.

2. **Forensic specimens.** Many states use forensic specimen kits that provide detailed instructions for the collection, storage, and transport of forensic specimens. Some specific comments about specimen collection include:
   a. Clothing worn during the assault should be preserved in a paper bag (not plastic, which promotes deterioration of secretions on the clothing and mold growth). Blood and other stains, possible semen, and so forth should be left undisturbed.
   b. Photographs of specimens and of injuries sustained by the victim (e.g., bruises, lacerations) are often helpful. Such photographs must be carefully labeled and separate consents for photography are usually beneficial. These consents may not be required in child abuse situations.
   c. Combing the pubic hair of the victim may collect hair transferred from the assailant. A sample of the victims hair should be plucked from the victim for comparison.
   d. Permanent slides should be fixed as for Papanicolaou (PAP) smears, not air dried, and should be clearly marked for identification with the victim's name, the date, and the initials of the examiner. Special slide holders should be used to protect specimens from being rubbed off.
   e. Wet mounts should be obtained with saline moistened swabs placed in body temperature normal saline solution. Motile sperm may be seen up to 72 hours following an assault and nonmotile sperm may be seen for

several days thereafter. This examination is useful only if accompanied by a history of consensual and/or non-consensual sexual activity in the week preceding the assault. The examination is of less value from a forensic standpoint after 72 hours have elapsed from the time of the assault.

f. Acid phosphatase reflects the presence or absence of ejaculate only. It may be especially useful in the case of an assailant who has had a vasectomy.

g. Colposcopy may be used in the assessment of the child who is a suspected sexual abuse victim. The reliability and acceptability in court of evidence obtained by this procedure is increasingly recognized. Some physicians believe that this is the only method that can detect trauma to the vaginal wall that would otherwise remain unnoticed.

D. **Medical management.** Figure 18.6 (Management Plan) presents the outline of management.

1. **Antibiotic therapy for STD for adults.** All adult victims should be offered prophylactic antibiotic treatment with a full explanation of the risks and benefits of treatment and refusing treatment. Recommended regimens include:

   a. **General recommendation**
   Oral **tetracycline** (500 mg q.i.d.), or oral **doxycycline** (100 mg b.i.d.), for 7 days.

   b. **For pregnant women or victims allergic to tetracyclines**
   Oral **amoxicillin** (3 g in a single dose) plus **probenecid** (1 g as a single p.o. dose), followed by oral **erythromycin** base (500 mg q.i.d. for 7 days) or oral erythromycin ethylsuccinate (800 mg q.i.d. for 7 days).

   c. In areas with a prevalence rate greater than 1% for antibiotic resistant strains of *Neisseria gonorrhoeae,* **ceftriaxone** (250 mg for one dose) followed by doxycycline (100 mg p.o. b.i.d. for 7 days) is recommended.

   d. All victims should be treated for any identified STD in either the victim or assailant.

2. **Antibiotic therapy for STD for children.** All child victims should be offered prophylactic antibiotic treatment if there is evidence that the assailant is infected, if follow-up compliance is suspected to be poor, if there are signs or symptoms of infection, or if the assault was by a stranger. In other cases, prophylactic therapy is usually not indicated, although in each case an individual clinical judgement is indicated. Such treatment is, of course, preceded by a full explanation of the risks and benefits of treatment and refusing treatment. Recommended regimens include:

   a. **General recommendation**
   Oral **amoxicillin** (50 mg/kg of body weight as a one-

time dose), plus oral **probenecid** (25 mg/kg of body weight to a maximum dose of 1 g).

b. **For penicillin allergic children and in geographic areas with a high prevalence of penicillinase-producing or chromosomally mediated resistant gonococci** IM **spectinomycin** (40 mg/kg of body weight) or, IM **ceftriaxone** (125 mg as a one-time dose) either followed by oral **tetracycline** or **erythromycin** (50 mg/kg body weight for 7 days). Tetracycline should not be used in children under 8 years old.

c. All victims should be treated for any identified STD in either the victim or assailant.

3. **Postcoital contraception.** At present there is no FDA-approved medication for postcoital contraception. The victim should understand that there is an estimated 1% to 2% chance of pregnancy after rape and a 1% failure rate for the postcoital medications that are available. Some victims may choose to take these medications after a full explanation of their risks and benefits. They should understand that the medications are teratogenic and that a therapeutic abortion is recommended in the 1% of cases where pregnancy occurs despite treatment. Other victims may choose to have a therapeutic abortion if they become pregnant. In many states, a woman who becomes pregnant as the result of sexual assault may obtain public assistance for a therapeutic abortion. Recommended regimens include:

   a. **Diethylstilbestrol (DES),** 25 mg p.o. b.i.d. twice a day for 5 days.

   b. **Ethinyl estradiol,** 5 mg p.o. q.i.d. for 5 days. (**Note: Prochlorperazine,** 10 mg p.o. q8 h, should be given on a non-p.r.n. basis with either postcoital medication to treat the nausea that will ensue.)

   c. 0.05 mg ethinyl estradiol and 0.5 mg norgestrel (Ovral), two tablets b.i.d. for 1 day.

4. **Tetanus toxoid** should be administered if indicated.

5. **Tranquilizers and sleeping medications** are not usually needed if the appropriate emotional treatment steps are taken in the acute phase. If such medications are provided, they should be prescribed in limited amounts.

**E. Discharge/follow-up plans**

1. Specific discharge plans should be given to the victim orally and in writing. This information should include a number where the patient may reach help at any time. This reinforcement is required for all victims because of the cognitive dysfunction common to them in the acute phase of rape trauma syndrome.

2. In the case of children, a determination must be made as to whether it is safe to allow the children to return home in the care of their parents. If there is question of ongoing abuse, or

the potential for abuse from the parents or guardians, consent for admission of the children should be sought from the parents, pending a more complete evaluation by appropriate child welfare agencies. If voluntary admission is declined by the parents, custody of the children should be obtained and child welfare authorities consulted about the possibility of foster home or other alternate placement pending a more complete investigation. In some cases this action will engender considerable unpleasantness, but a careful and respectful explanation to all involved is the best response by the health care team. In some cases, parents will allow hospitalization for observation, avoiding the need for legal action.

## IV. Legal issues of sexual assault and abuse

A. **Responsibilities of the health-care team** are primarily good medical and psychosocial care for the victim. These are congruent with their responsibilities to society, as dealing with the legal system is beneficial for victims regardless of whether or not the victim decides to proceed with action against the assailant. It is important for all members of the health-care team to remember that they are health-care providers, not law enforcement officers or prosecutors.

1. **The collection of forensic specimens.** The team's responsibility is to label forensic specimens carefully (just as they do with all medical specimens) and to keep track of them until turned over to law enforcement officials. The latter activity is called the "chain of evidence," and simply means that the specimens need to be kept safe (either in someone's direct care or locked away) from the chance of tampering until turned over to police.
2. **Court appearance.** Most health professionals dread appearing in court, in part because it is such a foreign arena compared to the health-care setting and also because they may feel their expertise is under "question." If the health-care professional remains calm and assured, responding to questions as asked, the appearance will usually be straightforward and often gratifying. It is important to use language that the layman can understand while nevertheless not appearing condescending.

B. **Responsibilities of the victim.** The victim's primary responsibility is to himself or herself within the context of recovery from the assault. This will make great demands upon the personal strengths and resources of the victim and may often require the use of outside available resources for counseling, support, and advice. The victim also has a responsibility to society to help in the apprehension and conviction of assailants.

C. **Responsibilities of the law enforcement officials.** Police and prosecutors share with health-care providers a strong desire for the victim's welfare but in addition have a responsibility to society to apprehend and convict assailants. At times these responsibilities may not seem congruent, but by working together, health-care professionals and law enforcement officials can smooth most areas of superficial disagreement.

## V. Follow-up, evaluation, and management of sexual assault victims

A. **Initial follow-up** should be arranged within 24 to 48 hours of the first care, either by a phone call to the victim or by an office visit. This will provide opportunity to discuss physical and emotional issues, identifying any problems that require immediate attention (e.g., suicidal ideation, rectal bleeding, safety and immediate child care) and those issues that will be dealt with in subsequent visits.

B. **The 6 weeks' visit—medical evaluation.** Victims should be seen 6 weeks after initial care for a medical evaluation. This should include physical examination, repeat cultures for STDs, and a repeat reactive plasmid reagent. Any further treatment indicated by the results of these examinations may be scheduled.

C. **Psychosocial follow-up and care.** Each victim should receive as much counseling and support as is necessary to her or his situation. This is best done by a multidisciplinary team, especially the team with whom she or he had initial care. If no program is available at the site of initial care, referral should be made to an appropriate local resource that may include a rape trauma organization; a local mental health agency; or an individual social worker, psychologist, psychiatrist, gynecologist, or pediatrician with special expertise in the psychosocial issues involving sexual assault and abuse.

*(Bibliography is on p. 313.)*

## Patient Information Form

Site of initial sexual assault/abuse care:

______________________________________________

Presentation of patient:

How did patient arrive?______________________________

Was patient accompanied? If so, by whom? What is their relationship to the patient?______________________________

______________________________________________

Time elapsed from time of incident to presentation of care:__________

Does the patient have any immediate concerns about someone else's welfare (family, children, etc.)? If so, specify the concerns and indicate action taken, when, and by whom:______________________________

______________________________________________

Does the patient wish anyone notified/called at the time of presentation? If so, whom?______________________________

______________________________________________

Date and time this was accomplished and response:______________

______________________________________________

Previous care for this problem:

Has the patient seen another health-care provider or been to another health-care facility for this problem? If so, where and when? If yes, has release of information been requested of the previous health-care provider/facility?______________________________

______________________________________________

Police/child welfare agency notification:

Police notification—when, by whom, to whom?______________

______________________________________________

Police report number:______________________________

Child welfare agency notification:

Telephone report—when, by whom, to whom?______________

______________________________________________

*(Continued)*

## Patient Information Form *(Continued)*

Written report—when, by whom, to whom?____________________

________________________________________

Financial status:

Health-care insurance:____________________________

Public aid:___________________________________

Private insurance:______________________________

HMO/PPO:____________________________________

Does the patient have an established health-care provider? Does the patient wish him/her notified? Date and time this was accomplished:_____

____________________________________________

____________________________________________

## Sexual Abuse/Sexual Abuse History Form

Date and time of abuse/assault incident:____________________

Place of abuse/assault incident (home, work, etc.):____________________

________________________________________

Time elapsed from abuse/assault to presentation for care:____________________

If known, identity, sex, race, and relationship to patient of assailant(s):__

________________________________________

| | Yes/no/not known | Where and with what |
|---|---|---|
| Does the patient report that he/she was: | | |
| struck | | |
| bound | | |
| strangled/choked | | |
| abused with a foreign object in any way | | |
| given or forced to take drugs or alcohol | | |
| Were others: | | |
| threatened or hurt<br>if so, who and how | | |
| given or forced to take drugs or alcohol<br>if so, who and how | | |
| Did assailant make contact with patient's | | |
| vulva/vagina | | |
| penis | | |
| anus | | |
| thigh(s) | | |
| breast(s) | | |
| mouth | | |
| buttocks | | |
| other | | |

Summary of other pertinent information:

## Patient Sexual and Medical History Form

Age: ______________________________

Sex: ______________________________

Race: ______________________________

| | Yes/No/Not Known | When | Pertinent Data |
|---|---|---|---|
| Since the assault/abuse has the patient: | | | |
| been unconscious | | | |
| consumed any drugs or medications | | | |
| consumed alcohol | | | |
| washed face | | | |
| washed hands | | | |
| washed genitals | | | |
| bathed/showered | | | |
| douched | | | |
| defecated | | | |
| urinated | | | |
| applied make-up | | | |
| changed clothes | | | |

Sexual history:

Has the patient been sexually active within 1 week before the assault/abuse? ______________________________

______________________________

Has the patient been sexually active since the assault/abuse? __________

______________________________

Has the patient been a victim of sexual abuse/assault previously? ______

If so, give description and summary: ______________________________

______________________________

______________________________

Has the patient frequented prostitutes or been prostituted? ____________

Do any of the victim's sexual contacts belong to groups identified as at high risk for human (acquired) immunodeficiency syndrome (AIDS) infection (drug users, those who have required multiple blood product transfusions, those of Haitian or African background, male or female prostitutes, gay or lesbian life-style)? ______________________________

Medical history:

Allergies: ______________________________

______________________________

*(Continued)*

## Patient Sexual and Medical History Form *(Cont'd)*

Major medical problems: ______________________________

______________________________

Current medications: ______________________________

______________________________

Previous diagnosis of and treatment for sexually transmitted disease—if so, give date: ______________________________

______________________________

Previous hospitalizations: ______________________________

______________________________

Previous surgery: ______________________________

______________________________

Obstetric/gynecologic history:

Age of menarche: ______________________________

Menses:

regular/irregular ______________ (interval in days) ______________

usual flow: duration ______________________________

amount ______________________________

date of last menstrual period ______________________________

date of previous menstrual period ______________________________

date of last bleeding of any kind ______________________________

Does patient think she is now pregnant? ______________________________

If so, how many weeks? ______________________________

Obstetric history:

Pregnancies ______________ Abortions ______________

Miscarriages ______________ Other ______________

Is the patient using a birth control method? ______________________________

If so, what and for how long? ______________________________

List the patient's social supports (parents, husband/wife, family, friends)

| Name | Relationship | Address/phone number |
|---|---|---|
| | | |

## Physical Examination Form

Give description and summary of the patient's overall demeanor (appearance, emotional state, orientation, verbal style, etc.):__________

________________________________________

________________________________________

________________________________________

Blood pressure _____/_____ Pulse ________ Respirations ________
Temperature ________ Height ________ Weight ________

General physical examination: (Each form should have a full figure front and back diagram and male and female genital diagrams to the indication of size and locations of lacerations and abrasions and other pertinent physical findings.)

HEENT:

Neck:

Back:

Breasts:

Chest:

Abdomen:

Extremities:

Skin:

Genital examination:

Female:

Mons:

Vulva:

Clitoris:

Urethra:

Perineum:

*(Continued)*

## Physical Examination Form *(Continued)*

Genital examination *(Continued)*

Introitus:

Vagina:

Cervix:

Uterus:

Adnexae:

Rectovaginal:

Male:

Pubis:

Penis:

Scrotum:

Rectum and anus:

# Laboratory Evaluation Form

| SPECIMEN | SITE(S) | SPECIMEN INCLUDED IN EVIDENCE KIT | RESULTS IF KNOWN |
|---|---|---|---|
| Appropriate and required: | | | |
| Cytopathology (PAP) smear | | | |
| Cultures: | | | |
| Gonorrhea | | | |
| Chlamydia | | | |
| Wet (saline) preparation | | | |
| Fluid for acid phosphatase | | | |
| Foreign material | | | |
| Reactive plasmin reagent | | | |
| Pregnancy test for all menstrual females: | | | |
| Urine | | | |
| β-hCG if indicated by clerical status of patient | | | |
| Blood type/Rh | | | |
| Hepatitis screen | | | |
| Where clinically appropriate: | | | |
| Herpes culture | | | |

Fingernail scrapings

Pubic hair combings

Pubic hair sample

Other

Urinalysis

Urine C & S

CBC

HIV (HTLV-III) antibody titre

Drug and toxicology screen:
  Urine
  Serum
Radiographs

Ultrasound

---

*Note:* PAP = Papanicolaou smear; β-hCG = beta-human chorionic gonadotropin; C&S = culture and sensitivity; CBC = complete blood count; HIV = human immunodeficiency virus.

## Therapeutic Management Plan Form

Medical treatment plans:

Antibiotic therapy for sexually transmitted disease (STD)

Treatment as appropriate for any diagnosed STD

Prophylactic treatment for STD according to Center for Disease Control guidelines

Postcoital contraceptive medication

Trauma treatment

Other

Discharge and follow-up plans:

Upon discharge you are planning to go to ______________________ with ______________________.

An appointment was made for you at ______________________ for follow-up care on ______________________, __/__/__, at ______ AM/PM.

Additional counseling has been arranged for you with ______________________ at ______________________, on ______________________, __/__/__, at ______ AM/PM.

If you have problems or questions in the interim, you may obtain help by calling ______________________.

Patient information:

You have received or did not receive the following care after a full explanation of the indications for each and the risks and benefits of each: Yes/no

Treatment for STD

Prophylactic treatment for STD

Postcoital medication (to prevent unwanted pregnancy) and an antiemetic (antinausea medication)

You received the following prescriptions with instruction on how to take the medications as well as their indications and possible side-effects:

1.

2.

3.

Release of information permission:

______________________ ______________________

Patient signature Date Witness signature Date

## BIBLIOGRAPHY

Abarbanel G. Helping victims of rape. Social Work 1976; 21:478.

Burgess A, Holstron G, Lytle L. Rape trauma syndrome. Am. J. Psychiatry 1974; 131:981.

Conte J. Progress in treating sexual abuse in children. Social Work 1984; 29:258.

Finklehor D. Child Sexual Abuse: New Theory and Research New York: The Free Press; 1984.

Fox S, Scherl D. Crisis intervention with victims of rape. Social Work 1972; 21:27.

Glaser J, Hammerschlag M, McCormack W. Sexually transmitted diseases in victims of sexual assault. N Eng J Med 1986; 315:625.

McCombie S. The Rape Crisis Intervention Handbook. New York: Plenum Press; 1980.

Russell D. Incidence and prevalence of intrafamilial and extrafamilial sexual abuse of female children. Child Abuse Neglect 1983; 7:133.

Sgroi S. Handbook of Clinical Intervention in Child Sexual Abuse Lexington, Mass: Lexington Books; 1985.

Sutherland S, Schrel D. Patterns of response among victims of rape. Am J Orthopsych 1970; 40:503.

# CHAPTER 19

# Sexually Transmitted Diseases and Pelvic Inflammatory Disease

**Jessica L. Thomason**
**Janine A. James**
**Frederik F. Broekhuizen**

The incidence of sexually transmitted diseases (STDs) is rising in the United States. Although some of the increase is secondary to a change of sexual mores, the use of certain contraceptive methods and the lack of antibodies to STD agents in young women contribute to the high incidence. Currently, human papillomavirus (HPV) is the most frequent viral STD whereas *Chlamydia trachomatis* is the most frequent bacterial STD. In the past, gonorrhea was more frequently reported. With the development of recent microbiologic technology, allowing rapid testing for STDs, clinical decisions can be made frequently within hours of patient examination, thereby preventing serious sequelae. However, a knowledge of the possible microbiologic organisms present and empiric institution of antibiotic therapy will significantly reduce morbidity and protect reproductive potential. Keys to effective management include rapid, accurate diagnosis; institution of appropriate therapy; re-evaluation of the patient for cure; treatment of the sexual partner; and patient education about the disease.

## *CHLAMYDIA TRACHOMATIS*

### I. Organism characteristics and microbiology

A. **Classification.** The genus of the organism is *Chlamydia.* There are two species, *C. trachomatis,* a human pathogen, and *Chlamydia psittaci,* a pathogen of birds and lower animals. Serotypes of *C. trachomatis* include:
   1. **A, B, C:** Associated with trachoma, the most frequent cause of neonatal blindness in third world countries.
   2. **D through K:** Associated with female and male genital tract infections and antenatal infections.
   3. **L1, L2, L3:** Associated with lymphogranuloma venereum (LGV).

B. **Life cycle.** *C. trachomatis* is an obligate intracellular organism that shares properties of both viruses and bacteria. The organism prefers the squamocolumnar cells of the transitional zone and endocervix where it reproduces itself by parasitizing adenosine triphosphate (ATP) of the infected cell. Unlike viruses, however, *Chlamydia* contains both deoxyribonucleic acid (DNA) and ribonucleic acid (RNA), divided by binary fission, and has cell walls similar to the gram-negative bacteria. The life cycle of the organism involves an infectious stage (elementary body) and a noninfectious stage (reticulate body). The elementary body attaches to the host cell and is ingested. The reticulate body (also known as "initial" body) is the reproductive stage during which the *Chlamydia* divide and replicate into hundreds of particles. *C. trachomatis* reproduces itself many times over 8 to 36 hours, thereafter causing the host cell to burst, releasing the infective organism.

**II. Incidence and epidemiology.** *C. trachomatis* is the most frequent bacteriologic and most damaging STD in the United States and Sweden. Annually, three to four million men and women acquire *Chlamydia*. Approximately 4% to 5% of sexually active women harbor *Chlamydia* in their cervix. Most sexual contacts of patients with culture proven *C. trachomatis* are asymptomatic (both men and women). However, asymptomatic patients can develop significant damage to the reproductive tract. Annually, *Chlamydia* accounts for one-quarter to one-half of the recognized cases of pelvic inflammatory disease (PID). *C. trachomatis* infections are believed to contribute significantly to the increasing number of women who develop ectopic pregnancy and infertility. The risk of transmission to women from men with nongonoccocal urethritis is 30% to 70%. *Chlamydia* is associated concomitantly with gonorrhea in 25% to 50% of women.

## III. Clinical disease

**A. In women, *C. trachomatis*** causes many diseases, including:

1. **Mucopurulent cervicitis** (MPC). A pus-like discharge drains from the endocervix, often appearing just as gonococcal cervicitis.
2. **Urethritis (acute urethral, dysuria-pyuria syndrome).** Patients with chlamydial urethritis complain of dysuria, have increased number of white blood cells in their urine, and yet have a negative urine culture. Chlamydia does not grow on standard urine culture media. Cell culture methods similar to those used to recover viruses are required to diagnose infection at this site.
3. **Salpingitis (PID).** Acute salpingitis is often associated with cervicitis and endometritis. Inflammation of the ovaries and parovarian structures may also be present. Acute salpingitis is identified in approximately 10% of women with chlamydial cervicitis and is a major cause of ectopic pregnancy and infertility.
4. **Endometritis.** The signs of endometritis include menorrhagia, menometrorrhagia, or mild pelvic discomfort. Diagnosis by endometrial biopsy with culture for *C. trachomatis*

can be performed through double or triple lumen catheters.

5. **Perihepatitis (Fitz-Hugh–Curtis syndrome).** Inflammation involves an acute localized fibrosis with subsequent scarring of the anterior surface of the liver and adjacent posterior peritoneum causing a perihepatitis. Fitz-Hugh–Curtis syndrome was previously believed to be secondary to gonorrheal infection. However, it is currently thought to more frequently occur secondary to chlamydial infections.
6. **Postpartum endometritis.** Endometritis that develops 7 or more days after delivery can be associated with *C. trachomatis.*
7. **Proctitis.** Manifestations include discharge, pain, diarrhea, hematochezia, and ulcerations. Particularly reported in homosexual men, it can also be experienced in women. It should be distinguished from *Neisseria gonorrhoeae* and herpes simplex virus proctitis.
8. **Pharyngitis.** Reported infrequently, pharyngeal pain and erythema should be evaluated in sexually active patients by culture if pharyngitis does not remit to conventional antibiotic therapy.
9. **Conjunctivitis (trachoma).** This infection is not sexually transmitted. Trachoma, a chronic inflammation of the conjunctiva, is the leading cause of blindness in underdeveloped countries. The infection may be spread by indirect contact with infected materials. Early symptoms include follicular conjunctivitis that may not be painful. Besides blindness, the sequelae of trachoma is lid distortion, trichiasis (misdirection of lashes), and entropian (inward deformation of the lid margin). Lid deformities can cause corneal ulceration and subsequent blindness.

   Inclusion conjunctivitis is also caused by *C. trachomatis.* This infection is caused by genital tract secretions into the eyes of infected infants. Chronic infections result in mild scarring and pannus formation but not usually blindness if left untreated. The serotypes causing inclusion conjunctivitis differ from those causing trachoma.
10. **Lymphogranuloma venereum (LGV).** If undiagnosed and untreated, LGV progresses through three stages, each more serious than the previous one. The primary lesion consists of papules, erosions, or ulcers that appear on the genitals 3 to 30 days after exposure. These lesions are generally painless, disappear in a few days, and may go unrecognized. The bubonic stage, marked by regional lymphadenopathy, follows. The buboes may suppurate and develop draining fistulas. The third stage consists of rectal fissures and lymphatic obstruction. Lymphogranuloma venereum is caused by *C. trachomatis* strains that differ biologically and serologically from those producing other chlamydial infec-

tions. These organisms are more invasive and virulent, infecting primarily lymphoid tissue rather than columnar epithelium. Lymphogranuloma venereum is a common problem in tropical or subtropical climates.

11. **Infertility.** Patients with infertility should be screened routinely for *Chlamydia*. Patients with tubal occlusion have serologic evidence of *C. trachomatis* infection three to seven times more frequently than the normal population.

B. **In neonates,** attack rates of 60% to 70% for infection in infants can be expected in women with cervical chlamydial infection.
   1. **Conjunctivitis.** Thirty-five percent to 50% of infants exposed to *Chlamydia* develop conjunctivitis, which manifests itself from 5 to 12 days after delivery.
   2. **Pneumonia.** Ten percent to 20% of infants exposed to *Chlamydia* develop pneumonia 3 to 11 weeks after delivery.

C. **Males** commonly present with **nongonococcal urethritis** and **acute epididymitis-orchitis** when infected with *Chlamydia,* although they may be asymptomatic. They may also have proctitis, conjunctivitis, pharyngitis, and LGV.

## IV. Diagnosis

A. **Culture.** Culturing remains the most definitive standard for diagnosis. Disadvantages include cost, complex sample preparation, need for special culture medium, expedient transport, refrigeration, and freezing. The laboratory test process demands a skilled and experienced technician. The cost and complexity of culture has discouraged its widespread use, especially since 2 to 6 days are required to complete the process making this method of identification less clinically useful than the more rapid tests listed below.

B. **Monoclonal fluorescent antibody test.** Various monoclonal antibody tests are currently available. The 2-hour test has 85% to 90% sensitivity and approximately 95% specificity. This test is currently marketed by several companies. Advantages include the ability to evaluate specimen adequacy and the rapidity with which the test can be performed. Specimens may also be "batched" for subsequent analysis. Disadvantages are that a fluorescent microscope must be used and a highly skilled individual is required for test interpretation.

C. **Enzyme immunoassay (EIA) methods.** The collection of specimens from the urethra, endocervix, and conjunctiva just as for cytology is used. A cotton swab is placed into premeasured transport solution killing any infective organisms. The assay detects both dead and live organisms reducing the risk of false negative results. Results can be available within a few hours. The EIA is as sensitive and accurate as a first-pass culture. Although this test is preferred for screening because of its relatively low cost and minimal technologic training, there are false positives.

D. **Cytology.** Cytologic identification of *C. trachomatis* on Papanicolaou (PAP) smear has a high false-positive and false-negative rate. It is not recommended.

E. **Serology testing** is not clinically useful except for research purposes. Immunoglobulin M (IgM) testing is available but is currently useful only in neonatal disease.

## V. Treatment

### A. Drug regimens of choice

1. Tetracycline HCI, 500 mg p.o. q.i.d. x 7 days
2. Doxycycline, 100 mg p.o. b.i.d. x 7 days. (**Note**: Both tetracycline and doxycycline are contraindicated in pregnant patients.)

### B. Alternative regimens

1. Erythromycin base or 500 mg p.o. q.i.d. x 7 days.
2. Erythromycin base 250 mg p.o. q.i.d. x 14 days or amoxicillin 500 mg t.i.d. x 7 days (in pregnant patients).
3. Sulfisoxizole, 2 g q.d. x 7 days (only use when testing for cure).

C. **Sexual partners.** Test partners or institute antibiotic therapy simultaneously with the treatment of female patients.

D. **Test of cure.** Repeat cultures or other diagnostic tests should be done 7 to 14 days post-therapy.

## CONDYLOMA ACUMINATA

**I. Viral characteristics.** Condyloma are caused by a DNA human papillomavirus (HPV) that cannot be grown on tissue culture. There are over 58 different subtypes:

A. HPV 16, 18 are associated with cervical intraepithelial neoplasia (CIN). These are found in dysplasias and carcinomas from all external regions of the male and female genital tract.

B. HPV 1, 4 are associated with plantar warts.

C. HPV 2 is associated with common warts (verruca vulgaris).

D. HPV 3, 10 are associated with flat warts.

E. HPV 6, 11 are associated with laryngeal papilloma, condyloma of the vulva and anal canal, and papillomas of the lower one-third of the vagina.

F. HPV 31, 33, 35, 39, 45, 51, 52, 56 are associated with high-grade genital dysplasias and carcinomas.

G. HPV 41, 42, 43, 44 are found in benign papillomas.

## II. Incidence and epidemiology

A. **Prevalence.** Precise data on the prevalence of HPV is unknown because HPV is not a reportable sexually transmitted disease, and a test has not been developed for detection of subclinical infection. Data compiled from numerous urban STD clinics over the last 10 to 15 years suggests an estimated annual incidence of genital warts in the range of 500 000 to 1 000 000 cases. Estimates of HPV infection include at least 30% of sexually active women and 10% as having clinically apparent disease.

B. **Risk factors of acquiring HPV** include local trauma, multiple sexual partners, oral contraceptive use, cigarette smoking, early age coitus, and alterations in cellular immunity.

C. **Transmission** is by direct skin to skin contact. Sexual transmission of genital warts occurs in 60% to 66% of partners exposed to warts after an incubation period of 3 weeks to 8 months (average: 3 months). Latency before cytologic, histologic, or clinical evidence of the virus can be present for years. Neonatal transmission can occur at the time of delivery of infected mothers.

D. **Disease patterns.** Cell mediated responsiveness is the key to resolution of HPV. Fifty percent of women with **vestibular** warts also have **cervical** warts and 70% of women with **perianal** warts also have **rectal** involvement. Other STDs occur concomitantly in 60% of patients.

E. **Carcinogenesis.** HPV infection alone is probably insufficient to induce carcinoma in an immunocompetent host. This conclusion is based on the long latent period between initial exposure, infection, eventual malignant conversion, and by spontaneous regression of many primary lesions. Malignant transformation may occur after HPV is exposed to additional etiologic agents such as physical agents (ultraviolet light, x-rays), chemical carcinogens (dietary components, hydrocarbons), and chronic irritation or inflammation. Possible cofactors within the lower genital tract include tobacco products, infection by other microbial agents, and immunosuppression.

## III. Clinical disease

### A. Physical appearance

1. **Venereal warts** (classic condyloma acuminata) are exophytic lesions that are papular, 2 to 3 mm in diameter, discrete or clustered on epidermal and mucosal surfaces with each papule covered by multiple finger-like projections (papillae). These tumors are pink, whitish, and vascular. They occur primarily in moist areas, especially those exposed to coital friction. In nonmucosal areas, condylomas may be more keratotic and less papilliferous.
2. **HPV-induced papular lesions** consist of small (3–7 mm), smooth, flat papules. These lesions may be pigmented or nonpigmented. The features frequently are multiple, sometimes coalescing to produce a larger area of disease resembling a cauliflower-like appearance.
3. **Flat or micropapillary plaques** of leukoplakia. Such lesions are usually noted on the cervix.

B. **Subclinical HPV infection.** Most genital HPV infections are subclinical, becoming grossly apparent only after the application of acetic acid producing "acetowhitening." Vulvar squamous papillomatosis involves the vulvar vestibule. Some papillae, usually 1 to 2 mm, are teardrop shaped especially on the inner, upper one-third of the labia minora. Rod-shaped papillae are more common on the thinner epithelial surfaces just outside of the hymen.

C. **Sites of HPV infection involvement** in women include the entire lower genital tract. The absence of gross macroscopic or colposcopically detected lesions does not exclude the presence of HPV virus.
   1. **Genital areas of involvement** include the urethra, clitoris, vulva, vestibule, posterior fourchette, perineal area, peri-anal/rectal area, vagina, cervix, and groin.
   2. **Oral involvement** occurs in areas of squamous epithelium (i.e., tongue, buccal mucosa).
   3. **Skin lesions** may occur anywhere on the body.

D. **Neonatal infection**
   1. **Laryngeal papillomatosis** (condyloma on the vocal cords) can occur in children born to infected mothers.
   2. Anogenital lesions may appear later in the neonatal period. However, first rule out sexual abuse in all cases.

## IV. Diagnosis

A. **Gross inspection** (as above).

B. **Colposcopy** of genital areas delineates the extent of disease involvement. Particularly in the male, the use of colposcopy reduces the likelihood of missing small lesions that might otherwise go undiagnosed.

C. **Biopsy of macroscopic lesions.** Biopsy larger or pigmented lesions to rule out coexisting malignancy. Avoid biopsy within 4 weeks after treatment with biochemical agents. The histology of chemically treated lesions can be confused with malignancy.

D. **PAP smear.** Cytologic diagnosis by smear is the most convenient way to diagnose HPV infection but is less accurate than DNA typing. Features of koilocytosis, dyskeratocytosis, and associated diagnostic criteria are used to diagnose HPV infection. Koilocytosis is a large cavity or vacuole surrounding an atypical appearing nucleus. Keratocytosis consists of small superficial cells occurring mainly in three-dimensional clusters with features of premature keratinization in the form of a densely eosinophilic cytoplasm. Nuclei appear opaque, hyperchromatic, and irregular. Binucleation or multinucleation, condensed filaments, and keratocytotic granules are diagnostic criteria commonly associated with infection, but not pathognomonic.

## V. Therapy

A. **Biochemical agents.** Topical cytotoxic agents can be applied every 2 to 3 days. With no improvement after two applications, a different agent or mode of therapy should be used. In general, warts of "new onset" respond better than "old" warts. Cytotoxic agents include:
   1. **Trichloroacetic (or bichloroacetic) acid,** 50%, 85% solution.

2. **5-fluorouracil 5% cream (Efudex).** Should not be used in pregnancy.
3. **Podophyllin,** 10% or 25%
   a. Contraindicated in pregnancy and children.
   b. Higher failure rate.
   c. Drug may be absorbed into the vascular system, producing neurologic problems, and death has been reported. Podophyllin applications should be avoided for lesions located in the vagina or on perianal skin.

B. **Cryosurgery,** if used, should be limited to lesions involving the cervix. Cryosurgery provides an uncontrolled depth of tissue destruction. Vaginal treatments with cryotherapy should be avoided because scarring and strictures may result.

C. **Laser surgery,** while more expensive, is preferred for larger (>1 cm) and more extensive lesions, and especially in women requiring therapy during pregnancy. Viral particles are present in surrounding normal-appearing skin and are responsible for early recurrences after such therapy. Use of this method requires a sophisticated operator with colposcopic skills.

D. **Surgical excision.** Laser therapy has basically replaced this form of therapy.

E. **Immunotherapy.** Interferon can be injected directly into lesions. Significant side effects limit the general use of this therapy.

F. **Subclinical disease** is not treated unless the patient suffers from dyspareunia, vulvodynia, or pruritis.

G. **Treatment for HPV** is not designed to eradicate the virus but to eradicate tissue that is at greater risk of becoming malignant.

H. **Examination and treatment of male partners** is essential to reduce disease recurrence.

## *NEISSERIA GONORRHOEAE*

### I. Bacterial characteristics and microbiology.

*N. gonorrhoeae* is a gram-negative diplococcus that prefers columnar and pseudostratified epithelium. Different strains of gonorrhea exist with some more virulent strains having pili allowing for easier attachment to mucosal surfaces. Human beings are the sole hosts of gonorrhea.

### II. Incidence and epidemiology

A. **Adult infection.** Transmission risk from an infected male to a woman is 70%. The rate of transmission from an infected woman to her male partner can be as low as 20% with one exposure, but rises to 80% to 90% after four sexual encounters. Seasonal variation occurs with highest incidence rates in the late summer and lowest in late winter. The rate of infection is highest in sexually active 15 to 19 year olds.

B. **Neonatal infection.** At least 20% of neonates delivered through an infected birth canal acquire the disease.

## III. Clinical disease

A. **In women and men.** Both women and men with gonorrheal infection are frequently asymptomatic.

1. **Women**

   a. **Site of infection.** The urethra, endocervix, upper genital tract, pharynx, or rectum are common sites of infection. Presenting symptoms include increased vaginal discharge, dysuria, and abnormal uterine bleeding.

   b. **Complications**

   (1) 20% to 40% of **PID** is gonorrheal associated.

   (2) **Premature rupture of the membranes and/or premature labor** have been linked to infected mothers.

   (3) **Disseminated disease** occurs most frequently when gonorrhea is acquired during the menses or during pregnancy. Common features of disseminated gonorrhea include tenosynovitis, skin lesions, fever, leukocytosis, polyarthralgias, hepatitis and mild leukocytosis, polyarthralgias, hepatitis and mild pericarditis. Less common manifestations of disseminated gonorrhea include meningitis, endocarditis, pneumonia, and osteomyelitis.

2. **Men.** In men, the urethra, epididymis, prostate, rectum, or pharynx are common sites of infection. Dissemination also can occur.

B. **In neonates,** gonococcal conjunctivitis or disseminated disease may occur.

## IV. Diagnosis

A. **Culture** for *N. gonorrhoeae* is the only reliable method to detect disease in women; however, numerous problems with culture can arise. Screening endocervical cultures detect only 65% to 85% of infected women. Factors contributing to inadequate diagnosis include technique used for specimen collection, lack of rapid transport to the laboratory, lack of accessibility of placing cultures into a $CO_2$ environment, and lack of incubation of cultures at 37°C prior to laboratory transport.

B. **Gram stains** of endocervical specimens are less reliable than culture for diagnosis. In men, however, Gram stain of urethral discharge can be used to accurately diagnose gonorrhea.

C. **Enzyme-linked immunosorbert assay (ELISA) tests** (e.g., gonozyme) currently are not useful in women.

## V. Treatment

A. Uncomplicated infections at the urethra, endocervix and rectum: ceftriaxone 250 mg IM plus doxycycline 100 mg b.i.d. x 7 days.

1. Alternative regimens all followed by doxycycline 100 mg b.i.d. × 7 days: spectinomycin 2 g IM, ciprofloxacin 500

mg p.o., norfloxacin 800 mg, cefotaxime 1 g IM, ceflizoxime 500 mg IM, cefuroxime axetil 1 g p.o.

2. If infections are caused by **nonpenicillin-resistant gonorrhea: amoxicillin** 3 g p.o. with 1 g probenecid orally.
3. If testing a *C. trachomatis* performed at the same time was negative, doxycycline is **not** needed.

B. **Pharyngeal gonorrheal infection.** Treat with ceftriaxone 250 mg IM or for patients who cannot be treated with ceftriaxone, give ciprofloxacin 500 mg p.o.

C. Test all patients for syphilis and offer HIV testing.

D. Treat persons exposed to gonorrhea within the preceding 30 days presumptively.

## HERPES SIMPLEX VIRUS

### I. Viral characteristics and microbiology.

The herpes simplex virus (HSV) is composed of DNA, making autoimmune elimination impossible. Once patients acquire HSV, it remains in their body throughout their lifetime, although the virus may remain in latent form producing no clinical signs or symptoms of disease. Other members of the herpes family include varicella-zoster (chicken pox, shingles), cytomegalovirus (CMV), and Epstein-Barr virus (mononucleosis). Different antigenic stains exist but are divided into two types: HSV-1 "oral," "above the waist" and HSV-2 "genital," "below the waist." Although HSV-1 and HSV-2 may occur and can be transmitted to either site, the majority of genital isolates are HSV-2, and the majority of oral isolates are HSV-1.

### II. Incidence and epidemiology

A. **Infection.** "Primary" infection usually occurs in childhood and is frequently asymptomatic. Following primary infection, the virus becomes latent. **Latent virus** resides in sensory neural ganglia and has been found in human trigeminal, sacral, and vagal ganglion. The reason for recurrent infections is unknown. From 50% to 100% of sampled adult populations have positive serologic evidence of HSV-1, and 20% to 80% have evidence of HSV-2.

B. **Transmission. Asymptomatic shedding** of HSV occurs and represents the hidden reservoir of infection. At any particular time, 0.75% to 5% of the general population shed HSV-1, and 0.38% to 8% shed HSV-2. Recurrence rates for HSV-2 are higher than for HSV-1 regardless of site of infection. Transmission occurs only by direct contact with viral particles. Aerosol transmission has never been proven. HSV is sensitive to minute amounts of chlorine and thus is not transmitted by water (i.e., hot tubs). **Autoinoculation is possible**; thus, good hygiene (i.e., handwashing) should be emphasized and the wearing of contact lenses during acute attacks should be discouraged.

**III. Clinical disease.** Although steps may be skipped, the usual sequence of disease is painful papules followed by vesicles, ulceration, crusting, and healing. Symptoms usually are more severe in women than men.

- **A. Primary episodes** of HSV have more systemic manifestations than recurrent episodes, although some infections may be asymptomatic. The incubation period averages 6 days but may range from 2 to 14 days. In primary infection, fever and lymphadenopathy frequently occur and viral shedding may be prolonged (average: 12 days). Healing of lesions may be prolonged (average: 3 weeks).
- **B. Recurrent episodes** of HSV frequently have a prodromal period signaling active virus replication. Lesions are often localized. The length of viral shedding is less than with primary episodes (average 7 days) and healing occurs more rapidly (average 5 days). Most recurrences are caused by reactions of latent virus rather than reinfection.

## IV. Diagnosis

- **A. Tissue culture** is the best method for diagnosis, but it is lengthy and costly. Diagnosis by cytopathologic effect (CPE) of the virus in tissue culture can be made as early as 18 to 24 hours, but the median time from inoculation to development of CPE is 4 days. Sixty-five percent of virus isolates are identified by 5 days and 90% within 10 days. The sensitivity of culture varies with the type of lesions. In general, vesicles are most likely to be culture positive.
- **B. Rapid diagnostic tests**
  1. **Indirect immunoperoxidase staining** of a tissue sample (not a scraping of lesion) has 70% sensitivity.
  2. **ELISA testing** (Herpes Sure Cell®, Kodak; Herpazyme®, Abbott Laboratories) has a 70% sensitivity compared to culture.
  3. **Direct immunofluorescent staining** of a tissue sample is dependent upon the number of cells present in the specimen and subsequently in the "collector." Vesicular lesions offer the best results. In good specimens, it is 75% as sensitive as culture.
  4. Neither a negative smear nor a negative culture exclude HSV disease.

**V. Treatment.** There is no effective treatment that eradicates HSV infection. Acyclovir is effective in alleviating symptoms and is recommended.

- **A. Acyclovir**
  1. **Oral acyclovir therapy**
     - a. First clinical episode: 200 mg five times per day for 7 to 10 days significantly shortens viral shedding and time to healing.

b. Suppression of recurrent infections: 200 mg five times per day of 80 mg b.i.d. Both regimens should be given for 5 days.
c. Daily suppressive therapy is needed if ≥ 6 episodes occur per year. Give 200 mg two to five times per day or 400 mg b.i.d. After 6 months to 1 year of therapy, discontinue the medication to assess recurrence.
d. The resumption of recurrence is not influenced by prior use of continuous acyclovir suppression.
e. Avoid continuous suppression therapy in women who may conceive during the treatment period.

2. **IV acyclovir therapy.** IV acyclovir therapy is recommended for immunocompromised patients, for severe symptoms or complications requiring hospitalization. Give 5 mg/kg every 8 hours for 5 to 7 days. Recurrences are not prevented.
3. **Acyclovir—5% ointment** applied twice a day is useful in men but not in women.

## SYPHILIS

I. **Organism characteristics and microbiology.** *Treponema pallidum* is a motile, tightly coiled spirochete that cannot be grown. Other treponemal spirochetes not endemic to the United States cause yaws and pinta. The spirochete can invade intact mucous membranes or areas of abraded skin.

II. **Incidence and epidemiology.** The incidence of syphilis is rising. Thirty percent of patients exposed acquire the disease. However, in infected patients receiving no therapy, 60% have immunodefenses sufficient to control the infection whereas approximately 40% develop late or tertiary complications of syphilis.

III. **Clinical disease**

A. **Early syphilis.** Early syphilis is the only infectious stage. It is divided into two clinical stages:

1. **Primary syphilis.** A **chancre** is the hallmark of primary syphilis, occurring from 10 to 90 days (average: 3 weeks) after exposure. It occurs at the site of inoculation. Although painless, the chancre can produce some discomfort at the site and regional lymphadenopathy.
2. **Secondary syphilis** occurs as mucocutaneous skin lesions a few weeks to 6 months (average: 6–8 weeks) after original inoculation. Alopecia, hepatitis, and nephrotic syndrome occur rarely. Up to 25% of patients have intermittent recurrent skin lesions over a 2 year period.

B. **Latent syphilis** is characterized by serologic evidence of disease but no clinical signs or symptoms. Most patients are not infectious but 25% of these patients may have a recent history of mucocutaneous eruptions. Arbitrary division of this stage has been made but has no clinical significance with regard to therapy (early latency: disease < 4 years from initial infection, late latency: disease > 4 years from initial infection).

C. **Late syphilis** is not infectious and occurs 5 to 30 years (mean: 8 years) after inoculation. There are three divisions.
   1. **"Benign" disease.** Lesions (gummas) occur in vital organs during this stage and can be life threatening if they compromise organ functions.
   2. **Cardiovascular disease.** Involvement of the heart and aorta are frequent and may cause significant cardiovascular dysfunction.
   3. **Neurological disease.** Three clinical syndromes of neurologic involvement are:
      a. **Asymptomatic disease.** Cerebrospinal fluid analysis is abnormal, yet no patient neurologic symptoms are manifest.
      b. **Meningovascular disease.** The common manifestation is paresis (tabes dorsalis).
      c. **Parenchymatous disease.** Dementia is the common manifestation.

## IV. Diagnosis

A. **Serologic testing** is divided into two types of tests: nontreponemal-specific tests (rapid plasma reagin [RPR] test, Venereal Disease Research Laboratory [VDRL] slide test) and treponemal-specific tests (flourescent treponemal antibody-absorbed [FTA-ABS] test, microhemagglutination assay for *T. pallidum* [MHA-TP]).

B. **Nontreponemal-specific tests** identify antibodies (called "reagin" antibodies) developed by the body in response to nonspecific antigens due to the immunologic inflammatory response to the spirochete. These tests are quantitated and reported in titers (i.e., 1:8, 1:64). The higher the titer, the higher the inflammatory reaction to infection. **False-positive tests** occur and are seen with chronic diseases (e.g., leprosy), autoimmune disease (e.g., lupus erythematosus), pregnancy, and in drug addiction.

C. **Treponemal-specific tests** identify specific antibody directed against *T. pallidum.* A positive result indicates either active disease or previous exposure to syphilis. MHA-TP is frequently used in testing neonates, whereas FTA-ABS is the standard adult test.

D. **Darkfield microscopy.** This is useful with lesions that have active motile spirochetes (primary and secondary lesions). The skin lesion should be scraped and the exudate touched to a glass slide, covered, and sealed at the edges with petroleum jelly. Spirochetes remain motile for hours in an anaerobic environment.

## V. **Treatment** for syphilis is based on clinical and serologic staging of the disease.

A. **Antibiotic therapy**
   1. **Early disease (primary or secondary stage) or latent disease less than 1-year duration**
      a. Benzathine penicillin 2.4 million units IM.
      b. Penicillin-allergic patients: Doxycycline 100 mg b.i.d. or tetracycline HCl 500 mg p.o. q.i.d. for 15 days.
   2. **Latent disease greater than 1 year duration or late disease**
      a. Benzathine penicillin 2.4 million units IM weekly for 3 weeks, **or**
      b. Penicillin-allergic patients: tetracycline HCl 500 mg p.o. q.i.d. for 30 days.

B. **Follow-up evaluation after treatment.** Patients should be reevaluated with nontreponemal quantitative tests at 3 and 6 months post-therapy. A four-fold rise in titer indicates inadequate treatment or reinfection and requires retreatment.

C. **Neurosyphilis.** Consultation with an infectious disease expert is required.

## MYCOPLASMAS

### I. Organism characteristics and microbiology.

Mycoplasmas consist of DNA and RNA and are the smallest free-living organisms. They are classified as bacteria but lack cell walls and therefore do not stain with Gram stain or respond to antibiotics that inhibit cell-wall synthesis. Mycoplasmas are affected by agents that inhibit protein synthesis. Only three species cause disease in humans: *Mycoplasma pneumoniae* causes atypical pneumonia, *Mycoplasma hominis* and *Ureaplasma urealyticum* are isolated from the genital tract. *Ureaplasma* can usually be isolated from 70% to 90% (range, 40%–95%) and *M. hominis* can be isolated from 40% to 60% of sexually active women.

### II. Incidence and epidemiology.

Colonization can occur with little demonstrable pathogenicity and occurs primarily following puberty, increasing as the number of sexual contacts rises. Neonatal colonization is transient.

### III. Clinical disease

A. **Pelvic involving mycoplasmas in women**
   1. **Pelvic inflammatory disease.** Usually isolated concomitantly with other organisms, *Mycoplasma* sp. is found in 10% to 15% of patients with PID. *M. hominis* is isolated more frequently than *U. urealyticum.*
   2. **Vaginitis.** *M. hominis* is usually associated with bacterial vaginosis.
   3. **Postabortion endometritis.** The incidence of *Mycoplasma* sp. postabortion endometritis is unknown, but is seen more frequently with *M. hominis* than *U. urealyticum.*
   4. **Postpartum fever** is usually associated with other concomi-

tant organisms; *M. hominis* is seen more frequently involved than *U. urealyticum.*

5. **Chorioamnionitis.** Mycoplasma associated chorioamnionitis is usually caused by *U. urealyticum.*
6. **Low birth weight/prematurity.** The data are conflicting as to the role mycoplasmas have on either complication of pregnancy.
7. **Infertility.** Mycoplasmas may play a role in infertility; but this issue remains controversial.
8. **Recurrent pregnancy loss.** Like infertility, the role of mycoplasma in pregnancy loss remains controversial.

B. **Diseases involving mycoplasmas in men.** Diseases in men include nonspecific urethritis, prostatitis, epididmymitis, and Reiter's disease.

## IV. Laboratory diagnosis.

**Laboratory diagnosis.** Culturing for mycoplasma is the most accurate method of laboratory diagnosis. Transport media is commercially available and is necessary to prevent overgrowth of specimens by other cervicovaginal flora. The best recovery rates are obtained if specimens are kept refrigerated prior to transport to the laboratory. Serologic testing is not useful for the diagnosis in genital tract mycoplasma.

## V. Treatment

A. **Antibiotic therapy of choice.** Drugs of first choice are the tetracyclines.

1. **Tetracycline HCl**, 500 mg p.o. q.i.d. for 7 days for *M. hominis.*
2. **Doxycycline**, 100 mg p.o. b.i.d. for 7 days.
3. **Clindamycin** 600 mg p.o. qd for 14 days for *M. hominis.*

B. **Second drugs of choice**

1. **Erythromycin**, 500 mg p.o. q.i.d. for 7 days for *U. urealyticum.*
2. **Lincomycin**, 500 mg p.o. t.i.d. for 7 days for *M. hominis.*

# PELVIC INFLAMMATORY DISEASE (PID)

## I. Incidence and epidemiology.

**Incidence and epidemiology.** By the year 2000, one out of every three office visits will be for the diagnosis, treatment, or sequelae of PID. Fifteen percent of women with PID currently fail initial antibiotic therapy, and 20% of women have at least one recurrence during their reproductive years.

## II. Risk factors

A. **Adolescence.** Sexually active adolescents have a one in eight chance of developing PID by age 20.

B. **Contraceptive methods.** Contraception may work either to protect against or facilitate the development of PID.

1. **Intrauterine devices (IUDs).** These devices carry a two to nine times risk for development of PID, regardless of the

length of time the IUD has been in place or type of IUD used.

2. **Oral contraceptive pills.** Although previously thought to protect, theories suggest the protective effects ascribed to oral contraceptives may have been overemphasized. Oral contraceptives are related to cervical ectropion, allowing STDs easy access to columnar epithelium, where they thrive. In addition, hormonal changes may allow more rapid proliferation of *C. trachomatis*.
3. **Barrier methods** of contraception (e.g., condoms, diaphragm) offer protective effects from all STDs.

C. **Multiple sexual partners.** Multiple sexual partners significantly increase the risk of PID.

D. **Association of PID with gonorrheal or chlamydial lower genital tract infection.** Endocervical infection, with gonorrhea or *C. trachomatis* increases the risk of upper genital tract infection.

E. **Previous PID.** A previous history of PID increases the likelihood of subsequent development of PID, ectopic pregnancy, and infertility.

## III. Diagnosis

A. **Clinical diagnosis.** Thirty percent of the time the diagnosis of PID is inaccurate when clinical signs are relied upon. The clinical diagnosis of PID is most accurate when all of the following are present:

1. Temperature > 38° C (100.4° F)
2. Cervical motion tenderness on bimanual examination.
3. WBC > 10 000 $mm^3$.
4. Abdominal pain.
5. In addition, one of the following should be present:
    a. Elevated sedimentation rate.
    b. Purulence retrieved by culdocentesis.
    c. Sonographic evidence of an adnexal mass consistent with an abscess or tubo-ovarian complex (caused by PID-associated pelvic adhesions).

B. **Laparoscopy.** Diagnostic laparoscopy is the most reliable method for the diagnosis of PID. Staging of disease so that infertility risk can be discussed subsequently with patients and adequate culturing of the site most reflective of disease (the fallopian tubes) is possible using this method for diagnosis.

C. **Staging of PID.** PID should be staged in all cases whether diagnosed clinically or laparoscopically, because it reflects the chance of future fertility. Tables 19.1 and 19.2 include staging protocols.

D. **Culture.** The endocervix should be cultured for STDs (*C. trachomatis*, gonorrhea, mycoplasmas) but should not be cultured for aerobes and anaerobes. Aerobes and anaerobes from this area do not reflect the microbiology of upper genital tract disease.

E. **Wet prep microscopic examination** of the vagina is inexpensive and has excellent specificity.

**Table 19.1. Grading of Pelvic Inflammatory Disease by Clinical Examination**

| | |
|---|---|
| Uncomplicated: | Limited to tube(s) and/or ovary(ies)<br>Without pelvic peritonitis<br>With pelvic peritonitis |
| Complicated: | Inflammatory mass or abscess involving tube(s) and/or ovary(ies)<br>Without pelvic peritonitis<br>With pelvic peritonitis |
| Spread: | To structures beyond pelvis (i.e., ruptured tubo-ovarian abscess) |

From Hager WD, Eschenbach DA, Spence MR. Criteria for diagnosis and grading of salpingitis. Obstet Gynecol 1983; 61:113–114. Reprinted with permission from the American College of Obstetricians and Gynecologists.

1. Examine the vaginal secretions for *Trichomonas vaginalis, Mobiluncus* sp., and clue cells.
2. If the number of epithelial cells is greater than the number of white blood cells (WBCs) per high powered field, the patient cannot have PID.
3. If WBCs > epithelial cells per high powered field, the patient may have PID. Verify diagnosis by other diagnostic criteria.

## IV. Treatment

A. **Polymicrobial infection.** The etiology of PID is polymicrobial and therefore treatment should be with a broad spectrum antibiotic. Remember that anaerobes always outnumber aerobes, *C. trachomatis* is isolated in 20% to 50% of infections, *N. gonorrhoeae* is isolated in 20% to 50% of infections, anaerobes and aerobes are isolated in 50% of infections, and mycoplasmas are isolated in 10% of infections.

B. **The decision to treat a patient with PID as an inpatient or outpatient** basis depends on a number of factors. Failure or delay to treat PID can result in pelvic adhesions and infertility.

**Table 19.2. Grading Severity of Pelvic Inflammatory Disease by Laparoscopic Examination**

| | |
|---|---|
| Mild: | Erythema, edema, no spontaneous purulent exudate*; tubes freely moveable. |
| Moderate: | Gross purulent material evident; erythema and edema more marked. Tubes may not be freely moveable, and fimbria stoma may not be patent. |
| Severe: | Pyosalpinx or inflammatory complex; abscess† |

*The tubes may require manipulation to produce purulent exudate.
†The size of any pelvic abscess should be measured.
From Hager WD, Eschenbach DA, Spence MR. Criteria for diagnosis and grading of salpingitis. Obstet Gynecol 1983; 61: 113–114. Reprinted with permission from the American College of Obstetricians and Gynecologists.

1. **Outpatient therapy.** Use the same regimen as that for the treatment of patients with gonorrhea. In addition, use tetracycline 500 mg q.i.d. or doxycycline 100 mg b.i.d. for 10 days of total therapy. (Determine that the patient is not pregnant.) It is critical that patients be re-examined within 72 hours after initiating therapy to evaluate responsiveness. If there is no clinical improvement, hospitalization is indicated. Criteria for hospitalization include:
   a. Noncompliant patient
   b. Temperature > 100.4° F (38° C)
   c. Questionable diagnosis
   d. Pregnancy
   e. Tubo-ovarian abscess
   f. Inability to take oral medications
   g. Upper peritoneal signs
   h. IUD in place
2. **Inpatient therapy**
   a. **Doxycycline** 100 mg IV b.i.d. or **tetracycline** 500 mg IV q.i.d. plus **cefoxitin** 2 g IV every 6 hours for at least 4 days or 48 hours after the patient improves clinically. Therapy should be continued as an outpatient with a tetracycline (500 mg p.o. q.i.d.) to complete 10 to 14 days of total therapy.
   b. **Clindamycin** 900 mg IV every 8 hours plus an **aminoglycoside** (i.e., gentamycin 2 g/kg in three divided doses) IV q8 h followed by 1.5 mg/kg IV, t.i.d. in patients who have normal renal function. Therapy should be continued as an outpatient with clindamycin (450 mg p.o. q.i.d.) to complete 10 days of total therapy.

C. **Surgical therapy.** The decision to surgically intervene should be made for questionable diagnosis, failure to respond to adequate antibiotic therapy, or a tubo-ovarian mass that is failing to resolve or decrease in size.

## V. Sequelae of PID

A. **Ectopic pregnancy** (was previously 1/200, now 1/20 pregnancies).

B. **Infertility.** Early diagnosis and treatment are crucial to preserve future fertility. There is a 10% risk of infertility after one episode of PID, 25% risk after two episodes, and 50% risk after three or more episodes. The risk of infertility increases with more severe disease noted at laparoscopy. There is a 6.1% risk of infertility with mild disease, a 13.4% risk with moderate disease, and a 3.0% risk with severe disease.

C. **Chronic pelvic pain** due to tubo-ovarian abscess, adhesions of omentum and to the bowel.

D. Peritonitis

E. Ruptured tubo-ovarian abscess

F. Sepsis

G. Bowel obstruction

## BIBLIOGRAPHY

Gibbs RS, Amstey MS, Sweet RL, Mead PB, Sever JL. Management of genital herpes infection in pregnancy. Obstet Gynecol 1988; 71:779–790.

Sweet, RL, Gibbs RS, eds. Infectious Diseases of the Female Genital Tract. Baltimore, MD: Williams and Wilkins; 1985.

Koutsky LA, Galloway DA, Holmes KK. Epidemiology of genital human papillomavirus infection. Epidemiol Rev. 1988; 10:122–163.

1989 Sexually transmitted diseases: Treatment guidelines. Morbidity and Mortality Weekly Report, Vol 38: No. S-8.

Wasserheit JN, Bell TA, Kiviat NB, Wolner–Hanssen P, Zabriskie V, Kirby BD, Prince EC, Holmes KK, Stamm WE, Eschenbach DA. Microbial causes of proven pelvic inflammatory disease and efficacy of clindamycin and tobramycin. Ann Intern Med 1986; 104:187–193.

# Part III

# Gynecologic Endocrinology and Infertility

# CHAPTER 20

# Amenorrhea and Hyperprolactinemia

**Eldon D. Schriock**

Hyperprolactinemia is a common gynecologic problem that usually presents with secondary amenorrhea, but may also result in oligomenorrhea, infertility, amenorrhea, and galactorrhea. However, amenorrhea may result from a wide range of gynecologic conditions. The diagnosis of both hyperprolactinemia and amenorrhea requires a combination of endocrine and radiologic evaluation. Prolactin-secreting pituitary adenomas are a common cause of hyperprolactinemia but must be differentiated from other physiologic, pharmacologic, and pathologic etiologies of hyperprolactinemia. The work-up of the hyperprolactinemic patient must also rule out other causes of anovulation.

I. **Incidence.** One-third of women with otherwise unexplained amenorrhea have hyperprolactinemia. Not all patients with hyperprolactinemia have galactorrhea and conversely, not all patients with galactorrhea have hyperprolactinemia. Elevated levels of prolactin may be found in women with regular menses, although these women may have inadequate luteal function. The incidence of prolactin-secreting microadenomas may be as high as 22% of the general population, based on autopsy studies. Although this incidence remains controversial, it does indicate that the majority of adenomas may be clinically benign.

II. **Pathogenesis and pathophysiology.** Prolactin-secreting pituitary adenomas are the most common pathologic entity associated with hyperprolactinemia. The process that causes or permits pituitary adenomas to develop has not yet been established. The major hypotheses explaining the development of pituitary adenomas include (a) a deficiency of dopamine secretion, which is normally responsible for suppressing prolactin secretion, (b) an inability of the adenomatous tissue to respond to dopamine, (c) a vascular defect isolating part of the pituitary from the dopamine-rich portal circulation allowing hyperplasia and adenoma formation. Once hyperprolactinemia has been established, it appears ovulation is inhibited by a decrease in pulsatile gonadotropin-releasing hormone (GnRH) secretion resulting in decreased pituitary and ovarian function.

III. **Morbidity.** Infertility is the major morbidity related to amenorrhea. The absence of menses, by itself, is not a cause of morbidity. An example is amenorrhea while taking oral contraceptives. The morbidity and mortality associated with amenorrhea must be viewed from two perspectives; first, morbidity that is directly related to the etiology of amenorrhea; and second, morbidity that is secondary to alterations in normal reproductive physiology. Table 20.1 presents morbidity related to specific causes of amenorrhea.

## IV. Etiology of hyperprolactinemia

### A. Common causes

1. **Physiologic causes** of elevated prolactin include sleep disorders, prolonged strenuous exercise, stress, pregnancy, and breast-feeding.
2. **Hormonal causes of elevated prolactin**
   a. Primary hypothyroidism results in marked increases in thyrotropin-releasing hormone (TRH) release. The TRH stimulates not only thyrotropin (TSH) but also prolactin. These patients can appear clinically similar to patients with prolactin-secreting adenomas because they also present with amenorrhea, galactorrhea, elevated prolactin, and an enlarged pituitary secondary to thyrotroph hyperplasia.
   b. Estrogen may cause the increase in prolactin concentrations found in pregnancy and during estrogen administration, for example, oral contraceptives.
   c. Hypoglycemia stimulates the release of several pituitary hormones including prolactin. This is used diagnostically as the insulin tolerance test.
3. **Drugs** associated with hyperprolactinemia include dopamine receptor blockers (metoclopromide), catechol depleting agents, catechol reuptake blockers, anesthetics, opiates, and antihistamines. Most drugs that stimulate prolactin release do so by interfering with the tonic inhibition of prolactin by dopamine. The mechanism of prolactin release induced by endogenous (stress-induced endorphin release) or exogenous opiates is unknown.
4. **Pituitary adenomas.** Prolactin-secreting pituitary adenomas are the most common pituitary tumor. The clinical course of these tumors is usually benign, although some tumors invade locally. Metastasis essentially never occurs. The size of the tumor is directly, although not absolutely, related to the serum concentration of prolactin. Pituitary

**Table 20.1. Causes of Amenorrhea and Associated Morbidity**

| ETIOLOGY | MORBIDITY |
|---|---|
| Hyperprolactinemia | Related to etiologic factor(s) (see section IV) |
| Hypoestrogenism | Loss of secondary sexual characteristics, osteoporosis |
| Unopposed estrogen | Endometrial hyperplasia and carcinoma |
| Hyperandrogenism | Hirsutism, acne, masculinization, decreased high-density lipoproteins, insulin resistance |
| Presence of Y chromosome | Malignant tumor |
| Pituitary adenoma | Headache, visual loss |
| Ovarian or adrenal tumor | Possible malignancy |
| Imperforate hymen or other Müllerian defect | Retrograde menstruation and endometriosis |
| Adrenal or ovarian steroid enzyme defect | Hypertension, electrolyte imbalance, ambiguous genitalia |
| Hyper- or hypofunction of adrenal or thyroid | Medical complications related to adrenal or thyroid gland |
| Anorexia nervosa | Starvation |
| Premature ovarian failure | Autoimmune disorders |
| Kallman's syndrome | Anosmia |
| Obesity | Multiple health risks |
| Vaginal agenesis | Unable to have intercourse |

adenomas of $\leq 1$ cm are classified as microadenomas, and those $> 1$ cm are called macroadenomas.

**B. Uncommon causes**

1. **Hypothalamic-pituitary tumors (craniopharyngioma)** cause elevated prolactin by a "stalk-effect." The tumor blocks the dopamine-rich portal blood from reaching the pituitary by impinging on the pituitary stalk. Prolactin release is then uninhibited.
2. **Empty sella syndrome** is a clinical condition that results from an intrasellar extension of the subarachnoid space. This results in compression of the pituitary gland and an enlarged sella turcia. Patients are usually hormonally normal, with hyperprolactinemia being the most common pituitary hormone abnormality present. Headache is the most common symptom.

3. **Renal failure.** Hyperprolactinemia can occur in patients with renal disease as a result of decreased metabolic clearance and an increased production rate, the pathophysiology of which is unknown.
4. **Ectopic prolactin production.**

## V. Differential diagnosis.

In addition to hyperprolactinemia, other causes of amenorrhea must be considered in the differential diagnosis.

### A. Common diagnoses

1. **Pregnancy.** All patients of reproductive age who present with amenorrhea should have a pregnancy test performed.
2. **Hypothalamic amenorrhea (HA)** is a diagnosis of exclusion. These women have no apparent abnormalities of the pituitary-ovarian axis or other endocrine function. A stressful situation in a woman's life is often associated with this diagnosis. An increasingly frequent cause of HA is excessive weight loss and/or exercise. A classic example of HA is that associated with anorexia nervosa. Clinically these women have low or normal gonadotropins and fail to bleed after a progestin challenge test indicating low endogenous estrogen production. A decrease in pulsatile GnRH secretion causes pituitary-ovarian failure in HA.
3. **Polycystic ovarian disease (PCOD)** represents a poorly defined spectrum of clinical disorders having oligo-ovulation or anovulation and hyperandrogenism as common features. There is no single, universally accepted biochemical or clinical definition. Clinical findings usually include anovulation resulting in irregular uterine bleeding, infertility, androgen excess resulting in hirsutism, acne, and obesity. The pathophysiology involves altered functions of the hypothalamus, pituitary, ovary, adrenal, and insulin action resulting in failure of folliculogenesis to regularly proceed to ovulation. Tonic estrogen and androgen production are present. The endocrine abnormalities can be linked together in a chain of events that perpetuate the syndrome. The cause of the initiating event remains enigmatic.

### B. Uncommon diagnoses

1. **End organ causes of amenorrhea**
   a. **Asherman's syndrome** or intrauterine adhesions obliterate the endometrial cavity and thereby produce secondary amenorrhea. The most common etiology of this condition is a vigorous, traumatic endometrial curettage immediately following a pregnancy.
   b. **Müllerian agenesis** is the second most common cause of primary amenorrhea behind gonadal dysgenesis. Ovarian function, growth, and development are nor-

mal. Associated urinary tract and skeletal abnormalities may be present. Various degrees of agenesis may be present involving uterus, cervix, and vagina.

c. **Testicular feminization.** These patients present with primary amenorrhea, a blind vaginal pouch, no uterus, and normal female secondary sexual characteristics. They are male pseudohermaphrodites with XY karyotypes. The disorder is transmitted by means of an X-linked recessive gene and is caused by a congenital insensitivity to the action of androgens. The gonads must be removed because of the high risk of tumor formation (gonadoblastoma).

d. **Imperforate hymen.** The classic presentation of this disorder is that of a pubertal girl who presents with an abdominal mass associated with monthly episodes of severe abdominal pain. Inaccurate diagnosis leading to inappropriate laparotomy may be disastrous to the patient's future fertility. In addition these patients have associated endometriosis.

e. **Tuberculosis** is rarely seen in this country as a cause of amenorrhea, but is more commonly seen in third world countries.

2. **Ovarian causes of amenorrhea**

a. **Ovarian failure.** Irradiation to the pelvis and chemotherapy can cause premature ovarian failure, but usually the etiology is unknown. The age of onset is variable and can occur in teenagers. Rare and sporadic resumption of ovarian function prevents the prediction of absolute sterility. Autoimmune and/or genetic disorders may also be involved in the pathogenesis of the disease. In the majority of cases, the etiology of premature ovarian failure is unknown.

b. **Ovarian tumors**

(1) **Androgen-producing ovarian tumors** usually present with signs of virilization in addition to amenorrhea, including male-pattern baldness, clitoral enlargement, and lowering of the voice. Virilization secondary to an androgen producing tumor is usually rapid in onset, occurring over a few months time. Although these tumors are rare, the diagnosis must be ruled out in the presence of rapidly progressive masculinization, serum testosterone greater than 200 ng/dL, or a unilateral pelvic mass.

(2) Estrogen-producing tumors are extremely rare in reproductive-age women.

c. **Gonadal dysgenesis.** The most common form of gonadal dysgenesis is Turner's syndrome. The pure syndrome has a 45 XO karyotype. Some of the commonly associated physical characteristics include short stature, webbed neck, shield chest, and an increased carrying angle of the elbow. Mosaicism is common and the presence of a Y chromosome must be ruled out.

d. **17-hydroxylase deficiency.** This rare disorder is caused by an absence of 17-hydroxylase activity in both the adrenal gland and ovary. The patients lack secondary sexual characteristics and are hypertensive with high serum concentrations of progesterone.

3. **Pituitary/hypothalamic causes of amenorrhea**
   a. **Hypopituitarism.** Isolated gonadotropin deficiency is extremely rare; thus these patients usually present with multiple endocrine abnormalities.
   b. **Sheehan's syndrome** results from acute necrosis of the anterior pituitary gland secondary to postpartum hemorrhage and shock. The degree of pituitary hypofunction is variable.
   c. **Anorexia nervosa** presents with a variety of endocrine and metabolic alterations with the development of amenorrhea. Associated findings include bulimia, eating binges, and dieting. Physical findings may include hypotension, lanugo, and bradycardia. Lab findings are varied but typically include hypothyroidism and elevated cortisol.
   d. **Granulomatous disease,** for example, tuberculosis.
   e. **Head injuries**
   f. **Kallmann's syndrome** is an unusual hypothalamic cause of amenorrhea. There is a congenital absence of GnRH activity associated with anosmia. Patients present with severe hypothalamic amenorrhea with absent secondary sexual characteristics. Ovulation can be induced by pulsatile GnRH administration.
4. **Adrenal causes of amenorrhea**
   a. **Tumor.** Adrenal androgen-producing tumors are usually aggressive tumors and must be ruled out in every androgenized patient. Fortunately they are rare.
   b. **Cushing's syndrome.** Most protocols for the work-up of amenorrhea do not include a screening step for Cushing's syndrome. Thus, the clinician must be constantly alert to the signs and symptoms of Cushing's syndrome.
   c. **Adrenal hyperplasia.** Enzyme defects in the steroidogenic pathway to cortisol can result in elevated adrenal androgens and amenorrhea. Diagnosis is usually made early in life. Mild defects present as variants of polycystic ovarian disease.

## VI. Diagnosis

A. **Criteria for diagnostic work-up.** Amenorrhea as an isolated transient event is quite common. Amenorrhea warrants investigation in the following situations:

1. No menses by age 14 in the absence of growth or secondary sexual characteristics.
2. No menses by age 16 in the presence of growth or secondary sexual characteristics.
3. No menses for a duration of time equal to three of the woman's previous menstrual cycles or 6 months.

B. **History.** The patient should be questioned on complete menstrual history. Important facts include menarche, thelarche, adrenarche, previous menstrual irregularity, infertility, and sexual and contraceptive history.

C. **Signs and symptoms.** Headache is the most common symptom in patients with prolactin-secreting pituitary adenomas. Other signs, symptoms, and historical points related to hyperprolactinemia include: galactorrhea, visual loss (bitemporal hemianopsia), stress, frequent self-breast examination, and a positive drug or medication history. A history of previous pelvic surgery or family members with amenorrhea should be investigated. Other symptoms that can help establish the diagnosis include: marked weight gain or loss, a diet history including signs of anorexia or bulimia, recent stressful events, increased amounts of exercise, hot flushes, dry vagina, hirsutism, acne, and lowering of the voice. The most common cause of amenorrhea, pregnancy, should always be suspected.

D. **Physical examination** must be performed including assessment of nutritional status, blood pressure, secondary sexual characteristics (Tanner staging), hair pattern, galactorrhea, and signs of thyroid or adrenal disease. Important aspects of the pelvic examination include: size of the clitoris, adnexal mass, and an estimation of endogenous estrogen status (vaginal mucosa and cervical mucus).

E. **Laboratory evaluation and diagnostic procedure.** Figure 20.1 outlines the initial steps in the amenorrhea work-up. This work-up can be used for both primary and secondary amenorrhea. The work-up, as outlined, will lead to four diagnostic groups: (a) anovulation, (b) end-organ failure, (c) ovarian failure, (d) CNS-pituitary failure. The presence of certain signs and symptoms, that is, stigmata of Turner's syndrome or absence of the uterus, will alter the diagnostic approach.

1. **Pregnancy test** must be obtained in all patients of reproductive age who have been sexually active.
2. **Serum prolactin** must be ordered in all amenorrheic patients. Before the diagnosis of hyperprolactinemia is made, the serum prolactin should be repeated because transient elevation of prolactin in normal women is common. There is no concentration of prolactin below which a pituitary adenoma can be ruled out. A TRH stimulation test may be useful in differentiating a pituitary adenoma from other causes of hyperprolactinemia in patients whose prolactin concentration is less than 80 ng/mL. A doubling of

the baseline prolactin concentration after 500 μg of TRH injected intravenously, with rare exception, rules out a clinically significant pituitary adenoma. If the prolactin concentration is greater than 80 ng/mL the pituitary should be evaluated by computerized tomography or magnetic resonance imaging. Intrathecal injection of metrizamide can aid the diagnosis of empty sella syndrome.

3. **TSH** must be ordered in all amenorrheic patients. Hypothyroidism is a rare cause of amenorrhea, but is easily missed unless TSH concentrations are evaluated. Evaluation of TSH in hyperprolactinemic women is particularly important because primary hypothyroidism can clinically mimic a prolactin-secretory adenoma.
4. **Progestin challenge test.** The progestin challenge test evaluates endogenous estrogen production. The progestin can be given orally as medroxyprogesterone acetate (10 mg per day for 5 days) or intramuscularly as progesterone in oil (200 mg). Any vaginal bleeding represents a positive test. A positive test confirms the presence of some estrogen production, the presence of a uterus that is able to respond, and anovulation as the cause of the amenorrhea. The work-up is now complete if the history, physical, and laboratory data are otherwise normal.

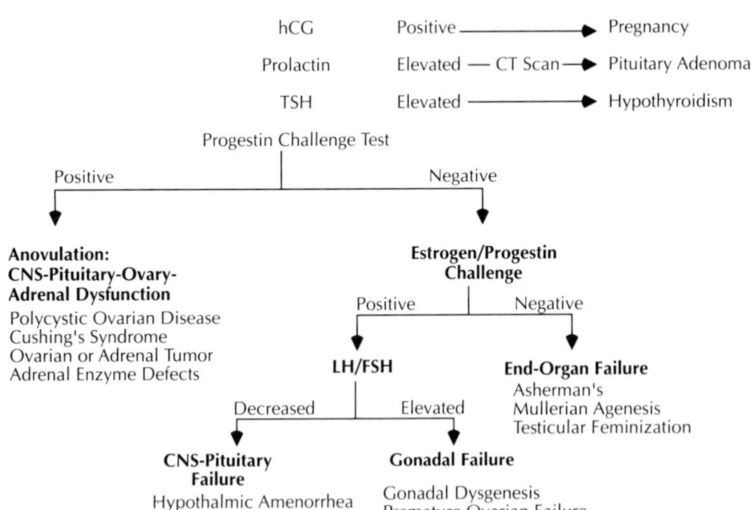


FIGURE 20.1 Work-up of amenorrhea with some common causes of amenorrhea. hCG = human chorionic gonadotropin; CT = computed tomography; TSH = thyrotropin; LH = luteinizing hormone; FSH = follicle-stimulating hormone.

5. **Hyperandrogenism.** Serum dehydroepiandrosterone sulfate (DHEAS) and testosterone should be evaluated if signs of hyperandrogenism (hirsutism or acne) or obesity are present.
   a. Measurement of testosterone assesses total androgen production from both the ovary and the adrenal. If serum concentrations of testosterone are greater than 200 ng/dL or signs of virilization are present, an androgen-secreting tumor must be suspected and pelvic ultrasonography, computed tomography (CT) scan of the adrenal, and possible selective venous catheterization must be ordered.
   b. **DHEAS.** Measurement of DHEAS assesses the adrenal contribution to the elevated serum androgen. If Cushing's syndrome is suspected an overnight dexamethasone suppression test should be performed. One milligram of dexamethasone is administered between 11 PM and midnight and an 8 AM plasma sample is obtained for measurement of cortisol. The cortisol level decreases to less than 5 μ/dL in patients without Cushing's syndrome. Elevated DHEAS concentrations should be evaluated by checking 17-hydroxyprogesterone (17-OHP) concentrations and if also elevated, corticotropin (ACTH) testing performed to diagnosis adrenal enzyme defects.
   c. **Other modalities.** Pelvic ultrasonography laparoscopy or laparotomy is not necessary to diagnose polycystic ovary disease.
6. **Tests to evaluate end organ failure.** If no bleeding follows the progestin challenge test either there is not enough estrogen production to proliferate the endometrium or there is a problem with the uterus or outflow tract. To make this differentiation, the patient is given all that is necessary to induce bleeding from a normal uterus: priming with estrogen followed by progestin withdrawal. This is accomplished by giving 2.5 mg of conjugated estrogens daily for 28 days with progestin (medroxyprogesterone acetone 10 mg) added during the final 14 days. No bleeding confirms end-organ failure. Biphasic basal body temperature charts with abnormalities on hysterosalpingography and/or hysteroscopy confirm the diagnosis of Asherman's syndrome. If no uterus is present, a karyotype is needed to differentiate between Müllerian agenesis and testicular feminization. Radiologic studies are indicated to rule out urologic and skeletal anomalies in patients with Müllerian agenesis.
7. **Test to evaluate ovarian failure.** Bleeding following the combined estrogen/progestin test indicates the presence of either a nonfunctional ovary or a normal ovary that is not

being stimulated. Elevated serum concentrations of luteinizing hormone (LH) and follicle stimulating hormone (FSH) confirm ovarian failure. All patients with ovarian failure under the age of 30 must have a karyotype to rule out the presence of a Y chromosome. A karyotype will differentiate the various forms of gonadal dysgenesis (XO, XY, XX, mosaic).

8. **Tests to evaluate CNS/pituitary failure.** This remaining group consists of patients with pituitary or hypothalamic failure. Pituitary failure is diagnosed by demonstrating no elevation of serum gonadotropin concentrations after prolonged pulsatile administration of GnRH. This differentiation is unnecessary unless GnRH is being considered for therapy. All patients with primary amenorrhea, a negative progestin challenge test and low gonadotropins should have a CT scan of the sella turcica to rule out a nonprolactin secreting tumor, such as, craniopharyngioma.

## VII. Management

A. **Estrogen progestin therapy.** Many amenorrheic women present to the physician to receive reassurance that their amenorrhea is not exposing them to any increased health risk. Reassurance alone without estrogen replacement is rarely indicated. All women who are hypoestrogenic, that is, negative progestin challenge test with a normal uterus and outflow tract, require estrogen replacement therapy. The minimum amount of estrogen required to prevent osteoporosis is 0.625 mg of conjugated estrogen daily. Higher doses of estrogen may be necessary to establish and maintain secondary sexual characteristics. If the uterus is present, intermittent progestin (10 mg medroxyprogesterone acetate for 10 to 14 days per month) should be added. All amenorrheic women who are progestin challenge test positive require intermittent (every 1 to 3 months) progestin therapy to prevent endometrial hyperplasia and carcinoma.

B. **Additional therapy according to cause of amenorrhea**

1. **Hyperprolactinemia.** Patients with hyperprolactinemia and/or galactorrhea, with no demonstrable pituitary tumor, should be followed by assessment of symptoms and prolactin concentrations every 6 months. Breast discharges that are bloody or greenish require a cytologic evaluation to rule out breast malignancy. Patients with breast discharge who are performing frequent breast examinations should be told to decrease self-exams to once per month. Therapeutic options for hyperprolactinemia and prolactin secretory tumors are:

   a. **Bromocriptine** is a potent dopamine agonist that inhibits prolactin secretion. All patients with hyperprolactinemia and/or galactorrhea, whether or not a prolactin-secreting adenoma is found, are candidates for bromocriptine therapy. Bromocriptine therapy is initiated with one tablet at night. Common side effects of nausea and postural hypotension can be minimized by initiating bromocriptine at night and gradually increasing the dose until prolactin concentrations are normalized. The usual effective dose is 2.5 mg b.i.d. Normal prolactin concentrations are obtained within a few days after reaching an effective dose. Ovulation occurs promptly after prolactin concentrations are normalized with the first menses occurring within 5 to 6 weeks. Bromocriptine is continued until a positive pregnancy test is obtained after the first missed menses. Approximately 80% of hyperprolactinemic women have achieved pregnancy with bromocriptine treatment. Women with pituitary adenomas who do become pregnant are followed very closely for symptoms of tumor growth including headache and visual symptoms. Following prolactin concentrations is not helpful because prolactin concentrations normally rise during pregnancy. Only 5% to 10% of women with microadenomas and 30% to 40% with macroadenomas will develop signs and symptoms of tumor growth during pregnancy. Symptoms of headache and visual disturbances, as well as tumor growth, are effectively treated during pregnancy with bromocriptine. If women remain asymptomatic during pregnancy without the addition of bromocriptine therapy, they may be allowed to breast-feed with continued observation for tumor growth. Most women have a recurrence of amenorrhea and hyperprolactinemia following the discontinuation of bromocriptine therapy. Thus, bromocriptine therapy may be required for the woman's entire reproductive life.

b. **Transphenoidal removal of prolactin-secreting pituitary adenomas** is successful in approximately 60% to 70% of patients with macroadenomas. A recurrence rate of 20% to 30% has decreased the attractiveness of this form of therapy. Presurgical therapy with bromocriptine will shrink the size of large tumors facilitating surgery.

c. **Irradiation for pituitary tumors** is usually reserved for medical and surgical treatment failures. Complications include the possibility of late onset of hypopituitarism.

2. **Hyperandrogenism.** Women with hyperandrogenism require symptomatic management of hirsutism and acne. Many of these women benefit from therapy with antiandrogens such as spironolactone, 50 mg b.i.d. and suppression of serum androgens by oral contraceptive therapy.

3. **Y chromosome.** All patients who have a Y chromosome must have their gonads removed. Patients with gonadal dysgenesis whose karyotype does not reveal a Y chromosome still require diligent yearly pelvic exams since remnants of the Y chromosome are not always found on routine karyotype, leaving them at risk for tumor development.
4. **Müllerian defects** resulting in retrograde menstruation must be surgically corrected to prevent the development of endometriosis. A vagina can be created in patients with vaginal agenesis either surgically or by using the Frank procedure, which consists of firm, intermittent pressure on the perineum with a dilator.
5. **Adrenal enzyme defects.** Symptoms related to adrenal enzyme defects can be successfully treated with glucocorticoid replacement therapy. This often results in normalization of elevated androgen levels and return of ovulatory menses. Other adrenal and thyroid disease is usually easily corrected by accurate diagnosis and treatment.
6. **Weight changes.** Amenorrhea associated with a change in weight can often be corrected by changes in the patient's life-style or diet. Small decreases or increases toward normalization of the patient's weight can result in resumption of menses.
7. **Ovulation induction.** Because anovulation is one of the most common causes of amenorrhea, ovulation induction is one of the most frequently requested therapies.
   a. **Medical therapy.** The three most commonly used medications for ovulation induction are clomiphene citrate, GnRH, and human menopausal gonadotropins (hMG).
      (1) **Clomiphene citrate** is a nonsteroidal estrogen with antiestrogenic properties. It remains the first choice for ovulation induction in most patients because of its relative safety, effectiveness, and low cost. It stimulates ovulation by inducing LH and FSH release from the pituitary, which initiates folliculogenesis, leading to ovulation. In the amenorrheic patient, the initial course of clomiphene citrate is easily remembered by the "rule of fives." After 5 days of progestin, the patient begins clomiphene citrate on the fifth day of bleeding. One 50 mg tablet of clomiphene citrate is taken for 5 days with intercourse beginning 5 days later in anticipation of ovulation. The dose of clomiphene citrate can be increased to 250 mg per day for 5 days. Alternative regimens and adjunctive therapies used with clomiphene citrate therapy include ultrasound, human chori-

onic gonadotropin (hCG), and progesterone suppositories. The most common side effect of clomiphene is flushing during the time of clomiphene citrate administration. The incidence of twins is increased to 5% to 10%. Almost 70% of patients treated with clomiphene citrate will ovulate and 40% will conceive.

(2) **Pulsatile GnRH therapy** is a new option for treatment of women who fail to ovulate with clomiphene citrate and bromocriptine and is an alternative to many women who currently receive human menopausal gonadotropin. For pulsatile GnRH therapy to be effective, both a functional pituitary and ovary need to be present, in contrast to hMG therapy where only a functional ovary is necessary. Thus, pulsatile GnRH therapy can be thought of as an artificial hypothalamus. The major advantages of GnRH therapy over hMG therapy are decreases in hyperstimulation and multiple birth. An infusion pump is used to administer GnRH intravenously or subcutaneously every 60 to 120 minutes.

(3) **Human menopausal gonadotropin** is one of the most potent and successful medications used for ovulation induction. The use of hMG is complex, and potential complications can be quite severe. Human menopausal gonadotropin is a purified extract prepared from the urine of postmenopausal women containing 75 U each of LH and FSH. The presence of an ovary capable of responding to gonadotropin is all that is necessary for successful hMG therapy. Human menopausal gonadotropin is the only therapy available for patients with no pituitary function. It is given as a daily IM injection until a pre-ovulatory follicle is developed. Ovulation is then induced by an IM injection of hCG. Follicular development is monitored by daily assessments of serum estradiol concentrations and ultrasound examinations. Ovulation can be induced in 60% to 90% of women with hMG therapy. Overstimulation of the ovaries is an unavoidable potential complication of hMG therapy. Patients present with abdominal discomfort and enlarged ovaries. Patients can become severely ill when large amounts of fluid migrate from the intravascular space into the abdominal cavity. Pelvic exams should never be performed if hyperstimulation is suspected because the enlarged ovaries are ex-

tremely susceptible to rupture. Multiple births and hyperstimulation can be held to a minimum with meticulous monitoring of therapy.

b. **Surgical therapy.** Ovarian wedge resection and ovarian cauterization for the treatment of amenorrhea in polycystic ovarian disease are therapies of last resort. All forms of medical therapy should be tried first. Surgical therapy can result in resumption of menses in approximately 60% of patients. This success, however, tends to be temporary and resumption of amenorrhea is often common. Patients also have a significant chance of developing adhesions secondary to these procedures that can then lead to infertility.

**VIII. Prognosis.** The prognosis for a patient with amenorrhea is directly related to the etiology. Certain forms of amenorrhea can be completely reversed. Examples include the resection of an adrenal or ovarian androgen-secreting tumor, surgical correction of an imperforate hymen, and correction of adrenal or thyroid dysfunction. Patients who have had previously normal menstrual periods frequently have a spontaneous return of normal menstrual function. Patients with other functional causes of amenorrhea including weight loss or exercise-induced amenorrhea also have a good prognosis. Polycystic ovarian disease is a disorder that tends to be present throughout the woman's reproductive life and can only be treated symptomatically.

Long-term studies of patients with microadenomas demonstrate that enlargement is uncommon and that some of these tumors will regress spontaneously. Only about 2% will show evidence of enlargement. Thus, many microadenomas do not require treatment if the patient is not experiencing amenorrhea or galactorrhea. For macroadenomas, long-term suppression is successful.

## BIBLIOGRAPHY


Blackwell RF, Chang RJ. Report of the National Symposium on the Clinical Management of Prolactin-Related Reproductive Disorders. Fertil Steril 1986; 45:607–610.

Goldzieher JW. Polycystic ovarian disease. Fertil Steril 1981;35: 371–394.

Griffin JE, Wilson JD. The syndromes of androgen resistance. N Engl J Med 1980; 302:198–209.

Jones HW, Rock JA. Reparative and Constructive Surgery of the Female Generative Tract. Baltimore Md: Williams & Wilkins; 1983.

Martin MC, Schriock ED, Jaffe RB. Prolactin-secreting pituitary adenomas. West J Med 1983; 139:663–672.

McDonough PG. Amenorrhea—etiologic approach to diagnosis. Fertil Steril 1978; 30:1–15.

Rebar RW, Erickson GF, Yen SSC. Idiopathic premature ovarian failure: Clinical and endocrine characteristics. Fertil Steril 1982; 37:35.

Simpson JL. Gonadal dysgenesis. In: Simpson JL ed. Disorders of Sexual Differentiation, Etiology and Clinical Delineation. New York: Academic Press; 1976: 259–302.

Speroff L, Glass RH, Kase NG. Clinical Gynecologic Endocrinology and Infertility. Baltimore Md: Williams & Wilkins; 1989.

Yen SSC, Jaffe RB. Reproductive Endocrinology. Philadelphia Pa: WB Saunders; 1986.

# CHAPTER 21

# Anovulation and Dysfunctional Uterine Bleeding

**Paul G. Stumpf**

Dysfunctional uterine bleeding (DUB) is defined as increased abnormal, uterine bleeding for which no specific organic cause can be established after careful evaluation. Therefore, the diagnosis of DUB is first and foremost a diagnosis by exclusion. Anovulation, the absence of regular, cyclic release of an egg by the ovary, is the most common reason for abnormal uterine bleeding without organic cause. The term anovulatory bleeding is sometimes used synonomously with DUB.

I. **Incidence.** DUB is most frequently encountered at the beginning and near the end of reproductive function, specifically in adolescence and around menopause. Anovulation and DUB are common problems in gynecologic practice.

II. **Morbidity and mortality** may result from anemia, or from the procedures or medications used to evaluate and treat anovulation or DUB. In modern practice, mortality related to anovulatory bleeding would be extremely rare.

III. **Etiology.** By definition, organic causes of bleeding must have already been excluded before the diagnosis of DUB can be established. The etiology of DUB is the failure of regular ovulation, and thus the absence of normal cyclic production and release of estrogen and progesterone. The ovulatory disturbance is most often a result of hypothalamic-pituitary dysfunction.

IV. **Pathogenesis and pathophysiology.** Normal cyclic menstrual bleeding results from the effects on the endometrium of the tightly controlled sequential production and release of steroid hormones by the ovary. Prior to ovulation, the developing follicle produces increasing amounts of estrogen (principally estradiol) that causes proliferation of the endometrium. Following ovulation, the follicle, now converted to a corpus luteum, produces relatively large amounts of progesterone, which induces differentiation of the endometrial cells. After about 12 days, progesterone production begins to fail and circulating levels of progesterone decrease. The decreasing levels of progesterone are insufficient to "maintain" the endometrial lining, so breakdown and sloughing begin. This sloughing of the endometrium is manifest as normal menstrual bleeding. Anything that interferes with this sequence of endometrial proliferation-differentiation-sloughing will produce abnormal or dysfunctional bleeding. Thus, disturbance of normal follicular maturation and conversion of corpus luteum (such as, oligo-anovulation) may result in DUB.

## V. Differential diagnosis

### A. Common problems

#### 1. Complications of pregnancy

a. **The evaluation** of vaginal bleeding for any woman within the reproductive years must first exclude the possibility of pregnancy. This evaluation consists of:
   (1) General medical history.
   (2) Gynecologic history (including contraceptive use, menstrual history, symptoms of pregnancy, vaginal passage of tissue).
   (3) General physical examination.
   (4) Gynecologic examination (including color and consistency of cervix, particularly status of cervical os; size, shape, position and consistency of uterus; masses or tenderness in adnexa).
   (5) Laboratory tests (e.g., hemogram, pregnancy test).
   (6) Judicious use of ultrasound examination.

b. **The following possible pregnancy complications** are specifically evaluated:
   (1) **Abortion.** Threatened abortion (os closed), inevitable abortion (os open), incomplete abortion (some tissue passed), or complete abortion (all gestational tissue passed, with or without significant residual bleeding) are complications of pregnancy and must be ruled out (Chapter 11—Abortion).
   (2) **Postpartum or postabortal.** Although a moderate amount of residual bleeding is normal following elective abortion, spontaneous abortion, or delivery, excessive amounts require evaluation for retained products of conception (fetal or placental), and infection (endoparametritis).
   (3) **Gestational trophoblastic disease (hydatidiform mole, invasive mole, or choriocarcinoma).** Quantitative human chorionic gonadotropin (hCG) titers and ultrasound examination are essential for the diagnosis (Chapter 33—Gestational Trophoblastic Disease).

(4) **Ectopic pregnancy** is a life-threatening pregnancy complication that must be considered when the pregnancy is complicated by first trimester vaginal bleeding or pain. Quantitative hCG titers, serum progesterone and ultrasound examinations are essential (Chapter 12—Ectopic Pregnancy).

2. **Malignancies.** Investigation of vaginal bleeding at any age must include an evaluation for possible malignancy with at least visual inspection of the entire perineum, external genitalia, vaginal epithelium, and cervix. The use of colposcopy, biopsies, and/or endometrial sampling must be considered. Attention is focused on the following specific areas to exclude malignant disease:
   a. **Vulva and perineum.** Superficial bleeding may be perceived and reported as vaginal bleeding by the patient (see Chapter 27—Vulvar Dysplasia and Carcinoma).
   b. **Vagina.** Painless vaginal bleeding is the most frequent presenting symptom of vaginal malignancy, which occurs most commonly in the menopausal age group between ages 50 and 60 (see Chapter 28—Vaginal Dysplasia and Carcinoma).
   c. **Cervix.** The "classic" early symptoms of cervical cancer include painless intermenstrual vaginal bleeding, and postcoital bleeding or bloody discharge, which becomes progressively heavier, more frequent, and of longer duration, thus mimicking DUB (Chapter 29—Carcinoma of the Cervix).
   d. **Uterus.** Endometrial cancer typically presents with abnormal vaginal bleeding, which may be unpredictable both in timing and amount. Furthermore, women with a history of anovulation are at increased risk for DUB and may be at increased risk for developing endometrial cancer. The distinction between anovulatory DUB and bleeding as a result of endometrial cancer can only be made on the basis of histologic examination. Therefore, endometrial sampling is mandatory in the evaluation of bleeding in all women over age 35 (Chapter 30—Carcinoma of the Uterus).
   e. **Ovaries.** Abnormal uterine bleeding is one of the late symptoms of ovarian cancer. Moreover, it has been reported that women with ovarian dysfunction manifested by premenstrual syndrome, heavy menstruation, breast tenderness, spontaneous abortions, infertility, and nulliparity may be at greater risk of ovarian cancer. Thus, in all patients with abnormal bleeding, but especially those who are over age 40 or have coexisting abdominal symptoms, meticulous attention to evaluation of the ovaries at pelvic examination is essential. Further testing, such as transvaginal ultrasound, and tumor marker determination is performed when indi-

cated (Chapter 32—Carcinoma of the Ovary). The role of these diagnostic modalities in "ovarian tumor screening" is not well-documented.

3. **Anatomic abnormalities.** Structural abnormalities of the uterus may produce abnormal bleeding, presumably on a mechanical basis.
   a. **Leiomyomata** are the most common benign uterine tumors in women, and most are asymptomatic. When abnormal bleeding occurs, it is usually in the form of hypermenorrhea or menorrhagia (excessively heavy but regular menstrual bleeding). Submucus and intramural leiomyomata can be associated with irregular or intermenstrual bleeding, as a result of:
      (1) Venous distension
      (2) Interference with the normal hemostatic mechanism
      (3) Thinning of the overlying endometrium

   Because growth of leiomyomata may be influenced by elevated or unopposed estrogen levels, women with previous true DUB may also later manifest clinically significant fibroids. Usually, the presence of leiomyomata will be suspected from findings at pelvic examination, but documentation may require pelvic examination under anesthesia, ultrasound, hysterosalpingography, or hysteroscopy. As endometrial hyperplasia is more common in those patients with leiomyomata, endometrial sampling should be used liberally. In general, attempts at hormonal control of bleeding, except with GnRH agonist therapy, is usually unsuccessful when secondary to significant leiomyomata.
   b. **Polyps.** Uterine bleeding secondary to endometrial polyps is classically postmenstrual spotting lasting 4 to 5 days, but may also be intermenstrual spotting or menometrorrhagia. The diagnosis may be made using hysterosalpingography, hysteroscopy, endometrial biopsy, or dilation and curettage (D & C). Because hormonal management will usually be unsuccessful and because of the possibility of coexisting endometrial cancer, treatment is always polyp removal by hysteroscopy, or more commonly, D & C. Polypectomy may be used if the polyp has prolapsed through the cervix.
4. **Infectious diseases.** Any of a number of infectious diseases may produce abnormal uterine bleeding due to edema, inflammation, and increased superficial vascularity.
   a. **Cervicitis** is associated with postcoital bleeding or bleeding after douching. Considerable controversy has occurred over the term chronic cervicitis, and it is certainly used much less frequently today than in the past. This diagnosis can only be made by biopsy and must eliminate the possibility of cervical malignancy. Once

the diagnosis is confirmed, local therapy with vaginal antibiotic or antiseptic creams, suppositories, or douches may be used but are often unsuccessful. Systemic antibiotics (tetracycline 500 mg p.o. q.i.d. for 7 days) is the treatment of choice for mucopurulent cervicitis secondary to a chlamydial infection. Cryosurgery, cautery, laser ablation, and cervical conization may be necessary in the most refractory cases, but thorough evaluation must be done to completely eliminate the possibility of cervical cancer (Chapter 6—Benign Diseases of the Cervix and Vagina).

b. **Endometritis.** Chronic infection or inflammation of the endometrium may result in irregular shedding of the uterine lining. Therefore, variable intermenstrual spotting or bleeding or menorrhagia may occur. The diagnosis is made by endometrial biopsy or D & C. Chronic endometritis is treated with tetracycline (doxycycline 100 mg/d for 7 to 10 days) to cover anaerobes and chlamydia.

5. **Exogenous treatments**
   a. **Steroid medications.** Administration of natural or synthetic estrogen or progestin may produce irregular endometrial shedding and anovulation.
   b. **CNS drugs.** A variety of psychotropic medications (for example, chlorpromazine, thioridazine, chlordiazepoxide, diazapam) may interfere with cyclic production and release of gonadotropins and thus produce anovulation. Usually, this causes amenorrhea but may occasionally produce DUB. Prolactin levels may be and should be evaluated.
   c. **Intrauterine devices** (IUD) are associated with an increase in both duration and amount of menstrual flow. However, some patients experience intermenstrual bleeding of varying amounts. Evaluation for possible pregnancy complications is indicated when an IUD is present.

**B. Less common problems**

1. **Systemic diseases**
   a. **Clotting disorders** are usually associated with profuse menorrhagía. Other manifestations of the underlying disorder, such as ability to bruise easily or delayed clotting after minor trauma, must be sought. Testing includes laboratory and clinical evaluation of the clotting mechanism. Obviously, the underlying disease should be treated if possible.
   b. **Endocrinopathies** such as diabetes, Cushing's syndrome, or thyroid disorders (both hypothyroidism and hyperthyroidism) may occasionally be associated with

irregular or increased vaginal bleeding due to oligo-ovulation or anovulation.

c. **Liver diseases** may produce increased vaginal bleeding in two ways. First, metabolism of estrogens and other steroids may be impaired, resulting in inappropriate hypothalamic-pituitary feedback. Second, disturbance in liver production of clotting factors can increase bleeding as outlined above.

d. **Significant obesity** is often associated with anovulation. Increased conversion of androstenedione to estrone in peripheral fat results in abnormally high, acyclic, unopposed total circulating estrogens. Because such patients are at increased risk for endometrial hyperplasia and adenocarcinoma, endometrial biopsy is indicated. When the obesity itself is refractory to treatment, cyclic progestin (medroxyprogesterone acetate 10 mg daily for 10 to 14 days every 1 to 3 months) should be administered to provide controlled withdrawal bleeding and prevent endometrial hyperplasia.

## VI. Diagnosis

A. **Signs and symptoms.** Patients with DUB present with excessive uterine bleeding, which may be increased in duration or amount (menorrhagia, hypermenorrhea), increased in frequency (polymenorrhea), or simply irregular (menorrhagia).

B. **Physical examination**

1. Vital signs in a lying, sitting, and standing position are checked to evaluate for tachycardia or postural hypotension. Overall appearance is noted, especially in reference to obesity or signs of Cushing's syndrome.
2. General physical examination is conducted to evaluate overall health and the specific disorders discussed above.
3. Pelvic examination is important to detect signs of any pelvic abnormalities or malignancies, as outlined above.

C. **Laboratory examination and diagnostic procedures**

1. Complete blood count to evaluate possible anemia or infection.
2. Pregnancy test.
3. Papanicolaou smear for cervical malignant or premalignant cells or infection.
4. Endometrial sampling to rule out malignancy should be done on all patients who are 35 years or older, and at a younger age if the patient has a long history of anovulation. The distinction between anovulatory DUB and bleeding as a result of endometrial cancer only can be made on the basis of histologic examination. A D & C can be used both as a diagnostic and therapeutic procedure when the patient has anemia in the face of persistent bleeding.

5. Basal body temperature (BBT) graphs and serum progesterone may help document ovulatory status, especially in patients who desire pregnancy.
6. Clotting studies should be obtained when indicated by history or physical examination.
7. Liver function tests or endocrine studies, as appropriate.
8. Hysterosalpingography or hysteroscopy for possible endometrial polyps, or submucosal leiomyomata when the history is suggestive, or in the patient with a persistent abnormal bleeding pattern.

VII. **Management.** Appropriate therapy for anovulation and DUB depend on the immediate medical goals, as well as the wishes and desires of the patient. The following clinical categories are examples of this individualized approach.

A. **Patients with profuse bleeding** associated with hypotension, tachycardia, dizziness, or severe anemia generally require D & C that will simultaneously stop the acute bleeding episode, while providing tissue for histologic evaluation. Unfortunately, except for specific problems such as endometrial polyps, a D & C is generally not curative of the underlying problem, which is unopposed estrogen, and therefore dysfunctional bleeding will usually recur.

B. **For clinically stable patients** the acute bleeding episode may be discontinued by:

1. **Administration of oral estrogen, followed by progestin.** Conjugated estrogens may be started at 2.5 mg b.i.d.; if bleeding continues after 2 days, the dose of conjugated estrogens is increased to 2.5 mg q.i.d. (For patients in whom bleeding has not stopped after 2 days at the higher dose, D & C is necessary.) Medical therapy is continued at the effective dose for a total of 21 days. Medroxyprogesterone acetate at a dose of 10 mg/d is added for the last 7 to 10 days of the regimen. Controlled withdrawal bleeding will occur in 5 to 10 days following cessation of these drugs.
2. **Combination oral contraceptives.** For patients who have difficulty complying with the sequential estrogen/progestin regimen, use of a combination oral contraceptive may be easier, and appears to be equally effective. Numerous treatment regimens have been described. One example is Enovid 5 μg (norethynodrel 5 mg with mestranol 75 μg per tablet), taken b.i.d. for 21 days. If bleeding does not stop after 2 days at this dose, the dose may be increased to two Enovid 5 mg tablets b.i.d. As above, if bleeding has not stopped after 2 days at the higher dose, D & C is indicated. Therapy is continued at the effective dose for 21 days. Withdrawal bleeding will follow predictably within 5 to 10 days after completing the course.

Another regimen consists of giving an oral contraceptive such as Ortho-Novum 1/35 (Norethindrone 1 mg, ethinyl estradiol 35 μg), or Lo-Ovral (Norgestrel 0.3 mg, ethinyl estradiol 30 μg) in a decreasing dose regimen (1 q.i.d. × 1 day, then t.i.d. × 1 day, then b.i.d. × 1 day, then q.d. for the remaining 12 days.). A second 21 day pack may be started immediately, to delay the withdrawal bleeding for another month if the patient remains anemic.

3. **Intravenous administration of conjugated estrogens** is also effective, especially if the patient requires hospitalization. The recommended dose is 25 mg conjugated estrogen IV every 4 hours until bleeding slows to a maximum of three to six doses, after which the patient may be switched to one of the oral regimens outlined above (see management section, VII-B-1, 2). Obviously, persistent bleeding unresponsive to this hormonal therapy requires D & C.

C. **Follow-up regimens.** To produce regular controlled bleeding after the initial episode has been treated, cyclic progestins, with or without cyclic estrogens, are used. Medroxyprogesterone acetate 10 mg/d for 10 to 14 days each month is prescribed. Controlled withdrawal bleeding occurs each month 5 to 10 days after the progestin is completed. This dose of progestin is probably adequate to produce secretory differentiation of the endometrium and thus decrease the risk of developing endometrial hyperplasia or adenocarcinoma. Note that this treatment regimen will not necessarily suppress ovulation, so the patient requires contraception. Oral progestins should not be administered if pregnancy is a possibility. Combined oral contraceptives may also be used to produce controlled cyclic bleeding, and have the advantage of providing effective contraception simultaneously, but carry the disadvantage of oral contraceptive associated side effects. Furthermore, oral contraceptives are considered a relative contraindication in patients over age 35 to 40, especially in the presence of other risk factors such as obesity, hypertension, diabetes, or cigarette smoking.

D. **In patients who have completed their child-bearing,** and where complete amenorrhea is desirable, such as with coagulopathy, the medroxyprogesterone acetate depot may be used at a dose of 150 mg IM every 3 to 4 weeks. Many patients will experience some, usually light, breakthrough bleeding during the initial months of therapy, which then resolves as therapy is continued.

E. **Patients attempting pregnancy,** who are anovulatory, require ovulation induction. Clomiphene citrate is generally the first line of therapy and is begun at an initial dose of 50 mg/d p.o., taken from the fifth to the ninth day after the start of a menstrual bleed. The patient is evaluated at about 14 days after finishing the 5-day course for signs of ovarian enlargement, and documentation of ovulatory response by BBT graph and measurement of serum progesterone. The dose is then continued, or adjusted, as appropriate. (**Note:** The use of ergot derivatives is not effective in the treatment of dysfunctional bleeding, and is therefore contraindicated.)

**VIII. Prognosis.** The overall outcome depends upon the specific goals of therapy, the wishes of the patient, and the individual clinical situation. The adolescent woman with anovulatory bleeding can expect to ovulate more regularly in the future and may only require temporary treatment. The infertile woman can expect an ovulatory response to appropriate treatment with clomiphene citrate in about 75% of cases. The perimenopausal woman is unlikely to resume spontaneous ovulation and will require cyclic progestins until her endogenous estrogen level decreases below about 30 pg/mL.

## BIBLIOGRAPHY

Arronet GH, Arrata WFM. Dysfunctional uterine bleeding: A classification. Obstet Gynecol 1967; 29:97.

Askel S, Segar-Jones G. Etiology and treatment of dysfunctional uterine bleeding. Obstet Gynecol 1974; 44:1.

Dysfunctional Uterine Bleeding—American College of Obstetricians and Gynecologists Technical Bulletin. Washington, DC: American College of Obstetricians and Gynecologists; No. 134, October, 1989.

Israel R, Mischell D, Labudovich M. Mechanism of normal and dysfunctional uterine bleeding. Clin Obstet Gynecol 1970; 13:386.

Kempers RD. Dysfunctional uterine bleeding. In: Sciarra JJ, Speroff L, Simpson JL, eds. Gynecology and Obstetrics. Philadelphia, Pa, 1984; Harper and Row.

Nilsfon L, Rybo G. Treatment of menorrhagia. Am J Obstet Gynecol 1971; 110:713.

Sheppard BL. The pathology of dysfunctional uterine bleeding. Clin Obstet Gynecol 1984; 11:227.

Strickler R. Dysfunctional uterine bleeding: Diagnosis and treatment. Postgrad Med 1979; 66:135.

# CHAPTER 22

# Menopause and the Climacteric

**Vivian Lewis**

Menopause is an isolated event that occurs as part of the climacteric, a transitional phase between the reproductive and the nonreproductive years. This chapter examines the physiology of the natural menopause, the indications and contraindications of hormone replacement therapy, and some of the principles of patient management.

I. **Incidence.** The mean age of menopause is 51.4 years, and, according to recent census figures, it is estimated that there are nearly 40 million women over the age of 50. Current projections are that by the year 2000, about 30% of women will be postmenopausal, a reflection of the aging trend in the American population.

II. **Morbidity and mortality.** There are systemic, gynecologic, and emotional changes that are associated with the menopausal and postmenopausal years. Some of these changes are specifically related to the tremendous decrease in estrogen levels, whereas others are simply related to the aging process.

A. **Gynecologic morbidity**

1. **Abnormal vaginal bleeding** is in part due to the increased frequency of anovulatory menstrual cycles, that occurs during the perimenopausal years. However, there is also an increased frequency of symptoms from organic pathology. For example, uterine myomas, endometrial and endocervical polyps, and most importantly endometrial cancer or adenomatous hyperplasia can be the cause of abnormal bleeding. Therefore, in this age group, abnormal bleeding should always be investigated either by endometrial biopsy or by dilation and curettage (D & C). Both are accurate in excluding either endometrial carcinoma or hyperplasia (Table 22.1).

2. **Gynecologic malignancies.** As with many other common malignancies, gynecologic malignancies become more common during the sixth and seventh decades of life. Con-

**Table 22.1. Accuracy of Outpatient Methods of Detection of Endometrial Carcinoma or Hyperplasia**

| METHOD | ACCURACY (%)* | |
|---|---|---|
| | CARCINOMA | HYPERPLASIA |
| Vaginal ectocervical smear | 42.8 | 26.0 |
| Endocervical aspiration | 72.8 | 26.0 |
| Endometrial aspiration | 88.7 | 100.0[†] |
| Endometrial lavage | 81.6 | |
| Endometrial brush | 87.4 | |
| Jet washer | 81.7 | 25.0 |
| Vabra curettage | 98.0 | |
| Vakutage | 100.0 | 94.0 |
| Endometrial biopsy | 90.0 | 85.7 |

*Mean values based on a survey of available literature.
[†]A single study.
Adapted from Ferenaczy A. Methods for detecting endometrial carcinoma and its precursors. In: Sciarra JJ, ed. Gynecology and Obstetrics. Philadelphia, Pa: Harper & Row; 1984. Reprinted with permission.

sideration should be given to the signs and symptoms of cervical, uterine, vulvar, and breast carcinomas. Appropriate cancer screening tests should be performed, including a Papanicolaou (PAP) smear, mammography, and colorectal screening (see Chapters 4—Diseases of the Breast, 27—Vulvar Dysplasia and Carcinoma, and 29—Carcinoma of the Cervix).

3. **Pelvic relaxation.** Symptomatic cystoceles and rectoceles, as well as uterine desensus are common in the menopausal and postmenopausal years (see Chapter 9—Pelvic Relaxation).
4. **Sexual dysfunction.** Estrogen deprivation has direct effects on the vaginal mucosa, that may result in discomfort during intercourse primarily the result of vaginal dryness. In addition, psychosocial factors may also have an effect (see Chapter 16—Sexual Problems).

B. **Systemic morbidity**

1. **Cardiovascular disease.** Prior to age 50, these problems are much more common among men than women. Starting at age 50, the incidence among women starts to increase, although mortality rates remain higher in men than women. Epidemiologic data demonstrate that estro-

gen protects women from these problems possibly modified by estrogen's positive effects on high-density lipoprotein (HDL) and low-density lipoprotein (LDL) cholesterol. However, the protective effects of estrogen seem to be negated in women who smoke. This may affect not only overall health, but also a decision to treat menopausal symptoms with hormone replacement therapy.

2. **Diabetes mellitus.** Unlike cardiovascular diseases, there is no difference between the sexes in the incidence of diabetes. For both sexes, it is more common over the age of 50. Diabetes may predispose to certain gynecologic conditions (i.e., endometrial carcinoma, sexual dysfunction, candidal infections). In addition, like cardiovascular disease, diabetes may affect a decision to treat with hormone replacement, because progestins may affect control of diabetes.
3. **Osteoporosis.** Although symptoms of this disease do not generally occur until the late 60s, bone mass peaks at age 35 and is lost at an accelerated rate starting in the early postmenopausal years. Risk factors for development of osteoporosis include:
   a. Female
   b. Caucasian or oriental
   c. Thin body habitus
   d. Decreased bone mass at menopause
   e. Sedentary life-style and the use of tobacco and alcohol
   f. Early menopause
   g. Family history of osteoporosis. Several studies show the importance of estrogen in the maintenance of bone mass. Osteoporosis is largely a preventable problem, if the physician and patient are aware of its significance and begin a preventive program including estrogen replacement therapy, dietary modifications, and exercise.

C. **Psychological problems**

1. **Emotional lability** may accompany the physical symptoms of estrogen withdrawal. For many women, more symptoms gradually abate with the successful treatment of physical symptoms by estrogen replacement therapy. However, emotional problems are frequently more complex and not simply the result of estrogen deprivation. Further evaluation of the patient's emotional health is indicated if symptoms persist despite estrogen replacement therapy.
2. **Depression.** Like emotional lability, this is frequently seen along with the physical symptoms of menopause. It is also a multifactorial problem that may be exacerbated by estrogen deprivation.

## III. Etiology

A. **Natural menopause** is a normal part of the aging process. The average age at which menopause occurs has remained remarkably constant despite the gradually decreasing mean age of puberty. The mean age of menopause among cigarette smokers is lower than nonsmokers.

B. **Surgical menopause.** Oophorectomy is not uncommon for diseased ovaries, as a prophylactic measure to prevent ovarian carcinomas or in women undergoing hysterectomy for chronic pelvic pain or infection. The incidence varies from about 17% to 34% of women according to ethnicity, education, and time of birth.

C. **Premature menopause.** Anyone with ovarian failure prior to the age of 40 is considered to have premature menopause, or premature ovarian failure. This may be due to a variety of causes.

1. **Idiopathic** menopause is the most common etiology. For unknown reasons, some women exhaust their supply of oocytes at an earlier age than others. It is not known whether this occurs because of an accelerated rate of atresia (loss of oocytes) or whether the initial supply of oocytes is smaller than normal.
2. **Familial.** Autosomal dominant transmission of menopause before age 40 has been suggested by some studies.
3. **Autoimmune.** Some patients have been found to have circulating antibodies to ovarian tissue. This may be associated with other autoimmune diseases in 18% to 30% of premature ovarian failure patients. Some of the associated diseases include Graves' disease, Addison's disease, myasthenia gravis, pernicious anemia, and hyperparathyroidism.
4. **Radiation or chemotherapy.** Premature ovarian failure is one of the common late side effects of these treatments given for various malignancies, Hodgkin's disease and childhood leukemia being two of the more common.
5. **Infection.** The ovaries may be involved in bacterial infections leading to severe pelvic inflammatory disease or pelvic abscesses, sometimes necessitating their surgical removal. Recently, it has been suggested that mumps infection in adults may affect the ovaries and predispose to early menopause.
6. **Environmental toxins** are more a theoretical than proven cause. Animal studies have suggested that sterility may occur or may affect developing oocytes predisposing to spontaneous abortion. Further study is needed to define the magnitude of this etiology in humans.
7. **Galactosemia.** This is a rare inherited disorder resulting from a deficiency of the enzyme galactose-1-phosphate uridyl-transferase. It may result in a decreased number of oocytes and possibly interfere with germ cell migration.

## IV. Pathogenesis and pathophysiology

A. **The climacteric.** The total complement of oocytes is a fixed number determined before birth. Degeneration of follicles or atresia begins at about 20 weeks of gestation in utero and continues throughout the lifetime of the individual. It is not known why some women seem to lose follicles more rapidly than others nor is it known what determines the absolute number of follicles with which an individual starts life. It is estimated that most females have about 6 to 7 million follicles present at 5 months' gestation. By the time of the climacteric, only about 400 follicles remain (Fig. 22.1). It is unknown which factors determine protection of those follicles from atresia, and why these follicles are less responsive to higher levels of gonadotropins. Clinically, this could explain the greater frequency of luteal phase defects and anovulatory cycles seen in the perimenopausal age woman. This could also result in changes in menstrual cycle length and flow patterns as well as a gradual decline in fecundity. As further depletion of follicles occurs, there is diminished steroidogenesis in response to physiologic levels of gonadotropins, resulting in further output of follicle-stimulating hormone (FSH) and luteinizing hormone (LH) as the pituitary senses this deficiency. Eventually this causes the pathognomonic elevation of gonadotropins (especially FSH) that we associate with the menopausal state.

B. **Menopause**

1. **Ovarian function.** Although menopausal ovaries are depleted of follicles and grossly appear small and atrophic, they are by no means inactive. The ovarian stroma continues to respond to gonadotropin stimulation. The principal products of this stimulation are androstenedione and testosterone, which may be converted peripherally to estrone, a relatively weak estrogen.
2. **Sources of sex steroids**
   a. The **ovaries and adrenals** both produce androgens (androstenedione and testosterone), which may act as substrates for the aromatase enzyme in the production of estrogens (Fig. 22.2). The total amount from these sources should remain in the postmenopausal range; if not one must suspect an ovarian neoplasm.
   b. The **conversion of androgens to estrogens** may be influenced by several factors. First, the efficiency of this conversion increases with age in both sexes. Teleologically, we can consider it a compensatory mechanism for the menopausal loss of estrogens. Second, the aromatase enzyme is found in many tissues, most notably skin and fat. Therefore, obese women will have greater levels of the aromatase enzyme and consequently more endogenous estrogens. Compared to slender women, they are less likely to suffer from estrogen deprivation and osteoporosis, but more like-

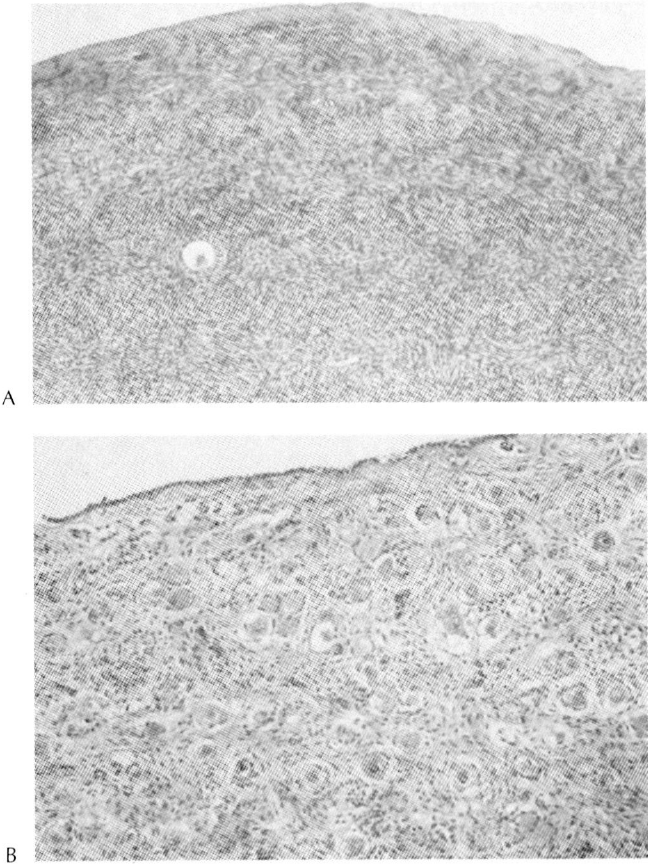

FIGURE 22.1. **Histologic sections of normal human ovaries.** A representative section from a perimenopausal woman's ovary (A) shows only one atretic follicle. By contrast, the section from the ovary of a newborn baby (B) shows multiple primordial follicles. Magnification is 125X. Courtesy of Dr. Wadi Bardawil, Department of Pathology, University of Illinois at Chicago.

ly to get endometrial hyperplasia or cancer. Various other medical conditions may also increase the efficiency of this enzyme, namely hyperthyroidism, compensated congestive heart failure, and liver disease, which should be kept in mind during clinical assessment of a patient's endogenous estrogenization.

## V. Differential diagnosis

### A. Natural menopause

1. **Common problems.** There are few diseases that can be confused with the natural menopause. Hyperthyroidism

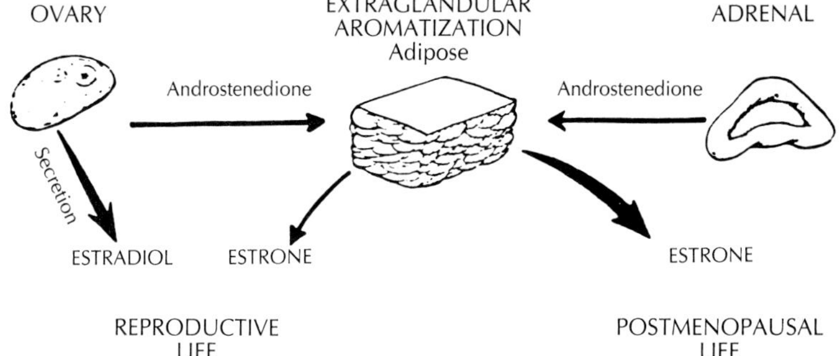


FIGURE 22.2. Endogenous sources of estrogens in premenopausal and postmenopausal women. Reprinted with permission from Carr BR, McDonald PC. Estrogen treatment of postmenopausal women. In: Stollerman GH, ed. Advances in Internal Medicine. Vol 28. Copyright© 1983 by Year Book Medical Publishers, Inc., Chicago, Ill.

may cause irregular vaginal bleeding and heat intolerance. However, the patient would also tend to have weight loss, tachycardia, and skin changes. Serum gonadotropins would either be normal or show an elevated LH/FSH ratio as a result of the hyperestrogenic state sometimes seen with hyperthyroidism.

2. **Uncommon problems**
   a. **Carcinoid syndrome** may cause episodes of flushing and vasomotor instability, usually as a result of 5-hydroxytryptophan secretion. These tumors usually have other associated symptoms: telangiectasia, diarrhea, tachycardia, and episodic bronchoconstriction. The diagnosis may be made by the finding of an elevated urinary 5-hydroxyindoleacetic acid, a serotonin metabolite. Gonadotropins should be normal or low.
   b. **Tuberculosis** is classically associated with night sweats. Amenorrhea may occur but is uncommon unless tuberculosis is far advanced. The diagnosis can be made by skin testing and appropriate radiologic and bacteriologic studies. Gonadotropins should be normal or low.
   c. **Medullary thyroid carcinoma** is usually asymptomatic and detected by palpation of a mass on examination of the thyroid. Although these tumors are known for secretion of calcitonin, they can sometimes secrete vasoactive substances such as corticotropin (ACTH), serotonin, and vasoactive intestinal protein (VIP), which may cause the patient to experience hot flushes. There is usually a family history of this prob-

lem. The diagnosis can be made by serum calcitonin levels and thyroid scan.

**B. Premature menopause**

1. **Natural menopause.** The differential is the same as for natural menopause (reached at the usual age).
2. **Resistant ovary syndrome** results in hypergonadotropic amenorrhea. In this condition, there are numerous viable follicles in the ovaries that for some reason do not respond to endogenous gonadotropins. It is not known whether this is due to gonadotropin receptor abnormalities, biologically inactive gonadotropins, or yet another mechanism. This condition is important to recognize in patients who actively desire pregnancy. Previously, the recommendation was to perform ovarian biopsy to look for viable follicles. However, because the prognosis is independent of this finding, biopsy is no longer done. Instead patients may be offered a trial of gonadotropin therapy (Pergonal) with or without initial gonadotropin-releasing hormone (GnRH) agonist therapy for down-regulation.

## VI. Diagnosis

**A. Signs and symptoms**

1. **Vasomotor instability,** the most common symptom accompanying the menopause, is experienced by 70% to 85% of menopausal women. Most women describe the hot flush as a sudden feeling of warmth in the face and neck that spreads to the chest. This feeling lasts several minutes and may be accompanied by diaphoresis, palpitations, and a visible reddening of the skin of the face. Objective correlates of this sensation include a rise in the skin temperature, changes in skin impedance and a sudden spike of LH release from the pituitary (Fig. 22.3). For most women, these episodes spontaneously subside after 1 to 2 years, even without treatment. However, some women continue to experience flushes for many years. The exact mechanism of these flushes is unknown, although it is known that the anterior hypothalamus contains the temperature regulation centers and a large number of neurons that contain GnRH in addition to many estrogen receptors.
2. **Irregular bleeding.** Because of waning ovarian function during menopause, the endometrium responds with less predictable shedding. However, intrinsic uterine pathology (especially uterine myomas or hyperplasia of the endrometrium) may also be manifested in this way. Therefore, any woman with prolonged, excessive or more frequent bleeding should have an endometrial biopsy for tissue diagnosis, whereas skipped menses are not necessarily an indication for endometrial biopsy.

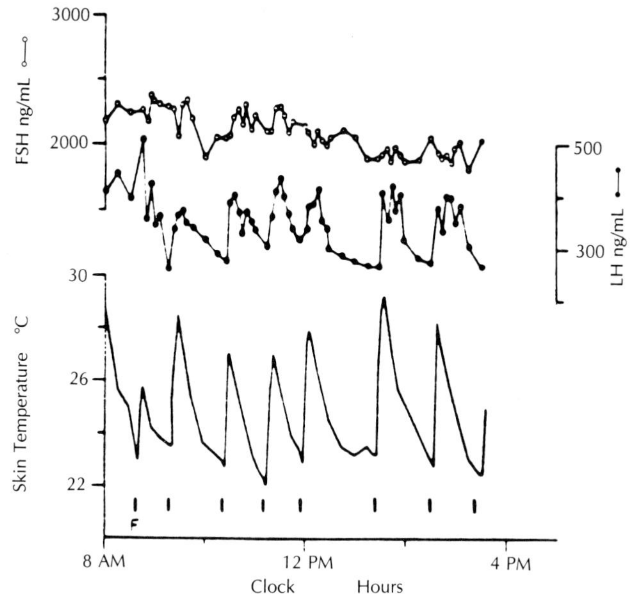


FIGURE 22.3. Changes in skin temperature and serum gonadotropins during an 8-hour study in a postmenopausal woman. Verticle bars (F) indicate onset of subjective symptoms of a hot flush. Note the close temporal relationship between symptoms, temperature spike, and serum luteinizing hormone (LH) levels. FSH = follicle-stimulating hormone. Adapted from Tataryn IV, Meldrum DR, Lu KH, Frumar AM, Judd HL. LH, FSH, and skin temperature during the menopausal hot flash. J Clin Endocrinol Metabol 1979; 49: Reprinted with permission.

3. **Vaginal mucosal atrophy.** The vaginal mucosa is extremely sensitive to estrogens. Vaginal cytology, blood flow, acidity, and flora are all influenced by estrogens (Fig. 22.4). The postmenopausal vagina may become dry and friable, which may result in irritation, pruritis, dyspareunia, and vaginal bleeding.
4. **Urinary tract symptoms.** The urethra and bladder trigone are sensitive to estrogens. In postmenopausal women, loss of estrogen may cause dysuria, urinary frequency, and sterile cystitis.
5. **Psychological symptoms.** Many women experience nervousness, anxiety, irritability, and depression as part of the menopausal syndrome. It is difficult to know how many of these symptoms can be attributed to aging, stress, or various social factors. The role of hormones is unclear. Lack of sleep associated with nocturnal hot flushes may be an additional exacerbating factor.

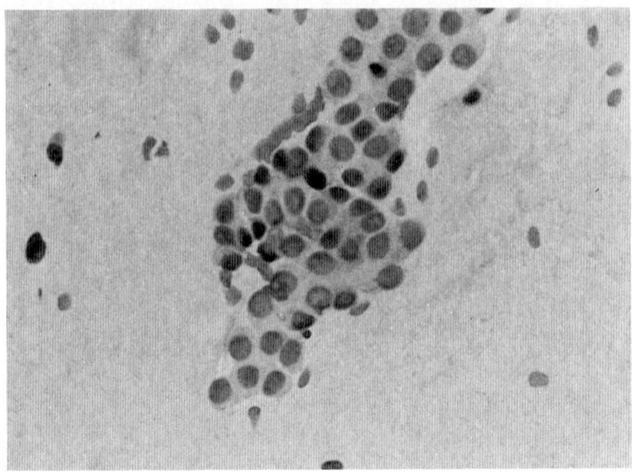

FIGURE 22.4. Cervical vaginal cytology from a prostmenopausal woman. The predominance of parabasal cells is consistent with a hypoestrogenic state. Photographed 400x. Courtesy of Dr. Richard DeMay, Department of Pathology, University of Illinois at Chicago.

6. **Musculoskeletal pain.** Vague back and musculoskeletal pain are more properly related to aging than to hormonal changes. Osteoporosis, a common problem in postmenopausal women, is usually asymptomatic until far advanced. Beginning at menopause, bone is lost at an accelerated rate. Women who start this period of bone loss with diminished bone mass are more likely to cross the threshold for fractures. In general, bone is initially lost from the spine, which results in vertebral compression fractures, a loss of height, and eventually acquisition of the so-called "Dowager's hump." In the later postmenopausal years, women are also prone to fractures of the radius or femoral neck after only minimal trauma.

**B. Physical examination**

1. **Evaluation of estrogenicity**
    a. **Body habitus.** Small, thin women are more likely to be hypoestrogenic.
    b. **The vaginal mucosa** should be observed for color, moistness, and presence or absence of rugae.
    c. **The vulva** also undergoes thinning and atrophy as a result of a lack of estrogen.
    d. **The breasts** may become atrophic and undergo reduction in amount of adipose tissue and lobules in the postmenopausal woman.
2. **Pelvic examination** should focus on the evaluation for an adnexal mass, cystocoele, rectocoele, and so on.

C. **Lab tests/diagnostic procedures**
   1. **Perimenopausal women**
      a. **FSH and LH.** The FSH/LH ratio is greater than 1.0 in ovarian failure, and may be used to confirm the clinical suspicion of ovarian failure. An FSH > 40 mIU/mL is considered postmenopausal.
      b. **Endometrial biopsy.** Aspiration biopsy of the endometrium should be performed for any intermenstral, postmenopausal, or other abnormal bleeding patterns.
      c. **Progestin challenge.** If the endometrium has been primed with estrogens and progestin is given, the patient should experience vaginal bleeding after the progestin is withdrawan. The patient who has endogenous estrogens will bleed after 5 days of treatment with oral medroxyprogesterone acetate 10 mg or one dose of progesterone in oil 150 mg IM. If a patient who is not on estrogen replacement therapy bleeds in response to a progestin challenge after at least 1 year of amenorrhea, this is of concern. There may be an undiagnosed source of endogenous estrogen. If the patient is still perimenopausal and bleeds after progestin administration, she is still producing her own endogenous estrogens. Such a patient can be treated with progestins alone, or estrogen combined with progestin for relief of menopausal symptoms.
   2. **Postmenopausal women.** Menopause is generally a clinical diagnosis based on a history of at least 1 year of amenorrhea with or without accompanying symptoms of estrogen deprivation. No laboratory confirmation is necessary unless the patient is under the age of 40 or has had a previous hysterectomy without oophorectomy. A combination of low serum estradiol (< 25 pg/mL) and elevated serum FSH (> 40 mIU/mL) is diagnostic of ovarian failure.
      a. **Cancer screening.** PAP smear for cervical cytology and stool specimen for occult blood should be part of the annual physical exam.
      b. **Mammography** should be done yearly in women over the age of 50.
      c. **Endometrial biopsy** should be performed in patients with abnormal bleeding but is not necessary for every patient prior to beginning hormone replacement therapy.
      d. **Lipid profile.** The National Heart, Lung, and Blood Institute suggests that all patients ≥ 20 years of age should have their blood cholesterol levels checked as a part of the regular health examination (Table 22.2).

**Table 22.2. Serum Cholestrol Levels: Appropriate Follow-up and Therapy**

| TOTAL CHOLESTEROL LEVEL (mg/dL) | LDL COUNT (mg/dL) | RECOMMENDATIONS | |
|---|---|---|---|
| | | RETEST | TREATMENT |
| ≤200 | — | 5 years | — |
| 200–239* | | | |
| No heart disease risk† | — | Yearly | Dietary information |
| Risks for hear disease present | ≤130 | 5 years | Dietary information |
| | 130–159 | 4–6 wks, 4X first year then 2X yearly | Diet, cholesterol-lowering drugs if diet fails |
| | ≥160 | 4–6 wks, 4X first year then 2X yearly | Diet, cholesterol-lowering drugs if diet fails |
| ≥240 | ≤130 | 5 year | Dietary information |
| | 130–159 | 4–6 wks, 4X first year then 2X yearly | Diet, cholesterol-lowering drugs if diet fails |
| | ≥160 | 4–6 wks, 4X first year then 2X yearly | Diet, cholesterol-lowering drugs if diet fails |

*Fractionate high-density (HDL) and low-density (LDL) lipoproteins. HDL should be ≥35 mg/dL, with an LDL ≤130 mg/dL.
†Risks include male sex, obesity, family history of heart disease, smoking, and hypertension.

3. **Premature menopause**
   a. **Progestin challenge.** This test can be used to assess estrogenization of the endometrium or the lack thereof.
   b. **Karyotype assessment.** About 20% of patients with premature ovarian failure have abnormal karyotypes. XX/XO mosaicism is the most common variant, although other abnormalities of the X chromosome are also found, including XX/XY mosaics. In cases in which a Y chromosome is found, prophylactic oophorectomy should be performed because of the high incidence of gonadoblastomas.
   c. **Serial gonadotropin measurements.** Both the LH and FSH should be measured on more than one occasion to determine if there is any ovarian activity, which is manifest by an FSH/LH ratio less than 1. There are reports of hypergonadotrophic amenorrhea in which subsequent ovulation and pregnancy occur. If this

does occur, it typically occurs as a result of a decrease in the FSH/LH ratio following estrogen replacement therapy.

d. **Autoimmune disease evaluation.** Autoimmune screen, erythrocyte sedimentation rate, albumin/globulin ratio, rheumatoid factor, antinuclear antibody, and thyroid function tests (T4, thyroid stimulatins hormone and antihydroglobulin, and antimicrosomal antibodies) should all be checked. Antiovarian antibody measurements are not commercially available; however, if the patient has any of the other autoantibodies, an autoimmune cause of ovarian failure is possible.

e. **Adrenal and parathyroid function screening.** Screening of adrenal and parathyroid function may be done with morning and night cortisol measurements as well as serum calcium and phosphorus.

## VII. Management

**A. Combination hormone replacement therapy.** Combined estrogen and progestin therapy is the mainstay in the treatment of menopausal symptoms.

1. **Indications.**
   a. **Relief of symptoms** associated with estrogen deficiency and aging (see diagnosis section, VI-A).
   b. **Prevention of osteoporosis.** Several studies have shown that estrogen, if started during the first 3 to 5 years after menopause, can prevent osteoporosis. Whether it is beneficial to treat someone who is more than 6 years past menopause is highly controversial. Indeed, not every woman is equally at risk of developing osteoporosis. Patients at greater risk for developing osteoporosis include Caucasians, Orientals, small, thin women, women with a family history of osteoporosis, smokers, and women who have a sedentary life-style. For lower risk patients, a program of physical exercise and increased dietary calcium may be sufficient to prevent severe bone loss.
   c. **Prevention of cardiovascular disease.** Most studies suggest a risk-lowering effect of estrogen replacement therapy on cardiovascular disease. This is becoming an indication for instituting therapy in all patients unless a contraindication is present.
2. **Contraindications**
   a. Undiagnosed abnormal vaginal bleeding.
   b. Previous breast cancer.
   c. Severe hypertension may rarely be exacerbated by hormone replacement therapy. Most hypertensive patients do well on low doses of hormone replacement.
   d. Chronic liver disease may be a relative contraindica-

tion to oral estrogen therapy; transdermal estrogen may be preferred for such patients.

e. Gall bladder disease is a relative contraindication, but is somewhat more common in patients on hormone replacement because estrogen can increase the cholesterol fraction of bile, a predisposing factor for stone formation. A patient with such a history may do better on transdermal estrogen by avoiding the "first pass phenomenon" of liver metabolism. Patients should be clinically monitored for signs and symptoms of cholecystitis.

f. Previous thromboembolic disease is a relative contraindication because estrogen may change hepatic synthesis of certain clotting factors (e.g., Factors VII, IX, X, and antithrombin III). Theoretically, transdermal administration of estrogen should lessen the estrogenic effect on hepatic function. In general, estrogen replacement therapy should not be withheld in this group of patients.

**3. Pharmacology**

a. **Doses** used should generally be as low as possible. Most patients experience relief of symptoms with a daily dose of 0.625 mg to 1.25 mg of conjugated estrogens. In the patient with a uterus present, progestins are generally given for 10 to 14 days with the estrogens. Medroxyprogesterone acetate is usually given in a dose of 10 mg daily for 10 to 14 days, or 2.5 or 5.0 mg daily throughout the cycle. Equivalencies with other steroids may be found in Table 22.3.

b. **Schedule.** The regimens listed here are widely accepted. First, conjugated estrogen (0.625 mg) daily with

**Table 22.3. Dose Equivalence of Some Commonly Used Oral Estrogens and Progestins**

| | DOSE (mg) |
|---|---|
| Estrogen | |
| Conjugated estrogens | 0.625 |
| Ethinyl estradiol | 0.015 |
| Mestranol | 0.02 |
| Estradiol-17β | 1.00 |
| Dienestrol | 0.10 |
| Estropipate | 0.75 |
| Progestin | |
| Medroxyprogesterone acetate | 10.00 |
| Norethindrone acetate | 5.00 |
| Norgestrel | 0.15 |
| Dydrogesterone | 5.00 ng |

progestin on days one to ten of each month. Conjugated estrogen can also be given on days 1 to 25, with the progestin on day 15 to 25. A newer regimen consists of daily conjugated estrogen (0.625 mg) with medroxyprogesterone acetate 2.5 mg given daily. This later regimen has been shown to be effective while at the same time preventing endometrial hyperplasia. This regimen has the advantage of having less withdrawal bleeding.

c. **Interactions with other medications.** The most common problem occurs with phenobarbital or one of the other anticonvulsants.

d. **Routes of administration**

(1) The oral route is the most common, least expensive and, for most patients, the most acceptable. Oral administration has the advantage of a possible beneficial effect on serum lipids, which is not seen with other forms of estrogen replacement.

(2) Vaginal creams are a popular means of administering estrogens for atrophic vaginitis and/or urethritis. Note that estrogen is well absorbed through the vaginal mucosa and thus the risk of systemic side effects is the same with topical drug administration as with systemic drug administration.

(3) Transcutaneous administration of estrogen (Estraderm) delivers a proportionally lower concentration of steroid to the liver (e.g., absence of the "first-pass" effect), which is desirable in some patients with hepatic problems and is preferred by women who dislike taking pills. The 0.05 twice weekly dose is equivalent to the 0.625 daily oral dosing schedule.

(4) Parenteral administration is costly, inconvenient, and potentially dangerous because of its prolonged action. Therefore, it should rarely be used.

e. **Side effects.** Perhaps the most disturbing side effect to the patient is a resumption of monthly vaginal bleeding upon progestin withdrawal. Withdrawal bleeding can be essentially stopped with daily progestin administration as compared with cyclic progestin therapy. Other symptoms may include bloating, weight gain, and breast swelling and tenderness.

**4. Monitoring therapy** is done primarily by clinical means. Patients should be seen 1 or 2 months after therapy initiation to check symptomatology and blood pressure. Thereafter, visits can be made every 12 months at which time symptom review, blood pressure check, and breast and pelvic examination should be performed. Any episode of abnormal vaginal bleeding should be promptly investigated by either endometrial biopsy or D & C.

B. **Alternatives to combination hormone replacement therapy**
   1. **Progestin therapy only.** Progestin therapy is effective in reducing vasomotor symptoms in about 75% to 90% of women. Oral progestins (10–30 mg of medroxyprogesterone acetate daily) or depomedroxyprogesterone acetate (150–200 mg IM every 3 months) may be used. In addition to symptom relief, some studies have demonstrated a beneficial effect on calcium metabolism. Note, however, that progestins may have adverse effects on carbohydrate and lipid metabolism as well as a mild elevation in blood pressure.
   2. **Alpha-adrenergic agonists** are less effective than progestins for treatment of vasomotor symptoms. However, for patients with severe hypertension or heart disease, they may be a reasonable alternative. They are given in very low doses, which usually do not affect blood pressure (i.e., 25 to 50 μg daily of clonidine hydrochloride).

C. **Calcium replacement therapy** is an important complement for hormone replacement therapy. The addition of approximately 1.0 g of calcium to the normal dietary intake of ½ g will provide the recommended daily intake of 1.5 g.
   1. **Calcium replacement regimen**
      a. Five Tums® antacid tablets per day, each of which will provide 200 mg of elemental calcium.
      b. Two Caltrate® tablets per day, each of which will provide 600 mg of elemental calcium.
   2. A history of calcium nephrolithiasis is a contraindication to calcium replacement therapy.

VIII. **Prognosis.** The major disease groups that cause morbidity and mortality during the climacteric or menopause will be examined briefly, in particular, concerning whether there is a difference in morbidity or mortality with hormone replacement therapy.

A. **Reproductive cancers**
   1. **Endometrial cancer.** There is a well-established causal relationship between prolonged, unopposed estrogen therapy and endometrial cancer. However, this risk can be prevented by co-administration of progestins for 10 to 14 days each month.
   2. **Breast cancer.** The causal relationship between estrogen replacement therapy and breast cancer has also been extensively studied. Certainly, hormonal factors may play a part because many tumors contain receptors for estrogen and clinically, late menopause is a risk factor for breast cancer. However, most studies have failed to show any increased risk of breast cancer in women receiving exogenous estrogen replacement.

**B. Cardiovascular disease.** Most studies suggest that estrogen replacement therapy lowers the risk of cardiovascular disease, probably by lowering total and LDL cholesterol and increasing HDL cholesterol. However, there are few long-term studies on the effects of combined estrogen-progestin therapy, which is important because progestins can reverse the beneficial effects of estrogen on the lipid profile. Nonetheless, currently available data do not suggest that combined estrogen-progestin therapy has any deleterious effect on the risk of cardiovascular disease.

**C. Diabetes mellitus.** Patients with diabetes are known to be adversely affected by the high doses of sex hormones found in birth control pills. However, the much smaller doses of sex hormone used for replacement therapy in menopausal women has no significant effect.

**D. Osteoporosis.** Estrogens have been shown to reduce the incidence of fractures in postmenopausal women. Progestins can also help reduce the loss of calcium in the urine of postmenopausal women. For a population at risk, hormone replacement therapy, especially in combination with calcium supplementation and exercise can help prevent osteoporosis. Calcium supplementation and exercise can also prevent osteoporosis. However, there are no long-term studies comparing the relative benefits of these therapies in the prevention of osteoporosis.

## BIBLIOGRAPHY

Buchsbaum HJ, ed. The Menopause. New York: Springer Verlag; 1983.

Carr BR, MacDonald PC. Estrogen treatment of postmenopausal women. In: Stollerman GH, ed. Advances in Internal Medicine. Vol 28. Chicago, Ill: Year Book Medical Publishers; 1983.

Gambrell RD. Clinical use of progestins in the menopausal patient. J Reprod Med 1982; 27:531.

Judd HL, Meldrum DR, Deftos LH, Henderson BE. Estrogen replacement therapy. Ann Intern Med 1983; 98:195.

Korenman SG, Sherman BM, Korenman JC. Reproductive hormone function: The perimenopausal period and beyond. Clin Endocrinol Metabol 1978; 7:625.

Mishell DR. Menopause: Physiology and pharmacology. Chicago, Ill: Year Book Medical Publishers; 1987.

Nachtigall LE, Nachtigall RH, Nachtigall RD, Beckman EM. Estrogen replacement therapy I: A 10-year prospective study in the relationship to osteoporosis. Obstet Gynecol 1979; 53:277–281.

Petersdorf RG, Adams RD, Braunwald E, Isselbacher KJ, Martin JB, Wilson JD, eds. Harrison's Principals of Internal Medicine. 10th ed. New York: McGraw–Hill; 1983.

Rebar RW. Hypergonadotropic amenorrhea and premature ovarian failure. J Reprod Med 1982; 27:179–186.

# CHAPTER 23

# Hirsutism, Defeminization, and Virilization

**Gretajo Northrop**

Exposure of the female to excessive levels of male sex hormone results in increasing hirsutism followed by virilization and defeminization. The magnitude of these changes are related to the concentration and duration of hormonal exposure. **Hirsutism,** female hairiness, is characterized by excessive hair growth (usually unwanted) on one or more regions of the body. **Virilization** can encompass not only hirsutism but also more severe androgen-induced changes such as lowering of voice pitch, recession of temporal scalp hair, and clitoral hypertrophy. Sometimes the term **defeminization** is used to denote loss of female body characteristics such as menstrual disturbances, decrease in breast size, excessive muscular development, and loss of female hair pattern. Although hirsutism is usually the initial event and represents the effect of mild hyperandrogenemia, there is no set sequence of the pattern of excessive hair growth. Commonly, the face (including the neck), abdomen, and/or thighs are the most likely regions to become hirsute and if excessive androgen exposure continues these areas will demonstrate the thickest and most rapid rates of hair growth. The sequence of the other androgen-induced clinical signs is not fixed, but clitoromegaly and alteration in voice pitch only result when androgen exposure has been of long duration and at high levels. In contrast, **hypertrichosis** is the abnormal growth of hair on nonandrogen-dependent regions such as ears, forehead, top of the nose, and interphalangeal joints. Clinical signs of hyperandrogenemia are summarized in Table 23.1.

## I. Prevalence

**A. Occurrence.** Hirsutism occurs in about one-third of Caucasian American women who are between the ages of 15 and 44 years. With advancing age the amount of body hair (including axillary and pubic hair) decreases although facial hair becomes more prevalent. Seventy-five percent of postmenopausal women, 60 years or older, have facial hirsutism. Other hyperandrogenemia-associated problems are less common. Hair patterns were observed in a study of 830 Caucasian women attending a general

**Table 23.1. Clinical Signs of Hyperandrogenemia**

Hirsutism

- Increased body hair
- Increased facial hair

Virilization

- Lowering of voice pitch
- Recession of temporal scalp hair
- Clitoral hypertrophy
- Defeminization
    - Menstrual disturbance
    - Decrease in breast size
    - Excessive muscular development
    - Loss of female fat distribution

medicine clinic and a university student health service. These patterns are represented in Table 23.2.

There is a wide variation in acceptance of body and facial hair as well as the amount of hair that is usually present in Caucasian women of different ethnic backgrounds. Caucasian women whose roots derive from northern European countries and England appear in general to possess less body and facial hair than their Welsh, Irish, and Mediterranean counterparts. Although people of both sexes and all races have the same total number of hair follicles, descendants of the American Indian, black, and Oriental races demonstrate significantly less body and facial hair than Caucasians. The reason for these ethnic differences in body and facial hair patterns is not related to altered blood levels of androgens. Studies of androgen receptor numbers and their physiology at the target sites are not yet reported but may provide some information about these differences.

The magnitude of hirsutism and its threat to a woman's femininity is rarely recognized by the physician who may often belittle or ignore her complaint. Many young women are so concerned with their physical changes, particularly increasing body and facial hair, that their entire life-system is compromised. Their perceived loss of femininity results commonly in social

**Table 23.2. Effect of Aging on Face and Body Hair Patterns in Women**

| LOCATION OF HAIR GROWTH | PUBERTY TO MENOPAUSE | POSTMENOPAUSE |
|---|---|---|
| Leg and forearm | 86% to 51% | 14% to 30% |
| Thigh | 43% to 25% | 14% |
| Lower abdomen | 30% | 6% |
| Chest | 24% to 7% | 1% to 2% |
| Face | 30% to 55% | 80% |

withdrawal and occasionally in depression requiring psychiatric counseling.

## II. Etiology

Androgen production is elevated in virtually all hirsute women. A complete androgen profile as well as sex-hormone-binding globulin (SHBG) level are required for proper evaluation. Because of the pulsatile nature of steroid secretion, multiple samples may be required to identify the specific problem.

## III. Pathophysiology

**A. Androgen biochemistry and clinical correlation.** Sex steroids are secreted by the placenta, gonads, and adrenal glands. Testosterone (T) is transported in the blood primarily bound to a large protein molecule, SHBG. Only about 1% of the total plasma T concentration is unbound (free) and biologically active. Reduction of T by 5α-reductase produces dihydrotestosterone (DHT) which can be further reduced to 3 β-androstanediol. All of these androgens have great affinity for androgen receptors and thus cause the biologic response characteristic of the cell type that is stimulated. Androgens stimulate collagen formation in the skin and capsule of the ovary (and testes). Hyperandrogenemia results in stimulation of cutaneous structures that may lead to skin thickening, excessive oiliness, hyperhidrosis, and acne. The increased hair growth, increased sweat and sebum production, as well as stimulation of the external genital structures in the female leading to clitoromegaly, are the usual physiologic responses caused by increased androgen levels in the female. Acne is severe enough to require treatment by a dermatologist in one-quarter of teenagers in the United States.

**B. Androgen metabolism.** Normal women produce about 250 mg/d of T. T production in hirsute women and men often exceeds the metabolic capacity of the liver (approximately 400 mg/d), which results in increased androgen metabolism in peripheral (nonhepatic) cells. The increased T results in excessive DHT as well as increased hair growth and frequently increased sweating and/or sebum production with associated acne. As the peripheral androgen metabolism increases, plasma androgen levels are restored to normal unless the androgen production rate exceeds both hepatic and nonhepatic cellular metabolism, as in adult men and severely hirsute or virilized women. Whenever the androgen production rate exceeds the rate of metabolic clearance, plasma androgen concentrations increase. Elevated T levels also cause a decrease in SHBG that may result in a normal total plasma T concentration, although free T (biologically active T) is elevated. The elevation of free T in the patient in whom total T is normal offers one explanation for apparently normal (total) T levels in many hirsute women. The T production rate is elevated in virtually all hirsute women. Thus the nonpregnant, nonobese hirsute patient has excessive androgen release from either her ovaries or adrenal glands. When the rate of androgen production exceeds the hepatic clearance rate, extrahepatic metabolism takes place in multiple sites as described above. Obese patients both produce and metabolize excessive amounts of androgen and estrogen in their fat cells. If the metabolic clearance by the liver and adipose tissue keeps pace with the androgen production, no hirsutism occurs. In fact, due to adipose tissue clearance, plasma levels of androgen may be relatively low in obese women. However, if androgen production exceeds the capacity of the liver and adipose tissue to metabolize these steroids, the hair follicles are stimulated. Plasma levels of androgen may still remain normal due to clearance by the subcutaneous skin structures (hair follicles and glands). It is only when the androgen production rate exceeds the total metabolic rate of clearance that plasma androgen levels rise.

## IV. Diseases associated with hyperandrogenemia

### A. Diseases of the ovary

#### 1. Polycystic ovary disease (PCOD)

a. **Chronic anovulation** due to any cause in a woman with adequate pituitary hormonal reserve may lead to polycystic ovary disease (PCOD). The association of enlarged multicystic ovaries with obesity, hirsutism, and irregular menses, with or without infertility (the Stein-Levanthal syndrome), remains elusive even today. The rigid criteria that defined the syndrome has been relaxed so that currently almost any constellation of findings in a woman who has polycystic ovaries is diagnosed as PCOD. More than 90% of hirsute women have PCOD and nearly 100% of these women produce excessive androgens. Less than 50% of women with PCOD are obese or have menstrual abnormalities.

Polycystic ovaries may range from normal size to four or five times normal in size. They are enclosed by a thickened white capsule, with prominent, numerous capillaries and multiple cysts of varying size that may protrude through the capsule or remain subcapsular in location. Microscopic alterations observed are multiple small follicular cysts surrounded by hyperplastic theca interna cells and hypertrophy of the ovarian stroma. Evidence of ovulation, a corpus luteum, or corpora albicantia, may be present. Thus, morphology corroborates the biochemical findings of increased androgen production by theca cells associated with elevated luteinizing hormone (LH) and decreased aromatization of the androgen to estrogen in the ovary by the follicle-stimulating hormone (FSH)-sensitive granulosa cells because of a decreased concentration of this gonadotropin. Peripheral conversion of androgen to estrogen results in a relatively high, minimally fluctuating estrogen level that perpetuates the gonadotropin pattern of an LH-FSH ratio $> 2$.

Controversy continues over the issue of central vs. peripheral etiology of PCOD. Support for a primary central defect centers around several lines of evidence such as an abnormal timing (daytime release) of LH in girls with PCOD rather than nocturnal LH release as is usual in the teenage girl. Increase in sensitivity to gonadotropin-releasing hormone (GnRH) in women with PCOD has been well-documented. Recently reported are studies in women that suggest failure of hypothalamic inhibition (suppression of LH) by endogenous opiates as well as failure to prevent with dopamine infusion a naloxone-induced rise in LH as would be expected in normal women. Thus hypothalamic derangement in women with PCOD is well-documented, but whether this is the primary defect or is a secondary defect due to an altered peripheral hormonal millieu (excessive androgens and/or estrogens) remains unsettled.

b. **Endocrine diseases.** A variety of endocrine abnormalities may result in polycystic ovaries; thus, PCOD may be thought of as a final common pathway for expression of many endocrine disorders. Because hirsutism is associated with excessive androgen production in almost all women tested, and most hirsute women have PCOD, excessive androgen production remains the primary association with PCOD, particularly in those women who are hirsute.

2. **Ovarian hyperthecosis** cannot be distinguished from PCOD as a specific disease except by ovarian biopsy. Microscopically, nests of luteinized cells are seen in the hyperplastic ovarian stroma that otherwise appears as classic PCOD. Ovarian hyperthecosis may be familial. Women with ovarian hyperthecosis may be refractory to treatment with clomiphene as well as to wedge resection of the ovaries. Their hirsutism is often severe and unrelenting.
3. **Luteoma of pregnancy and stromal luteoma.** Luteinized thecal cells may become hyperplastic and develop into nodular masses during pregnancy (luteoma of pregnancy) or at other times, particularly menopause (stromal luteoma). Luteomas are probably due to elevation of chorionic gonadotropin or LH. Hirsutism or virilization usually resolves with termination of pregnancy and resolution of a luteoma of pregnancy. Lesions found at menopause are not malignant.
4. **Neoplasms of the ovary.** There are several neoplasms of the ovary that are associated with hyperandrogen-like clinical

presentations (see Chapter 32—Carcinoma of the Ovary).

a. **Granulosa-theca cell tumor**
b. **Sertoli-Leydig cell tumor (arrhenoblastoma)**
c. **Gynandroblastoma**
d. **Lipid cell tumor ("adrenal rests," hilum cell tumors)**
e. **Gonadoblastoma**
f. **Dysgerminoma**
g. **Rare androgen-secreting tumors**
    (1) Mucinous and serous **cystadenomas**
    (2) **Brenner tumor**
    (3) **Krukenberg tumor** (reported as a source of androgen in pregnancy)

**B. Diseases of the andrenal glands**

1. **Congenital adrenal hyperplasia (CAH)** is a group of hereditary diseases characterized by limited cortisol production due to compromised enzymatic activity at one of several steps leading to cortisol synthesis. Cortisol-directed negative feedback at the hypothalamic-pituitary axis is inadequate and the resulting increased corticotropin (ACTH) results in adrenal cortical hyperplasia. Cortisol precursors, as well as androgens and their precursors, accumulate behind the enzymatic block and are deficient after the compromised enzymatic step. Deficiency of 21- and 11-hydroxylase as well as 3-hydroxysteriod dehydrogenase may be noted in women presenting with hirsutism, virilization, and menstrual abnormalities. Nonclassic (late onset) 21-hydroxylase deficiency may occur in 1% of the non-Jewish Caucasian population and 3% of the Jewish population. In contrast to the classical neonatal presentation of 21-hydroxylase deficiency with salt-wasting and/or prenatal virilization of the external genitalia and biochemical evidence of at least increased 17-hydroxyprogesterone (17-OHP), the nonclassic 21-hydroxylase deficient patient has a normal phenotype and remains asymptomatic until early puberty or young adulthood. Often, the biochemical defect can be elicited only by stimulation with ACTH, which results in elevation of 17-OHP, thus permitting genotyping of the 21-hydroxylase deficiency. Because the gene for 21-hydroxylase regulation is closely related to the human leukocyte antigens (HLAs) on chromosome 6, HLA genotyping may be helpful both to the patient and other members of the family.
2. **Cushing's syndrome.** In contrast to CAH, in which cortisol production is decreased, Cushing's syndrome is characterized by excessive cortisol secretion. Patients with Cushing's disease in which excessive ACTH is of pituitary origin have a rather slow onset of both the symptoms of hyperandrogenemia and hypercortisolemia. Thus, the symptoms of cortisol excess may be helpful for diagnosis if accompanied by those of excessive androgen secretion. The symptoms of hypercortisolemia include: (see diagnosis section, V-C-3)

a. Redistribution of body fat so the limbs are thin as compared with the trunk.
b. Accumulation of fat pads, with the associated buffalo hump and moon facies.
c. Increased catabolism that results in muscle weakness and wasting.
d. Loss of elastic fibers in the skin resulting in thin skin, purple striae, and plethoric complexion.
e. Friable blood vessels and ability to bruise easily.
f. Mildly abnormal glucose tolerance.
g. Mild-to-moderate hypertension.

3. **Neoplasms of the adrenal glands**
   a. **Adrenal cortical adenoma.** Hirsute women with cortical adenomas have the clinical characteristics of Cushing's syndrome. These women experience a much more rapid onset and progression of their symptoms of hyperandrogenemia in contrast to the usual presentation of women with PCOD.
   b. **Adrenal carcinoma.** Women with adrenal carcinoma have rapid onset and progression of symptoms due to hyperandrogenemia and hypercortisolemia. These tumors are often bilateral and metastasize early.

C. **Other diseases occasionally associated with hirsutism or virilism.** (These conditions are rarely encountered as the sole etiology of hirsutism.)

1. **Anorexia nervosa and starvation.** Patients with anorexia nervosa are extremely thin; have fine lanugo hair over most of their body (not in the male pattern distribution); dry, rough, coarse skin; vital signs that are low (decreased heart rate, respiratory rate, blood pressure, and body temperature); amenorrhea; hyperactivity; and denial of any medical problem including thin body image.
   a. **Laboratory studies**
      (1) Thyroxine ($T_4$) is low normal.
      (2) Triiodothyronine ($T_3$) resin uptake ($T_3RU$) is normal.
      (3) $T_3$ is below normal.
      (4) Thyroid-stimulating hormone (TSH) is normal, and the response to the thyrotropin-releasing hormone (TRH) test is characteristically exaggerated and prolonged.
      (5) FSH and LH are low.
      (6) Estradiol and progesterone are low.
      (7) Cortisol and growth hormones are normal or elevated.
   b. **Treatment** is mainly psychiatric, with the results often discouraging.
2. **Hypothyroidism** frequently presents with complaints of fatigue, cold intolerance, weight gain, dry skin, constipation, and menorrhagia. Physical findings may include hypothy-

roid facies, heavy, thick, dry myxedematous skin, hoarse voice, as well as slow reflexes and mentation.

a. **Laboratory studies** and expected results include:
   (1) $T_4$ is low
   (2) $T_3$ is low
   (3) $T_3$RU is low
   (4) TSH is elevated. Occasionally in mild borderline hypothyroidism the TSH may be normal. However, the TRH test results are abnormal with an elevated TSH at 20 minutes.

b. **Treatment.** Replacement with synthetic levothyroxine.

3. **Intersexuality.** In intersex patients, the genotype (karyotype) does not harmonize with the phenotype (sexual characteristics).
   a. **Female pseudohermaphroditism** occurs when a fetus with ovaries and a female karyotype (45,XX) is exposed to excessive androgen in utero prior to gestational week 12 or 13 usually due to CAH, maternal production of androgens (tumor) or maternal ingestion of drugs (progesterone). Androgen exposure of the female fetus at this time results in loss of the classic female phenotype.
   b. **Male pseudohermaphroditism** occurs when the genotype includes a Y chromosome (46,XY), the gonads contain testicular tissue, and the phenotype reveals varying degrees of femaleness.
      (1) **Enzyme deficiencies.** The compromised enzyme resulting in CAH may result in deficient cortisol and/or sex steroid production (Fig. 23.1). Some enzyme deficiencies, if severe, result in death because cholesterol is never converted to the basic adrenal and gonadal steroid, pregenolone, whereas some enzyme deficiencies result only in impaired T production with development of male pseudohermaphroditism.
      (2) **Testosterone-receptor abnormalities.** Androgen-receptor abnormalities cause resistance at the cellular level to T with lack of male phenotypic differentation. **Testicular feminization** is characterized by a normal female phenotype with full breast development and absence of pubic and axillary hair. On examination, the vagina is shortened, the uterus is absent, and normal testes are located anywhere along the normal pathway of decent (intra-abdominal to labia majora). An incomplete form of androgen resistance may exist in which some receptors are normal; this results in varying amounts of hirsutism and of clitoromegaly at puberty.
      (3) **5α-Reductase deficiency.** This enzyme deficiency

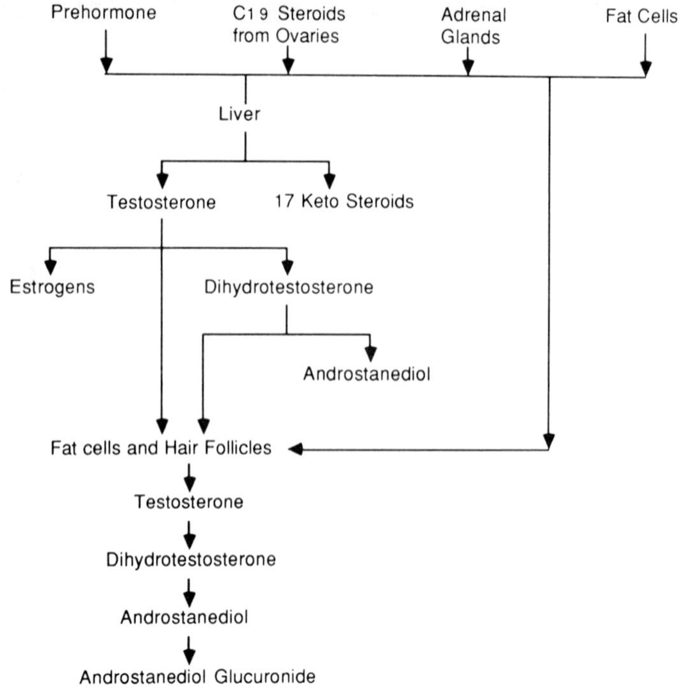


FIGURE 23.1. Summary of androgen formation and metabolism in women.

results in inadequate conversion of T to DHT, the androgen required by the urogenital sinus for differentiation into the male phenotype. It should be recalled that the female phenotype is basic and will develop unless domineered by testicular release of T at critical times in embryonic development. Failure to reduce T and DHT in utero results in severe hypospadias and a vagina of varying depth called "pseudovaginal perineoscrotal hyposadias." This deficiency is important to diagnose when the child is young because at puberty the high levels of T produced by the adult testes cause generalized masculinization and in most patients male psychosexual orientation, if socially possible.

(4) **Gonadal dysgenesis in genotypic 46,XY phenotypic females.** Sawyer's syndrome is characterized by a normal female phenotype, a normal male karyotype, and streak nonfunctioning gonads. These patients present at puberty with amenorrhea and sometimes hirsutism and/or clitoromegaly. Go-

nadoblastomas occur in 30% to 70% of these patients and, when present, may produce androgens that cause masculinization.

(5) **Transsexuals.** These patients are hormonally normal male or female patients who reject their gonadal and phenotypic sex but cannot reject their karyotypic sex. These adult patients may be in different stages of converting their phenotypic sex from male to female (male to male transsexual) or female to male (female to female transsexual). When fully treated, they are castrated, have the appearance and psychologic adjustment of the opposite sex of their karyotype, and are maintained on sex hormone replacement appropriate for the surgically acquired phenotypic sex. Male to female transsexuals have female breasts and a vagina and appropriately seek gynecologic care as women. They require exogenous estrogen replacement.

D. **Drugs** associated with hirsutism include:

1. ACTH
2. Methyldopa (Aldomet)
3. Minoxidil
4. Androgenic steroids (e.g., T, danzol)
5. Diazoxide
6. Phenytoin (Dilantin)
7. Glucocorticoids
8. Oral contraceptives
9. Phenothiazines
10. Spironolactone
11. Streptomycin
12. Cyclosporine

## V. Diagnosis

### A. History

1. **Age of onset.** The age of onset of symptoms may provide some help in diagnosis by association with the "classic" historical presentation of the various syndromes (Table 23.3).
2. **Symptoms.** The duration and rate of progression of symptoms may provide a clue about the level of hyperandrogenemia. Rapidly developing hirsutism and/or virilization is suggestive of a tumor.
3. **Reproductive history**
   a. **Menses.** The menstrual history is frequently abnormal with oligomenorrhea the most commonly reported abnormality. Menorrhagia and menometrorrhagia are less common and primary amenorrhea is rarely reported.
   b. **Fertility.** Reproductive performance is inversely related to the level of hyperandrogenemia. Fertility is frequently

**Table 23.3. Etiology of Hirsutism by Age Group**

| AGE | CAUSE OF HIRSUTISM |
|---|---|
| Birth to puberty | Genetic syndromes:<br>  Congenital adrenal hyperplasia (classical form)<br>  Leprechaunism<br>  Gangliosidosis<br>  Bird-headed dwarf of Seckel<br>  Cornelia de Lange's syndrome<br>  Hypertrichosis lanuginosa<br>Starvation syndromes<br>Precocious puberty:<br>  Idiopathic<br>  Tumors (see below)<br>Tumors:<br>  Pituitary<br>  Ovaries<br>  Adrenal glands<br>  Ectopic hormone-producing tumor sites:<br>      Lung<br>      Liver<br>      Pancreas<br>      etc.<br>Drugs:<br>  Hormone: oral contraceptives<br>  Phenytoin<br>  Diazoxide |
| Puberty to menopause | Polycystic ovary disease (PCOD)<br>Hyperandrogenemia without evidence of PCOD (hyperthecosis) |

| | |
|---|---|
| | Genetic syndromes:<br>  Intersex problems<br>  Male pseudohermaphroditism including the androgen-resistant syndromes<br>Gonadal dysgenesis<br>Congenital adrenal hyperplasia (nonclassical form)<br>Pregnancy: luteoma<br>Tumors:<br>  Pituitary<br>    Adenomas associated with Cushing's disease and acromegaly<br>  Adrenal glands<br>  Adenomas and carcinomas<br>Drugs:<br>  Hormone: oral contraceptives ACTH, anabolic steroids, androgens, progestogens<br>  Phenytoin<br>  Diazoxide, rarely in adults<br>  Streptomycin<br>  Cyclosporine<br>  Minoxidil, methyldopa<br>  Phenothiazines<br>Miscellaneous: Conditions of localized hypervascularity may be associated with localized hirsutism i.e., chronic skin irritation, chronic osteomyelitis, severe varicose veins, and stasis ulcers. Increased localized hair growth following inguinal lymphadenectomy for melanoma. Unilateral facial hair growth was reported associated with ipsilateral phenytoin sodium (Dilantin) induced gingival hyperplasia and in another woman to have occurred without known cause. |
| Postmenopause | Ovary: With aging, number of ova and presumably granulosa cells decline. Excessive theca to granulosa cell numbers result in an elevated androstenedione to estradiol ratio. The extragonadal metabolism of androstenedione (principally in adipose tissue) accounts for increases in estrone and 3α-androstanediol glucuronide as well as the more biologically active androgens, testosterone, and dihydrotestosterone. |

Adapted from Northrop G. Hirsutism, defeminization and virilization. In: Ellis, JW, Beckmann RB, eds. A Clinical Manual of Gynecology. East Norwalk, Conn: Appleton-Century-Crofts; 1983: 506.

impaired with the occurrence of spontaneous abortion, especially following medically assisted conceptions.

4. **Nongonadal and metabolic history**
   a. **Obesity** is present in more than 50% of hirsute women. The degree of obesity may be estimated by clinical presentation or by comparison of the patient's weight to her "ideal weight," which in women may be estimated by assigning 100 pounds for 60 inches in height with the addition of five pounds for every additional inch in height. The anabolic effect of androgens results in positive nitrogen balance that can lead also to increased muscle mass.
   b. **Hypothyroidism** may lead to decreased 5α-reductase with impaired metabolic clearance of testosterone.
   c. **Nutrition.** Malnutrition including anorexia nervosa or severe illness leading to the low $T_3$ syndrome may also result in reduced 5α-reductase.
   d. **Liver disease,** and porphyria cutanea tarda, causes a decrease in 5α-reductase.
5. **Hereditary factors**
   a. **CAH.** Hereditary factors are well-documented in CAH.
   b. **PCOD.** The existence of a genetic basis for PCOD is as yet unproven. However, hirsute women often have a positive family history for one or more of the following:
      (1) Father with excessive hairiness.
      (2) Mother or sisters who are hirsute, obese, have menstrual irregularity or are subfertile.

**B. Physical findings associated with hyperandrogenemia**

1. **Skin**
   a. **Hair** in normal women is distributed in the female terminal hair pattern (eyebrows, eyelashes, axillary, and pubic areas). Stimulation by male hormones (androgens) may result in development of the usual male hair pattern (face, neck, chest, back, shoulders, abdomen, and presacral areas with heavy growth present on the arms and legs extending on to the dorsums of the hands and feet, respectively). A decrease or absence of scalp hair may be noted, as thinning or balding in the frontal or temporal regions.
   b. **Acne** is occasionally noted on the face of many women as a few pimples part or all of the time. In addition, deep, painful cysts may cover the face, chest, shoulders, and back. Boils and abscesses may be noted in the axillary and inquinal areas as well as in other skin folds.
   c. **Hyperhidrosis,** excessive sweating, may be noted particularly in the axillary and inquinal areas.

d. **Acanthosis nigricans** is a black, velvet-like pigmentation that is predominantly found in the flexor skin folds of the neck, axilla, antecubital, and inquinal areas. In young, obese women without signs of malignancy, PCOD and insulin resistance are likely present.

2. **Breast.** The size of the breasts may decrease in women with hyperandrogenemia.
3. **Clitoris.** Enlargement of the clitoris is associated with high levels of androgen exposure. Androgens also increase clitoral sensitivity.
4. **Ovary.** Enlarged ovaries are noted in many hirsute women.
5. **Muscle.** An increase in muscle mass, particularly when the normal female fat distribution is absent, is likely to be associated with hyperandrogenemia of long duration.

C. **Laboratory examination and diagnostic procedures**

1. **General principles of the laboratory evaluation of suspected hyperandrogenemia.** The primary reason for failure to diagnose and successfully treat the hirsute patient is inadequate laboratory evaluation.

A detailed and comprehensive protocol for sequential diagnostic evaluation of the hirsute or virilized female is presented in Figure 23.2. If the protocol is strictly followed the correct diagnosis is unlikely to be missed. However, appropriate laboratory examination of most young hirsute women should minimally consist of a complete blood androgen screen (see Fig. 23.3) as well as gonadotropin levels. Steroids with androgenic activity are pictured in Figure 23.3. Information that may be gathered from these tests is summarized in Table 23.4.

Most women between 13 and 45 years of age who seek help from the endocrinologists or gynecologist because of minimal to moderate hirsutism, with or without menstrual problems, do not require the above detailed evaluation if they report

(a) The gradual onset of hirsutism and/or acne over a relatively long time.
(b) Absence of suspicious drug use.
(c) A negative history for CAH. Because Cushing's syndrome and hypothyroidism are rare causes of the common complaint of hirsutism, clinical evaluation is usually sufficient in most women.

Virtually all women with hirsutism have excessive androgen production. Difficulties arise in interpretation of laboratory data when both the ovaries and the adrenal glands are secreting the same androgen excessively, a problem encountered in about one-third of hirsute women. It is now well-documented that dynamic testing protocols for localization of the source of androgen secretion are ineffective.

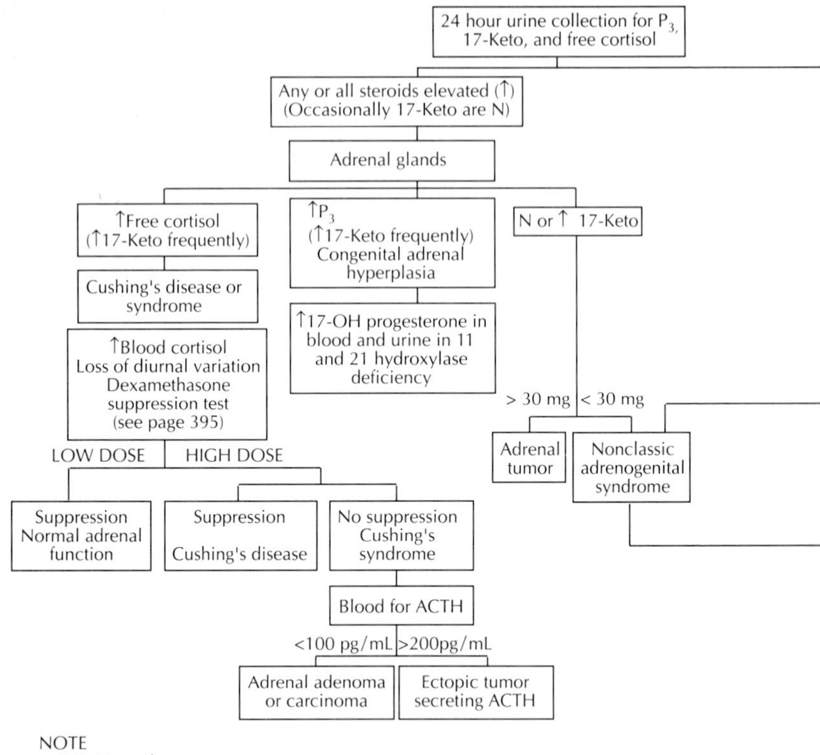


FIGURE 23.2. A protocol for diagnostic evaluation of the hirsute or virilized female. Additional studies for localization must be employed when a tumor is suspected. LH = luteinizing hormone; FSH = follicle-stimulating hormone; DHEAS = hydro-epiandrosterone sulfate; A = androstenedione; T = testosterone; DHT = dihydrotestosterone; $E_2$ = estradiol; hCG = human chorionic go-

Suppression of adrenal cortex with dexamethasone followed by stimulation of the ovaries with human chorionic gonadotropin (hCG) while the adrenal glands remain suppressed, is not helpful because unfortunately, the ovaries may respond to ACTH by secreting androgens, and adrenal tumors have responded to stimulation of hCG.

2. **Distinguishing nonclassic congenital adrenal hyperplasia from PCOD.** There is growing evidence that hirsute women

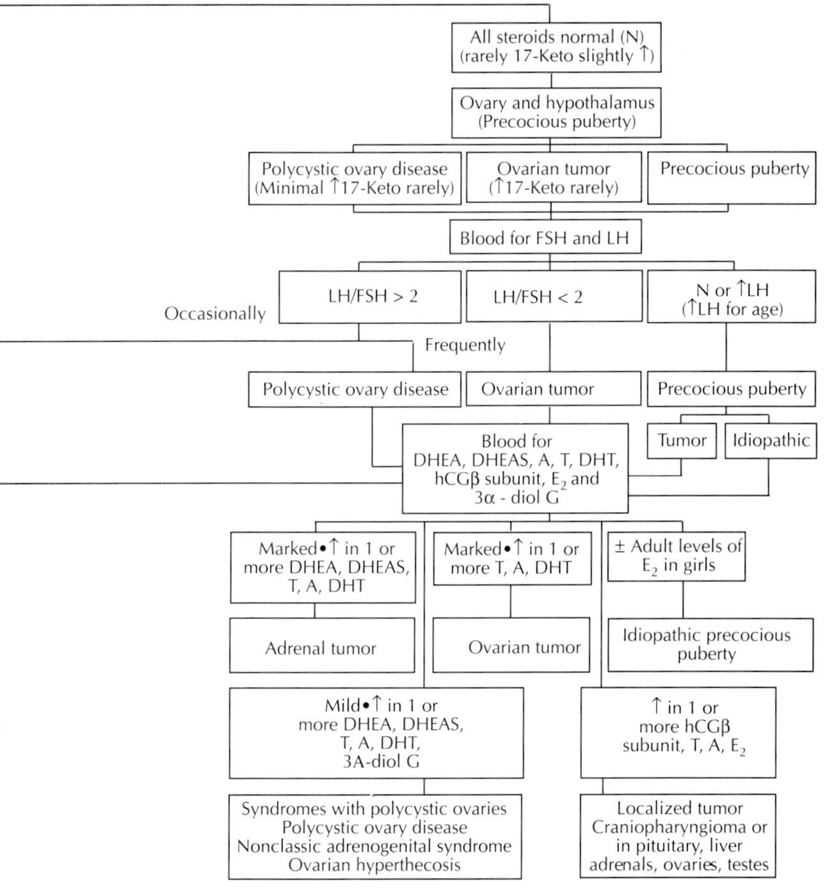


nadotropin; 3α-diol G = 3α-androstanediol; ACTH = corticotropin. From Northrop G. Hirsutism, defeminization, and virilization. In: Ellis JW, Beckmann RB, eds. A Clinical Manual of Gynecology. East Norwalk, Conn: Appleton-Century-Crofts; 1983: 522–523. Reprinted with permission.

with nonclassic CAH may be difficult to distinguish from women with PCOD without apparent genetic or adrenal abnormalities. Patients with nonclassic CAH have subtle deficiencies in adrenal enzymes required for cortisol synthesis. This causes decreased cortisol production, which results in a compensatory increase in ACTH-mediated cortisol synthesis required to maintain normal plasma concentrations of cortisol. Enzyme deficiencies thus far reported to be associ-

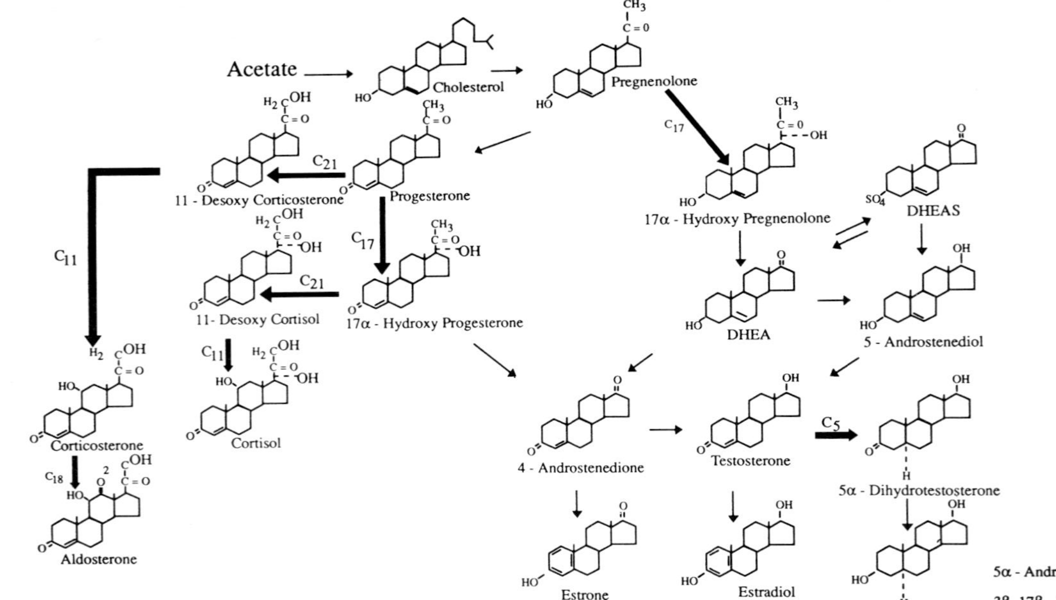


FIGURE 23.3. Common steroid metabolic pathways in the ovaries, testes, and adrenal glands. Names of steroid molecules that exhibit varying degrees of androgen activity in women are underlined. Enzymatic steps (arrows), and sites of hydroxylation or reduction on the steroid molecule are labeled for ease in recognition as follows: $C_3$ = 3β-hydroxylation plus isomerase; $C_{17}$ = 17α-hydroxylation; $C_{11}$ = 11β-hydroxylation; $C_{21}$ = 21β-hydroxylation; $C_{18}$ = 18-dehydrogenation; $C_5$ = 5α-reduction. Molecules of cyclopentanophenanthrene rings (i.e., androstenedione, testosterone, dihydrotestosterone, DHEAS, and DHEA) exhibit varying degrees of androgen activity in the human female.

**Table 23.4. Clinical Significance of Elevation of Androgens in Peripheral Blood**

| BLOOD TEST | ABBREVIATION | SIGNIFICANCE OF EVALUATION IN PERIPHERAL BLOOD |
|---|---|---|
| DHEA | D | Usually excessive adrenocortical secretion |
| DHEAS | DS | |
| Androstenediol | A | Either excessive adrencortical or ovarian secretion |
| Testosterone | T | |
| Dihydrotestosterone | DHT | Excessive conversion of D, DS, A, or T by tissue 5α-reductase |
| 3α-androstanediol | 3α-diol G | Excessive conversion of androgens in tissues peripheral to hepatic metabolism |
| Luteinizing hormone/follicle-stimulating hormone | LH/FSH | Ratios 2 or 3 are suggestive of PCOD (Excessive androgen production and hirsutism are commonly associated with PCOD) |
| Sex-hormone-binding globulin | SHBG | Low concentrations permit a greater percent of the total T or DHT to remain unbound and be biologically active (free) |

DHEA(S) = dehydroepiandrosterone sulfate; PCOD = polycystic ovary disease.

ated with nonclassic CAH are 21-hydroxylase, 3β-hydroxysteroid dehydrogenase, and rarely 11-hydroxylase. These subclinical enzyme deficiencies may be revealed by an accumulation in the blood of the steroid intermediate, prior to the compromised enzyme when cortisol synthesis is maximally stimulated with ACTH (cortrosyn 0.25 mg administered IV over 1 to 3 minutes). Elevation of 17-OHP, after ACTH administration, suggests 21-hydroxylase deficiency.

3. **Distinguishing Cushing's syndrome**
   a. Physical characteristics that are frequently visualized in patients with Cushing's syndrome (see diseases associated with hyperandrogenemia section, IV-B-2).
      (1) Truncal obesity. Fat deposits are frequently described by location that gives the patient a characteristic appearance (moon facies, buffalo hump, and prominent abdomen). Most women with buffalo humps do not have Cushing's syndrome, but are obese.
      (2) Thin muscle wasted extremities.
      (3) Plethoric facies.
      (4) Pink striae.
      (5) Thin skin (loss of subcutateous fat).

**Table 23.5. Dexamethasone Suppression Test**

| DAY | DEXAMETHASONE ORAL DOSE EVERY 6 HOURS | 17-HYDROXYCORTICOSTEROIDS (mg/24-HOUR URINE) | REMARKS |
|---|---|---|---|
| 1 | None | Twelve or less | Normal |
| 2 | 0.5 mg* | No collection | |
| 3 | 0.5 mg* | Three or less | Normal |
| 4 | 2.0 mg | No collection | |
| 5 | 2.0 mg | Suppression $>50\%$ of the baseline | Normal<br>Cushing's disease |
| | | Suppression $<50\%$ or no suppression compared to the baseline | Cushing's syndrome |

*Weight-adjusted dose of dexamethasone, 20 μg/kg of actual body weight, may improve discrimination.
From Northrop G. Hirsutism, defeminization, and virilization. In: Ellis JW, Beckmann RB, eds. A Clinical Manual of Gynecology. East Norwalk, Conn: Appleton-Century-Crofts; 1983: 519–520. Reprinted with permission.

b. Laboratory evaluation of Cushing's syndrome.
   (1) Plasma cortisol in excess of 10 pg/dL at 8 AM with less than a 50% decrease or in excess of 10 pg/dL at 8 PM.
   (2) Urinary free cortisol (complete urine collection) in excess of 100 pg/24 hours. A 24-hour urine for analysis of free cortisol has the usual disadvantages associated with the mechanics of obtaining a complete collection, but provides an integrated reflection of cortisol secretion. The free urinary cortisol concentration (normally less than 100 pg/24 hours) is not affected by body surface area (which is increased in obesity), or hepatic metabolism, (which is altered by hepatic disease, drugs, and thyroid disease).
   (3) **Dexamethasone suppression test.** The short dexamethasone suppression test (8 AM plasma cortisol below 5 pg/dL following 1 mg of oral dexamethasone the previous night at midnight) is falsely negative in 30% of the patients with Cushing's syndrome. The long dexamethasone suppression test is clearly the more useful in separating patients with Cushing's disease and syndrome from normal individuals. The long oral dexamethasone suppression test is performed as shown in Table 23.5.

Further separation of patients with Cushing's syndrome is gained by obtaining blood ACTH levels. Patients with autonomous adrenal secretion of cortisol (adrenal adenomas or carcinomas) suppress pituitary ACTH levels to less than 100 pg/mL. Ectopic secretion of ACTH from a tumor generally results in blood ACTH levels greater than 200 pg/mL.

Results recently reported from an overnight 8 mg oral dexamethasone test show that suppression of the morning plasma cortisol to less than 50% of baseline occurred in 92% of patients with Cushing's disease. No patients with tumors (adrenal adenomas and carcinomas or ACTH-producing tumors) suppressed the morning cortisol levels as far as 50% of baseline. This procedure may become the best method to separate patients with Cushing's disease from those with Cushing's syndrome.

c. **Ultrasonography** is useful in evaluation of pelvic structures, providing information on size and density of one or both ovaries. Solid tumors, when detected, can be distinguished from cysts.

d. **Computerized tomography (CT)** is used for examination of both the head and body for seeking and delineating a tumor. Suprasellar extension of a tumor or an empty sella can also usually be determined. Detection of cervical, thoracic, and abdominal masses including bilateral adrenal hyperplasia provides objective information and is a noninvasive technique.

e. **Magnetic resonance imaging (MRI)** provides the newest method of scanning the head or body for tumor. Imaging is related to nuclear cell density so another avenue of differentiation of one group of cells from another is provided. Radiologists differ on which scan, CT or MRI, is best to detect sellar lesions. Because high resolution CT scanners are more readily available, the MRI scan may be used when additional information would be helpful, or in patients in which masses have not been detected by CT scanning but are clinically suspected.

f. **Selective catheterization** for obtaining blood for hormone analysis from both adrenal glands and ovaries by the femoral vein. When peripheral blood levels of androgen are in excess of two times normal, and localization of excessive androgen secretion is desired, catheterization of the femoral vein is helpful for obtaining blood from both the adrenal glands and ovaries for hormone analysis. This procedure is helpful when noninvasive techniques have failed and tumor is suspected.

g. **Laparoscopy** is used alone or in combination with laparotomy when visualization (and biopsy) of the ovaries or other tissues is desired. This is particularly helpful in women with severe hirsutism and PCOD when the ovaries are extremely different in size. Unfortunately, small tumors, such as lipid cell tumors, have been missed when ovarian biopsy by the laparoscope has been performed.

## VI. Management

Most hirsute women have hyperandrogenemia and PCOD, which usually responds to medical management. In general, most drugs prescribed for treatment suppress either the ovaries or adrenal glands by acting as an exogenous source of the regulating hormone from the gland that is being suppressed. Thus, by negative feedback, the hypothalamic-pituitary axis is inhibited, the trophic hormone is not released, and the target gland is not physiologically stimulated. This form of treatment is not effective when the gland is functioning autonomously or a tumor is present.

### A. Corticosteriods

1. **Congenital adrenal hyperplasia.** Prednisone is one of several glucocorticoids that may be used. The dose is based on the body surface area and suppression of blood or urinary levels of 17-hydroxyprogesterone to normal. An approximate starting dose of prednisone is 6.5 mg/m$^2$ every 8 hours.

2. **PCOD**
   a. **Treatment.** PCOD associated with elevated dehydroepiandrosterone sulfate (DHEA or DHEAS) and normal levels of plasma cortisol is treated with oral prednisone, or other glucocorticoids, because the adrenal glands are the primary ($>90\%$) source of these $C_{19}$ steroids detected in the plasma. Patient compliance can be increased by providing adequate prednisone (5 mg at bedtime) to inhibit the spontaneous nightly ACTH release, plus a small morning prednisone dose (2.5 mg) each day that provides further duration of blockade of ACTH release as well as supports the patient physiologically on rising in the morning. Adequate adrenal suppression is maintained without need for midday medication.
   b. **Treatment effect.** Prolonged suppression of the adrenal cortex with exogenous glucocorticoids is expected to result in delayed synthesis of endogenous glucocorticoids such as cortisol. Thus, while in a suppressed state, or shortly thereafter, any significant stress, for example, surgery, tooth extraction, common cold with a fever, is a cause for careful observation. Temporary administration of additional glucocorticoid medication is likely appropriate.
   c. **Toxicity.** Significant toxicity, except rarely for gastric irritation, should not be encountered at physiologic replacement levels with glucocorticoids. At higher doses, symptoms of Cushing's syndrome are dependent upon the dose and duration of treatment.

B. **Oral contraceptives** are used for treatment of excessive androgen secretion of ovarian origin (plasma levels of DHEA, DHEAS, and cortisol are normal) when neoplasm appears unlikely. These drugs cause decreased gonadotropin secretion and elevation of SHBG. Androgens cause a decrease in SHBG, which results in relatively more free (biologically active) levels of androgens. Thus, for a normal level of total T in the blood, there is relatively more free (biologically active) T when the concentration of SHBG is decreased. Oral contraceptives elevate SHBG so that the level of free T is decreased.
   1. **Choice of oral contraceptive.** As a general rule, an oral contraceptive containing the least amount of estrogen compatible with regular uterine withdrawal bleeding (absence of breakthrough bleeding) is appropriate. There is dispute over potency between ethinyl estradiol and mestranol, the two synthetic estrogens employed in oral contraceptives. However, ethinyl estradiol appears to exert more biologic activity than mestranol based on weight in most protocols studied. It is reported that the biologic activity of 0.05 mg of ethinyl estradiol approximates 0.08 mg of mestranol.
   2. **Cautions in the use of oral contraceptives.** Recently the **pro-**

**gestogen** component of oral contraceptives has come under close scrutiny, principally due to their atherogenic properties. Rarely in some women, progestogens (19-nortestosterone derivatives) may be metabolized as androgens resulting in increased hirsutism. The use of oral contraceptives primarily because of the estrogen component is either inappropriate or must be given careful consideration in women with:

a. History of thrombophlebitis or thromboembolic disease.
b. Cerebral vascular or coronary artery disease.
c. Estrogen-dependent headaches, neoplasms, hypertension.
d. Diabetes mellitus when controlled with oral hypoglycemic agents or diet.

Breakthrough bleeding or amenorrhea is not an indication to stop oral contraceptives, but the patient should be re-evaluated and probably have her medication changed. Two factors that are associated with increased hazard of consuming oral contraceptives are smoking and increasing age.

C. **Oral contraceptives and prednisone.** When both the adrenal glands and ovaries are secreting excessive amounts of androgens, suppression with a single drug may only partly inhibit hair growth. The addition of a second suppressive agent is frequently required so that both ovarian and adrenal gland suppression is accomplished. Combining oral contraceptives with prednisone, even when the adrenal gland is the primary source of androgen secretion, may prove helpful because estrogens increase SHBG and thus lower biologically active T and DHT.

D. **Additional drugs recently used for treatment of hirsutism**

1. **Medroxyprogesterone acetate** (MPA, Depo Provera, 100–200 mg IM weekly) may provide some ovarian suppression. However, treatment of hirsutism has been disappointing with this and other progestogens. Recent investigators have reported that MPA, in addition to 19-nortestosterone derivatives, cause the blood lipoprotein, high-density lipoprotein (HDL)-cholesterol, to be decreased. In particular, the beneficial subfraction, $HDL_2$ cholesterol, is suppressed. Thus, according to current thinking, progestogens may, in addition to androgens, be atherogenic and thus detrimental.
2. **Spironolactone** (50 to 200 mg per day in individualized dosages) may be used as the only drug in women who are poor candidates for oral contraceptives for ovarian suppression, or, in combination with oral contraceptives, may provide yet another avenue for reduction in hair growth. This drug blocks the target receptor (receptor on the hair follicle) and thus decreases the effect of circulating androgens on the target cells. Data from recent studies suggest that spironolactone may also partly inhibit adrenal androgen synthesis. When spironolactone is combined with oral contra-

ceptives, the high frequency of polymenorrhea is reduced and the rate of hair growth appears to decrease in some patients.

E. **Clomiphene citrate** (Clomid), an antiestrogen, stimulates the ovary by increasing pituitary gonadotropins. Clomiphene citrate is useful for induction of ovulation and should be used in hirsute women primarily for this purpose. Ovarian stimulation by clomiphene citrate frequently results in excessive androgen secretion with potentiation of hirsutism often accompanied by regular ovulatory menses.

F. **Hair removal.** Mechanical alterations or removal of excessive hair is effective in women with minimal hirsutism. Most women who are successful in the use of peroxide for bleaching hair or plucking or wax removal methods, are not identified by the physician. Women in whom hair growth is too rapid for the above methods resort to shaving and electrolysis. Dermatologists claim shaving does not stimulate hair growth. Electrologists claim hair removal is more difficult in areas in which it has previously been removed by wax or plucking. Certainly, electrolysis kills the hair follicle. However, if excessive androgen production continues, new terminal hair will replace previously removed hair. Thus, the effective control of hair growth, continued suppression of excessive androgen secretion coupled with electrolysis is mandatory. After hair follicles have been destroyed, continued medical suppression is usually required to prevent continued stimulation of androgens.

G. **Surgery**

1. **PCOD.** Ovarian wedge resection is usually reserved for women who desire pregnancy and have failed to ovulate while taking clomiphene citrate. Hirsute women not desiring immediate pregnancy, refractory to adrenal suppression, and unable to take oral contraceptives may also be considered for ovarian wedge resection. Removal of ovarian stromal tissue results in decreased T or androstenedione in the ovarian veins, decreased peripheral conversion of T to estradiol, normalization of the plasma LH:FSH ratio, decreased urinary 17-ketosteroids, subsequent ovulation, and a decrease in hirsutism, in that order, in most women.
2. **Neoplasms.** The treatment of hirsutism and/or virilism associated with neoplasms is surgical removal, followed by chemotherapy and/or radiation when required.

VII. **Prognosis.** The majority of hirsute women do not have life-threatening malignancy, but most hirsute women feel they have a life-disturbing problem. Excessive body and facial hair in women is unwelcomed in most societies. Successful treatment of the majority of hirsute women depends upon the correct diagnosis, as well as diligent and chronic treatment with excellent results expected in most patients. When treatment is initiated prior to involvement over extensive areas of the body, the cosmetic effect is maximal. When large areas of the body are involved, long hours of electrolysis time is required. With effective suppression of androgen production, additional follicles do not produce terminal hairs, and only a minority of the established hair-producing follicles remain active, making 5 to 15 minutes of electrolysis necessary two or three times per year. Some form of suppressive therapy is usually required indefinitely.

In patients with tumor-related hirsutism, the rate of hair growth relates to management of the tumor. Hair growth present for greater than 1 year is unlikely to remit spontaneously with androgen removal or pharmacologic blockade. Electrolysis for follicle destruction should be effective and required only until the active hair-producing follicles are destroyed.

## BIBLIOGRAPHY

Coney P. Polycystic ovarian disease: Current concepts of pathophysiology and therapy. Fertil Steril 1984; 42:667–682.

Kirschner MA. Hirsutism and virilism in women. Special Topics in Endocrinology and Metabolism 1984; 6:55–93.

New MI, Levine LS. Recent advances in 21-hydroxylase deficiency. Ann Rev Med 1984; 35:649–663.

Rittmaster RS, Loriaux L. Hirsutism. Ann Intern Med 1987; 106:95–107.

Tyrrell JB, Findling FW, Aron DC, Fitzgerald PA, Forsham PH. An overnight high-dose dexamethasone suppression test for rapid differential diagnosis of Cushing's syndrome. Ann Intern Med 1986; 104:180–186.

Yen SSC, Jaffe RB. Reproductive Endocrinology. 2nd ed. Philadelphia Pa: WB Saunders; 1986.

CHAPTER 24

# Normal and Abnormal Sexual Differentiation and Development

**Ira M. Rosenthal**

An understanding of developmental anatomy facilitates the evaluation and management of abnormalities of sexual differentiation. Such abnormalities can be effectively diagnosed and treated with knowledge of the underlying pathophysiology. This chapter discusses normal and abnormal sexual differentiation and development.

## I. Normal sexual development and physiology

### A. Normal female differentiation

1. **Ovaries.** In the female fetus, the indifferent gonad develops into an ovary during the 13th and 16th week of gestation. Two X chromosomes are necessary for normal fetal ovarian development. The absence of one X chromosome (i.e., 45,X) results in the deterioration of ova with resultant streak gonads.
2. **Internal reproductive organs.** Most of the internal reproductive tract, (i.e., fallopian tubes, uterus, and the superior portion of the vagina) is formed from the Mullerian ducts. The remainder of the vagina is formed from the urogenital sinus. The Wolffian ducts degenerate except for a small caudal portion, which forms the Gartner duct and a small cranial portion, which forms the epoöphoron.
3. **External genitalia.** The clitoris is formed from the genital tubercle, the labia minora develop from the urethral folds, and the labia majora are derived from the genital swellings.

### B. Normal male differentiation

1. **Testicular development.** The indifferent fetal gonads in the male begin to develop into testes at the seventh week of gestation under the influence of the Y chromosome. It appears that the testis determining factor (TDF) gene of the Y chromosome is essential for the differentiation of the testes.

2. **Müllerian duct regression.** Anti-Müllerian duct hormone (AMH), a polypeptide secreted by the Sertoli cells of the fetal testes, results in regression of the Mullerian ducts except for the most cranial portion which persists as the appendix testes. The process begins at 7 weeks of fetal life and is completed by 10 weeks.
3. **Wolffian duct differentiation.** Testosterone is responsible for the differentiation of the Wolffian ducts into epididymides, vasa deferentia, and seminal vesicles. Five enzymes are involved in the synthesis of testosterone from cholesterol. Three of these enzymes (20,22-desmolase, 3β-hydroxysteroid dehydrogenase, and 17α-hydroxylase) are also present in the adrenals. Therefore, a deficiency in any one of these enzymes can result in a defect of glucocorticoid and/or mineralocorticoid production, as well as in the production of testosterone. Two of the enzymes necessary for testosterone synthesis (17,20-desmolase and 17β-hydroxysteroid oxidoreductase) are present primarily in the testes. Dihydrotestosterone (DHT) is apparently not necessary for Wolffian duct differentiation.
4. **External genitalia.** Testosterone is reduced in the genital tubercle and urogenital sinus by 5α-reductase to form DHT. Male external genital differentiation is dependent on DHT. The prostate, which develops from the prostatic bud, an outpocket of the urogenital sinus, is also dependent on DHT for its development.

C. **Role of pituitary gland in sexual development**

1. **Function of FSH and LH in gonadal development.** The hypothalamic-pituitary-gonadal axis begins functioning during fetal life. Follicle-stimulating hormone (FSH), luteinizing hormone (LH), and human chorionic gonadotropin (hCG) play important roles in sexual differentiation by stimulating gonadal growth and by helping to maintain sex steroid synthesis and secretion by the gonads. FSH plays a synergistic role with LH in the development of LH receptors on Leydig cells. The stimulation of hCG-LH receptors on Leydig cells is necessary for the fetal testes to produce testosterone.
2. **Function of FSH and LH at puberty.** FSH and LH are elevated at birth, but by 2 years of age low values characteristic of prepubertal children are reached. Gonadotropin secretion is regulated by complex interactions of the central nervous system, the hypothalamus, the pituitary, and feedback regulation of these centers by both estrogens and androgens. At the onset of puberty there is increased secretion from the hypothalamus of gonadotropin-releasing hormone (GnRH). The events that trigger increased GnRH secretion remain unknown. LH is first produced in nocturnal surges followed by smaller episodic increases in FSH production. An adult pattern of LH release (pulsatile

throughout the 24-hour period) is reached late in puberty in females. In females FSH rises during the early stages of puberty until a plateau is reached about the time of menarche. LH values remain lower than FSH values until about a year before menarche, when higher values are present. In the female, FSH stimulates follicle development and, along with LH, is part of the ovulatory surge. LH also supports corpus luteal function.

3. **Function of DHEA and DHEAS.** Ordinarily about 2 years before the rise in GnRH secretion, adrenal androgen secretion, primarily dehydroepiandrosterone (DHEA) and its sulfate (DHEAS), increases. These compounds play a role in the development of pubic hair and axillary hair. The exact control of this process is not completely understood.

D. **Nutrition and sexual development.** Nutrition is important in the onset of puberty. The progressively earlier menarche that has occurred in Western countries since 1850 reflects better nutrition. For the past 3 decades, a critical weight of 46 kg has been associated with menarche. This weight is usually attained between 12.5 and 13 years of age.

II. **Intersexuality.** Abnormalities of sexual differentiation may result from virilization of a genetically female fetus, from incomplete masculinization of a genetically male fetus, the presence of both ovarian and testicular tissue in a fetus genetically 46,XX or 46,XY and from the presence of certain sex chromosome abnormalities (i.e., 45,X/46,XY). Early diagnosis is necessary to designate the proper sex rearing, to institute immediate therapy when indicated, and to devise plans for later treatment.

A. **Female pseudohermaphroditism (virilization of genetic females)** occurs when the genitalia are partially masculinized, the gonads are ovaries, and the karyotype is 46,XX.

1. **Congenital adrenal hyperplasia (CAH)** are autosomal recessive inherited abnormalities where affected genetic females have varying degrees of virilization of the external genitalia. A urogenital sinus is usually present, although there may be separate urethral and vaginal orifices; occasionally the urethra may penetrate the clitoris. Virilization results from excessive testosterone production in individuals with 21-hydroxylase or 11-hydroxylase deficiency and from increase in DHEA production in 3β-hydroxysteroid dehydrogenase deficiency. Normal Mullerian-derived organs are present. These patients have the potential for normal fertility if treated properly. Virilization is progressive if proper therapy is not instituted and maintained.

a. **21-hydroxylase deficiency.** Over 90% of patients with virilizing CAH have a deficiency in the enzyme 21-hydroxylase. These patients have elevated serum levels of 17α-hydroxyprogesterone and testosterone. The clitoris is enlarged at birth, and there is usually an urogenital sinus and occasionally a clitoral urethra. In more than half of the patients, there is an electrolyte disturbance characterized by low serum sodium and elevated potassium (salt-wasting type), probably resulting from a deficiency of aldosterone synthesis. The electrolyte deficiency is usually manifested by day 4 to 10 after birth with symptoms of vomiting, lethargy, and signs of dehydration. Hypoglycemia may also be present. Simple virilizing cases do not have salt wasting. Note that 21-hydroxylase deficiency in females may occur without the development of pseudohermaphroditism (nonclassic cases). Such patients may manifest virilization later in childhood or in adult life and may suffer from severe acne. In cryptogenic cases no symptoms are present. The enzyme 21-hydroxylase is coded on the short arm of chromosome 6, close to the sites for the human leukocyte antigen (HLA) complex. This has made it possible to use HLA typing for genetic studies of this disease. Specific abnormalities in the DNA coding for 21-hydroxylase have been identified.

(1) **Diagnosis** of 21-hydroxylase deficiency is suspected from the clinical presentation. The karyotype is 46,XX and there is marked elevation of plasma **17-hydroxyprogesterone (17-OHP)** levels. Serum testosterone and androsteanedione levels are also elevated. After the first few days of life in patients with an electrolyte disturbance, serum sodium is decreased and potassium is increased. Abnormalities in the electrocardiogram may develop. Urinary 17-ketosteroids and pregnanetriol (a metabolite of 17-OHP) are elevated. The increase in pregnanetriol may not be manifest during the first few weeks of life. Screening of all newborns by measurements of 17-OHP on blood spots collected on filter paper has proven to be successful and appears to diminish the mortality from undiagnosed cases.

(2) **Therapy.** Patients with simple virilizing 21-hydroxylase deficiency and no associated electrolyte disturbance are treated with oral glucocorticoids from the time of diagnosis. The glucocorticosteroid dose must be increased as the child becomes older. In case of stress, the dose of this medication must be increased temporarily, and it may be necessary to use the parenteral route for administration. It has been suggested that in some cases, use of mineralocorticoids may reduce the dose of glucocorticoids neces-

sary for adequate control. Infants with associated electrolyte disturbance, in addition to glucocorticoids usually require IV fluids with sodium chloride and glucose at the time of initial therapy. They may initially require parenteral hydrocortisone. In addition, they require mineralocorticoid treatment with 9α-fluorocortisol (Florinef). Extra oral sodium chloride is required. The blood pressure of these patients should be carefully monitored, and if elevated, the amount of mineralocorticoids and sodium chloride should be decreased appropriately. Corrective surgery to the genitalia (clitoroplasty) and reconstruction of the urogenital sinus is required in most cases of 21-hydroxylase deficiency, and is performed in the first few years of life.

b. **11-hydroxylase deficiency** is a rare disorder affecting less than 5% of the patients with virilizing CAH. In most cases hypertension develops in time possibly because of excessive synthesis of desoxycorticosterone (DOC). Hyponatremia and hyperkalemia do not occur. The gene for 11β-hydroxylase is located on chromosome 8. There is no association with the HLA antigen. As in 21-hydroxylase deficiency, mild, late onset and cryptogenic forms of 11-hydroxylase deficiency occur.

(1) **Diagnosis** of 11-hydroxylase deficiency is established by increased urinary excretion of tetrahydro-11-desoxycortisol (THS) and tetrahydrodesoxycorticosterone (THDOC). There is a mild elevation of serum 17-hydroxyprogesterone and increased concentration of 11-desoxycortisol (S) and DOC.

(2) **Therapy** of 11-hydroxylase deficiency consists of glucocorticoid replacement. Hypertension, if present, usually disappears with proper therapy. Clitoroplasty is usually required and can be performed after late infancy.

c. **3β-hydroxysteroid dehydrogenase deficiency.** Virilization of genetic female infants with 3β-hydroxysteroid dehydrogenase deficiency is mild. There are variable degrees of labial fusion. In severe deficiency cases the electrolyte disturbance is marked since there is impairment of mineralocorticoid as well as glucocorticoid synthesis. Less severely affected infants and older individuals with "late onset" of this abnormality occur. Such cases appear to be more common than the severe form. There is no association of the gene for this enzyme with the HLA complex.

(1) **Diagnosis** of 3β-hydroxysteroid dehydrogenase

deficiency is confirmed by elevated serum levels of 17-hydroxy-5-pregnenolone and DHEA. Urine contains large amounts of delta-5-steroids such as 5-pregnenetriol and 16-pregnenetriol.

(2) **Therapy** is similar to that for 21-hydroxylase deficiency with electrolyte disturbance. The prognosis is guarded in severe cases. Corrective genital surgery may be required. Mild cases with simple virilization may only require hydrocortisone p.o.

2. **Virilizing maternal tumor.** The arrhenoblastoma is the most common virilizing tumor occurring in women during pregnancy. Other maternal tumors that can virilize the fetus include Leydig cell tumors, adrenal rest tumors, Krukenberg tumors, and mucinous cystadenomas. Luteomas of pregnancy, not true neoplasms, are solid hCG-dependent tumors that can also be associated with virilization of the female fetus; they disappear after pregnancy. Infants of mothers with virilizing tumors during pregnancy can be born with an enlarged clitoris. Virilization of such infants, however, is not progressive.
   a. **Diagnosis** of virilizing maternal tumors is usually made from history, physical findings, analysis of maternal blood samples, and after surgery, from histology of the maternal tumor.
   b. **Therapy.** The infant may require no therapy as regression of the virilization usually occurs after delivery. In some cases, however, surgery is required to correct a genital abnormality.
3. **Ingestion of virilizing medication during pregnancy.** A number of progestational agents, 19-nor compounds, were implicated in causing fetal virilization during the period that this type of medication was used for the treatment of threatened abortion. The most common drug implicated, at that time, was 19-norethesterone (Norlutin). Only a small percentage of female fetuses exposed to these medications developed virilization. This problem is rarely encountered now as most physicians are aware of the virilizing effects of such medications and avoid their prescription during pregnancy.
   a. **Diagnosis.** A history of ingestion of virilizing substances during early pregnancy is obtained. Physical examination of the infant whose mother ingested virilizing medication during pregnancy discloses enlargement of the clitoris and some fusion of the labia.
   b. **Therapy.** Virilization following medication is not progressive. Female sex should be assigned. Plastic surgical correction of the genital abnormality has been required in some cases.

4. **Special nonadrenal female pseudohermaphroditism.** Nonadrenal female pseudohermaphroditism is associated with abnormalities of the upper urinary tract such as hydronephrosis, and with imperforate anus, anorectal atresia, and fistulae between lower urinary tract and vagina; a double uterus is common. The cause of this genital abnormality is not known.
   a. **Diagnosis** is made by examination of internal and external genitalia, presence of a karyotype 46,XX, and the presence of other anomalies. Plasma steroid levels and urinary metabolites are normal.
   b. **Therapy.** Surgical correction of genital abnormalities is usually required.
5. **Idiopathic nonadrenal female pseudohermaphroditism.** Masculinization of external genitalia, no progressive virilization, and no other somatic abnormalities characterize idiopathic nonadrenal female pseudohermaphroditism.
   a. **Diagnosis** is made from examination of genitalia and exclusion of known causes, including maternal luteoma.
   b. **Therapy.** Surgical correction of genital abnormalities is required.

B. **True hermaphroditism** is characterized by the presence of ovarian and testicular tissue in the same individual. An ovotestis may be present on each side of the body. There may be an ovotestis on one side and a testis on the other, or an ovotestis on one side and an ovary on the other. In some cases there is an ovary on one side and a testis on the other. The karyotype is usually 46,XX. Mosaicism (i.e., 46,XX/46,XY) may be present. It is unusual to have 46,XY pattern. Although almost all cases of true hermaphroditism have been sporadic, there have been a few reports of familial occurrence. Gynecomastia and menstruation in individuals reared as males may be presenting symptoms.
   1. **Diagnosis.** True hermaphroditism is suspected from the clinical presentation. The degree of male differentiation depends on the capacity of the fetal testicular tissue to secrete testosterone and anti-Mullerian hormone. There is considerable variation in the development of the phallus and in the configuration of the external genitalia. A uterus and vagina are usually present, but the fallopian tube is generally absent on the side in which testicular tissue is present. Sexual maturation at puberty is dependent on the functional capacity of the ovarian and testicular tissue. About 70% of cases have breast development. Karyotype may be 46,XX (58.2%), 46,XX/46,XY (13.4%), 46,XY (11.6%), 46,XY/46,XXY (6.4%), 45,X/46,XY (4.0%), other mosaics (6.4%). The diagnosis of true hermaphroditism is dependent on biopsy of both gonads and histologic studies.

2. **Therapy** depends upon the sex assignment. After diagnostic studies are complete, a decision is made regarding sex assignment based in large part on the functional capacity of the genitalia for sexual relations. Fertility is ordinarily not a consideration because these patients are sterile.
   a. **Assigned female sex.** In most infants, female sex is assigned. Testicular tissue is removed and reconstructive surgery of the genitalia is performed.
   b. **Assigned male sex.** If male sex is assigned, ovarian tissue is removed. If gender role and sex identity are established at the time of diagnosis, the assigned sex is generally maintained and appropriate surgical therapy instituted with removal of inappropriate gonadal tissue. Intra-abdominal testicular tissue, which cannot be brought into the scrotum, should be removed to avoid tumor formation. True hermaphrodites may require replacement of sex hormones at puberty and thereafter consistent with the assigned sex.

C. **Incomplete masculinization of the genetic male.** Patients with male pseudohermaphroditism have testes, but male differentiation of the external genitalia is incomplete or there may be persistence of Müllerian structures. The basic causes include abnormality of fetal testicular tissue, unresponsiveness of the fetal Leydig cells to hCG and LH, inborn errors of testosterone biosynthesis, end-organ unresponsiveness to testosterone and an abnormality in the production or action of anti-Müllerian hormone. The karyotype of these patients is 46,XY.

1. **Inborn errors of testosterone synthesis.** Of the five enzymes necessary for the synthesis of testosterone from cholesterol, three are present in both adrenals and testes and affect the production of glucocorticoids and mineralocorticoids. In all five enzyme defects, the degree of intersexuality present varies considerably and is dependent upon the degree of enzyme deficiency. Müllerian duct development does not occur in these patients. Testes are usually underdeveloped and are frequently intra-abdominal. The defects are inherited as autosomal recessive traits.
   a. **20-22 desmolase deficiency.** In 46,XX and XY infants with this disease, also known as **congenital lipoid adrenal hyperplasia,** the genitalia are female. In 46 XY infants a blind vaginal pouch is present with no uterus or fallopian tubes. Testes that are undescended are present. Because neither glucocorticoids nor mineralocorticoids are synthesized, there are severe electrolyte disturbances with early Addisonian crisis. There is lipid accumulation in adrenal and Leydig cells. All patients have had a severe deficiency, and there has been a high mortality rate.
      (1) **Diagnosis** is made upon demonstration of low or absent urinary 17-ketosteroids and 17-hydroxy-

corticosteroids. Karyotype and pelvic ultrasound are helpful in diagnosis. Enlarged adrenals may be demonstrated radiologically.

(2) **Therapy** includes glucocorticoid and mineralocorticoid replacement. In 46,XY patients who survive, testes should be removed surgically during infancy. Appropriate female sex hormone substitution would be necessary in case of survival to the normal age of puberty.

b. **3-β-hydroxysteroid dehydrogenase deficiency.** There are varying degrees of hypospadias and incomplete pseudovaginal hypospadias in this disease. Biosynthesis of delta-4-steroids is blocked with insufficiency of glucocorticoids and mineralocorticoids. Electrolyte disturbance is usually severe, and mortality may be high despite therapy, although some patients manifest little electrolyte disturbance; late onset of the syndrome has also been described. In surviving patients at puberty, gynecomastia develops, probably resulting from high estrogen production. Arrest of spermatogenesis is found.

(1) **Diagnosis** is made upon demonstration of a karyotype 46,XY and low cortisol and aldosterone levels. (See female pseudohermaphroditism, section II-A, with same defect for biochemical findings.)

(2) **Therapy.** Glucocorticoid and mineralocorticoid replacement is essential to therapy. If male sex is assigned, surgical correction of the genital abnormalities is indicated. In individuals with severe enzymatic deficiency, the external genitalia have a female appearance. Female sex assignment with removal of testes should be recommended in such cases.

c. **17-α-hydroxylase deficiency.** Patients with 17-α-hydroxylase deficiency of the severe type have external genitalia of the female phenotype, whereas in the partial deficiency, there may be variable degrees of phallic development with hypospadias. These patients may demonstrate some signs of spontaneous secondary sex development, and gynecomastia has occasionally been seen. In complete deficiency, however, secondary sexual characteristics do not develop, and the patients have normal-appearing female external genitalia. Hypertension and hypokalemia, common in older patients, are due to excessive production of DOC.

(1) **Diagnosis** is made upon demonstration of elevated serum levels of pregnenolone, progesterone, DOC, and corticosterone with low serum levels

of cortisol and aldosterone. Hypokalemia occurs, renin is low. Serum gonadotropins are elevated.

(2) **Therapy.** Sex of rearing is dependent upon the ability to function sexually as an adult. Female sex is usually assigned. Glucocorticoid replacement lowers elevated blood pressure. Appropriate sex hormone replacement at the time of puberty is necessary. Corrective genital surgery may be necessary.

d. **17-20 desmolase deficiency.** Mineralocorticoid and glucocorticoid deficiencies do not occur in patients with 17-20 desmolase deficiency. There are abnormalities of phallic development and hypospadias.

(1) **Diagnosis.** Increased urinary pregnenetriol and 11-keto-pregnenetriol are found in this syndrome. Serum testosterone and delta 4-androstenedione are low. No significant rise in testosterone occurs following hCG injection. Plasma gonadotropins are elevated.

(2) **Therapy.** Replacement sex hormones are needed at the time of puberty. Surgery to render the external genitalia appropriate to the sex assignment may be necessary. Most patients have male sex assignment. If the sex assignment is female, orchiectomy and vaginoplasty are indicated.

e. **17-β-hydroxysteroid dehydrogenase deficiency (17-ketosteroid reductase deficiency).** Patients with 17-β-hydroxysteroid dehydrogenase deficiency are seldom identified until puberty. Because of the limitation of this enzyme to the testes, neither salt loss nor Addisonian crisis occurs. The external genitalia at birth are usually female in character, with a blind vaginal pouch, and testes can be palpated in the inguinal canals. At the time of puberty hirsutism and phallic growth occur and usually gynecomastia is evident.

(1) **Diagnosis.** At puberty, marked elevation of plasma concentrations of delta-4-androstenedione is present, associated with low levels of testosterone. LH levels are high whereas FSH levels are less constantly elevated. In prepubertal subjects, daily hCG administration for 5 days with subsequent measurement of testosterone and delta-4-androstenedione levels is diagnostic. Studies demonstrate relatively high levels of androstenedione. The karyotype is 46,XY. Family studies for genetic pedigrees may be helpful.

(2) **Therapy.** If female sex is assigned at birth, removal of the testes, corrective plastic surgery, and administration of estrogens at puberty are

indicated; vaginoplasty may be necessary. If recognized at birth from family studies, male sex can be assigned and corrective surgery performed on the genitalia. Virilization at puberty can be anticipated.

2. **Inborn error of testosterone metabolism: 5-α-reductase deficiency.** There is inadequate conversion of tetosterone to dihydrotestosterone in this condition. Dihydrotestosterone is necessary for normal penile and prostate development and later for growth of facial hair, male-pattern baldness, and acne. Genetic males with 5-α-reductase deficiency lack Müllerian structures and have a blind vaginal pouch with varying degrees of phallic development. Seminal vesicles are present, and the excretory ducts empty into the vagina. Hypospadias is present. Virilization and penile growth occur at puberty. Gynecomastia does not occur. Formation of spermatozoa is impaired. Clinically expressed 5-α-reductase deficiency is inherited as an autosomal recessive condition limited to males. Genetic females with the full enzymatic defect are normal and fertile.
   a. **Diagnosis.** Laboratory values in this disorder include a high serum testosterone/DHT ratio in adults. In prepubertal patients this can be demonstrated after hCG administration. Gonadotropins are not elevated. Definitive diagnosis is established by finding decreased 5-α-reductase activity in genital skin obtained at biopsy.
   b. **Therapy.** If good phallic development is present, the sex of rearing should be male, because virilization occurs at the time of puberty. Surgical repair of the hypospadias is necessary. If the phallus is poorly developed, sex assignment can be female. Orchiectomy and plastic surgery of the genitalia is then indicated. Treatment with female sex hormones at the time of puberty is indicated. In patients assigned female sex but not recognized until virilization occurs at puberty, psychiatric evaluation is indicated to determine if a change in sex assignment is indicated. Appropriate surgical, medical, and psychiatric therapy depends on the sex assignment.
3. **End-organ insensitivity to androgens.** There is considerable variation in these end-organ insensitivity syndromes, depending on the degree of insensitivity affecting the receptor. The receptor disorders can be classified as complete testicular feminization, incomplete testicular feminization, the Reifenstein syndrome, and the infertile male syndrome.
   a. **Complete testicular feminization** is characterized by female external genitalia, blind vagina, underdevel-

oped labia, female habitus, full breast development, sparse or absent axillary and pubic hair, X-linked recessive transmission.

(1) **Diagnosis** is made by clinical features, 46,XY karyotype, normal or high plasma levels of testosterone, high plasma levels of estrogen (for males), elevated LH levels.

(2) **Therapy** consists of female sex assignment, removal of testes (possibility of malignancy), and estrogen administration.

b. **Incomplete testicular feminization** is characterized by enlarged clitoris, partial fusion of labioscrotal folds, female habitus, breast development, normal pubic and axillary hair for females, no uterus, and no fallopian tubes. Partially developed Wolffian ducts that connect to the vagina are noted. Testes are usually cryptorchid in this syndrome, with X-linked recessive transmission.

(1) **Diagnosis** is made by clinical findings, normal or high plasma testosterone, estrogen levels higher than in normal males, elevated LH levels, and 46,XY karyotype.

(2) **Treatment.** Removal of testes, plastic surgical genital correction, and estrogen administration are indicated.

c. **Reifenstein syndrome** is characterized by male phenotype with perineoscrotal hypospadias, breast enlargement at puberty, normal pubic and axillary hair, scanty beard, no uterus, no fallopian tubes, and often by cryptorchidism. The Wolffian ducts are usually developed in the syndrome with X-linked recessive transmission.

(1) **Diagnosis** is made by clinical findings, 46,XY karyotype, normal or high plasma testosterone, high plasma levels of estrogens for males, and elevated LH levels.

(2) **Treatment.** Surgery to correct genitalia and gynecomastia and male sex assignment are indicated.

4. **Testicular unresponsiveness to hCG and LH.** Synergistic effects of hCG and LH are necessary for Leydig cells to secrete testosterone in fetal life. In cases with poor response to these hormones, the physical abnormalities are dependent on the functional capacity of the Leydig cells. More severely affected individuals show a female pattern of pubic hair, normal-size clitoris, and have a short vaginal pouch. There is no breast development. No Müllerian structures are present.

a. **Diagnosis.** Definitive tests include 46,XY karyotype, elevated serum LH and gonadal biopsy with demonstration of absent Leydig cells. Low testosterone levels are noted.

b. **Therapy.** Sex assignment should depend on the nature of the external genitalia, which in turn depends on the degree of Leydig cell dysgenesis. Replacement hormones are necessary at the time of puberty to induce appropriate secondary sex characteristics. Plastic surgery is necessary in the patient with female sex assignment to enlarge the vaginal orifice and produce a functional vagina.

5. **Persistence of Müllerian duct derivatives.** In this syndrome phenotypic males are found to have a uterus and fallopian tubes due to a defect in the synthesis of anti-Müllerian hormone or in its receptors. There are two anatomical forms. In one (male) type one testis and ipsilateral fallopian tube and uterus enter the inguinal canal. Traction can bring the contralateral testes and tube into the same canal. Transverse testicular ectopia may be present. In a more uncommon form (female type) the uterus is found in the pelvis maintained by round ligaments and the testes are in the position normally occupied by ovaries. These abnormalities may be discovered in the course of hernia surgery. In most patients bilateral undescended testes are present. These patients virilize normally at puberty.

   a. **Diagnosis** is made by demonstration at surgery of Müllerian duct derivatives in males. The karyotype is 46,XY.

   b. **Therapy.** Because the vas deferens are usually found on each side on the posterior surface of the uterus, to prevent damage to these structures it has been suggested that a total hysterectomy not be performed to preserve the potential for fertility. Partial hysterectomy is indicated with the preservation of the cervix and the vas deferens on each side. Orchidopexy, after freeing dissection, should be performed if the testes are not descended. If orchidopexy cannot be done, orchiectomy should be considered.

6. **Abnormalities of fetal testicular formation**

   a. **46,XY pure gonadal dysgenesis.** Patients with pure gonadal dysgenesis are phenotypically female, of normal stature and lack female secondary sex characteristics. Minimal phallic development may be present. A vagina is present. TDF has been present in most, but not all, cases.

      (1) **Diagnosis** is made upon clinical findings and the demonstration of streak gonads bilaterally. The karyotype is 46,XY.

      (2) **Therapy.** Female sex should be assigned. Streak gonads should be removed because of their high

incidence of tumor formation. Replacement sex hormones are necessary at the time of puberty.

7. **Mixed gonadal dysgenesis (45,X/46,XY).** Patients with this mixed karyotype combine features of Turner's syndrome with male pseudohermaphroditism. Understature is present. There is considerable variation in the sexual phenotype, with varying degrees of male differentiation depending on the capacity of the fetal testicular structures to synthesize and secrete testosterone and anti-Müllerian hormone.
   a. **Diagnosis.** The karyotype is 45,X/46,XY. At laparotomy a streak gonad is frequently found on one side and a dysplastic testes on the other.
   b. **Therapy.** Female sex assignment with removal of gonads is recommended for many of these patients. Plastic surgical treatment to the genitalia may be indicated depending on the appearance of the genitalia. Replacement sex hormones are necessary at the time of puberty. If the phenotype is definitely male, sex assignment is in accordance with the phenotypic sex. Surgical removal of streak gonads is indicated. Plastic surgical correction of the genitalia may be required. Because of the 45,X line, understature should be anticipated. Treatment with growth hormone can be considered.

D. **Abnormalities of the Y chromosome.** The pericentromeric region of the short arm of the Y chromosome contains genes related to testicular differentiation. Loss of the short arm of the Y chromosome will result in phenotypic females with streak gonads, probably due to loss of TDF. Male differentiation occurs with deletion of the long arm of the Y chromosome although there may be abnormalities of the genitalia.

1. **Diagnosis.** Failure of sex maturation in phenotypic females with characteristic karyotype is diagnostic. Abnormality in genitalia of phenotypic males with abnormal karyotype relative to the Y chromosome occurs.
2. **Therapy.** Removal of streak gonads is indicated. In phenotypic females, replacement sex hormone therapy is started at puberty. Phenotypic males may require corrective surgery and replacement hormonal therapy at puberty.

III. **Precocious puberty** is defined as the development of secondary sexual characteristics before the age of 8 years. Precocious puberty has been subclassified into true precocious puberty and pseudoprecocious puberty. In **true precocious puberty** the hypothalamic-pituitary-gonadal axis is activated. In **pseudoprecocious puberty** the secondary sexual characteristics develop either from an exogenous source of hormones or from endogenous sex hormone production without activation of the hypothalamic-pituitary-gonadal system. Precocious puberty is defined as **isosexual** if development is in accord with the phenotypic sex and as **heterosexual** if discordant with the phenotypic sex. **Premature thelarche** and **premature adrenarche** are benign conditions that mimic precocious puberty.

A. **True precocious puberty.** In females, true precocious puberty is usually idiopathic. An underlying cause has been found in only about 15% of patients, but studies with newer imaging techniques may raise this figure. Etiologies include trauma, septo-optic dysplasia, brain infection, and tumors such as hamartomas. In all patients, physical examination should include a complete neurologic evaluation. The patient is usually tall for her age, and her bone age is advanced. Computerized tomographic (CT) films and/or magnetic resonance films of the skull are indicated in most cases.

1. **Idiopathic true precocious puberty**

a. **Diagnosis.** The presumptive diagnosis of idiopathic precocious puberty is made if no other etiology can be identified. The diagnosis is thus one of exclusion. Bone age is advanced, serum FSH, LH, and estrogen levels are elevated for chronological age, the response in GnRH is similar to normal puberty, and increased LH and FSH concentrations are noted during sleep. CT scanning and/or magnetic resonance studies of the skull and ultrasound studies of the pelvis are indicated.

b. **Therapy.** In idiopathic true precocious puberty, therapy with oral or intramuscular medroxyprogesterone acetate prevents menstruation and may cause regression of breast development. There is, however, little or no effect on the advancement of bone age. Cyproterone acetate and danazol may arrest gonadotropin secretion, but they do not affect advance in bone age. These forms of treatment are being replaced by therapy with analogs of GnRH that are more potent and have longer duration of action than the native hormone. Elevated levels of these compounds inhibit the release of gonadotropins by the pituitary. The treatment is effective because to maintain release from gonadotropins, gonadotropic cells need intermittent periods of relief from stimulation by GnRH. Advance in bone age appears to be arrested. Modest clothing should be worn to discourage sexual molestation. It should be stressed that although the child is advanced in physical appearance, her behavior is in accord with chronologic age.

2. **Familial constitutional true precocious puberty** is a relatively rare syndrome that can be a sex-limited autosomal dominant trait. A family history of early onset of menarche of mother, aunts, and sisters can be diagnostic.

a. **Diagnosis.** Same as precocious puberty section, III-A-1-a.

b. **Therapy.** Same as precocious puberty section, III-A-1-b.

3. **Trauma, infection, or tumor.** Head trauma, encephalitis, meningitis, hydrocephalus, or brain surgery may predispose to precocious puberty. Neurologic signs and symptoms may indicate the possibility of brain tumor.
   a. **Diagnosis.** Bone age is advanced and gonadotropins are elevated. CT scans are useful, and other studies such as angiography may be indicated.
   b. **Therapy.** If a brain tumor is diagnosed, treatment should be directed toward its removal if possible or toward x-ray therapy. Shunting procedures may be indicated if there is hydrocephalus. Otherwise the treatment is as in section precocious puberty III-A-1-b.
4. **Systemic illness associated with precocious puberty**
   a. **Tuberous sclerosis and von Recklinghausen disease.** Both of these syndromes are transmitted as autosomal dominants although spontaneous mutations do occur. Examination of parents may reveal stigmata of these conditions.
      (1) **Diagnosis.** Signs of precocious puberty and characteristic dermatologic findings pathognomonic for these conditions are found.
      (2) **Therapy.** Same as precocious puberty section, III-A-1-b.
   b. **Silver's syndrome** is associated with understature, characteristic facies, clinodactyly, and often with hemihypertrophy. Sexual precocity rarely occurs.
      (1) **Diagnosis.** Signs of the syndrome in association with precocious puberty are noted.
      (2) **Therapy.** Same as precocious puberty section, III-A-1-b.
   c. **Hypothyroidism** is occasionally associated with precocious puberty. Understature may be present. Breast development is present, but pubic and axillary hair are sparse. Menstruation occurs, and galactorrhea may be present. Linear growth is slow.
      (1) **Diagnosis.** Laboratory findings include low serum thyroxine, high thyroid stimulating hormone (TSH), elevated prolactin, FSH, and LH. An enlarged sella may be present. Ultrasonography may show multicystic ovaries.
      (2) **Therapy.** Appropriate thyroid replacement, preferably levothyroxine, can result in dramatic improvement. Galactorrhea, if present, usually subsides within 2 or 3 weeks. The elevated TSH level may not return to normal for several months.

## IV. Isosexual pseudoprecocity

A. **McCune-Albright syndrome** is a sporadic disease characterized by pigmented skin lesions and polyostotic fibrous dysplasia, often associated with endocrine dysfunction including Cushing's syndrome, growth hormone hypersecretion and hyperprolactinemia. A common abnormality is isosexual precocious puberty. Most cases have autonomous ovarian hyperfunction.

1. **Diagnosis.** Morphologic ovarian abnormalities can be demonstrated by ultrasound. Advanced bone age is present.
2. **Therapy.** Treatment with testolactone has recently been reported to control precocious puberty.

B. **Ovarian and adrenal tumors.** Functional ovarian and adrenal tumors are rare in children. The most common tumor that produces isosexual precocity is the **granulosa cell tumor.** Physical examination usually reveals an adnexal mass. Ultrasonography can reveal the tumor. Other less common ovarian tumors to be considered are **luteomas, thecomas, teratomas,** and **choriocarcinomas.** Gonadal sex cord tumors may occur in Peutz-Jeghers syndrome. Rarely, **adrenal neoplasms** cause isosexual pseudoprecocity.

1. **Diagnosis.** Advanced bone age and tall stature occur with the presence of female secondary sex characteristics. Vaginal bleeding may occur. A vaginal cytologic smear for estrogenic effect is positive. Serum and urinary estrogens are increased and serum LH may be elevated, reflecting a high hCG level found in patients with choriocarcinoma. Except for this condition, serum FSH and LH values are low. Urinary 17-ketosteroids are low unless an adrenal tumor is present. Ovarian tumors may often be palpable. Sonograms and abdominal CT scanning may be diagnostic.
2. **Therapy.** Surgical extirpation, if possible, is indicated. After surgery, treatment depends on the type of tumor. If all tissue is removed, some regression of secondary sex characteristics may occur. If bone age is advanced, true sexual precocity may develop.

C. **Exogenous sources of estrogens.** Foods and certain cosmetics contaminated with estrogens or oral contraceptives may cause pseudoprecocity.

1. **Diagnosis** is suspected from history. Examination of suspected products for the presence of estrogens may be indicated. Low serum gonadotropins are noted.
2. **Therapy.** Discontinuance of exposure to estrogens.

## V. Heterosexual pseudoprecocity

A. **Exogenous androgens.** Occasionally ingestion or local application of androgens may cause heterosexual pseudoprecocity.

1. **Diagnosis.** History and examination of the product involved.
2. **Treatment.** Stop exposure to product responsible.

B. **Adrenal and ovarian causes.** Aberrant adrenal function, either tumor or virilizing adrenal hyperplasia, is the usual cause. Patients with CAH may manifest this condition. In some patients the virilization from this condition may not be noted at birth, but becomes manifest later in childhood or early adult life. Ovarian causes are rare in children. They include arrhenoblastoma, lipoid cell tumor, and hyperthecosis. Evaluation of patients with heterosexual precocity should include careful family history, because some cases are familial. Physical examination may reveal increased muscularity, deep voice, acne, receding hairline, enlarged clitoris, and hirsutism.

1. **Diagnosis.** Bone age is advanced. Laboratory tests should include serum testosterone, FSH, LH, 17-α-hydroxyprogesterone, and cortisol. Urinary excretion of 17-ketosteroids and pregnanetriol should be measured. To help distinguish virilizing CAH from adrenal tumor, dexamethasone suppression may be used. Dexamethasone causes a marked suppression of plasma 17-OHP and of urine 17-ketosteroids in patients with hyperplasia, but not in adrenal virilizing tumors. Sonograms and body CT scanning are useful in the detection of tumors. Angiography is sometimes useful in localization.
2. **Therapy.** Adrenal or ovarian tumors should be removed surgically. Some regression of virilization may be anticipated. Further treatment for the tumor may be indicated. Virilizing adrenocortical hyperplasia should be treated with adrenocorticoid steroids. Patients with salt loss also require additional sodium chloride and sodium-retaining hormones such as fludrocortisone acetate.

## VI. Precocious thelarche.

**VI. Precocious thelarche.** Isolated breast development in precocious thelarche may be due to enhanced estrogen receptor activity in the breast anlage, or to slightly elevated circulating levels of estrogens for the age of the patient.

A. **Diagnosis.** Bone age is not advanced. Serum FSH and LH levels are prepubertal and sexual hair and menarche do not appear early. The breast enlargement may spontaneously regress without treatment.

b. **Therapy.** Reassurance of parents, modest dress, and follow-up examination every 6 months is indicated.

**VII. Precocious adrenarche** is the presence of pubic hair with or without axillary hair, due to early adrenal activation and presumably to the production of DHEA and its sulfate. There is no clitoral enlargement.

A. **Diagnosis.** Bone age is normal or slightly advanced. Height and weight percentile rankings are not abnormal. Serum FSH and LH are prepubertal. Serum testosterone is normal. Urinary 17-ketosteroids are normal for age. Serum DHEA may be elevated.

B. **Therapy.** No therapy is required. Follow-up at 6-month intervals is recommended.

## VIII. Incomplete sexual precocity.

**VIII. Incomplete sexual precocity.** Incomplete sexual precocity marks intermittent or unsustained puberty. Thelarche with growth acceleration, mild advancement of bone age, and pubic hair without progression are found. The disorder is probably caused by elevated serum estrogens of autonomous ovarian origin.

**IX. Delayed adolescence.** A phenotypic female who has not shown any secondary sexual characteristics by 13 years of age or has not had menarche by the age of 16 should be evaluated for delayed adolescence.

A. **Constitutional delay of adolescence.** The most common condition associated with sexual infantilism at the normal age of puberty is constitutionally delayed adolescence. Understature is commonly found with a growth spurt finally developing with the onset of puberty. A family history including the ages of sexual maturation and menarche should be obtained.
   1. **Diagnosis** is based on clinical findings, a normal female karyotype, delayed bone age, and normal hypothalamic, pituitary, and gonadal function. Serum FSH and LH values are prepubertal.
   2. **Therapy.** The prognosis is good. Patients usually have normal pubertal progression and are fertile so that drug therapy in general is not indicated. Reassurance to the patient and her parents is essential. Rarely, usually for psychologic reasons, hormone replacement therapy is indicated.

B. **Systemic disease.** Serious systemic disease can result in delayed adolescence. Among the conditions to be considered are Crohn's disease, ulcerative colitis, and celiac disease. Severe renal disease, cardiac disease, liver disease, hypothyroidism, sickle cell disease, and thalassemia may also cause delayed adolescence. Short stature is frequently found in these conditions, and bone age may be delayed.
   1. **Diagnosis** is made upon consideration of the possibility of systemic disease in cases of delayed adolescence.
   2. **Therapy** should be directed at the underlying systemic disease.

C. **Nutritional factors.** In addition to gastrointestinal dysfunction, anorexia nervosa, bulimia, and food aversion may delay sexual maturation and menarche. Emotional stress, not associated with anorexia, may also delay puberty.
   1. **Diagnosis.** Evident from history and physical examination.
   2. **Therapy.** Psychiatric management and improved nutrition is required for anorexia nervosa. Better nutrition and less

exercise is required for athletes and dancers with delayed adolescence to permit normal sexual development.

D. **Drugs.** Heavy marijuana smoking can cause delayed adolescence. Discontinuance of the habit ensures normal development.

E. **Hypothalamic dysfunction.** Patients with delayed adolescence associated with hypothalamic dysfunction may also have labile temperature control, abnormal appetite, and behavioral problems. Serum FSH and LH are prepubertal, but a rise is found after stimulation with GnRH.

1. **Prader-Willi syndrome** is characterized by varying degrees of hypogonadism, hyperphagia with marked obesity, hypotonia, understature, mental retardation, and small hands and feet. A history of feeding difficulties in infancy is frequently obtained. The exact etiology is unknown, but hypothalamic dysfunction has been postulated. The condition occurs sporadically in both females and males. There is a deletion of a small segment of chromosome 15 in many cases.
   a. **Diagnosis** is based on clinical findings. Chromosomal studies are indicated using prophase chromosomes.
   b. **Therapy.** Dietary restriction is usually required. Sex hormone replacement may be necessary. Many patients appear to respond to growth hormone.
2. **Laurence-Moon-Biedl syndrome** is transmitted as an autosomal recessive trait. It is believed to have a hypothalamic component. The syndrome is characterized by hypogonadism, understature, polydactyly, obesity, retinitis pigmentosa, and varying degrees of mental retardation.
   a. **Diagnosis.** Based on clinical findings and history.
   b. **Therapy.** Sex hormone replacement if delayed adolescence is prolonged.
3. **Kallmann's syndrome** is characterized in some cases by anosmia or hyposmia as well as delayed adolescence and delayed menarche secondary to hypothalamic hypogonadism. A familial history is noted in 50% of cases, possibly autosomal dominant. Midline facial defects, such as cleft lip and palate have been reported. Color blindness and eighth nerve deafness occur in some cases. The syndrome is more common in males. Growth is usually normal.
   a. **Diagnosis** is based on the characteristic clinical findings. Evaluation of olfactory function is required. Low gonadotropins and prepubertal response to GnRH are noted.
   b. **Therapy.** Sex hormone replacement may be necessary if sexual maturation is delayed or is incomplete. Ovulation can be induced in many patients with clomiphene citrate. Pulsatile therapy with GnRH can also induce ovulation.

F. **Pituitary dysfunction**

1. **Isolated gonadotropin deficiency.** In some cases isolated gonadotropin deficiency may be hypothalamic in origin. These patients have normal stature, but remain sexually infantile.
   a. **Diagnosis.** Serum gonadotropins are low and remain low as the patient reaches late teenage years. The response to GnRH by gonadotropins is lower than normal.
   b. **Therapy.** Replacement therapy with estrogens and progestational agents is indicated.
2. **Isolated growth hormone deficiency.** An isolated deficiency of growth hormone is characterized by understature, delayed bone age, and late appearance of secondary sex characteristics. Sexual maturation and menarche may not appear until the third decade of life.
   a. **Diagnosis** is by clinical presentation. Failure of growth hormone elevation after provocative tests such as clonidine, L-dopa, insulin, sleep, exercise, or arginine is noted.
   b. **Therapy.** Treatment is with growth hormone. With growth, gain of weight, and advancement of bone age, sexual maturation and menarche will develop. Early replacement with sex hormones may diminish the ultimate height attained.
3. **Panhypopituitarism.** Secretion of gonadotropins, growth hormone, and frequently TSH and corticotropin (ACTH) is diminished in panhypopituitarism. In some cases secretion of antidiuretic hormone is also reduced. The problem is occasionally congenital. Craniopharyngioma is the most common cause, although histiocytosis X, hemochromatosis, sarcoidosis, and trauma are other causes. Sexual infantilism is present. Sexual maturation and function is arrested if onset of disease of the pituitary occurs after puberty.
   a. **Diagnosis.** Clinical findings are supplemented by low serum FSH and LH with poor or no response to GnRH. TSH is often low with poor response to TRH. Serum cortisol levels are low, with good response to ACTH. Low levels of growth hormone with poor response to provocative tests.
   b. **Therapy.** Replacement with thyroxine and hydrocortisone as indicated. Growth hormone is necessary for understature. At the age of puberty, estrogens and progestational agents are required for replacement therapy.

G. **Gonadal dysfunction.** Gonadal disorders associated with delayed or absent secondary sexual development include Turner's syndrome, 46,XY gonadal dysgenesis, 46,XX pure gonadal dysgenesis, and damaged or extirpated gonads as the result of trauma, surgery, irradiation, or tumor.

1. **Turner's syndrome** patients may present with understature, edema of feet in infancy, pterygium colli, short fourth metacarpals, congenital heart disease (primarily coarctation of the aorta), and other abnormalities. Sexual infantilism is usually found, although in some cases there is some breast development and occasional menstrual periods. Sex chromosome abnormalities are found in all cases. The most common chromosomal abnormality is 45,X, although mosaicism, ring X-chromosomes, iso-X-chromosomes, and other abnormalities have been found.
   a. **Diagnosis** is based on clinical findings, abnormal karyotype, and elevated FSH and LH. Gonadotropins may be high in infancy, decline after 2 to 3 years and then achieve high levels at the usual time of elevation of gonadotropins in normal subjects.
   b. **Therapy.** Appropriate sex hormone replacement beginning with very low doses of estrogens at about the age of 13 years, followed by cyclic therapy with estrogens and progestational agents. In unusual cases with normal sexual maturation and menses, therapy may be delayed. Growth in these patients may be enhanced with growth hormones given before replacement sex hormone therapy is administered. Removal of streak gonads is not necessary.
2. **46,XX pure gonadal dysgenesis.** Patients with 46,XX pure gonadal dysgenesis are of normal stature. The lack of breast development and primary amenorrhea are the reasons for seeking medical assistance. None of the other stigmata of Turner's syndrome are present. Family history may be helpful, because transmission appears to be autosomal recessive. Normal Mullerian duct differentiation occurs.
   a. **Diagnosis.** Elevated gonadotropins and a 46,XX karyotype are found in this syndrome. Ultrasound may indicate streak gonads.
   b. **Therapy.** Replacement therapy for sexual development is with estrogens and progestational drugs. Removal of ovarian streaks is not indicated.
3. **46,XY gonadal dysgenesis.** Findings are similar to 46,XX gonadal dysgenesis but the karyotype is different. Streak gonads should be removed surgically because of potential for malignant change. Replacement therapy for normal female sexual development is indicated.
4. **Rokitansky syndrome** is characterized by failure to achieve menarche. There is a rudimentary or bicornate uterus. Fallopian tubes and ovaries are normal as is breast development. The vagina may be completely absent or the lower portion may be present as a blind shallow pouch. Occasional cases are familial with affected sisters.

a. **Diagnosis.** The characteristic physical findings are diagnostic. Ultrasound studies are useful for the evaluation of internal defects. The karyotype is 46,XX.
b. **Therapy.** Surgical construction or reconstruction of the vagina is required.

## BIBLIOGRAPHY

Burgoyne PS. Mammalian sex determination: thumbs down for zinc finger. Nature 1989; 342:860–862.

Guerrier D, Dien Tran JM, Vanderwinden SH, Van Outryve L, Legeal L, Bouchard M, Van Fliet G, De Laet MH, Picard JY, Kahn A, Josso N. The persistent mullerian duct syndrome: A molecular approach. Clin Endocrinol Metabol 1989; 68:46–52.

Hopwood NJ. Pathogenesis and management of abnormal puberty. In: Cohen MP, Foa PP, eds. Special Topics in Endocrinology and Metabolism. Vol 7. New York: Alan R Liss 1985: 175–236.

Josso N. The Intersex Child. Pediatric and Adolescent Endocrinology. Vol 8. Basel, Switzerland: S. Karger; 1981:1-273.

McGillivray BC. Testicular differentiating factor, current concepts. Growth, Genetics and Hormones 1989; 5:1–3.

Wilson JD: Sexual differentiation. Ann Rev Physiol 1978; 40:279.

# CHAPTER 25

# Infertility

**William L. Gentry**
**John E. Buster**

Infertility is the inability to conceive or complete the reproductive goals of a couple. Primary infertility is defined as failure to conceive after 1 year of unprotected intercourse in a couple trying to achieve a pregnancy for the first time. During this year, approximately 90% of all couples who are attempting conception will conceive. Patients with secondary infertility are those who have been pregnant at least once before but have been unable to conceive again. It is the intent of this chapter to provide a guide for the evaluation and treatment of the infertile couple.

I. **Incidence.** Approximately 10% to 20% of all married couples in the United States are infertile. The need for infertility services has been increasing over the past decade. This has been attributable to the decrease in the number of babies for adoption, postponement of marriage and attempts at childbirth, the increase in sexually transmitted diseases (STDs), and improvements in the provision of contraceptive and family planning services. Also, infertile couples today are more knowledgeable about fertility issues and may desire earlier intervention.

II. **Morbidity and mortality.** Physical morbidity usually stems from the cause of the infertility and not the infertility itself. However, psychological morbidity from infertility may be severe and can cause depression, anxiety, marital discord, and even divorce.

III. **Evaluation and etiology.** The evaluation of the infertile couple should be as complete and rapid as possible but also take into account the couple's age, history, and personal desires. For example, a young couple 20 years of age who are using vaginal lubricants and inappropriate timing for intercourse would be counseled differently than a 39-year-old patient with a 10 year history of infertility.

All couples should have a complete history and physical examination in an attempt to rule out any illnesses that may be related to infertility. Sexual history should include frequency and timing of intercourse, use of lubricants or douches, use of tobacco, alcohol, and other drugs, and pelvic infections.

There are three main requirements for pregnancy. These include egg availability, sperm availability, and a functional transport system for egg, sperm, and embryo. The following pages describe the infertility work-up based on these requirements.

**A. Ovulation (egg availability)**

**1. Documentation of normal ovarian function**

a. **History.** Following a complete history and physical examination, the presumptive documentation of ovulation should be made. The likelihood is high that an infertile woman with a history of predictable monthly menstrual cycles with premenstrual molimina and a normal physical examination is ovulating, especially in the presence of dysmenorrhea.

b. **Ancillary tests** to document presumptive ovulation include (Table 25.1):

(1) **Basal body temperatures (BBT).** Under the influence of progesterone and its action on the hypothalamus, the BBT rises following ovulation. The rise is from 0.4° to 1.0° F. However, BBT does not always increase even with other evidence of ovulation. A rise in BBT is helpful in documenting presumptive ovulation and the length of the luteal phase, but is not helpful in timing intercourse for that cycle. It is also important that the patient take her temperature each morning before rising to insure that the results are truly basal.

(2) **Serum progesterone.** A single serum progesterone value above 3 ng/mL in the mid-luteal phase can be considered as evidence for presumptive ovula-

**Table 25.1. Methods Used to Detect Presumptive Ovulation**

| METHOD | ADVANTAGES | DISADVANTAGES |
|---|---|---|
| Basal body temperature | Inexpensive | Predictive only 60% of the time, requires daily commitment by patient |
| Serum progesterone | Reliable | Cannot be used for timing intercourse |
| Endometrial biopsy | Reliable | Cannot be used for timing intercourse |
| Urinary luteinizing hormone detection kits | Useful for timing intercourse | Requires patient to interpret dipstick results |
| Follicular monitoring with ultrasound | Most reliable | Expensive, inconvenient |

tion. However, levels greater than 10 ng/mL are desired because of fluctuations in the level associated with pulsatile secretion. If the sample is obtained too early or too late in the luteal phase, the results may be low due to the rise and fall of progesterone in a normal cycle. Therefore, a good time to draw a serum progesterone is 1 week following the rise in BBT.

(3) **Endometrial biopsy.** Another way of providing presumptive evidence of ovulation is an endometrial biopsy in the late luteal phase within 2 or 3 days of the next menses. Histologic evidence of ovulation and its associated progesterone effect on the endometrium can be observed by the presence of secretory changes in the endometrial glands. When the changes in the endometrium and the day in the menstrual cycle differ by more than 2 days, a so-called luteal phase defect may exist. This implies there may be an inadequate amount of progesterone secreted by the corpus luteum. However, to document this, at least two cycles must be biopsied, each showing greater than 2 days difference between the histology and date of the cycle (see evaluation and etiology section, III-D-2).

(4) **Urinary (LH) kits.** Recently, commercially available home urinary LH kits have been used to detect the LH surge prior to ovulation. These have been shown to predict ovulation approximately 80% of the time and are useful to time intercourse.

(5) **Ultrasonography.** The most accurate predictor of presumed ovulation is serial monitoring of follicle size by ultrasonography. Although this is the most reliable way of establishing ovulation, it is not as useful in predicting when ovulation will occur as are the urinary LH detection kits. Also, ultrasound monitoring is more inconvenient and expensive to the patient.

2. **Abnormalities of anovulation/oligo-ovulation.** Ovulatory dysfunctions are a common cause of female infertility. They present clinically as irregular or absent menses. The only absolute confirmation of ovulation is pregnancy. Although most women with predictable, cyclic menses ovulate, objective evidence is still required.

When anovulation or oligo-ovulation is suspected, further work-up is indicated (Figure 25.1). Initial evaluation includes a progestin challenge to induce withdrawal bleeding. This is done by giving medroxyprogesterone acetate (Provera) 10 mg daily for 5 days. If there is menstrual bleeding, all that is needed are thyroid function tests (thyroid stimulating hormone, thyroxine) and a serum prolactin. Hypothyroid-

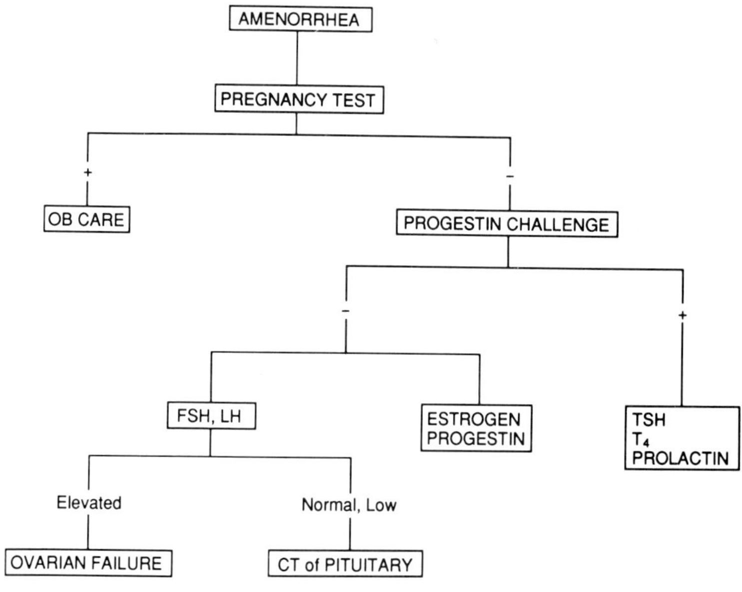


FIGURE 25.1. Evaluation of anovulation. OB = obstetric; TSH = thyroid stimulating hormone; $T_4$ = thyroxine; FSH = follicle-stimulating hormone; LH = luteinizing hormone; CT = computed tomography.

ism and hyperprolactinemia may cause anovulation. When hirsutism (sign of androgen excess) is present, measurement of serum testosterone and dehydroepiandrosterone sulfate (DHEAS) is indicated. Anovulation in the presence of androgen excess is most consistent with polycystic ovarian disease (PCOD). If the progestin challenge test is negative (no withdrawal bleeding), then serum follicle-stimulating hormone (FSH) should be drawn. FSH levels ≥ 40 mIU/mL are indicative of ovarian failure. Levels in the normal or low range may indicate hypothalamic-pituitary pathology. Therefore, radiographic examination of the sella turcica is indicated. Also, to rule out an end-organ (uterine) cause for the negative progestin challenge, conjugated estrogens (Premarin) 2.5 mg daily for 21 days followed by medroxyprogesterone acetate 10 mg daily for 5 days may be given. Withdrawal bleeding following this regimen assures an intact uterus.

Note that anovulation may also be caused by extreme weight loss or gain, anorexia nervosa, or intense physical conditioning. Except for extreme weight gain, these conditions cause anovulation by depressing gonadotropin secretion (Fig. 25.2).

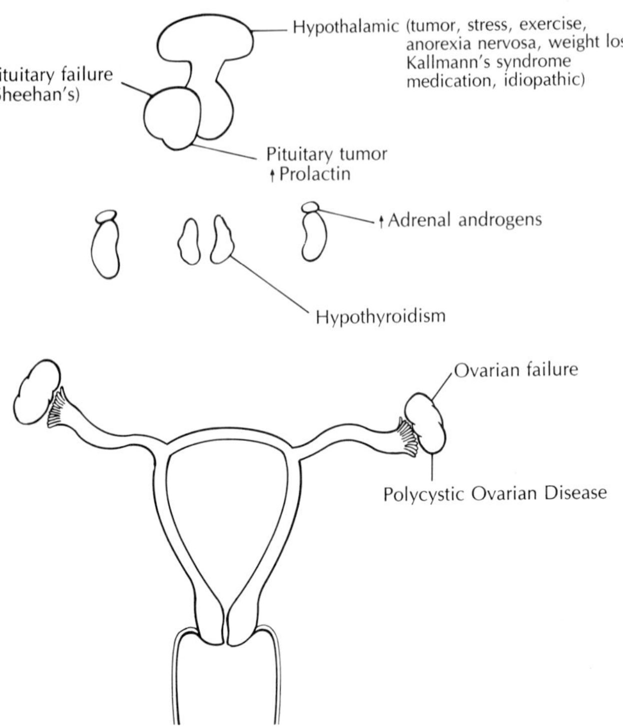


FIGURE 25.2. Causes of anovulation.

Rarely, serial ultrasound fails to demonstrate follicular collapse consistent with ovulation in spite of luteal phase serum progesterone levels consistent with ovulation. This has been termed luteinized unruptured follicle syndrome. The significance of this observation is controversial.

**B. Sperm availability ("male factor")** (Fig. 25.3). Overall approximately 40% of infertility may be attributed to male factor. This diagnosis can usually be made from the history and physical examination and the semen analysis. Occasionally additional tests such as a sperm penetration assay (SPA), antisperm antibody test (immuno-bead test), or hormonal assays may be helpful. Documentation of normal function should include:

1. **History.** No infertility evaluation is complete without an evaluation of the male partner's reproductive function. Historical evidence of fatherhood, testicular injury, or mumps orchitis are all important. Information concerning family history of male infertility may also be helpful. The following drugs may adversely affect sperm count.
   a. Heavy marijuana use
   b. Chemotherapeutic agents

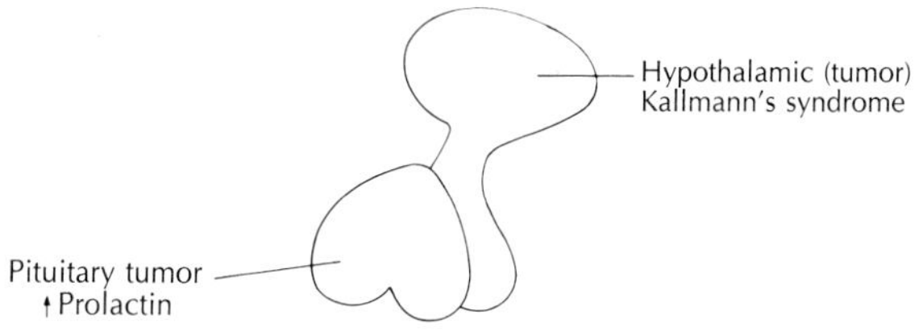


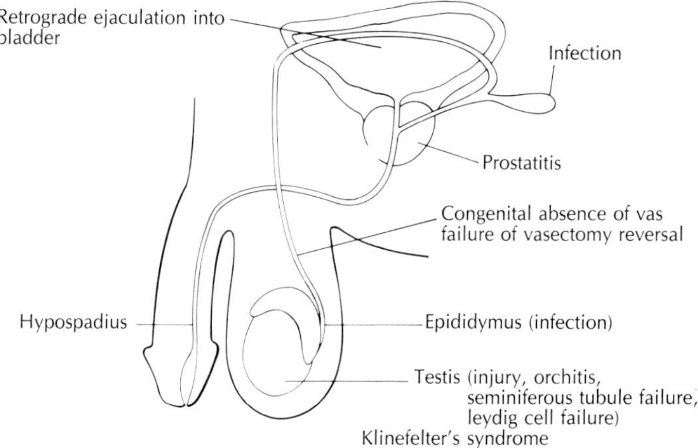


FIGURE 25.3. Causes of male infertility.

   c. Cimetidine
   d. Spironolactone
   e. Nitrofurantoin (Furodantin)

2. **Physical examination** of the male reproductive organs may provide evidence of testicular atrophy, hypospadius, or the presence of a varicocele.
3. **Laboratory evaluation.** No matter what the history and physical examination reveals, a semen analysis is always essential. Other tests may be helpful and are included in this section.
   a. **Semen analysis.** Specimens may be collected in a clean glass container at home or at the office or clinic by masturbation. If collected at home, the specimen must be kept warm and rapidly transported (within 1 hour) to the lab to insure accurate results. An abstinence period of 2 to 3 days prior to collection is optimal. Most of the spermatozoa are in the first portion of the ejaculate, patients should be cautioned not to spill any of the specimen and should not produce the specimen by withdrawal. Normal values are shown in Table 25.2. Although sub-

**Table 25.2. Normal Semen Values**

| | |
|---|---|
| Volume | 2 to 6 mL |
| Count | >20 million per mL |
| Motility | >50% |
| Swimming speed | >30 μm per second |
| Morphology | >50% normal forms |
| Viscosity | Liquefaction within 60 min |

normal values do not imply absolute sterility, they may indicate a significant decrease in the chances of conception in any given month. Repeat semen analysis should be performed for any abnormal values. Oligospermia implies less than 20 million sperm per mL of semen. Azoospermia means no sperm are present in the sample.

b. **Sperm penetration assay** (Fig. 25.4). Further evaluation of the functional capacity of sperm may be done by performing an SPA. This test may be performed when the semen analysis is abnormal, or when the infertility work-up reveals no obvious cause. The SPA involves sperm capacitated in vitro and hamster ova from which the zona pellucida have been removed. The percent hamster ova penetrated by the patient's sperm is compared to the percent penetrated by fertile donor sperm. In most laboratories, greater than 10% penetration would be considered normal.

c. **Other tests** (Table 25.3). Occasionally, enzyme and hormonal evaluations are helpful. Absence of fructose in the semen implies congenital absence of the vas deferens and is associated with azoospermia. Testosterone, gonadotropin, or prolactin levels may be abnormal in certain instances.

d. **Testicular biopsy.** On rare occasions, testicular biopsy may be indicated to differentiate primary damage to the testes from outflow obstruction.

C. **Transport of sperm and egg.** For fertilization to occur, sperm deposited in the vagina must meet the egg that has been released by the ovary. Sperm must, therefore, migrate through the cervix, uterus, and into the ampulla of the fallopian tube. The egg must be picked up by the fimbria and transported to the ampulla of the tube. It has been estimated that a defect in this transport system may account for 30% to 40% of female infertility.

1. **Document normal ability to transport sperm and egg**

a. **History.** A careful history should be taken concerning infections of the cervix, uterus, or fallopian tubes, and symptoms of endometriosis including painful intercourse and menses. Questions concerning uterine or renal anomalies should be asked as well as obtaining a personal or family history of endometriosis.

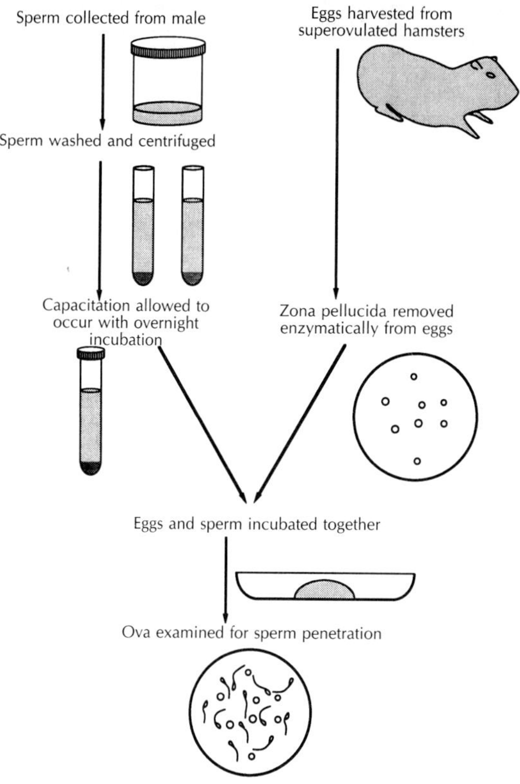


FIGURE 25.4. Sperm penetration assay.

**Table 25.3. Evaluation of the male**

I. History and physical

II. Laboratory evaluation

- A. Semen
  1. Semen analysis
  2. Sperm penetration assay
  3. Antisperm antibody assay
- B. Blood
  1. Luteinizing hormone, follicle-stimulating hormone, prolactin, testosterone
  2. Hypothalamic-pituitary test
  3. Karyotype
- C. Radiology
  1. Ultrasound
  2. Vasography
  3. Pituitary computed tomography or magnetic resonance imaging

b. **Laboratory evaluation**

(1) **Postcoital test (PCT).** This test evaluates sperm-cervical mucus interaction. It is performed by aspirating mucus with a tuberculin syringe from the cervical os 2 to 8 hours after the couple has had intercourse. This mucus is then examined grossly and under the microscope. Spinnbarkeit (stretchability) of the cervical mucus can be tested by placing the mucus on a slide, covering it with a cover slip and then lifting the cover slip. It should stretch 8 to 10 cm at midcycle. Microscopically, motile sperm indicate appropriate timing of the cycle when cervical mucus is thin and watery (under estrogen influence), and confirms proper coital technique. However, even when no sperm are seen, pregnancies have been reported, and sperm have been recovered from peritoneal fluid. If the sperm are shaking back and forth or are clumped together, antisperm antibodies are suspected. These antibodies may have come from the cervical mucus or the male reproductive tract. The role of antibodies in human reproduction is still largely unknown. Most cases in which no sperm are visualized on the PCT are due to inappropriate timing of the test and inadequate estrogen influence on the cervical mucus.

(2) **Hysterosalpingography (HSG)** is a radiographic procedure that involves injecting either a water- or an oil-based contrast media into the uterus and fallopian tubes transcervically under fluoroscopic visualization. This enables visualization of the intrauterine contour as well as patency of the fallopian tubes. Drawbacks of this test include the false-positive blockage of the isthmic-cornual junction and the inability to determine the presence of peritubal and periovarian adhesions that may impair ovum pick-up. However, distal tubal occlusions and intrauterine lesions such as adhesions, polyps, submucosal myomas, and septums can be reliably diagnosed. This test should be performed in the follicular phase of the cycle (after menses but before ovulation).

(3) **Laparoscopy.** Although an invasive procedure usually performed under general anesthesia, laparoscopy has developed into a valuable diagnostic and therapeutic tool. Pelvic adhesions, endometriosis, and tubal occlusion can be diagnosed and treated through the laparoscope using multiple punctures and adjunctive instruments. Laparoscopy should be performed when HSG reveals tubal abnormali-

ties or when the work-up so far has been unrevealing as to the etiology of the infertility. As with all tests of tubal function, laparoscopy should be performed in the follicular phase of the cycle.

2. **Investigate abnormalities of egg and sperm transport** (Fig. 25.5)
   a. **Cervical factors.** The cervical mucus must be thin and watery at the time of ovulation to be receptive to sperm. It is the estrogen effect on mucus that makes this possible. Sperm, which can live in cervical crypts for several hours and still be functional, must have an environment free of infections, antibodies, or white blood cells.
   b. **Uterine factors.** Lesions in the uterus may be detrimental for either gamete migration or embryo implantation. These include endometritis, Müllerian anomalies, synechiae, and submucosal myomas. Although the role of these uterine lesions in infertility is undetermined, they may be diagnosed by HSG or hysteroscopy.
   c. **Tubal or pelvic factors** may contribute to as much as 30% of female infertility. Peritubal or periovarian adhe-

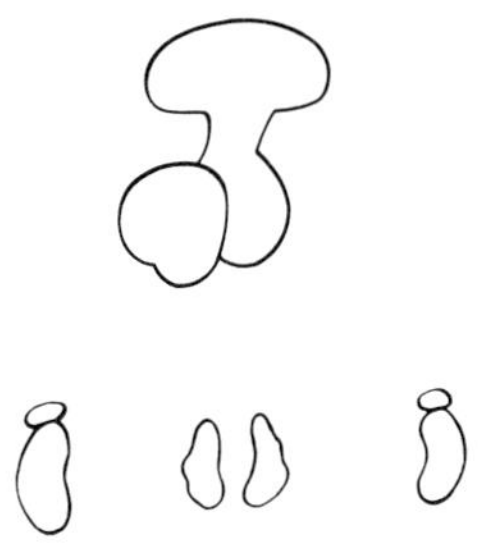

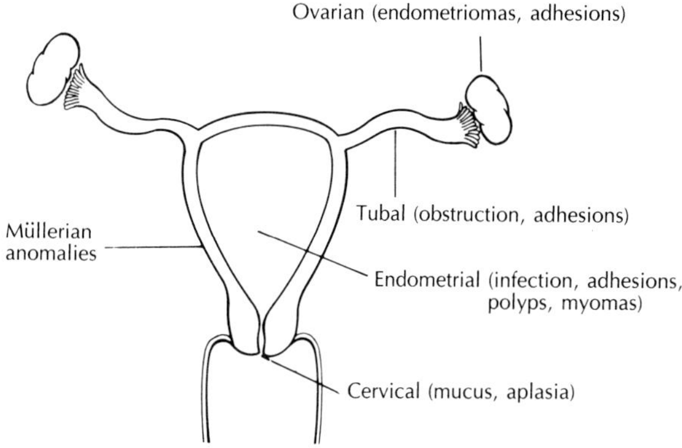


FIGURE 25.5. Locations of gamete transport defects.

sions cause infertility by preventing egg pick-up and transport. Tubal occlusions prevent pregnancy by blocking sperm and egg from meeting and allowing fertilization to occur.

Pelvic adhesions and tubal obstruction may be sequelae to pelvic inflammatory disease (PID). A history of PID may be elicited in 50% of cases of pelvic adhesions. After a single episode of pelvic infection, up to 23% of women are infertile due to tubal disease. With each episode of infection, the incidence of infertility increases.

HSG may reveal tubal blockage either at the isthmic-cornual junction or distally creating a hydrosalpinx. Cornual occlusions may be caused by fibrosis, salpingitis isthmica nodosum, or endometriosis.

Laparoscopy is the most reliable means of evaluating the pelvis for adhesions, tubal blockage, and endometriosis. Tubal blockage is assessed by injecting dilute indigo carmine or methylene blue through a cannula placed in the cervix and then visually observing spillage of dye from the fimbrial end of the tube.

d. **Ovarian factors.** Adhesions involving the surface of the ovary interfere with fertility by preventing egg pick-up by the fimbrial end of the fallopian tube. These can only be diagnosed by direct vision through a laparoscope. Also, endometriomas (endometriotic cysts) may be seen in association with endometriosis and infertility.

e. **Peritoneal factors.** Endometriosis is the most common peritoneal factor along with inflammatory adhesions. Endometriosis can only be diagnosed by direct visual observation or biopsy at laparoscopy or laparotomy. Although endometriosis is common among fertile patients, there is an association between endometriosis and infertility. All endometriosis found at laparoscopy should be staged according to the revised American Fertility Society Classification System.

Symptomatic endometriosis usually presents as either pelvic pain and/or infertility. While it is easily understood how mechanical obstruction caused by endometriosis can cause infertility, it is not understood how mild or moderate endometriosis can cause infertility. However, various investigators have observed increased pelvic macrophages and sperm phagocytosis, which leads one to suspect that the immune system may play a role.

**D. Establishing other causes when infertility is unexplained.** The evaluations will provide a diagnosis approximately 70% of the time (Fig. 25.6). However, given a negative evaluation up to this point, the following investigations and etiologies may be suggested.

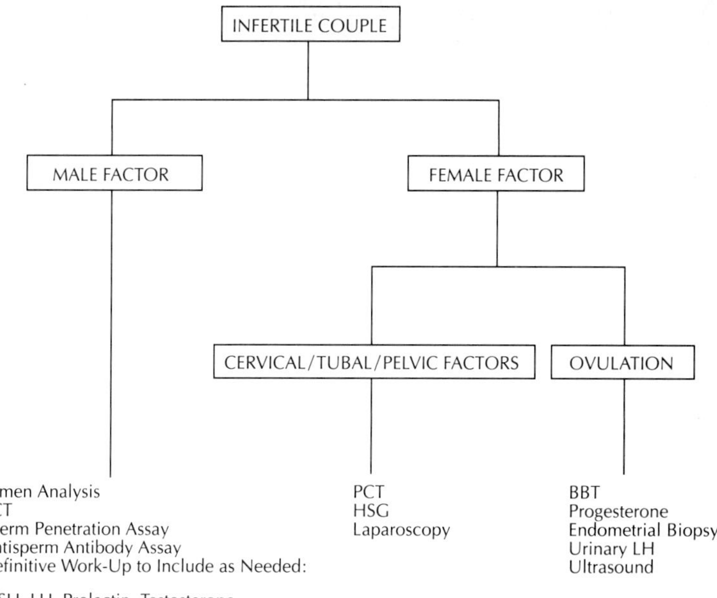


FIGURE 25.6. Evaluation of the infertile couple. PCT = postcoital test; FSH = follicle-stimulating hormone; LH = luteinizing hormone; CT = computed tomography; MRI = magnetic resonance imaging; HSG = hysterosalpingography; BBT = basal body temperature.

1. **Infections.** While cervicitis may be cause for cervical factor infertility and abnormal PCT, the role of *Mycoplasma* in causing infertility is unknown. Other organisms, such as *Chlamydia,* may be responsible for causing upper tract infections with sequelae such as pelvic adhesions and tubal blockage. Treatment with appropriate antibiotic therapy is indicated only when cultures are positive.
2. **Luteal phase defect.** As described earlier, the endometrial biopsy may be used as evidence for presumptive ovulation. When the biopsy results are greater than 2 days different than the day of the cycle, the diagnosis of luteal phase defect may be entertained. To document this, two cycles must be sampled that show greater than 2 days difference in histology and day of the cycle. Because normal fertile women have been shown to have "out of phase" endometriums, the significance of luteal phase defects in causing infertility is in question.

3. **Antibodies.** Along with endometriosis, immunologic causes of infertility have been suggested. Antisperm antibodies have been implicated in inhibiting sperm migration in the female reproductive tract and interfering with sperm–egg interaction in the process of fertilization. The sharing of human leukocyte antigens (HLA) by the couple may be a contributing factor to the couple's infertility.
4. **Intrauterine abnormalities** such as adhesions, Müllerian defects, and myomas have been blamed for infertility, but again, no controlled studies have proven this. Even with all present day capabilities, 10% to 20% of infertility is still unexplained.

## IV. Management

### A. Ovulation defects (Table 25.4)

1. **Clomiphene citrate.** In patients with oligo-ovulation, ovulation occurs less frequently than is optimum for conception. If initial studies are normal and the patient shows no signs of androgen excess, one may proceed directly to clomiphene citrate.
   a. **Mechanism of action.** Clomiphene is both an antiestrogen and a weak estrogen. It acts by competing with estradiol for estrogen-binding sites in the hypothalamus. Therefore, it blocks the negative feedback of estradiol in the hypothalamus, permitting increased release of gonadotropin releasing hormone (GnRH) which stimulates the pituitary to increase FSH and LH production and release. Clomiphene also acts directly on the pituitary and the ovary. It does not cause ovulation to occur but sets in motion the processes that eventually lead to ovulation.
   b. **Administration.** Clomiphene may be used to induce ovulation similarly in anovulatory patients. Following a negative pregnancy test, 5 days of medroxyprogesterone acetate 10 mg/d are given to induce withdrawal bleeding. With the first day of bleeding called day 1, clomiphene may be started at the dose of 50 mg/d on day 3 or day 5 and continued for 5 days. If started on day 5, ovulation usually occurs 11 to 13 days after the

**Table 25.4. Drugs Used to Induce Ovulation**

| DRUG | INDICATION |
|---|---|
| Clomiphene citrate | Anovulation/oligo-ovulation |
| Dexamethasone | Suppress adrenal androgens |
| Bromocriptine | Hyperprolactinemia |
| Human menopausal gonadotropins | Pituitary failure<br>Clomiphene failure |
| Gonadotropin-releasing hormone | Hypothalamic hypogonadism |

first dose on day 16 or 17. Menses should occur 2 weeks later if ovulation occurred. If no menses, either the patient did not ovulate or is pregnant. Therefore, a pregnancy test is performed. If she is not pregnant, then 5 days of medroxyprogesterone acetate is given to induce bleeding and another cycle of clomiphene is given but at 100 mg/d for 5 days. Until ovulation occurs, the dose may be increased to 200 mg/d. However, the likelihood of doses higher than 150 mg/d inducing ovulation are low. Presumptive evidence of ovulation may be shown by measuring a midluteal phase serum progesterone or a late luteal phase endometrial biopsy. The latter may be helpful in assuring that the development of the endometrium in the luteal phase is in phase with the date in the menstrual cycle. In phase endometrium would then suggest that the ovulatory dysfunction had been corrected and that folliculogenesis was proceeding normally.

c. **Additional measures.** Most pregnancies conceived on clomiphene do so during the first 3 or 4 months of treatment. However, even though 80% of ovulatory women will ovulate on clomiphene, only about 40% conceive and deliver. Therefore, after 3 or 4 months of ovulatory cycles, an appropriately timed PCT may be indicated. If this reveals thick hostile mucus with no sperm, this may be due to the antiestrogen effect of clomiphene. Instead of adding midcycle conjugated estrogens, consideration may be given to human menopausal gonadotropins (hMG).

   There is no increased risk of congenital anomalies during clomiphene treatment. However, as with other drugs, one should not give this drug if the patient is pregnant. Patients should also be counseled concerning the 5% to 8% increase in multiple gestation pregnancies. Also patients may develop ovarian cysts on therapy. Hypoestrogenic women, those who do not have withdrawal bleeding after progestational agents, rarely respond to clomiphene therapy.

2. **Dexamethasone.** In patients with PCOD and elevated adrenal androgens who do not ovulate on maximum doses of clomiphene, the addition of 0.5 mg dexamethasone at bedtime may be helpful. This will lower serum DHEAS, and an occasional patient will ovulate.
3. **Bromocriptine (Parlodel).** In anovulatory patients with elevated serum prolactin levels and a normal thyroid stimulating hormone, radiographic examination of the sella turcica is warranted. If no tumor is visualized or if the size is $< 1$ cm (microadenoma), treatment with bromocriptine is indicated. If the pituitary tumor is $> 1$ cm (macroadenoma), then referral to a neurosurgeon may be wise.

Patients with elevated prolactin often have associated galactorrhea. Drugs may be the most common cause of elevated prolactin, especially those that block or deplete CNS dopamine such as phenothiazines. Hypothyroidism, chest trauma, nipple stimulation, herpes zoster, acromegaly, and Cushing's disease have also been implicated.

Bromocriptine lowers prolactin by direct effect on the pituitary and has a dopamine agonist effect on the hypothalmus. The recommended dose is 2.5 to 7.5 mg/d, but higher doses may be needed. The most common side effect is nausea, and bedtime doses may be helpful. The effects of the drug are temporary, and often prolactin levels increase after bromocriptine is discontinued. Long-term studies on the natural history of prolactin producing pituitary tumors reveal that some regress on their own. Serum prolactin levels and radiographic monitoring of these tumors are, therefore, indicated.

4. **Human menopausal gonadotropins (Pergonal).** Women with hypogonadotropic hypogonadism and those not responding to clomiphene are candidates for hMG. Human menopausal gonadotropin is a purified preparation extracted from the urine of postmenopausal women. Each ampule contains 75 IU of FSH and 75 IU of LH. It is not expected to be successful in inducing ovulation in patients with ovarian failure. The use of hMG for ovulation induction should only be performed by one experienced in its use, preferably a reproductive endocrinologist, and requires careful monitoring of the serum estradiol levels and ultrasound monitoring of ovarian follicles. When one to three follicles reach 16 mm in mean diameter, ovulation is triggered by 5000 to 10 000 IU of human chorionic gonadotropin (hCG). Ovulation is expected 32 to 36 hours later.

   Benefits of this therapy include high ovulation rates and high pregnancy rates in patients with anovulation. Risks include hyperstimulation of the ovaries, multiple gestation pregnancies (20% to 25%), high cost of therapy, and inconvenience.
5. **Urofollitropin.** Recently, a new gonadotropin preparation has been marketed. This is urofollitropin (Metrodin). This product is prepared by removing LH from hMG. It is more costly and its exact role and efficacy are unclear until more studies are completed.
6. **GnRH.** In patients with hypothalamic causes of anovulation, GnRH will induce ovulation. GnRH may be given IV or SQ by a pump with doses given every 60 to 90 minutes. It is not helpful in patients with pituitary failure. Advantages include safety, low risk of hyperstimulation, and decreased multiple gestation pregnancies. A major disadvantage is inconvenience.

7. **Ovum donation.** Recently ovum donation has been used to treat patients with egg unavailability such as ovarian failure or surgical absence of the ovaries. Eggs are removed from fertile women, fertilized in vitro, and then transferred into the uterus of the infertile woman. Another technique, uterine lavage, involves placing a special catheter in the uterus and retrieving a blastocyst that has not yet implanted. This blastocyst can then be placed into the hormonally synchronized uterus of the infertile woman.

B. **Lack of sperm availability.** When subnormal semen parameters are present, any obvious etiology must be identified. Environmental problems or chronic illnesses should be removed and treated whenever possible. Drugs that may be harmful to spermatogenesis should be discontinued. Lubricants and douches should be avoided. Male reproductive tract infections, evidenced by white blood cells in the semen, should be aggressively treated.

1. **Medical therapy.** In oligospermia or asthenospermia, treatment with thyroid replacement, testosterone, hCG, corticosteroids, and clomiphene have not been shown in controlled studies to be of major benefit.
2. **Intrauterine insemination.** With severe male factor, < 20 million sperm per mL, intrauterine insemination of sperm has not been helpful in improving pregnancy rates. However, insemination with frozen donor sperm of proven quality, has produced monthly fecundity of 8% to 12%. Due to the prevalence of STDs, including acquired immunodeficiency syndrome, only quarantined frozen sperm should be used for donor insemination.
3. **Vasectomy reversal.** Approximately 50% of men who have had vasectomy reversals subsequently father children. A major complication for these infertile patients is antisperm antibodies that are often produced when the so-called blood-testis barrier is violated. These antibodies produce severe clumping of spermatozoa that may inhibit sperm migration as well as fertilization.
4. **In vitro fertilization.** Recently the treatment of choice for severe male factor infertility has become in vitro fertilization (IVF). This procedure involves transvaginal oocyte retrieval under IV sedation, insemination of oocytes with sperm in vitro in the laboratory, documentation of fertilization, and transfer of multiple embryos at the two to four cell stage 48 hours after egg retrieval. IVF was first introduced in England in 1978 with the birth of the first infant and now has been instituted in many fertility centers worldwide.

   It is felt that it requires fewer spermatozoa to fertilize oocytes in the laboratory than naturally through the female reproductive tract. Not only is this procedure a therapeutic option, but is also provides diagnostic information concerning absence or presence of fertilization. The patient and her partner also have the option of allowing the use of donor sperm at the same time. If the husband's sperm does not fertilize the wife's eggs but donor's sperm does, this provides strong evidence that the infertility is secondary to the husband's sperm. Therefore, at this point, donor insemination or adoption would be the logical choice of treatment. Current research concerning the dilemma of male factor infertility has involved the use of micromanipulative techniques. Using animal models, the technique of zona drilling using acid Tyrode's solution has increased fertilization with fewer spermatozoa. Similar experiments have been performed injecting sperm into the ooplasm and the perivitelline space. More recently in humans, investigators have used micro needles to slit the zona pellucida, and have shown increased fertilization rates compared to controls.

C. **Defect in gamete transport**

1. **Cervical factors** are thought to represent about 5% to 10% of all female infertility. Anatomical congenital anomalies, such as cervical aplasia, are quite rare and not readily treated. The most common difficulty lies with the cervical mucus. If the lack of mucus is due to a previous surgery or trauma to the cervix, little in the way of treatment is helpful to improve the quality of the mucus. However, most poor quality mucus, as judged by postcoital tests, is due to poor timing. That is, the PCT was not done just prior to ovulation when estrogen levels are highest and estrogen effect on mucus is greatest. This may be corrected by more accurate timing using urinary LH detection kits. Other causes, such as cervicitis and infection may be corrected by antibiotic treatment. Poor PCT results may also be due to male factor reasons. Their treatments have been discussed in the above section.

   Cervical mucus–sperm interaction difficulties thought to be secondary to immunologic causes may benefit from intrauterine insemination (IUI). In fact, IUI may be the treatment of choice for cervical factor infertility and has been shown to be efficacious in treating infertility with this diagnosis.

2. **Tubal/pelvic factors.** Pelvic adhesions and tubal occlusions are a major cause of infertility. With the changing sexual mores and the increasing incidence of STDs, these factors will most likely increase in prevalence.

   a. **Surgical (laparotomy and laparoscopy)**

      (1) **Adhesive disease.** Treatment depends on extent of pathology and its location. The best prognosis can be made when only peritubal or periovarian adhesions are present, and both tubes are patent. Many of these patients can be treated through the laparoscope with salpingolysis accomplished by additional puncture sites and the use of scissors or

laser. The worse prognosis is distally blocked tubes and hydrosalpinx formation. Surgical repair, usually through a laparotomy, requires opening the end of the tube and suturing the tube open with fine sutures. Recently, treatment with laparoscopic laser salpingostomy has been used. Future studies will indicate which techniques are superior. Although most techniques can open tubes, the ultimate result depends on mucosal damage inside the tube.

(2) **Tubal ligation reversal.** The one procedure that has proven to benefit from magnification and microsurgical techniques is tubal reanastomosis following previous tubal ligation. This success rate depends on length of remaining tube and site of anastomosis. Isthmic-isthmic reanastomosis with 5 cm or more of remaining tube is associated with 70% to 80% pregnancy rates.

The length of remaining tube is dependent on the previous type of sterilization. Hulka clip or ring sterilization causes the least tubal damage, while electrocautery tends to destroy a greater proportion of tubal length.

Isthmic-ampullary or ampullary-ampullary reanastomosis has decreased pregnancy rates but is still acceptable. Surgery involving the cornua or reimplantation has much lower pregnancy rates. Many would not consider surgery in these patients and would proceed directly to IVF.

b. **Transcervical catheterization.** Recently, new transcervical catheters have been developed to treat proximal fallopian tube obstruction. Results are promising in selected patients and this in time may prove to be a valuable therapeutic option. However, this technique is not suitable for distal tubal obstruction.

c. **In vitro fertilization/embryo transfer (IVF/ET).** The ultimate treatment for irreversible tubal disease is IVF/ET. In experienced centers, clinical pregnancy rates of 20% to 25% per embryo transfer are realized (Fig. 25.7).

3. **Uterine factors.** Lesions that occur in the uterus include synechiae, septae, and submucus myomas. There currently is controversy concerning the role of these lesions in infertility and recurrent pregnancy loss. However, these lesions may be diagnosed and treated by hysteroscopy.

**D. Endometriosis.** Because of its importance, a complete chapter (26) is devoted to its diagnosis and management.

**E. Unexplained infertility.** Ten percent to 15% of infertile couples have no diagnosis as to the cause of their infertility even after an extensive evaluation. At this time, their choices include either expectant management or empiric therapy. Empiric therapy usu-

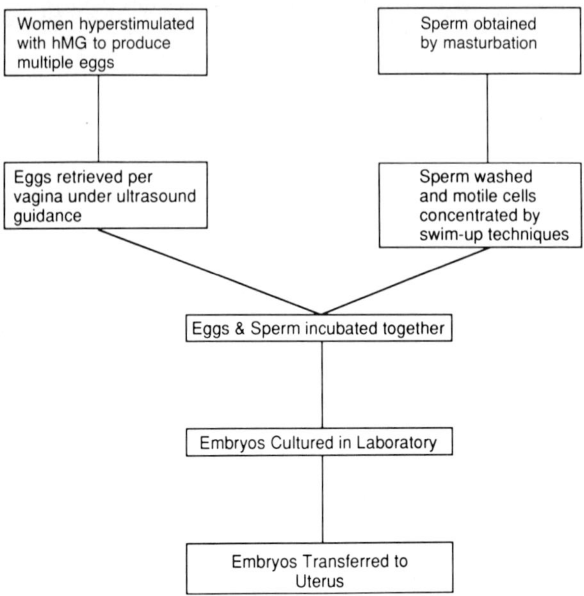


FIGURE 25.7. In-vitro fertilization and embryo transfer. hMG = human menopausal gonadotropin.

ally begins with controlled ovarian hyperstimulation with hMG and either timed intercourse or intrauterine insemination of washed sperm. Monthly fecundity with this treatment varies between 5% to 15%. If after three to six cycles and the patient still is not pregnant, more aggressive options include gamete intrafallopian transfer (GIFT) or IVF. However, these therapies are more invasive and expensive ($5000 to $7000 per treatment cycle). Expectant pregnancy rates per cycle varies between 20% to 30% for GIFT and 10% to 20% for IVF.

**V. Future trends.** It is increasingly clear in the face of ever-rising health-care costs, that future therapies for infertile patients must be both effective and cost efficient. They also must be consistent with the ethical values of the couple and society. Often, in our highly technological world, technology leads the way in front of society's answer to the questions this technology introduces. Nowhere is this more apparent than today's reproductive medicine.

With this in mind, tomorrow's therapies must be office or outpatient based with minimal anesthesia or analgesia. Improvements in ultrasound technology will enable reproductive specialists to perform many procedures transvaginally in the office setting. As the ability to culture embryos in the laboratory improves, pregnancy rates with alternate reproductive techniques will improve. Laparoscopic surgery will substitute for most laparotomies due to improved fiberoptics, cameras, microinstruments, suturing techniques, and laser. All in all, patients will receive better care with less invasive treatments that are most cost effective.

## BIBLIOGRAPHY

Adashi EY. Clomiphene citrate: Mechanism(s) and site(s) of action—A hypothesis revisited. Fertil Steril 1984; 42:331.

Asch RH. Laparoscopic recovery of sperm from peritoneal fluid in patients with negative or poor sim-Huhner test. Fert Steril 1976; 27:1111.

Contim E, Friberg J, Gleicher N. Transcervical balloon tuboplasty. Fertil Steril 1986; 46:963.

Coulam CB, Moore SB, O'Fallon W. Investigating unexplained infertility. Am J Obstet Gynecol 1988; 158:1374.

Daris OK, Berkeley AS, Naus GJ, Cholst IN, Freedman KS. The incidence of luteal phase defect in normal, fertile women, determined by serial endometrial biopsies. Fertil Steril 1989; 51:582.

Fraser IS. Successful pregnancy in a patient with congenital partial cervical atresia. Obstet Gynecol 1989; 74:443.

Gordon JW, Talansky BE. Assisted fertilization by zona drilling: A mouse model for correction of oligospermia. J Exp Zool 1986; 239:347.

Haas GG. How should sperm antibody tests be used clinically? Am J Reprod Immunol Microbiol 1987; 15:106.

Ho PC, Poon IML, Chan SYW, Wang C. Intrauterine insemination is not useful in oligoasthenospermia. Fertil Steril 1989; 51:682.

Hummel WP, Talbert LM. Current management of a donor insemination program. Fertil Steril 1989; 51:919.

Mann JR. Full-term development of mouse eggs fertilized by a spermatazoon microinjected under the zona pellucida. Biol Reprod 1988; 38:1077.

Muscato JJ, Haney AF, Weinberg JB. Sperm phagocytosis by human peritoneal macrophages: A possible cause of infertility in endometriosis. Am J Obstet Gynecol 1982; 144:503.

Revised American Fertility Society. Revised American Fertility Society Classification of Endometriosis. Fertil Steril 1985; 43:351.

Rogers BJ. The sperm penetration assay: Its usefulness re-evaluated. Fertil Steril 1985; 43:821.

Sauer MV, Macosa TM, Ishida EH, Giudice L, Marshall JR, Buster JE. Pregnancy following nonsurgical donor ovum transfer to a functionally agonadal woman. Fertil Steril 1987; 48:324.

Schlechte J, Dolan K, Sherman B, Chapler F, Luciano A. The natural history of untreated hyperprolactinemia: A prospective analysis. J Clin Endocrinol Metab 1989; 68:412.

Shoupe D, Mishell DR, LaCarra M, Lobo RA, Horenstein J, d'Ablaing G, Moyer D. Correlation of endometrial maturation with four methods of estimating day of ovulation. Obstet Gynecol 1989; 73:88.

Steptoe PC, Edwards RG. Birth after the reimplantation of a human embryo. Lancet 1978; 2:366.

Stone SC. Peritoneal recovery of sperm in patients with infertility associated with inadequate cervical mucus. Fertil Steril 1983; 40:802.

Thrumond AS, Rösch J, Patton PE, Burry KA, Novy M. Fluoroscopic transcervical fallopian tube catheterization for diagnosis and treatment of female infertility caused by tubal obstruction. Radiographics 1988; 8:621.

Walter HE, Cohen J. Partial zona dissection of the human oocyte: A nontraumatic method using micromanipulation to assist zona pellucida penetration. Fertil Steril 1989; 51:139.

# CHAPTER 26

# Endometriosis

**Steven J. Ory**

Endometriosis has fascinated clinicians since its original description by Rokitansky in 1860. Considerable debate regarding the etiology of the disease occurred in the early part of this century. Currently, great controversy regarding its role in infertility and preferred modes of treatment exists. Endometriosis is the occurrence of ectopic endometrial tissue outside of the uterine cavity. Endometriosis was previously referred to as endometriosis externa in distinction to adenomyosis or endometriosis interna. Although the latter represents the occurrence of endometriosis within the uterine myometrium, it appears to be a distinctly different entity.

I. **Incidence.** The true incidence of endometriosis is not known since laparoscopy or laparotomy is necessary for confirmation of diagnosis. In large surgical series, endometriosis has been incidentally encountered in 8% to 30% of pelvic laparotomies. One group of investigators reported it in 80% of cases. Most patients with endometriosis present in their twenties and thirties, but postpubertal teenagers and menopausal women may also be affected.

II. **Morbidity.** Endometriosis is not usually a lethal disease but may result in considerable morbidity. Malignant degeneration of endometriosis has been reported in 0.8% of cases. The true incidence of infertility is unknown, but infertility is attributed to endometriosis in 30% to 40% of affected patients. Pelvic pain is a more common morbidity and may vary from mild vague pelvic discomfort to an acute surgical abdomen subsequent to rupture of an endometrioma. Significant impairment of quality of life may arise from dysmenorrhea and dyspareunia. Less common associations include rectal pain or bleeding, bowel obstruction, urinary tract involvement with suprapubic discomfort, frequency, dysuria, hematuria, ureteral obstruction, and/or cyclic hemoptysis.

III. **Etiology.** There have been several theories proposed regarding the etiology of endometriosis. No single theory accounts for all cases of endometriosis.

A. **Sampson's theory,** published in 1927, suggests that endometriosis is a consequence of retrograde menstruation. This material contains viable endometrial tissue that may superficially implant on dependent tissue and proliferate. The ectopic endometrium may respond to cyclic ovarian hormone production. Recent studies demonstrating a higher frequency of menstrual reflux than previously anticipated suggest that reflux menstruation alone is not a critical determinant in the development of endometriosis. Impaired immunologic surveillance is presumed to contribute to the development of disease.

B. **Meyer's** proposed the theory of coelomic metaplasia as an explanation for the histogenesis of endometriosis. He postulated that the peritoneal mesothelium could undergo metaplastic transformation to endometriosis if exposed to a chronic irritant such as menstrual debris.

C. **Meigs** suggested that Müllerian metaplasia could be induced by hormonal influences such as prolonged estrogen exposure. The occurrence of endometriosis in women treated with diethylstilbestrol supports this theory.

D. **Halban** postulated that endometriosis could be spread by hematogenous or lymphatic dissemination. The rare occurrence of endometriosis in lung and kidney supports this notion.

E. **Other factors**

1. **Genetic.** The incidence of endometriosis is documented to be higher within affected families suggesting a predisposition.
2. **Immunology.** There is preliminary data suggesting an immunologic role. Lymphocyte-mediated cytotoxicity to endometrial cells in vitro is reduced in endometriosis patients compared with controls, and serum concentrations of certain complement components are elevated in women with endometriosis.

IV. **Pathogenesis and pathophysiology of infertility and pelvic pain.** Both the incidence of infertility and degree of pelvic pain are generally correlated with the extent or stage of disease. However, there are many exceptions and it is not rare to encounter a fertile, pain-free patient with extensive endometriosis incidentally diagnosed during an unrelated surgical procedure. The appearance of blood in the peritoneal cavity from bleeding endometrial implants or from reflux menstruation may be associated with pelvic pain, and the subsequent inflammation may be associated with infertility.

A. **Mechanical distortion.** Extensive endometriosis may produce marked scarring and distortion of anatomy including tubal occlusion and periovarian adhesions. Scarring may also result in fixation of pelvic structures and pain from distending endometriomas and nerve entrapment.

B. **Endocrine factors**

1. **Anovulation.** Most women with endometriosis have normal ovulatory activity, but 17% have persistent anovulation.
2. **Luteal dysfunction.** Several investigators have reported an association of endometriosis with luteal phase deficiency and abnormal uterine bleeding. Less frequently, hyperprolactinemia and galactorrhea may be associated as well.
3. **Prostaglandins** are produced by ectopic endometrial tissue, have multiple actions, and are capable of inducing the ischemic changes producing dysmenorrhea. Elucidating the role of prostaglandins produced by ectopic endometrium in the pathogenesis of infertility has been complicated by their unique biochemical features including short half-life, variations throughout the menstrual cycle, and multiple biologic roles. Potential mechanisms by which they might produce infertility include interference with the mechanical process of ovulation, alterations of ovum pick-up, and tubal transport, impairing corpus luteum function, interfering with implantation, and stimulating uterine contractility.

C. **Immunologic studies**

1. Peritoneal macrophages are increased in women with endometriosis, and they have augmented phagocytic activity against both sperm and oocytes. A possible mechanism of infertility may involve the lethal injury of either the gamete or the early embryo by macrophages in the oviducts or peritoneal cavity.
2. Other immunologic studies have reported the presence of complement deposition in ectopic endometriosis glands, hemagglutination antibodies to endometrium in endometriosis patients, and the presence of the CA-125 antigen, an ovarian tumor marker, in patients with extensive endometriosis. The immunologic response in endometriosis patients is variable, and this may be a factor in fertility.

D. **Peritoneal fluid.** Other factors elaborated by endometriosis and presumed to be present in peritoneal fluid may contribute to infertility by impairing sperm motility and transport, fimbrial oocyte pick-up, and fertilization and embryo survival.

V. **Differential diagnosis.** Endometriosis may produce a variety of signs and symptoms and may mimic a variety of diseases.

A. **All other causes of infertility** should be included in the differential diagnosis of endometriosis. In 40% of patients, more than one factor may be elucidated (see also Chapter 25—Infertility).

1. Ovulatory dysfunction
2. Male factors
3. Cervical factors
4. Uterine factors

5. Tubal disease
6. Infectious causes

B. **Acute abdomen.** Endometriosis may present initially as an acute abdomen, and all other possible causes of acute abdomen should be considered. Other common causes of pelvic pain that may present in a manner similar to endometriosis are:
1. Pelvic inflammatory disease
2. Ectopic pregnancy
3. Appendicitis
4. Diverticulosis/diverticulitis

C. **Gastrointestinal or urinary tract disease.** Less frequently, patients may have predominantly gastrointestinal or urinary tract symptoms, and diagnosis may be more obscure. Also included in the differential list are:
1. Irritable bowel syndrome
2. Ulcerative colitis
3. Crohn's disease
4. Urinary tract infections
5. Pyelonephritis
6. Glomerulonephritis
7. Congenital abnormalities

D. **Malignancy.** On pelvic examination, endometriosis may be discernible as disseminated nodules with adnexal enlargement or dense scarring. Ovarian, endometrial, gastrointestinal, and other malignancies should be considered, and their potential existence necessitates confirmation of the diagnosis by direct visualization at laparoscopy or laparotomy.

VI. **Diagnosis.** There are no pathognomonic features of endometriosis.

A. **Signs and symptoms**
1. **Pelvic pain and dysmenorrhea** are the most common symptoms of endometriosis. The pain varies in location, occurrence in the menstrual cycle, and quality. It may be perceived as backache, pressure in the pelvic floor or perineum, or dull or sharp pain in the adnexa. Dyspareunia with deep penetration characteristically is more prominent during the premenstrual and menstrual phases of the cycle. Often the pain is localized in a circumscribed area. Dysmenorrhea is usually acquired rather than primary and may become progressively more severe over time. Typically, the pain begins prior to the onset of menses and gradually improves once the period ensues.
2. **Infertility** exists in 30% to 40% of women with known endometriosis. Because the true prevalence of endometriosis is unknown, the actual relative occurrence of infertility is unknown.
3. **Abnormal uterine bleeding** may occur in one-third of women with endometriosis. In a few cases, there may be

associated organic causes such as polyps or leiomyomas. In other cases, it is not known whether or not endometriosis produces abnormal bleeding directly, perhaps by impairing steroidogenesis.

4. **Other symptoms.** Less common symptoms may be encountered with involvement in unusual sites. Dyschezia, rectal bleeding, and intestinal obstruction have been noted with bowel involvement. Suprapubic pain, frequency, dysuria, and hematuria may occur with urinary tract implants. Flank pain and fever may result from ureteral involvement. Chest pain and cough accompanied by hemoptysis may exist with pulmonary lesions. Other patients have developed endometriosis in old surgical scars and experienced localized pain or bleeding.

B. **Physical examination.** The most characteristic physical examination feature of endometriosis is the presence of tender, nodular induration along the uterosacral ligaments, posterior uterus, and cul-de-sac. Uterine retroversion with decreased mobility is often present as well. These findings are most easily appreciated during the perimenstrual interval. Adnexal involvement may produce tender cystic ovaries or dense induration with fixation. Lesions in the lower reproductive tract may be grossly visible and appear as bluish cysts or red friable lesions. However, many patients with mild endometriosis, and a few with extensive disease, have no abnormal physical findings.

C. **Diagnostic procedures**

1. **Laboratory studies.** There are no laboratory tests that are conclusive in establishing the diagnosis of endometriosis. Some patients with endometriosis may have leukocytosis or an elevated erythrocyte sedimentation rate. CA-125 levels are often elevated in patients with endometriosis but are not diagnostic.

2. **Laparoscopy and laparotomy.** The definitive diagnosis is established by laparoscopy or laparotomy. Biopsy may be performed at either operation if there is uncertainty about the diagnosis, but it is not essential for diagnosis and may be inconclusive if the specimen is extensively distorted by scarring. Endometriosis usually appears as a red friable or raised blue punctate "powder burn" lesion, often associated with scarring and other lesions. Less commonly, it may be less obvious when present as unpigmented, clear, excrescences, or pink flame-like areas.

3. **Other tests**

   a. Patients with urinary symptoms, including hematuria or extensive disease, should have IV pyelograms and cystoscopy.

   b. Bowel involvement should be assessed with a barium enema and appropriate endoscopic studies with biopsy.

c. Ultrasound, computed tomography, and magnetic resonance imaging have not proven to be useful in the diagnosis of endometriosis.

## VII. Management

**A. Prophylaxis.** Because a comprehensive understanding of the etiology and pathophysiology of endometriosis is lacking, specific preventive measures with proven efficacy cannot be recommended. Individuals with affected first-degree relatives should be apprised of their increased risk of developing endometriosis. Patients with endometriosis are commonly advised to have children earlier and at shorter intervals in hopes of avoiding infertility and retarding the progression of disease. Patients at risk for developing endometriosis, and symptoms of endometriosis, are often prescribed oral contraceptives that are effective in reducing the amount of menstrual flow and, perhaps, refluxed tissue. However, their efficacy in preventing endometriosis is not documented.

**B. General management concepts.** It is critical to confirm the diagnosis and determine the stage of disease at laparoscopy or laparotomy before initiating therapy.

1. **Staging.** The Revised American Fertility Society Classification System is currently the favored staging scheme (Fig. 26.1). There have been several previous systems published and all have inherent limitations. A classification system allows comparison of results of different treatments among different clinicians. There are few prospective controlled studies using the same classification scheme that permit accurate comparison of one treatment modality to another. Important features of staging process include:
   a. Selection of optimal treatment plan.
   b. Opportunity to serially assess the effectiveness of therapy.
   c. Basis for offering prognosis to patients.
2. **Indications for treatment**
   a. **Age.** Patients over 35 may require more rapid evaluation and aggressive treatment, especially those who have been infertile and/or wish to become pregnant.
   b. **Pain.** Women experiencing significant pain attributed to endometriosis should receive treatment. In addition to treatment aimed at eradication or suppression of disease, analgesics and prostaglandin inhibitors may be helpful.
   c. **Patients with issues of fertility and conception.** Many women with minimal and mild endometriosis may spontaneously conceive without treatment. Several recent studies have shown 50% to 75% conception rates in patients managed expectantly for one year fol-

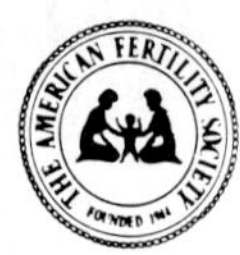


## THE AMERICAN FERTILITY SOCIETY
## REVISED CLASSIFICATION OF ENDOMETRIOSIS

Patient's Name ______________________ Date ______________________

Stage I (Minimal) - 1-5
Stage II (Mild) - 6-15
Stage III (Moderate) - 16-40
Stage IV (Severe) - >40
Total ______________

Laparoscopy ________ Laparotomy ________ Photography ________
Recommended Treatment ______________________
______________________
Prognosis ______________________

| | | | | |
|---|---|---|---|---|
| PERITONEUM | ENDOMETRIOSIS | <1cm | 1-3cm | >3cm |
| | Superficial | 1 | 2 | 4 |
| | Deep | 2 | 4 | 6 |
| OVARY | R Superficial | 1 | 2 | 4 |
| | Deep | 4 | 16 | 20 |
| | L Superficial | 1 | 2 | 4 |
| | Deep | 4 | 16 | 20 |

| | | | |
|---|---|---|---|
| | POSTERIOR CULDESAC OBLITERATION | Partial | Complete |
| | | 4 | 40 |

| | | | | |
|---|---|---|---|---|
| OVARY | ADHESIONS | <1/3 Enclosure | 1/3-2/3 Enclosure | >2/3 Enclosure |
| | R Filmy | 1 | 2 | 4 |
| | Dense | 4 | 8 | 16 |
| | L Filmy | 1 | 2 | 4 |
| | Dense | 4 | 8 | 16 |
| TUBE | R Filmy | 1 | 2 | 4 |
| | Dense | 4* | 8* | 16 |
| | L Filmy | 1 | 2 | 4 |
| | Dense | 4* | 8* | 16 |

*If the fimbriated end of the fallopian tube is completely enclosed, change the point assignment to 16.

Additional Endometriosis: ______________________

Associated Pathology: ______________________

To Be Used with Normal Tubes and Ovaries

L R

To Be Used with Abnormal Tubes and/or Ovaries

L R

FIGURE 26.1. The American Fertility Society revised classification of endometriosis.

lowing diagnosis. In general, conception rates following surgery are highest in the immediate 12 months following surgery. If surgery is elected, it should be performed at a time when patients are able to immediately initiate efforts at conception. Infertile patients should undergo complete infertility evaluations including assessment of ovulatory function, male factor, and tubal patency before beginning treatment. Significant findings may influence the choice and timing of treatment.

d. **Perimenopausal patients** with less severe pain approaching menopause may be followed without treatment. The vast majority of endometriosis patients will experience resolution of their disease during the climacteric.

e. **Second-look laparoscopy.** Although no studies conclusively document its value, many investigators recommend repeating laparoscopy after a course of medical therapy to assess response to therapy, this approach may ultimately expedite treatment and avoid additional progression of disease.

C. **Observant management.** After laparoscopic diagnosis, some patients feel better and seem to have regression of their disease. This clinical effect may reflect the benefit of laparoscopy, especially when combined with chromopertubation. Observant management should be considered for patients with minimal and mild disease for a pre-set length of time (6 to 12 months), with careful re-evaluation after that time. The nature of that evaluation will depend on the clinical course demonstrated by the patient.

D. **Endocrine therapy.** Although there is no comparative data citing improved outcome for patients treated with 17-alpha-ethinyl testosterone derivative (danazol) vs. other hormone therapy, it is currently the first-choice hormonal agent.

1. **Danazol**

a. **Major effects**

(1) Partial suppression of gonadotropin hormone-releasing hormone (GnRH) and possible direct suppression of pituitary release of luteinizing hormone (LH) and follicle-stimulating hormone (FSH).

(2) Direct suppression of ovarian steroidogenesis.

(3) Competitive interaction with progesterone and androgen receptors in endometriosis implants.

(4) Increased metabolic clearance rate of estradiol and progesterone.

(5) Suppression of endometriosis-associated autoantibodies.

b. **Advantages.** Nonsurgical

c. **Disadvantages**
   (1) Expense
   (2) Duration of therapy
   (3) High recurrence rate
   (4) Not effective for adhesions or large ovarian endometriomas

d. **Contraindications**
   (1) Pregnancy
   (2) Abnormal uterine bleeding
   (3) Breast-feeding
   (4) Abnormal hepatic, renal, or cardiac function

e. **Treatment regimen.** The standard recommended dose is danazol, 400 mg p.o. b.i.d. for 6 months, followed by clinical/surgical re-evaluation according to the patient's clinical response. Lower doses and shorter durations of treatment may also be effective, but data is inconclusive to date.

f. **Side effects**
   (1) Weight gain
   (2) Muscle cramps
   (3) Androgen effects (acne, hirsutism, decreased breast size, voice change)
   (4) Depression

**2. GnRH analogs.** Available GnRH analogs include leuprolide acetate, nafarelin acetate, and goserelin acetate. Preliminary data suggests comparable clinical efficacy to danazol.

a. **Major effect.** Marked suppression of LH and FSH release with consequent suppression of ovarian steroidogenesis to postoophorectomy levels, "medical oophorectomy."

b. **Advantages.** Potent medical therapy with more tolerable side effect profile.

c. **Disadvantages**
   (1) Expense
   (2) Sequelae of marked hypoestrogenism, including osteoporosis
   (3) Parenteral administration
   (4) Not effective for adhesions or ovarian endometriosis
   (5) High recurrence risk

d. **Contraindications.** Sensitization to GnRH analogs

e. **Treatment regimen**
   (1) **Leuprolide acetate.** 0.5 to 1.0 mg/d administered subcutaneously for 6 months or as a depot every 28 days.
   (2) **Nafarelin acetate.** One spray (200 mg) into one nostril in the morning and one spray into the other nostril in the evening (total 400 mg/d).

Recommended duration of therapy is 6 months.

(3) **Goserelin acetate.** 3.6 mg IM every 28 days for 6 months.

f. **Side effects**

(1) Hot flashes

(2) Vaginal atrophy

(3) Increased calcium excretion, with probable osteoporosis

(4) Depression

3. **Oral contraceptives ("pseudopregnancy" regimen)**

a. **Major effects**

(1) Induces a decidual reaction in implants with subsequent necrosis and resorption

(2) Spread of disease is limited by resultant anovulation and amenorrhea

b. **Advantages**

(1) Nonsurgical

(2) Less expensive than danazol and GnRH analogs

c. **Disadvantages**

(1) Less effective than danazol and GnRH analogs

(2) Side effects more common and more bothersome

(3) Duration of therapy

(4) High recurrence rate (approximately 17%)

d. **Contraindications**

(1) Large leiomyomata

(2) History significant for liver disease or abnormal liver function tests

(3) Previous estrogen-dependent neoplasia

(4) History of thrombophlebitis or pulmonary embolus

(5) Cardiovascular disease

e. **Treatment regimen.** Oral contraceptives (30–50 μg estrogen formulation) daily and continuously for 6 to 12 months, followed by clinical/surgical re-evaluation according to the patient's clinical response. Dose may be increased incrementally to three pills per day to control breakthrough bleeding.

f. **Side effects**

(1) Patients may initially experience increased pain before receiving clinical benefit

(2) Breakthrough bleeding

(3) Nausa

(4) Breast tenderness

(5) Fluid retention and weight gain

4. **Progestins** (medroxyprogesterone acetate)

a. **Major effect.** Induces decidualization and later atrophy and resorption of endometriosis

b. **Advantages**
   (1) Nonsurgical
   (2) Relatively inexpensive
   (3) May be used in individuals who cannot take danazol or oral contraceptives
c. **Disadvantages**
   (1) Limited clinical experience reported
   (2) Significant side effects
   (3) Long duration of action with parenteral formulation
d. **Contraindications**
   (1) History of thrombophlebitis or pulmonary embolism
   (2) Liver dysfunction
   (3) Breast malignancy
   (4) Undiagnosed vaginal bleeding or pregnancy
e. **Treatment regimen.** Medroxyprogesterone acetate (Provera) 10 mg p.o. t.i.d. for 3 months or depomedroxyprogesterone acetate 100 mg IM every 2 weeks, then 200 mg monthly after 8 weeks.
f. **Side effects**
   (1) Breakthrough bleeding
   (2) Depression

**5. Androgens** (methyltestosterone)
   a. **Major effect.** Unknown direct effect on endometriosis; most patients remain ovulatory on treatment
   b. **Advantages.** Nonsurgical and effective in relieving pain
   c. **Disadvantages**
      (1) Less effective in treating infertility
      (2) Side effects (see management section, VII-D-5-F)
      (3) Potential virilization of female fetus if taken during pregnancy
   d. **Contraindications**
      (1) Pregnancy (see management section, VII-D-5-C-3, above)
      (2) Hepatic dysfunction
   e. **Treatment regimen.** Methyltestosterone 5 to 10 mg sublingually daily
   f. **Side effects**
      (1) Hirsutism and acne
      (2) Virilization
      (3) Hepatocellular jaundice

**E. Surgery**

**1. Conservative surgery** means the removal or destruction of endometriosis by excision, laser vaporization, fulguration, or resection of severely affected tissues. Surgery also includes lysis of adhesions and restoration of anatomy with the intent of preserving fertility potential. Conservative surgery is often performed at laparoscopy using endoscopic instruments or laser and can be performed at laparotomy with microsurgical operative technique. Patients with minimal or mild disease may be treated with fulguration with cautery or laser at the time of diagnostic laparoscopy. All of these surgical techniques are acceptable treatment and no one technique has been shown to yield better clinical results.

a. **Advantages**
   (1) Unless postoperative hormonal therapy is used, or conception is contraindicated by ongoing medical therapy, patients are able to resume efforts at conception without a 6 to 9 month delay, which is incumbent with medical therapy.
   (2) Best option for patients with significant adhesions and significant endometrioma formation.

b. **Disadvantages**
   (1) Risks of major surgery
   (2) Recurrence rate of 14% to 41%

c. **Adjuvant to conservative surgical procedures.** Additional adjuvant surgical procedures that may be performed at the same time include presacral neurectomy, appendectomy, anterior uterine suspension, uterosacral plication, and various grafts to cover peritoneal surfaces. The advantage of each of the latter has not been clearly demonstrated.

2. **Definitive surgery.** Except in instances where there is extensive residual scarring or nerve entrapment, total abdominal hysterectomy and bilateral salpingo-oophorectomy are consistently effective in arresting progression of disease and relieving pelvic pain. Some patients will respond favorably if an ovary is not removed provided no endometriosis is left. Definitive surgery is best suited for older patients who do not wish to have additional children and for women with progressive pain refractory to hormonal regimens and conservative surgery. It is possible to perform embryo donation on patients following bilateral salpingo-oophorectomy if the uterus is retained.

3. **Medical adjuvant therapy**
   a. **Preoperative danazol or GnRH analog therapy** may improve outcome by reducing inflammation, lesion size, and tissue reaction at the time of surgery.
   b. Benefit of **postoperative danazol** is more controversial, but it appears to be helpful if concerns about residual endometriosis exist.
   c. **High molecular weight dextran** instilled into the pelvic cavity at the time of surgery and postoperative **steroids, antihistamines,** and **antiprostaglandins** have been used to retard adhesion formation.

**VIII. Prognosis.** Although endometriosis is rarely lethal, it does convey substantial morbidity. Relief from pelvic pain can usually be anticipated with all modalities. Subsequent fertility is much harder to gauge and depends on the stage of disease, duration, age of the patient, and presence of other fertility factors. The potential for recurrence of endometriosis and the need for additional therapy is high for all treatment modalities other than definitive surgery.

## BIBLIOGRAPHY


Bellina JH, Voros JL, Fick AC, Jackson JD. Surgical management endometriosis with the carbon dioxide laser. Microsurgery 1984; 5:197.

Buttram VC. Conservative surgery for endometriosis in the infertile female: A study of 206 patients with implications for both medical and surgical therapy. Fertil Steril 1979; 31:117.

Buttram VC, Reiter RC, Ward S. Treatment of endometriosis with danazol: Report of a six year prospective study. Fertil Steril 1985; 43:353.

Halban J. Metastatic hysteroadenosis. Wien Klin Wochenschr 37:1205, 1924.

Fox H, Backley CH. Current concepts of endometriosis. Clin Obstet Gynecol 1984; 11:279.

Kistner RW. Endometriosis and infertility. Clin Obstet Gynecol 1979; 22:101.

Kitchin JD. Endometriosis. In Sciarra JJ, ed. Gynecology and Obstetrics. Vol. 1, Philadelphia, Pa: Harper and Row Publishers; 1982:1.

Meils JV. Endometriosis: A possible etiological factor. Surg Gynecol Obstet 1938; 67:253.

Meyers R: Metaplasia theory with inflammation as a primary inducing factor: Adenomyosis, adenofibrosis and adenomyoma. In: Vonwalter H, ed. Viet-Stochel Hanbuch des Gynachologic. Munchen: Bergmann; 1930.

Nikkanen V, Punnonen R. External endometriosis in 801 operated patients. ACTA Obstet Gynecol (Scand) 1984; 63:699.

Pittaway DE, Woultz AC. Endometriosis and corpus luteum function. Is there a relationship? J Reprod Med 1984; 29:712.

Schmidt CL. Endometriosis: A reappraisal of pathogens and treatment. Fertil Steril 1985; 44:157.

Strathy JH, Molgaard CA, Coulam CB, Melton LJ. Endometriosis and infertility: A laparoscopic study of endometriosis among fertile and infertile women. Fertil Steril 1982; 38:667.

Wheeler JM, Malinak LR. Recurrent endometriosis: Incidence, management, and prognosis. Am J Obstet Gynecol 1983; 146:247.

# Part IV

# Gynecologic Oncology

# CHAPTER 27

# Vulvar Dysplasia and Carcinoma

**Daniel L. Clarke-Pearson**

Neoplasms of the vulva are relatively rare diseases. Often, success of treatment is diminished because of delay in diagnosis by both patients and physicians. Intraepithelial neoplasia of the vulva constitutes two discrete disease processes: carcinoma in situ of the squamous epithelium and Paget's disease. Invasive carcinoma of the vulva is predominantly squamous cell carcinoma, with melanoma, sarcoma, basal cell carcinoma, and adenocarcinoma comprising less than 10% of the remaining lesions. Radical vulvectomy and inguinal lymphadenectomy have been the cornerstone of treatment for vulvar cancer, although in recent years less radical surgical procedures have been suggested for patients with early invasive vulvar carcinoma.

## I. Incidence

**A. Intraepithelial neoplasia.** The incidence of intraepithelial neoplasms of the vulva is unknown; however, it appears that carcinoma in situ is increasing in frequency. It is also being diagnosed in increasingly younger women. Carcinoma in situ generally occurs in the third to fourth decade of life but may also be diagnosed in the postmenopausal years. Paget's disease, in contrast, is typically a disease of the postmenopausal patient and is a much rarer entity than carcinoma in situ.

**B. Invasive vulvar cancer** accounts for 3% to 4% of gynecologic malignancies. The treatment history of this disease is frequently characterized by delayed diagnosis secondary to hesitancy on the part of elderly women to present themselves to a physician for evaluation. Unfortunately, diagnosis has often been further delayed by the reluctance of the physician to obtain a biopsy for histologic confirmation of the disease process.

1. **Squamous cell carcinoma** accounts for 85% to 90% of all vulvar cancer. The median age at diagnosis is approximately 65 years, and many patients are in their eighth to ninth decade of life. In these older patients, concurrent medical conditions often complicate therapy. In recent

years younger women have been identified with invasive vulvar carcinoma; 15% of patients with vulvar cancer are under the age of 40 years. Melanoma arising primarily on the vulva accounts for 5% of vulvar malignancies and has the same characteristics as other cutaneous melanomas.

2. **Other malignancies** arising on the vulva include basal cell carcinoma (1.4%), adenocarcinoma (1.2%), and sarcomas (2%). Basal cell carcinoma and adenocarcinoma arise in the more elderly age group, whereas sarcomas most often occur in premenopausal women.

## II. Morbidity and mortality

### A. Intraepithelial neoplasia

1. **Mortality.** Intraepithelial neoplasia of the vulva carries an excellent prognosis with no expected mortality. The malignant potential of carcinoma in situ is uncertain although it has been associated with invasive carcinoma and therefore is treated as if it may progress to a frankly invasive carcinoma. Paget's disease alone has essentially no mortality, but when associated with underlying adenocarcinoma it has an associated mortality that is directly tied to the prognostic features of the adenocarcinoma.
2. **Morbidity** is primarily due to the local symptoms of pruritis, pain, or tenderness which these patients suffer if the disease is left untreated.
3. **Recurrence.** Both entities are associated with a variable incidence of recurrence after treatment, recorded as high as 30% in some series.

### B. Invasive vulvar carcinoma.

**Invasive vulvar carcinoma.** The modern treatment of invasive vulvar carcinoma is primarily surgical: radical vulvectomy and inguinal lymphadenectomy. The overall corrected survival for patients with vulvar carcinoma is approximately 75%.

1. **Survival** is closely linked to stage, size of primary lesion, inguinal lymph node metastasis, histologic grade of the tumor, and depth of invasion (see management section VII).
2. **Complications leading to operative mortality** occur in 1% to 2% of patients in modern series. Morbidity of the surgery for vulvar carcinoma includes significant changes in body image and sexual function. Inguinal and vulvar wound infection and disruption are reported in approximately 50% of cases. Some degree of leg lymphedema follows inguinal lymphadenectomy in approximately 50% of patients. Deep venous thrombosis and pulmonary embolism, inguinal lymphocyst, and secondary stress urinary incontinence are also frequent complications associated with radical vulvectomy.

## III. Etiology.

**Etiology.** The etiology of carcinoma in situ and invasive carcinoma of the vulva is poorly understood. An association with sexually transmitted diseases such as herpes, condylomata accuminata, and human papilloma virus (HPV) has been noted in many patients. There is an increasing body of evidence that the HPV is associated with vulvar and other genital carcinomas. The hypothesis of a viral etiology for this disease is further supported by the association of squamous intraepithelial neoplasia and invasive carcinoma in the vagina and cervix. Further, patients who are chronically immunosuppressed, such as those with a renal transplant or on chronic steroid therapy, have a much higher incidence of vulvar carcinoma in situ. The role of an intact immune system in combating a viral carcinogen is suggested by these findings. Paget's disease of the vulva has no known etiology.

## IV. Pathophysiology

A. **Carcinoma in situ.** The pathophysiology of carcinoma in situ is also poorly understood, although it is generally felt to be similar to that involved with the uterine cervix, that is, a course of variable progression from atypia (dysplasia) to carcinoma in situ and then further progression to invasive carcinoma of the vulva. The time course of the disease process and the actual incidence of progression from carcinoma in situ to invasive carcinoma is not known. Spontaneous regression of carcinoma in situ, especially multifocal carcinoma in situ or Bowenoid papulosis has also been reported. Carcinoma in situ is also associated with other vulvar dystrophies of both a hyperplastic and atrophic nature as well as being associated with other lower genital tract malignancies especially of the cervix and vagina. This relationship to other lower genital tract squamous cell carcinoma suggests a "field" effect of the carcinogen with varying sensitivity and transformation time in the different genital tract epithelium.

B. **Paget's disease.** The pathophysiology of Paget's disease is that of an indolent course with frequent recurrences following wide local excision. Paget's disease of the vulva occasionally is associated with an underlying adenocarcinoma, and the clinician must be diligent in examining the vulva and palpating subcutaneously for lesions suggestive of associated adenocarcinoma.

C. **Invasive carcinoma of the vulva** is usually localized and well-demarcated, with 70% arising on the labia. As compared to carcinoma in situ, invasive carcinoma is rarely multifocal except for the "kissing lesion" found on an abutting portion of the contralateral labia. Squamous cell carcinoma tends to be a slowly growing malignancy with local extension and late lymphatic metastases. Key to the successful treatment of squamous cell carcinoma is an understanding of the lymphatic drainage of the vulva. Lymphatic vessels drain the labia minora and majora anteriorly to the upper vulva and mons. Lymphatics then turn laterally, terminating in the inguinal and femoral lymph nodes (primarily the medial upper quadrant of the femoral nodes). The inguinal and femoral nodes actually arise in a superficial and deep set of nodes that are divided by the cribriform fascia. It is therefore the superficial nodes that are the first chain to be exposed to metastatic tumor emboli that then may metastasize to the deeper femoral nodes and then to the pelvic nodes. Cloquet's node, the last deep femoral node just beneath Poupart's ligament, has been traditionally considered the sentinel node prior to the beginning of the pelvic lymphatic chain. Direct drainage from the vulva, especially from the clitoral region, to the pelvic nodes has been demonstrated anatomically. However, this does not appear to be clinically significant. In most cases in which a clitoral primary lesion was found to be metastatic to pelvic nodes, involvement was also noted in inguinal lymph nodes. The collateral flow of lymphatics across the anterior vulva also allows for contralateral inguinal metastasis. In practicality, however, unilateral lesions nearly always metastasize to the ipsilateral lymphatic chain and it is highly unusual to have contralateral metastasis without concurrent ipsilateral metastasis. Tumor extension to the vagina, urethra, or anus also allows potential lymphatic drainage directly to the associated pelvic lymphatic chains.

D. **Other types of cancer of the vulva**

1. **Melanoma** of the vulva also appears to spread in a stepwise fashion to the inguinal-femoral lymphatics. Metastases of melanoma to these lymphatics carry a poor prognosis.
2. **Basal cell carcinoma** of the vulva tends to be locally progressive and rarely metastasizes to pelvic lymph nodes whereas adenocarcinoma and sarcomas spread by way of direct lymphatic extension.

## V. Differential diagnosis

A. **Nonulcerative vulvar lesions.** The differential diagnosis of nonulcerative vulvar lesions that might mimic carcinoma in situ or invasive carcinoma is listed in Table 27.1. The past confusion about descriptive terminology for vulvar lesions has been simplified, as is reflected in the table. Because any of the disease entities listed in Table 27.1 must be considered based on the gross appearance of a vulvar lesion, biopsy is required to establish a firm diagnosis. The pathologic evaluation of these lesions, as opposed to the clinical impression, is rarely confused.

B. **Exophytic, ulcerative, or mass lesions of the vulva.** Exophytic lesions of the vulva may be squamous cell carcinoma, verrucous carcinoma or benign condylomata. Ulcerative lesions may also be squamous cell carcinoma but may be benign conditions such as granuloma inguinale or lymphogranuloma venereum. Mass lesions of the vulva may be adenocarcinoma arising from Bartholin's gland, fibrosarcoma, lymphoma, or embryonal rhabdomyosarcoma, especially in children.

**Table 27.1. Nonulcerative Vulvar Lesions That May Mimic Carcinoma in Situ or Invasive Vulvar Cancer**

| | | |
|---|---|---|
| I. Red lesions | Reactive vulvitis<br>Candida<br>Squamous cell carcinoma<br>Tinea cruris | Psoriasis<br>Paget's disease<br>Carcinoma in situ<br>Vestibular adenitis |
| II. Hyperpigmented lesions | Carcinoma in situ<br>Hemangioma<br>Lentigo<br>Endometriosis | Nevi<br>Melanoma<br>Reactive hyperpigmentation<br>Seborrheic keratosis |
| III. White lesions | Lichen sclerosus<br>Mixed dystrophy<br>Vitiligo<br>Radiation reaction | Hypertrophic dystrophy<br>Carcinoma in situ<br>Condolymata accuminata |

C. **Metastatic lesions.** The vulva may also demonstrate metastatic malignancies, especially metastases from the cervix, rectum, endometrium, and choriocarcinoma.

## VI. Diagnosis

### A. Signs and symptoms

1. Patients with carcinoma in situ often complain of vulvar pruritus, a lump, or thickening of the vulvar skin. Approximately 50% of patients with carcinoma in situ are entirely asymptomatic and must be diagnosed on the basis of clinical observation by the gynecologist.
2. **Paget's disease** is usually associated with a more intense vulvar pruritus and extreme tenderness and pain.
3. **Squamous cell carcinoma** of the vulva generally presents with pruritus, pain, bleeding, discharge or the recognition of a mass or "lump." Patients may also complain of dysuria or dyspareunia.
4. **Melanomas** of the vulva may cause pruritus or pain or may only be recognized as a raised or dark lesion.
5. **Adenocarcinoma**, especially that arising in Bartholin's gland, may cause significant pain, a palpable mass, and dyspareunia.

### B. Physical examination

1. **Clinical evaluation.** Thorough clinical examination of the vulva should be done as part of a routine pelvic examination. Certainly a patient with vulvar symptoms must be examined for a proper diagnosis. Examination of the vulva is enhanced by adequate lighting and a careful inspection of the vulva and perianal skin. The location and size of the vulvar lesion as well as any involvement of adjacent structures such as urethra, vagina, or the anus should be noted.

Because the primary route of spread of vulvar carcinoma is to inguinal and femoral lymphatics, the inguinal chain should be palpated carefully. In cases in which adenocarcinoma or melanoma are found, other sites of primary disease should be considered.

a. **Colposcopy.** The colposcope or other magnification is often of assistance in identifying multifocal lesions. Colposcopic examination of the vulva, however, does not reveal the typical vascular patterns recognized on the cervix that are associated with cervical intraepithelial neoplasia. Colposcopic findings of vulvar carcinoma in situ are usually those of raised white or hyperpigmented lesions. The application of acetic acid (2%) to the vulva augments the recognition of white or hyperpigmented lesions.
b. **Evaluation of the perianal skin** is made with an anoscope, since carcinoma in situ frequently involves the anal canal.
c. **Toluidine blue (1%)** is used for the identification of carcinoma in situ on the vulva. Toluidine blue is a nuclear stain that, when applied, becomes concentrated in neoplastic areas with parakeratosis. Toluidine blue solution is applied liberally to the vulva and perianal skin and allowed to dry for 2 to 3 minutes. It is then washed off with 2% acetic acid solution and the vulva is reinspected. Areas of increased nuclear activity stain deeply blue and are therefore considered abnormal. This test is helpful in identification of multifocal lesions. However, hyperkeratotic lesions, even though neoplastic, rarely stain deeply blue because of their increased amounts of superficial keratin that prevent absorption of the dye. Excoriated or traumatic areas, despite their benign histology, often take up the toluidine blue stain leading to a false-positive diagnosis by this test.

**2. Clinical findings**

a. **Carcinoma in situ** of the vulva may have a variety of appearances ranging from white, hyperkeratotic islands, which occasionally are scaley, to red lesions appearing as papules or macules. Ten percent to 15% of carcinoma in situ lesions are hyperpigmented. Carcinoma in situ may be a single discrete lesion but often is multicentric, involving multiple discrete areas of the vulva, perineum, and perianal skin. This disease process must be thought of as an anogenital disease.
b. **Paget's disease** has a typical appearance of sharply demarcated, indurated, red lesions with superimposed white "sugar-coated" patches. These lesions may also be multicentric and include skin involving

the perirectal area, the buttocks, inguinal skin, mons, or vagina.

c. **Invasive carcinoma** should be suspected when an ulcerated endophytic lesion or a raised exophytic lesion arising on the labia, perineum, or mons is found. Palpation of the vulva may identify a mass especially near Bartholin's gland. Careful palpation should also be performed to ascertain fixation to underlying muscle or bone.

d. **Melanoma** of the vulva usually is pigmented and raised although it may present as an ulcerated bleeding lesion.

C. **Diagnostic procedures.** Paramount to the accurate diagnosis of vulvar lesions is the liberal use of vulvar biopsy. Biopsy of suspicious vulvar lesions may be easily accomplished under local anesthesia (infiltration with a local anesthetic such as 1% xylocaine) in the office. Discrete lesions may be widely excised with a scalpel or more diffuse lesions sampled by using a Keyes punch. Papanicolaou smear of suspicious lesions is of little value and should not be considered a screening test of significant reliability.

1. **Punch biopsy.** The site to be biopsied should be infiltrated with local anesthetic. A 4 or 6 mm Keyes punch, depending on the size of biopsy desired, is used to incise and remove the suspicious lesion (see Chapter 34—Common Office Gynecologic Procedures). The biopsy specimen is oriented on cardboard, sliced cucumber, or paper towel so that the pathologist may avoid tangential histologic sections. The orientation should be such that the subcutaneous portion of the specimen is in contact with the material to which it is attached and the epithelial surface is directed outward from the surface of the attachment material. Hemostasis of the biopsy site can usually be achieved with topical silver nitrate or Monsell's solution. A Gelfoam® plug applied to the biopsy site has also been used successfully. Rarely, an interrupted suture of 3-0 chromic cat gut is needed for hemostasis.
2. **Excisional biopsy** (see Chapter 34–Common Office Gynecologic Procedures) For lesions too large to biopsy with a Keyes punch or small enough to easily biopsy, a wide local excision should be made in a elliptical fashion, performed with the long axis of the biopsy oriented vertically on the vulva and horizontally on the perineum to obtain the best cosmetic and functional closure. These sites should be closed with interrupted 3-0 chromic cat gut sutures.
3. **Incisional biopsy from ulcerative lesions.** In patients with ulcerative lesions, an incisional biopsy from the lateral margin of the ulcer is often most helpful for identification of the invasive component. This location avoids necrotic tissue in the center of a tumor that may not be diagnostic.

Rarely is colposcopy, toluidene blue, or acetic acid of significant assistance in evaluating sites to biopsy in frankly invasive carcinoma.

4. **Pathologic evaluation** should not only make a diagnosis of invasive cancer but should also note depth of invasion, confluence of invasion (in early lesions), the degree of differentiation, and vascular space involvement. For melanomas, the depth of invasion based on Clark level and Breslow level should be reported as these features are directly related to prognosis.

D. **Staging**

1. **Staging.** The staging of vulvar carcinoma was established by the International Federation of Gynecology and Obstetrics (FIGO) in 1971 and was revised significantly in 1988 (Table 27.2). The former (1971) clinical staging system was fraught with error; especially in the evaluation of inguinal lymph nodes. Because assessment of lymph nodes was based on clinical evaluation rather than histology, a 15% false positive rate and a nearly 40% false negative rate was encountered. The revised staging system (1988) requires surgical removal and pathologic study of the nodes.
2. **Staging evaluations.** The staging studies for invasive vulvar carcinoma should include chest x-ray and IV pyelogram as well as complete blood count, liver function tests, and renal function tests. Cystoscopy and proctoscopy may be reserved for patients who have specific symptoms or disease located near the urethra or anus. Depth of invasion and lymph node metastases must be determined by surgical excision.

## VII. Management

A. **Intraepithelial vulvar lesions** are treated by excision or ablation of the intraepithelial lesion. Several treatment choices are available and should be selected based on the extent of the lesion as well as the patient's desires and need for cosmetic results and continued sexual function.

1. **Discrete vulvar lesions** may be widely excised under local, regional, or general anesthesia. Primary closure may usually be accomplished since the vulvar skin has significant elasticity and redundancy. The use of a rhomboid flap or split thickness skin graft to cover a larger area of excision may be necessary. A minimum of a 5 mm margin is suggested in an attempt to clear the margins of a purported carcinoma in situ.
2. **Multiple lesions (multiple sites of the same lesions by gross examination)**. Carcinoma in situ and Paget's disease in many patients is a more diffuse process involving multiple sites on the vulva, perineum, and perianal area. In these instances, more extensive therapy is required. Treat-

**Table 27.2. FIGO Classification and Staging of Carcinoma of the Vulva***

| | |
|---|---|
| **Stage 0** | |
| Tis | Carcinoma in situ, intraepithelial carcinoma |
| **Stage I** | |
| T1 N0 M0 | Tumor confined to the vulva and/or perineum—2 cm or less in greatest dimension. No modal metastasis |
| **Stage II** | |
| T2 N0 M0 | Tumor confined to the vulva and/or perineum—2 cm or less in greatest dimension. No modal metastasis |
| **Stage III** | |
| T3 N0 M0 | Tumor of any size with: |
| T3 N1 M0 | 1. Adjacent spread to the lower urethra and/or the vagina, or the anus, and/or |
| T1 N1 M0 | 2. Unilateral regional lymph node metastasis |
| T2 N1 M0 | |
| **Stage IVA** | |
| T1 N2 M0 | Tumor invades any of the following: |
| T2 N2 M0 | Upper urethra, bladder mucosa, rectal mucosa, pelvic bone and/or bilateral regional node metastasis |
| T3 N2 M0 | |
| T4, Any N, M0 | |
| **Stage IVB** | |
| Any T, Any N, MI | Any distant metastasis including pelvic lymph nodes |
| T | Primary Tumor |
| T1 | Tumor confined to the vulva and/or perineum—2 cm or less in greatest dimension |
| T2 | Tumor confined to the vulva and/or perineum—greater than 2 cm in greatest dimension |
| T3 | Tumor of any size with adjacent spread to the urethra and/or the vagina and/or the anus |
| T4 | Tumor invades any of the following: upper urethra, bladder mucosa, rectal mucosa, pelvic bone |
| N | Regional Lymph Nodes |
| N0 | No nodal metastasis (surgically proven) |
| N1 | Unilateral regional lymph node metastasis |
| N2 | Bilateral regional lymph node metastasis |
| M | Distant Metastases |
| M0 | No distant metastases |
| M1 | Distant metastasis including pelvic lymph nodes |

*The International Federation of Gynecology and Obstetrics (Revised, 1988).

ment options include simple vulvectomy, superficial vulvectomy with split thickness skin graft, or laser vaporization. Electrocautery or cryotherapy have also been used, but in general are discouraged because of pain, slowness of healing, and poor cosmetic results when compared to laser vaporization.

a. **Simple vulvectomy** was historically the treatment of choice for both carcinoma in situ and Paget's disease. This relatively simple surgical procedure can be done rapidly and the patient ambulated early following such surgery. Healing is usually prompt with minimal morbidity. The cosmetic results of simple vulvectomy, however, leave much to be desired and sexual function is certainly compromised following this procedure. For this reason, simple vulvectomy should be reserved for the elderly patient in whom an extensive surgical procedure or a lengthy period of bedrest postoperatively must be avoided.

b. **Superficial vulvectomy ("skinning vulvectomy") with split thickness skin graft** allows for extensive resection of involved skin while preserving subcutaneous tissue. The split thickness skin graft is easily obtained from the lateral thigh or buttocks and after its application to the dry surgical field is held in place by a bulky dressing for 6 days. During this period of time the patient must remain at bed rest while the skin graft begins to heal. Cosmetic and functional results of this surgical procedure are excellent. Over 90% of the skin graft heals by primary intention. Although recurrences have been noted in the skin graft, these are quite infrequent.

c. **Carbon dioxide laser** may be used to vaporize intraepithelial lesions of the vulva, especially carcinoma in situ. As this procedure is painful, adequate anesthesia must be achieved. For extensive vulvar lesions, either regional or general anesthesia may be necessary. Following laser vaporization the vulva is treated as a burn with sitz baths three times a day, a cleaning and drying regimen and application of 1% Silvadene® Cream (silver sulfadiazine) three times a day. Pain can usually be controlled with mild oral analgesics such as aspirin, acetaminophin, or codeine combinations of either. The cosmetic results of laser therapy are excellent and are significantly better than those achieved with electrocautery or cryotherapy. One disadvantage to laser therapy is that no pathology specimen is obtained and therefore extensive biopsies should be taken preoperatively to assure that no focal areas of invasion are present.

3. **5-fluorouracil ointment (Efudex 5%)** may also be used as topical chemotherapy for carcinoma in situ. A success rate of 60% to 70% is reported if Efudex is applied t.i.d. for 4 to 6 weeks. The success of this therapy is dependent upon a compliant patient who will tolerate the pain and discomfort as the skin becomes ulcerated by the Efudex therapy.

4. **Wide excision, vulvectomy, or superficial vulvectomy** with skin graft is the preferred treatment for Paget's disease of the vulva. In treating Paget's disease by wide excision, frozen section of margins is recommended, as this disease tends to be clinically occult significant distances from the primary lesion. Laser therapy to date has not been used extensively in this disease process.

B. **Invasive vulvar carcinoma**

1. **Radical vulvectomy**

a. **Radical vulvectomy with bilateral inguinal lymphadenectomy**. Standard treatment of invasive squamous cell carcinoma, melanoma, adenocarcinoma, and sarcoma of the vulva is a radical vulvectomy with bilateral inguinal lymphadenectomy. The extent of surgical excision of the mons and inguinal skin varies from one surgeon to another. The more radical excision is associated with a higher complication rate. The lateral vulvar incisions usually are made at the labiocrural fold, across the mons pubis superiorly and just superior to the anus inferiorly. The inner incision must encompass the lesion with adequate margin of 2 to 3 cm. Thus, the medial incision is usually at the hymenal ring, extending just anterior to the urethra but excising the clitoris. Excision of adenocarcinomas arising in the Bartholin's gland may require more extensive dissection in the ischiorectal fossa and/or possible excision of a portion of the distal rectum. The vulvectomy site is usually closed primarily, resulting in significant disfigurement potentially compromising sexual function. The sartorius muscle should be incised at its attachment to the iliac crest and mobilized to cover the exposed femoral vessels. Suction drains are placed in the subcutaneous inguinal region and the subcutaneous tissue closed over them. The use of suction drains and mobilization of the sartorius muscle has greatly diminished the incidence of lymphocysts and infection with subsequent necrosis of the femoral vessels. Nonetheless, inguinal wound infection with separation is a frequent complication. Plastic surgical procedures to cover widely excised inguinal skin include creation of a tensor fascia lata myocutaneous flap or split thickness skin graft. Reconstruction of the vulva has been moderately successful by using gracilis myocutaneous flaps.

b. **Modified radical vulvectomy**. Over the past decade several investigators have questioned the need for radical vulvectomy and inguinal lymphadenectomy for early invasive vulvar carcinoma. Although the term "microinvasive carcinoma" of the vulva has not been widely accepted, early invasive vulvar carcinoma is usually considered to be squamous cell carcinoma with the primary lesion 2 cm in diameter or less and invading less than 5 mm. These lesions have only a 5% to 10% incidence of metastases to the inguinal lymph nodes. In addition, the local recurrence rate is exceedingly small. Because of this favorable prognosis, several investigators suggest that these small lesions may be treated less radically while still achieving an excellent chance of cure, preserving vulvar anatomy, and reducing morbidity of complete inguinal lymphadenectomy. The surgical procedure suggested is a modified radical vulvectomy that radically excises unilateral disease while leaving the contralateral vulva intact. Because the prognosis for vulvar cancer is highly correlated with metastatic disease in the lymph nodes, the inguinal nodes, superficial to the cribriform fascia, are completely excised and studied. If there are no metastases in the superficial nodes, the deeper inguinal node dissection would seem to be unnecessary. On the other hand, if metastatic disease is in the superficial inguinal nodes, a complete inguinal lymphadenectomy is recommended. Although this therapeutic alternative is based on sound anatomic and clinical features, it has been applied to a limited number of patients and therefore must still be considered investigational.

2. **Exenteration with radical vulvectomy**. Advanced vulvar carcinoma involving the urethra, vagina, or anus is usually managed by exenterative surgery combined with radical vulvectomy. Careful patient selection is necessary and is often limited to younger patients with advanced disease.
3. **Pelvic lymphadenectomy**. In the past many surgeons also performed an extraperitoneal pelvic lymphadenectomy in combination with inguinal lymphadenectomy. This was especially advocated if inguinal lymph nodes were found to contain metastases. Others have advised whole pelvis radiation therapy in this setting, thus avoiding the morbidity of pelvic lymphadenectomy. Recently, the completion of a randomized trial has clearly demonstrated that whole pelvis radiation therapy is significantly more successful in the treatment of potential disease in pelvic lymph nodes, thus avoiding the extended surgical procedure of a pelvic lymphadenectomy.
4. **Radiation therapy** is generally poorly tolerated by the vulva and cannot be considered primary therapy in most cases of advanced vulvar carcinoma. However, some investigators have shown excellent treatment results for locally advanced vulvovaginal carcinoma by combining preoperative radiation therapy with a wide excision of the

remaining malignancy. In so doing these investigators have avoided exenterative surgery. However, preoperative radiation therapy does lead to increased operative complications, especially poor wound healing in the groin and vulvar incisions.

5. **Sexual rehabilitation** of the patient following radical vulvectomy may be augmented by plastic surgery procedures such as vulvar reconstruction with gracilis myocutaneous flaps or coverage of the inguinal region with tensor fascia lata flaps or skin grafts. Attention must be directed to the continued sexual rehabilitation of these patients and emotional support offered as necessary.

C. **Metastatic disease of the inguinal lymph nodes**. The best management of metastatic disease of inguinal lymph nodes is yet to be established, although it is clear that these metastases worsen the individual's prognosis. The prognosis is especially poor if the patient has more than three lymph nodes involved with metastatic tumor, and in this setting we would advise inguinal and whole pelvis radiation therapy. As was previously noted, whole pelvis radiation therapy is more effective than pelvic lymphadenectomy in treating patients with potential metastatic disease in the pelvic nodes. On the other hand, patients with one to three positive inguinal lymph nodes should have reasonably good survival and whether additional radiation therapy is of benefit has yet to be demonstrated.

D. **Recurrent vulvar carcinoma**. Approximately 80% of recurrent disease is noted within the first 2 years of follow-up. One-half of recurrences are localized to the vulva or inguinal regions and are usually associated with patients who had large primary malignancies or those with positive inguinal lymph nodes. Occasionally a vulvar recurrence may be widely resected with success or treated with interstitial radiation therapy. Recurrent disease in inguinal lymph nodes is much more difficult to treat. Wide local excision (if possible) followed by radiation therapy is recommended. The remainder of recurrences are at distant sites in pelvic and para-aortic lymph nodes or as pulmonary or bony metastases and are only palliated with chemotherapy regimens.

E. **Basal cell carcinoma** may be adequately managed by wide local excision, as this malignancy has a low propensity to metastasize to inguinal lymph nodes.

F. **Vulvar melanoma** has traditionally been treated with radical vulvectomy and inguinal lymphadenectomy, although more recently wide local excision of the melanoma has been advocated. The need for inguinal lymphadenectomy also must be debated as to whether this serves only as a prognostic staging tool or whether it is therapeutic. In most patients with metastatic disease to inguinal lymph nodes long-term survival is uncommon.

## VIII. Prognosis

A. **Intraepithelial vulvar lesions** (carcinoma in situ or Paget's disease). The prognosis for a patient with carcinoma in situ or Paget's disease should be excellent, as this is not an invasive carcinoma. Adenocarcinoma associated with Paget's disease, however, carries a poor prognosis, which is directly related to the size of the lesion and inguinal lymph node metastasis. Both carcinoma in situ and Paget's disease have a relatively high recurrence rate which is related to the adequacy and extent of primary therapy. Paget's disease, in particular, often extends well beyond the grossly visualized lesion, and positive surgical margins are frequently reported. Therapy for recurrent or persistent carcinoma in situ and Paget's disease is similar to primary therapy. Continued surveillance of the genital tract for other neoplasia is important. Carcinoma in situ of the vulva may coexist or precede carcinoma in situ or invasive carcinoma of the cervix or vagina. The rare association of Paget's disease with vulvar adenocarcinoma also warrants close long-term follow-up.

B. **Invasive vulvar carcinoma**. The overall survival for patients with invasive vulvar carcinoma is approximately 75% at 5 years (corrected survival). Prognostic features significantly associated with survival include primary tumor size, metastatic disease in inguinal lymph nodes, grade of tumor, depth of invasion, and invasion of lymphatic channels. Patients with stage I and II squamous cell carcinoma of the vulva enjoy approximately 90% corrected 5-year survival. Stage-related survival rates are shown in Table 27.3. Regardless of disease stage, if the patient has negative inguinal lymph nodes, survival is approximately 90%. On the other hand, if the patient has a inguinal lymph node metastasis, the overall survival decreases to approximately 35% at 5 years. The number of inguinal nodes affected also seems to be important; patients with three or less lymph nodes have approximately a 68% 5-year survival rate, whereas those patients with greater than three lymph nodes involved in the inguinal region rarely survive. Patients with known pelvic lymph node metastases have approximately a 20% 5-year survival rate.

**Table 27.3. Survival Related to Stage of Vulvar Carcinoma**

| STAGE | CORRECTED 5-YEAR SURVIVAL (%) |
|---|---|
| I | 81.4 |
| II | 56.6 |
| III | 37.6 |
| IV | 14.6 |

C. **Melanoma**. The overall corrected 5-year survival for patients with melanoma of the vulva is 36%. The most important prognostic features of melanoma of the vulva are its depths of invasion as reflected in the Clark's or Breslow's levels and whether there are regional lymphatic metastases.

## BIBLIOGRAPHY

Boronow RC. Therapeutic alternatives to primary exenteration for advanced vulvovaginal cancer. Gynecol Oncol 1973; 1:233–255.

Breslow A. Thickness, cross-sectional areas, and depth of invasion in the prognosis of cutaneous melanoma. Ann Surg 1970; 172:902–908.

Clark WH, From L, Bernardino, EA, Mihm MC. The histogenesis and biologic behavior of primary human malignant melanomas of the skin. Cancer Res 1969; 29:705–727.

Creasman WT, Gallager HS, Rutledge R. Paget's disease of the vulva. Gynecol Oncol 1975; 3:133–148.

Curry SL, Wharton JT, Rutledge F. Positive lymph nodes in vulvar squamous carcinoma. Gynecol Oncol 1980; 9:63–69.

DiSaia PJ, Creasman WT, Rich WM. An alternate approach to early cancer of the vulva. Am J Obstet Gynecol 1979; 133:825–832.

Friedrich EG, Wilkinson EJ, Fu YS. Carcinoma in situ of the vulva: A continuing challenge. Am J Obstet Gynecol 1980; 136:830–843.

Iverson T, Aalders JG, Christensen A, Kolstad P. Squamous cell carcinoma of the vulva: A review of 424 patients. 1956–1974. Gynecol Oncol 1980; 9:271–279.

Lenchter RS, Hacker NF, Voet RL, Berek JS, Townsend DE. Primary carcinoma of the Bartholin gland: A report of 14 cases and review of the literature. Obstet Gynecol 1982; 60:361–368.

Morley GW. Infiltrative carcinoma of the vulva: Results of surgical treatment. Am J Obstet Gynecol 1976; 124:874–888.

Morrow CP, DiSaia PJ. Malignant melanoma of the female genitalia: A clinical analysis. Obstet Gynecol 1976; 31:233–271.

Parker RT, Duncan I, Rampone J, Creasman W. Operative management of early invasive epidermoid carcinoma of the vulva. Am J Obstet Gynecol 1975; 123:349–355.

Podratz KC, Symmonds RE, Taylor WF, Williams TJ. Carcinoma of the vulva: Analysis of treatment and survival. Obstet Gynecol 1983; 161:63–74.

Rutledge F, Sinclair M. Treatment of intraepithelial carcinoma of the vulva by skin excision and graft. Am J Obstet Gynecol 1968; 102:806–818.

Way S. Malignant Disease of the Vulva. Edinburg, Scotland: Churchill-Livingston; 1982.

Wharton JT, Gallager S, Rutledge FN. Microinvasive carcinoma of the vulva. Am J Obstet Gynecol 1974; 118:159–162.

# CHAPTER 28

# Vaginal Dysplasia and Carcinoma

**Daniel L. Clarke-Pearson**

Carcinoma in situ of the vagina is a rare clinical entity that in many respects is similar to carcinoma in situ of the cervix or vulva. In fact, it is often found to be associated with other antecedent or coexistent intraepithelial or invasive neoplasia of the lower genital tract. Essentially asymptomatic, the lesion is usually detected initially by a Papanicolaou (PAP) smear. The multifocal nature of these lesions should guide investigation and treatment options which will preserve vaginal function when possible.

Invasive cancer of the vagina is one of the rarest gynecological malignancies. Squamous cell carcinoma, which accounts for approximately 95% of vaginal cancers, occurs primarily in postmenopausal women. Other vaginal malignancies include adenocarcinoma, melanoma, sarcoma, sarcoma botryoides, and endodermal sinus tumor.

## I. Incidence

A. **Carcinoma in situ.** The exact incidence of carcinoma in situ of the vagina is unknown, although it is clearly much less common than carcinoma in situ of the cervix or vulva. It usually occurs in women from the third decade of life on.

B. **Invasive vaginal cancer** accounts for 1% to 2% of all gynecologic malignancies.

1. **Squamous cell carcinoma** makes up approximately 95% of vaginal malignancies and occurs primarily in women 55 to 65 years of age. The incidence of vaginal squamous cell carcinoma is increased in patients who have been previously treated with pelvic radiation therapy and should be strongly considered in patients who develop abnormal genital cytology following pelvic radiotherapy.
2. **Adenocarcinoma** of the vagina accounts for only 2% of vaginal carcinomas. The identification of a cluster of young women with clear cell adenocarcinoma of the vagina led to studies that demonstrated in utero exposure to diethylstilbestrol (DES) as the etiologic factor. The inci-

dence of adenocarcinoma following DES exposure has been calculated to be 0.14 to 1.4 per 1000 female fetuses exposed. The median age of onset of clear cell adenocarcinoma of the vagina is 19 years. However, the age of onset has been described in patients as early as 7 and as late as 30 years of age.

3. **Melanoma** of the vagina accounts for approximately 2% of vaginal malignancies. Rarer still are the sarcomas (leiomyosarcoma and fibrosarcoma) arising primarily in the vagina. The rare entity, sarcoma botryoides (rhabdomyosarcoma) develops in children of a median age of 2 years.

## II. Morbidity and mortality

A. **Morbidity** associated with all invasive vaginal cancers is usually secondary to treatment modalities. Cancers arising in the vagina are difficult to treat and a higher morbidity is encountered because of the close anatomic association of the bladder and rectum. Radiation therapy, the primary treatment modality for most patients, leads to reasonably high complication rates associated with urinary tract or rectovaginal fistulae, vaginal radionecrosis, vaginal stenosis, and fibrosis. The surgical approach to this disease relies on radical hysterectomy and upper vaginectomy for lesions located in the upper vagina. Lesions located in the mid to lower third of the vagina require a more extensive surgical procedure such as pelvic exenteration, sometimes combined with radical vulvectomy. Morbidity and mortality from these radical surgical procedures can be significant.

B. **Mortality**

1. **Vaginal carcinoma in situ** has no morbidity or mortality, but it does have the potential for progression to an invasive vaginal carcinoma. Because the lesion is usually asymptomatic, morbidity must be considered in terms of therapy complications.
2. **Squamous cell carcinoma.** The overall 5-year survival for invasive squamous cell carcinoma of the vagina is approximately 51% (Table 28.1). This disease progresses by local invasion and metastasis to regional pelvic lymph nodes. Thus, recurrences are often in the pelvis and lead to death secondary to obstructive uropathy, bleeding, and infection.
3. **Clear cell adenocarcinoma.** The 5-year survival for patients treated for clear cell adenocarcinoma (related to DES exposure) is 80%. This is significantly better than that reported for squamous cell carcinoma. Identification of high risk population of women has led to earlier diagnosis and thus improved survival. Approximately 50% of recurrences are found in the vagina, and 36% in the lungs.

**Table 28.1. 5-Year Survival Rates for Squamous Cell Carcinoma and Clear Cell Adenocarcinoma of the Vagina (Diethylstilbestrol Exposure)**

| FIGO STAGE | SURVIVAL RATES (%) | |
|---|---|---|
| | SQUAMOUS CELL | CLEAR CELL ADENOCARCINOMA |
| I | 65 | 90 |
| II | 60 | 80 |
| III | 35 | 37 |
| IV | 39 | — |
| Overall | 51 | 80 |

FIGO = International Federation of Gynecology and Obstetrics.

4. **Melanoma.** Primary melanoma of the vagina is exceedingly rare. Limited reports suggest an overall survival of only 5%. In a group of patients treated by total pelvic exenteration, who have no metastasis to the pelvic lymph nodes, the survival may be as high as 50% at 5 years.

## III. Etiology

A. **Carcinoma in situ.** Although poorly understood, the etiology of carcinoma in situ of the vagina seems to be similar to that of intraepithelial lesions of the cervix or vulva. One-half to two-thirds of patients with carcinoma in situ of the vagina usually have an antecedent lesion or coexistent neoplasm of the lower genital tract. Because of its frequent association with antecedent or coexistent neoplasia of the cervix or vulva, the ''field-effect'' of a carcinogen must be strongly considered. The hypothesis pointing toward a viral etiology (human papilloma virus—HPV) of these lesions is most reasonable in view of current research.

1. **Carcinoma in situ following hysterectomy.** One to two percent of patients who undergo hysterectomy for carcinoma in situ of the cervix ultimately develop carcinoma in situ in the upper vagina. Whereas some of these lesions may be persistent disease from direct extension of the carcinoma in situ from the cervix to the upper vagina, other lesions develop subsequent to hysterectomy. This is one argument for yearly PAP smears after hysterectomy.
2. **Carcinoma in situ following radiation therapy.** Intraepithelial neoplasia of the vagina has also been reported to follow pelvic and vaginal radiation therapy for another gynecologic malignancy. These lesions clearly can progress to invasive carcinoma if left untreated.

B. **Squamous cell carcinoma.** The etiology of squamous cell carcinoma of the vagina is unknown. Because of its close association with malignancies arising in the cervix, or vulva, a "field" effect has been suggested and the possibility of a viral etiology (especially HPV) has been entertained. Some authors have shown an association between squamous cell carcinoma of the vagina and vaginal prolapse, pessary use, and prior pelvic radiation therapy.

C. **Clear cell adenocarcinoma** of the vagina arising in young women was described in 1971 by Herbst, who demonstrated a link with in utero exposure to DES, which was used to prevent premature labor. All women who have this association were exposed to DES before the 18th week of gestation, although the duration of therapy and dosage of DES exposure are not necessarily proportional to the likelihood of subsequent development of adenocarcinoma of the vagina in these young women.

D. **Melanoma, sarcomas, and sarcoma botryoides.** The etiology of melanoma, sarcomas, or sarcoma botryoides is unknown.

## IV. Pathogenesis/pathophysiology

A. **The course of carcinoma in situ** of the vagina is variable but it is assumed that if left untreated, carcinoma in situ may progress to invasive vaginal carcinoma. Dysplasia and carcinoma in situ of the vagina appear to be slowly progressive diseases and radical therapy (such as vaginectomy) should be withheld until all conservative measures have failed. Twenty-five percent of patients who develop carcinoma in situ of the vagina following pelvic radiation therapy progress to invasive carcinoma if untreated.

B. **The lymphatic drainage** of the vagina is complex and must be understood when considering the pathophysiology of cancer. The location of the carcinoma in the vaginal tube is important in order to identify regional nodes that may be at risk. The upper half of the vagina drains to the pelvic lymph nodes including the external iliac, obturator, hypogastric, and common iliac lymph nodes. Lesions located in the lower portion of the vagina may drain to lymphatic channels in a similar fashion as vulvar carcinoma; that is, the inguinal femoral lymphatics. Treatment of these lymphatics must be considered to successfully treat patients. Fifty-four percent of squamous cell carcinoma of the vagina is located in the upper third of the vagina, most often on the posterior wall. Fourteen percent of vaginal carcinomas are located in the middle third, whereas 32% are located in the lower one-third of the vagina.

C. **The spread pattern of squamous cell carcinoma** of the vagina is primarily by local extension and secondarily by lymphatic metastasis. Because the vesicovaginal septum and rectovaginal septum are relatively thin, local extension directly into the bladder or rectum is frequently encountered. Invasion into the paracolpos and extension to the pelvic sidewall may ultimately be identified in advanced cases. The exact incidence of lymph node metastasis is unknown, although it is assumed to be approximately the same as that of similar volumes of squamous cell carcinoma arising on the cervix.

D. **Adenocarcinoma** arising in association with DES exposure usually occurs in the upper half of the vagina and may be associated with adenocarcinoma of the cervix. Local extension and nodal metastasis are the primary means of spread of this carcinoma. In patients with stage I carcinoma, approximately 18% will be found to have metastasis in the pelvic lymph nodes; stage II disease has approximately 30% nodal metastasis rate (see diagnosis section, VI-G for discussion of staging).

E. **Sarcoma botryoides** usually arises from the anterior vaginal wall of young girls and infants and is often multicentric. The disease tends to be locally recurring, although it may spread to distant sites by hematogenous routes.

## V. Differential diagnosis.

**V. Differential diagnosis.** Histologic confirmation of vaginal lesions is mandatory prior to instituting therapy.

A. **Carcinoma in situ** must be considered when lesions that appear as red, ulcerated, or white hyperplastic epithelium are found on examination of the vagina. Such abnormal lesions may also be infectious in origin (herpes), traumatic (from forced sexual intercourse, foreign body, or tampon use), hyperkeratosis (secondary to chronic irritation, poorly fitted diaphragm), adenosis, or a chronically draining sinus tract from a permanent foreign body material such as Marlex® mesh or nonabsorbable suture used in prior pelvic surgery.

B. **Invasive vaginal carcinoma**

1. Lesions in the vagina that may be considered in the differential diagnosis in invasive carcinoma are:
    a. Squamous cell carcinoma
    b. Adenocarcinoma
    c. Sarcoma
    d. Melanoma
    e. Metastatic carcinoma
    f. Carcinoma in situ
    g. Adenosis
    h. Endometriosis
    i. Condylomata accuminata
    j. Traumatic lesions
2. **Metastatic lesions.** When malignancy is encountered, the possibility of the vaginal lesion being metastatic from another primary malignancy should be considered. Frequently encountered sources of metastasis to the vagina include carcinoma of the cervix, endometrium, vulva, colorectal carcinoma, ovarian carcinoma, choriocarcinoma, and urethral carcinoma.

## VI. Diagnosis

A. **Signs and symptoms**

1. **Carcinoma in situ of the vagina** is an asymptomatic disease and frequently is only detected by PAP smear. Vagi-

nal discharge, pruritus, or postcoital spotting may be associated with carcinoma in situ in a minority of cases.

2. **Squamous cell carcinoma of the vagina** is usually first detected when the patient develops vaginal bleeding or discharge. Patients are not usually detected in the asymptomatic stages by PAP smear because of the lack of uniform vaginal cytopathologic sampling. As the lesion progresses, and depending upon its location, the patient may also develop urinary tract symptoms, rectal pain or pressure, or lower extremity edema.
3. **Melanoma and adenocarcinoma**, like squamous cell carcinoma usually present with vaginal bleeding or discharge, although it appears that the screening of young women exposed to DES has been successful in identifying a larger proportion of patients who are asymptomatic with early stage clear cell adenocarcinoma.
4. **Vaginal sarcomas** often present with symptoms of a mass lesion, pressure, or pain. Bleeding may also occur if the sarcoma undergoes necrosis. Sarcoma botryoides usually presents as a bloody vaginal discharge or protruding masses of "grapelike" polyps noted at the introitus by the child's mother.

**B. Physical examination**

1. Inspection and palpation of the vagina is an integral part of the pelvic examination and the most important maneuver in the physical examination of suspected vaginal neoplasia. Unfortunately, the vagina is often inspected only visually in a cursory fashion, with much of the vagina not seen at all because it is hidden behind the blades of the speculum. The bimanual examination should include palpation of the vaginal canal. Routine inspection and palpation of the vagina will sometimes reveal evidence of carcinoma in situ. Occasionally a raised, whitened, hyperkeratotic lesion or an ulcerated lesion may be noted, which ultimately is found to be carcinoma in situ.
2. **Colposcopy.** Clinical examination must be aided by colposcopy and/or Schiller's staining of the vaginal mucosa to identify subclinical lesions. Examination findings in patients with vaginal carcinoma usually are those of an exophytic or ulcerative lesion that is friable. As previously noted, the carcinoma may be located anywhere in the vagina. By convention, if the cervix, urethra, or vulva is involved it is designated the primary site rather than the vagina. Palpation of the vagina is important to identify thickened or nodular mucosal areas that may represent other metastatic sites or may be the only primary site encountered in women exposed to DES.

**C. PAP smear** is usually the diagnostic method by which carcinoma in situ of the vagina is identified. Yearly PAP smears of the upper vagina should be obtained in all patients who have had previous hysterectomy for cervical intraepithelial neoplasia. Directed PAP smears from specific vaginal lesions may be obtained with a spatula. Prior to treatment of carcinoma in situ of the vagina the lesion must be confirmed histologically as well as its location identified.

D. **Colposcopy** is an excellent method for identification of carcinoma in situ when suspected from PAP smear results. Colposcopic examination of the vagina is time consuming and requires adequate exposure of all walls of the vagina as well as considerable expertise in colposcopy. Using the same technique as colposcopy of the cervix (inspection before and after application of 3% acetic acid, as well as utilization of a green light filter) will usually show white epithelium, punctation, and/or mosaic vascular patterns similar to those lesions observed on the cervix. In patients who have had previous hysterectomy, the upper apex of the vaginal vault should be closely inspected. Postmenopausal patients who are estrogen deficient should use estrogen vaginal cream nightly for 3 to 4 weeks prior to colposcopic examination. Direct application of estrogen to the vaginal mucosa is much more effective in maturing the epithelium, thus providing a sharper contrast between normal squamous epithelium and dysplastic epithelium. Note that carcinoma in situ of the vagina may be multifocal throughout the entire vagina. The whole vagina must therefore be carefully inspected by colposcopy and biopsies should be obtained of suspicious areas. The application of Schiller's solution to the vagina also greatly assists in identification of multifocal lesions.

E. **Vaginal biopsy** must be performed of all suspicious areas to rule out invasive carcinoma and to confirm the location of the carcinoma in situ. Biopsy may usually be performed in the outpatient setting without difficulty. Anesthesia is best achieved with a topical benzocaine gel applied to the vaginal mucosa prior to biopsy. Biopsies may be adequately obtained by a Kavorkian or Whittnauer biopsy forcep. Because of the pliability of the vaginal wall, traction and stabilization of the area to be biopsied with a sterile skin hook or tenaculum is often helpful. Bleeding after a biopsy is usually minimal, but if hemostasis is required, the application of silver nitrate or Monsel's solution is usually sufficient. Hemostatic suturing is rarely needed, but, if required, is best done with a fine taper (atraumatic) needle attached to 3-0 chromic suture.

F. **Endocervical and endometrial biopsy.** In patients with adenocarcinoma, especially elderly patients, metastasis from another primary site should be excluded and therefore endocervical and endometrial biopsies should be obtained. In addition the gastrointestinal tract, especially the stomach and colon, should be surveyed for the possibility of either as the site of primary adenocarcinoma. Melanoma may also be metastatic to the vagina from another primary site.

### G. Staging

1. **Staging procedures** for carcinoma of the vagina include investigation of local as well as distant metastasis in a fashion similar to that of carcinoma of the cervix. Radiographic studies advised include chest x-ray and IV pyelogram. Cystoscopy and proctosigmoidoscopy should be performed depending on the location of the lesion in the anterior or posterior vaginal wall. Lymphangiogram or computerized tomography may be of assistance in identifying metastases to pelvic lymph nodes. Computed tomography may also detect distant metastases.
2. The **clinical staging system** for carcinoma of the vagina.
   **Stage 0**: Carcinoma in situ.
   **Stage I**: Carcinoma limited to the vaginal mucosa.
   **Stage II**: Carcinoma involving the subvaginal tissue but not extending onto the pelvic wall.
   **Stage III**: Carcinoma extending onto the pelvic wall.
   **Stage IV**: Carcinoma extending into the mucosa of the bladder or rectum or distant metastases.
3. **Surgical staging** of vaginal cancer is rarely performed, except in conjunction with surgical therapy.

## VII. Management

### A. Carcinoma in situ

1. **Primary goals of therapy** for carcinoma in situ of the vagina is to achieve ablation of this intraepithelial lesion while at the same time preserving vaginal depth, caliber, and sexual function. As part of the treatment considerations, care must be taken to avoid injury to the bladder, urethra, and rectum especially if the lesion is located on the anterior or posterior vaginal wall.
2. **Lesion ablation.** Intraepithelial lesion ablation may be achieved by local excision (partial colpectomy) or laser vaporization. Both procedures may cause pain or bleeding although laser vaporization can usually be performed in the office if the lesion is not too extensive. Vaporization to a depth of 2 to 3 mm is sufficient to ablate the intraepithelial lesion in the vagina and also avoid penetration of an adjacent viscus. Following colpectomy and primary closure of the defect, vaginal intercourse or other trauma to the suture line should be avoided until the epithelium is healed. Following laser vaporization, agglutination of the vaginal walls must be avoided by the daily application of a triple sulfa cream (sulfathiazole, sulfacetamide, sulfabenzamide) high in the vagina of the premenopausal patient or estrogen cream (Premarin® vaginal cream) in the postmenopausal patient.
3. **5-fluorouracil cream (Efudex 5%)** is an alternative therapy that may also be used successfully in the treatment of carcinoma in situ of the vagina, especially if it is multifocal or

extensive. Two grams of 5-fluorouracil should be applied high in the vagina by vaginal applicator at bedtime for 10 consecutive nights. Prior to the application of 5-fluorouracil in the vagina, the patient should apply petroleum jelly to the vulva to minimize vulvar irritation. The 10-day 5-fluorouracil cycle should be repeated after a 14-day rest period. Follow-up with vaginal PAP smears should be reinstituted approximately 4 months following 5-fluorouracil treatment.

4. **Total or partial vaginectomy with application of a split thickness skin graft** over a vaginal mold or stint (McIndoe precedure) may be used for treatment of carcinoma in situ of the vagina following failure of the previously described treatment procedures. Vaginectomy with split thickness skin graft is a major surgical procedure requiring general anesthesia. Following the application of the skin graft, the vaginal mold must continue to be used for approximately 6 months to avoid vaginal stenosis, stricture, and scarring.
5. **Cryotherapy** is a poor method of ablating carcinoma in situ of the vagina because of the lack of control of depth of freeze and frequently poor contact of the cryotherapy probe to the undulating vaginal mucosa.
6. **Vaginal irradiation** with a vaginal cylinder has been used to treat carcinoma in situ but usually leads to unsatisfactory sexual function secondary to vaginal fibrosis and stenosis.

B. **Invasive vaginal carcinoma**. Management of invasive vaginal carcinoma may require more flexibility and ingenuity on the part of the physician than of any other gynecologic malignancy. In general the treatment plan is based on the size, location, and extent of the lesion in areas beyond the vagina.

1. **Squamous cell carcinoma** of the vagina has been treated by both surgical and radiotherapy approaches.
   a. **Radiation therapy** is the method by which the majority of patients are treated for vaginal squamous cell carcinoma because it allows conservation of the bladder and rectum. The goals of radiation therapy for stages I–III are to eradicate the local lesion, and to sterilize disease in the pelvic or inguinal lymph nodes. This is usually accomplished by the combined use of external beam teletherapy to the whole pelvis in conjunction with local application of brachytherapy. Brachytherapy may include the use of a vaginal "cylinder," or interstitial implant of radium needles or iridium "ribbons" in after-loading needles or tubes.
      (1) **Small lesions ($<$ 2 cm)** may be successfully treated with interstitial implants (radium or iridium$^{192}$ after-loading needles) or vaginal cylinder loaded with cesium.

(2) **Large lesions ( > 2 cm)** are treated with a combination of external beam radiotherapy delivered to the whole pelvis covering both the primary lesion as well as the lymph nodes on the pelvic sidewall. External beam therapy of 40Gy to 50Gy is delivered first to optimize shrinkage of the primary tumor. If anatomy allows, interstitial or intracavitary brachytherapy follows. Lesions located in the upper vagina are often treated like cervical carcinoma with Fletcher–Suit tandem and ovoids. Lesions of the mid and lower one-third are usually treated by interstitial implants of radium needles, after-loading iridium$^{192}$ needles, or a cylinder loaded with lesions. Lesions located in the lower one-third of the vagina must be considered potentially metastatic to the inguinal nodes, and inguinal lymphadenectomy is usually recommended prior to instituting radiation therapy.

b. **Surgical resection**. In selected surgical candidates, upper vaginal lesions may be treated by radical hysterectomy and upper vaginectomy combined with pelvic lymphadenectomy. Lower vaginal lesions, especially those involving the vulva, have been successfully treated with pelvic exenteration and radical vulvectomy. This mode of therapy obviously does not allow conservation of the bladder or rectum.

**2. Clear cell adenocarcinoma**

a. **Radical hysterectomy with upper vaginectomy**. Younger women with clear cell adenocarcinoma of the vagina usually have the lesion located in the upper one-half of the vagina. A desire to conserve ovarian and vaginal function is paramount. Most of these women have undergone radical hysterectomy with upper vaginectomy combined with pelvic lymphadenectomy for primary treatment. Preservation of ovarian function and vaginal pliability as well as prevention of long-term radiation therapy complications has been achieved.

b. **Radiation or exenterative surgery**. For larger lesions, advanced stage lesions, or those located in the lower half of the vagina, adenocarcinoma should also be treated with radiation therapy or exenterative surgical procedures.

**3. Melanoma** of the vagina should be treated with radical surgery if at all possible. Radiation therapy and chemotherapy have produced little effect in treating these lesions.

4. **Sarcoma botryoides** was treated in the past primarily with pelvic exenteration. This is an unpalatable procedure to consider in any patient but especially so in the young child. More recent reports suggest that wide excision combined with chemotherapy, such as multi-agent therapy with methotrexate, dactinomycin, and cyclophosphamide, can lead to sustained remissions and at the same time preserve the bladder and rectum.
5. **Leiomyosarcoma** in the vagina should be treated by wide excision if anatomy allows. Many of these lesions are sensitive to radiation therapy and therefore may be amenable to therapy similar to that recommended for squamous cell carcinoma (see diagnosis section, VII-B-1).

## VIII. Prognosis

A. **Carcinoma in situ** of the vagina, if left untreated, will usually progress to invasive carcinoma over a long period of time, sometimes many years. Successful treatment with colpectomy, laser vaporization, 5-fluorouracil cream, or vaginectomy should lead to an 80% to 95% cure rate. Certainly all patients who have had carcinoma in situ of the vagina should remain under close surveillance by inspection and PAP smears from all vaginal walls for the remainder of their lives. The cervix and vulva must also be part of careful surveillance, as intraepithelial and invasive lesions in these organ sites are often times associated with vaginal intraepithelial neoplasia.

B. **Invasive vaginal carcinoma**

1. Because of the varying treatment modalities for squamous cell carcinoma of the vagina, it is difficult to evaluate whether surgery or radiation therapy achieves a higher cure rate. Most survival statistics are presented as combined survival of both radiation therapy and surgically treated patients. Representative survival rates based on the International Federation of Gynecology and Obstetrics (FIGO) Stage are shown in Table 28.1. Survival for early stage adenocarcinoma (clear cell) in the DES exposed woman are shown in Table 28.1 as well. For earlier stage disease, the survival appears to be higher than that of squamous cell carcinoma, and the overall survival of 80% is considered better than the 51% for squamous cell carcinoma. The overall survival for melanoma of the vagina is approximately 5%. As with melanoma elsewhere in the body, it is directly related to depth of invasion and whether metastasis to lymph nodes has occurred. Reliable statistics for survival of leiomyosarcoma, fibrosarcoma, and rhabdomyosarcoma are difficult to present as these are rare tumors having been treated in a variety of treatment schemes.
2. **Recurrence** of squamous cell carcinoma of the vagina is similar to cervical cancer in its behavior with most recur-

rences occurring within 2 years of primary therapy. Most recurrences are localized in the pelvis. Treatment of recurrences following radiation therapy must be ultraradical surgery if the patient's medical condition and location of the tumor are favorable. Recurrence after surgical treatment, especially in the DES exposed female, may be treated with radiation therapy or more radical exenterative procedures.

3. **Distant metastasis** from squamous cell carcinoma or adenocarcinoma have occasionally responded to chemotherapeutic agents such as cisplatin, methotrexate, bleomycin, mitomycin C, and vincristine, although the optimal drug or treatment regimen has yet to be identified.

## BIBLIOGRAPHY

Ball HG, Berman ML. Management of primary vaginal carcinoma. Gynecol Oncol 1982; 14:154.

Barclay DL. Carcinoma of the vagina after hysterectomy for severe dysplasia or carcinoma in situ of the cervix. Gynecol Oncol 1979; 8:1.

Brown AR, Fletcher GH, Rutledge F. Irradiation of in situ and invasive squamous cell carcinoma of the vagina. Cancer 1971; 28:1278.

Flamant F, Chassagne D, Cossett JM, Gerbaulet A, Lemerle J. Embryonal rhabdomyosarcoma of the vagina in children–conservative treatment with curietherapy and chemotherapy. Eur J Cancer 1979; 15:527–532.

Herbst AL, Ulfelder H, Roskunzer DC. Adenocarcinoma of the vagina. Association of maternal stilbestrol therapy with tumor appearance in young women. N Engl J Med 1971; 284:878.

Hilgers R. Pelvic extenteration for vaginal embryonal and rhabdomyosarcoma. Obstet Gynecol 1975; 45:175.

Kanbour AI, Kilionsky B, and Murphy AI. Carcinoma of the vagina following cervical cancer. Cancer 1974; 34:1838.

Morrow CP, DiSaia PJ. Malignant melanoma of the female genitalia: A clinical analysis. Obstet Gynecol Surv 1976; 31:233.

Ortega JA. A therapeutic approach to childhood pelvic rhabdomyosarcoma without pelvic extenteration. J Pediatr 1979; 94:205.

Perez CA, Camel HM. Long-term follow-up in radiation therapy of carcinoma of the vagina. Cancer 1982; 49:1308.

Prempree T, Virauathana T, Slawson RG, Wizenberg MJ. Radiation management of primary carcinoma of the vagina. Cancer 1977; 40:109.

Pride GL, Buchler DA. Carcinoma of the vagina 10 or more years following pelvic irradiation therapy. Am J Obstet Gynecol 1977; 127:513.

Puthawala A, Syed AM, Nalick R, McNamara G, DiSaia PJ. Integrated external and interstitial radiation therapy for primary carcinoma of the vagina. Obstet Gynecol 1983; 62:367–372.

Rutledge FN. Cancer of vagina. Am J Obstet Gynecol 1967; 97:635.

Rutledge FN, Sullican M. Sarcoma botryoides. Ann NY Acad Sci 1967; 142:694.

# CHAPTER 29

# Carcinoma of the Cervix

**Guy I. Benrubi**

Invasive cervical carcinoma is a disease for which definite curable precursor lesions can be identified using a Papanicolaou's (PAP) smear as a screening test. Use of this screening test and diagnostic procedures such as colposcopy, colposcopically directed cervical biopsy, and endocervical curettage accounts for the significant decrease in the incidence of invasive cervical carcinoma. Although improvements in the treatment of invasive cervical carcinoma, especially in radiotherapy and radical surgical techniques, have increased the lifespan of victims with invasive cervical carcinoma, they have not significantly improved the cure rate. Early detection of precursor lesions can, however, prevent the progression from dysplasia to invasive carcinoma. Cervical carcinoma can become virtually eliminated if every woman is regularly and correctly screened with a yearly PAP smear.

## I. Incidence

A. **Cervical cancer** is no longer the most commonly diagnosed gynecologic malignancy, having been surpassed by both endometrial cancer and ovarian cancer. It is annually diagnosed in approximately 16 000 women in the United States, accounting for 20% of malignancies of the female reproductive tract. The median age for invasive cervical cancer is 45, and for carcinoma in situ it is 35. The median ages of both, however, are dropping.

B. **Cervical intraepithelial neoplasia**, a precursor lesion, is diagnosed in approximately 45 000 women annually. The incidence varies between ethnic and socioeconomic groups, being 15 per 100 000 in whites, as opposed to 34 per 100 000 in blacks.

## II. Morbidity and mortality.

Approximately 7000 women die annually in the United States from cervical cancer. There has been a drastic reduction of mortality, but all gains are due to improved screening and not to improved therapy. Invasive cervical cancer requires radical and aggressive modalities of therapy. Consequently, therapeutic morbidity is significant. In women that survive the disease, there is a loss of fertility caused by therapy. This has become an important consideration because preinvasive disease is being diagnosed in younger women and many women are electively postponing childbearing until their third decade.

III. **Etiology and risk factors.** Cervical carcinoma can be thought of as a venereal disease. Whether or not a carcinogenic factor is transmitted during intercourse is of question. The risk factors for venereal disease and cervical carcinoma are strikingly similar, and the woman who is most likely to develop a venereally transmitted malady is also the woman who is most likely to develop cervical dysplasia and, if untreated, invasive carcinoma of the cervix. The ultimate cause of invasive cancer is a failure of health-care delivery. If every woman in the country were properly screened and appropriately treated, invasive cervical cancer death would become as rare as mortality due to measles. The disease has a characteristic and orderly progression pattern, that can be interrupted at several early intervals by therapeutic modalities with acceptable morbidity. Epidemiologic risk factors include:

A. **Low socioeconomic status**

B. **Age at first intercourse.** A woman who first experienced sexual intercourse at age 16 or before has a fivefold greater chance of developing cervical carcinoma than does a woman whose first intercourse was age 24.

C. **Sexual activity.** Patients with more than one sexual partner have a greater propensity toward developing carcinoma of the cervix. This risk increases as the number of sexual partners increases.

D. **Viral agents.** Infections with herpes simplex type II and human papilloma virus (HPV) have been implicated in carcinogenesis in the cervix. Currently, data is conflicting but the developing consensus is that HPV infection is the necessary but not sufficient variable for the start of the process leading to dysplasias and, if untreated, to invasive cancer. Suspected promoters include herpes, smoking, and bacterial vaginosis, the latter because it produces nitrosamines in the vagina.

1. **HPV types 6 and 11** are associated with genital tract infections that do not progress to neoplasia. However, types 16, 18, and 31 are associated with lesions that histologically have abnormal mitoses and on hybridization studies reveal aneuploidy. These lesions are thought to be potentially progressive.
2. **A herpes-specific antigen** has been isolated and associated with invasive cancer. Preliminary studies have shown that titers of this antigen can be used to predict therapeutic response and possible recurrence. Further clinical trials are needed, however.

E. **Carcinogenic sperm.** It has been postulated that some male sperm may be carcinogenic. The histone:protamine ratio of the sperm may be the etiologic factor. Difficulty has been encountered in determining whether this is an independent variable because "carcinogenic sperm" seem to be more prevalent in lower socioeconomic males.

## IV. Pathology and pathogenesis.

**Pathology and pathogenesis.** Histologically, 90% of cervical cancers are squamous, and most of the remainder are adenocarcinomas. The practitioner must be familiar with certain cytologic and histologic terms and the pathologic progressions of cervical dysplasias to understand the pathogenesis of cervical cancer and its precursors.

A. **Squamous metaplasia** is a benign process that occurs in every woman in which areas of the cervix that were covered by columnar epithelium become covered by squamous epithelium. Controversy exists concerning the mechanism by which this transformation is accomplished, although it is probably done by the shedding of the columnar epithelium and its replacement by squamous cells, which differentiate from reserve or immature cells. This process is most active during the adolescent and early reproductive years.

B. **Squamocolumnar (S-C) junction.** The S-C junction is the line at which the columnar epithelium of the endocervix comes in contact with the squamous epithelium of the exocervix. During childhood the S-C junction is found on the portio of the cervix. As the process of squamous metaplasia exerts its effects and starts replacing the columnar epithelium with squamous epithelium, the S-C junction recedes past the os and up into the endocervical canal. In postmenopausal women, the S-C junction may be found high up in the endocervical canal.

C. **Transformation zone.** The area of the portio and endocervical canal originally covered by columnar epithelium but which, through the process of squamous metaplasia, becomes covered by squamous cells is called the transformation zone. It is essentially that part of the cervix between the initial S-C junction and the current S-C junction. Its size may vary from patient to patient. All dysplasias and, therefore, all cervical cancers arise in the transformation zone. As a result, adequate follow-up for an abnormal PAP smear can be done only if the entire transformation zone is meticulously evaluated. Because early age of initial intercourse is a high risk factor, and dysplasia and carcinoma arise in the area of the cervix that has undergone transformation, it is theorized that a carcinogen introduced by intercourse somehow interacts with the "reserve" or immature cells that cause the transformation and leads to dysplasia and carcinoma.

D. **Atypia.** Only one atypical cell is needed for the cytologic diagnosis of atypia. An atypical cell is one in which the nucleus has different characteristics from those of the nucleus of a normal cell. Its nucleus:cytoplasm ratio is greater, and it has a small amount of cytoplasm compared to a normal cell. An abnormal PAP smear (an examination of fixed cells on a slide) means that there are cells on the slide that appear atypical.

E. **Dysplasia.** Normal cervical epithelium, when seen under the microscope, has an orderly appearance, with no atypical cells. The cells closest to the basement membrane look different from those at the top of the epithelium. There is a precise orientation and maturation of the layers of cells as they progress up the epithelium. In dysplasia the cells are atypical and the well-organized, stratified orientation and maturation of the tissue are lost.
   1. **Degrees of dysplasia**
      a. **In mild dysplasia** the outer third of the epithelial tissue shows the above changes.
      b. **In moderate dysplasia** two-thirds of the tissue are involved.
      c. **In severe dysplasia** or **carcinoma in situ** the full thickness of the epithelium shows dysplastic changes.
   2. **PAP smear correlation.** Atypical cells shed from a dysplastic epithelium are found on the PAP smear. When a PAP smear reads as "class III or dysplastic" the pathologist notes that "There are atypical cells on this slide. Experience indicates that this degree of atypia is seen in cells that are shed from a moderately dysplastic epithelium." What must be kept in mind is that a PAP smear is a **cytologic screening tool.** A patient with a Class III smear may have moderate dysplasia or invasive carcinoma. However, these are histologic diagnoses, and they cannot be definitely made until the cervix is biopsied.

F. **Cervical intraepithelial neoplasia (CIN)** is the new terminology for describing dysplastic changes in the cervical epithelium. It implies that mild dysplasia is an early stage in a disease continuum, which, if untreated, will become invasive cancer.
   1. **CIN classifications** correspond approximately to the older descriptive classifications, and like them, are based on cytopathologic description.
      a. **CIN I** corresponds to **mild dysplasia**.
      b. **CIN II** corresponds to **moderate dysplasia**.
      c. **CIN III** corresponds to **severe dysplasia and carcinoma in situ**.

G. **Invasive cervical cancer**
   1. **Metastatic patterns**. The mechanism of spread for invasive cervical cancer is primarily by local extention and by lymphatic dissemination. From the cervix, entention is stepwise to the upper vagina, parametrium, lower vagina, and pelvic side wall. Lymphatic involvement is stepwise, with metastasis appearing first in obturator nodes followed by hypogastric, external iliac, common iliac, and para-aortic nodes. Prior to the use of percutaneous nephrostomy,

death was by ureteral obstruction and uremia. Now it is usually by infection, hemorrhage, lung metastasis, liver metastasis, or debility.

2. **Gross spread patterns**. Tumors may be exophytic and appear to be fungating from the cervix. Other tumors may be excavating and almost the whole cervix may necrose and slough and be replaced by a crater. Still others, especially adenocarcinomas and lesions arising within the endocervical canal, may be endophytic, and the whole diameter of the cervix will grow.

## V. Differential diagnosis.

**V. Differential diagnosis.** Any cervical lesion or process that causes pelvic scarring may be mistaken for cervical cancer.

**A. Common differential diagnoses**

1. Cervicitis
2. Cervical condyloma
3. Endometriosis
4. Other genital neoplasias, especially if metastatic to the cervix
5. Dysfunctional uterine bleeding

**B. Less common differential diagnoses**

1. Chronic pelvic inflammatory disease (PID)
2. Other cervical neoplasias
3. Foreign bodies, particularly neglected pessaries
4. Trauma

**VI. Diagnosis** will ultimately depend on proper interpretation and management of abnormal PAP smears or gross lesions of the cervix.

**A. Signs and symptoms**. Many patients with cervical carcinomas are asymptomatic, although the symptoms that may be caused by cervical cancer are protean. Unfortunately, in early disease these symptoms are often not alarming, resulting in a delay before the patient seeks medical care.

1. **Vaginal bleeding**. The most frequent symptom encountered in cervical cancer is postcoital vaginal bleeding. Unfortunately, patients are more likely to ignore this bleeding than they are to ignore irregular vaginal bleeding, which is also seen in cervical carcinoma.
2. **Vaginal discharge**. Although a vaginal discharge may be associated with cervical cancer of any stage, it is more often seen in large primary tumors with tissue destruction. Such a discharge is frequently associated with a distinct and often unpleasant odor.
3. **Symptoms associated with advanced disease**. In advanced disease, tumor may invade the bowel and/or bladder causing fistulae. The signs and symptoms of urinary and rectal fistulas are the passing of urine or flatus from the vagina. These may be the first symptoms sufficiently disturbing to cause the patient to seek care. With advanced metastatic

disease, systemic signs such as cachexia, weakness, shortness of breath become apparent.

B. **PAP smear**

1. **PAP smear technique**. The patient should be told not to douche prior to coming to the physician, and she should not be menstruating. A two-slide technique is preferable.
   a. A moist cotton swab is placed in the endocervix and is gently twisted.
   b. The swab is then taken out of the vagina and gently rolled over the slide; then the slide should be sprayed with fixative or placed in a fixative containing transport bottle within 10 seconds.
   c. Next, a PAP smear spatula is used to gently scrape the exocervix, and the spatula is scraped over a second slide.
   d. The second slide should be fixed in the same manner.
   e. Alternative sampling techniques such as the cytobrush and Bayne brush reportably aid in obtaining endocervical cells and in some laboratories obviate the need for two slides.
2. **Test accuracy**. There is a 10% to 15% false-negative rate with the PAP smear even under the best of circumstances.
3. **Frequency of PAP smear screening**. Every woman should have an annual pelvic examination with PAP smear from the time of menarche or the onset of sexual activity, whichever comes first. Note that there is currently some controversy as to the proper interval between PAP smears. According to the American Cancer Society: "The Society recommends that all asymptomatic women age 20 and over, and those under 20 who are sexually active, have a PAP test annually for two negative examinations and then at least every three years from age 20 to 40 and annually thereafter." However, the American Cancer Society qualifies this, saying that women at risk of cervical carcinoma should have more frequent PAP smears. One of the risk factors is defined as more than two sexual partners over a lifetime. It is the opinion of the author and editors that many women fall into the "at risk" group. Whereas some women are at lower risk than others, historical identification is often inaccurate, and in any event the false-negative rate for the properly done PAP smear makes repetition of this inexpensive test reasonable and prudent. Thus, as the PAP smear is an inexpensive and nonmorbid procedure, we recommend annual PAP smear examinations.
4. **Evaluation of abnormal PAP smears.** The best hope of preventing invasive carcinoma in a patient is to promptly and thoroughly evaluate an abnormal PAP smear. A common

mistake is to repeat the PAP smear. Because there is a 15% chance of obtaining a false-negative smear, repeating an abnormal smear will often be negative for the patient. The steps to evaluating an abnormal smear follow:

a. The clinician should review the smear with the cytologist to understand what is meant by the assigned classification of the observed abnormality. For example, if it is a Class II smear, are there only inflammatory changes, or is there atypia associated with dysplasia present on the slide? Are the atypical cells seen consistent with an adenomatous or a squamous lesion? By asking the cytopathologist such questions, the clinician gains a full understanding of the abnormal finding and information needed for the next steps of the evaluation.
b. If the abnormalities are thought to be purely inflammatory, the patient can be treated with an anitimicrobial drug and then have the PAP test repeated. To eliminate ambiguous terminology, a workshop was held at the National Cancer Institute in December 1988, and the Bethesda System for reporting cervical vaginal diagnosis was devised.

   The Bethesda System recommends that a cervical/vaginal cytopathology report address each of the following elements:
   (1) A statement of adequacy of the specimen.
   (2) A general categorization of the diagnosis.
   (3) The descriptive diagnosis.
c. Any smear demonstrating atypia that cannot be accounted for on the basis of inflammation must be evaluated further:
   (1) **Colposcopy** with colposcopically directed biopsies of abnormal-appearing areas and endocervical curettage is the next step in the evaluation. An adequate colposcopy presupposes that the colposcopist is well-trained, the colposcope is functioning, and the whole transformation zone (including S-C junction) is completely and thoroughly visualized.
   (2) **Cervical conization** is indicated if:
      (a) The S-C junction is not visualized colposcopically or if the entire transformation zone cannot be evaluated.
      (b) If the colposcopically directed biopsies show a microinvasive carcinoma of the cervix.
      (c) The endocervical curettage reveals dysplastic epithelium.
      (d) The PAP smear suggests the presence of a lesion that cannot be explained on the basis

of the colposcopically directed biopsies.

d. **Dilation and curettage (D & C)**. If an abnormal PAP is not explained on the basis of the colposcopic findings or by the cone biopsy, a fractional D & C should be performed to evaluate for endometrial carcinoma which may, on occasion, be the source of an abnormal PAP smear.

e. **Laparoscopy**. If there is still no explanation for the abnormal PAP smear, a laparoscopy is indicated because adnexal disease such as ovarian carcinoma may cause an abnormal PAP test.

C. **Physical examination** is the primary means of evaluation and clinical classification of cervical carcinomas, and must accomplish three goals.

1. **Assessment of local involvement**. Cervical carcinoma may be confined to the cervix, or it may involve the structures adjacent to the cervix (the parametria), the vagina, and/or the uterine corpus as it spreads by direct extension. Clinical estimation of the size, shape, and degree of extension of the tumor relative to the cervix, uterus, vagina, and structures about the cervix is of the greatest importance. This clinical evaluation must be done by an experienced examiner because the findings may at times be difficult to evaluate as the tumor spreads in an often irregular fashion. Evaluation of extension of tumor to the parametrium and possibly beyond to the pelvic side walls is accomplished by performing a rectovaginal as well as a vaginal bimanual examination. Vaginal bimanual examination alone is not adequate.

2. **Assessment of possible distant spread.** Cervical cancer metastases to distant sites primarily by spread along the lymphatic system and to a lesser extent by hematogenous routes.

   a. **Careful examination of the lymphatic nodes** (especially the groin and supraclavicular nodes) is important if advanced carcinoma is suspected.

   b. **Careful examination of the chest and lungs** is also of special importance because pulmonary involvement is common.

   c. **Examination of the abdomen** for evidence of liver involvement, ascites, or other signs of metastatic carcinoma is required.

3. **Assessment of medical status.** The ability of the patient to undergo either radical surgery or extensive radiation therapy must be evaluated.

D. **Laboratory and diagnostic procedures**

1. **Initial laboratory work-up** will depend on the therapeutic modality chosen. The patient needs to have a good hemoglobin regardless of the treatment selected. Patients should be screened with a complete blood count, serum chemis-

tries, and liver function studies. Pulmonary function studies are good indicators of respiratory health and are useful for those patients with evidence of respiratory compromise.

2. **An IV pyelogram (IVP)** must be done on all patients as extension of the cancer may obstruct the urinary tract. For example, if the ureters are blocked, patients would be inoperable and instead a candidate for other therapy such as radiation.
3. **Cystoscopy** should be considered in all patients because the bladder is a possible site of local spread and treatment is substantially different if it is involved.
4. **Proctoscopy** should also be considered because the rectum is also a site of local tumor spread.
5. **Barium enema (BE) or lower gastrointestinal series.** BE is an optional radiographic study, depending on the clinical findings. It is of greatest value in older patients, to rule out concomitant disease or pathology, such as colitis, that may preclude a particular therapeutic modality such as radiation.
6. **Computerized tomography (CT).** Magnetic resonance imaging and CT imaging is valuable in large or advanced lesions, especially in ruling out nodal and liver metastasis, and retroperitoneal disease. They are probably a waste of money in small early stage lesions.
7. **Lymphangiography** is being increasingly replaced by CT scanning, and is rarely indicated.
8. **Percutaneous needle biopsy**, often under ultrasound or CT scan guidance, is available in many centers. It can be used to demonstrate para-aortic node involvement, which would preclude surgery and mandate radiotherapy directed at a large radiotherapeutic field.

## VII. Clinical staging of cervical carcinoma

As with all carcinoma, management of invasive cervical cancer begins with, and is to a great extent, determined by proper clinical staging. The International Federation of Gynecology and Obstetrics (FIGO) classification of cancer of the cervix is as follows:

**Stage 0** Carcinoma in situ.

**Stage I** The carcinoma is strictly confined to the cervix (extension to the corpus should be disregarded).

**Stage IA** Preclinical carcinomas of the cervix; that is, those diagnosed only by miscroscopy.

**Stage IA1** Minimal microscopically evident stromal invasion.

**Stage IA2** Lesions detected microscopically that can be measured. The upper limit of the measurement should not show a depth of invasion of more than 5 mm taken from the base of the epithelium, either surface or glandular, from which it originates, and a second dimension, the horizontal spread, must not exceed 7 mm. Larger lesions should be staged at IB.

**Stage IB** Lesions of greater dimensions than stage IA2, whether seen clinically or not. Preformed space involvement should not alter the staging but should be specifically recorded so as to determine whether it should affect treatment decisions in the future.

**Stage II** Involvement of the vagina but not out to the sidewall.

**Stage IIA** Involvement of the vagina, but no evidence of parametrial involvement.

**Stage IIB** Infiltration of the parametria but not out to the sidewall.

**Stage III** Involvement of the lower third of the vagina but not out to the pelvic sidewall.

**Stage IIIA** Involvement of the lower third of the vagina but not out to the pelvic sidewall if the parametria are involved.

**Stage IIIB** Involvement of one or both parametria out to the sidewall.

**Stage IIIC** Obstruction of one or both ureters on IVP (urinary) without the other criteria for stage III disease.

**Stage IV** Extension outside the reproductive tract.

**Stage IVA** Involvement of the mucosa of the bladder or rectum.

**Stage IVB** Distant metastasis or disease outside the true pelvis. Note: Despite the new FIGO staging, most centers still use the Society of Gynecologic Oncology (SGO) concept of microinvasive disease. This is frequently defined as invasion limited to 3 mm below the basement membrane with no invasion into vascular or lymphatic spaces, and no deep tissue tongues.

## VIII. Management

**A. Management of CIN.** The management of CIN lesions is based upon the thorough evaluation of the abnormal PAP smear findings, either by complete satisfactory colposcopy (colposcopy with colposcopically directed biopsy if indicated) or cervical conization.

1. **CIN I (mild dysplasia)**
    a. **Excisional biopsy of a focal lesion.** If the lesion is focal, often all that is necessary is excisional biopsy under colposcopic direction.
    b. **Cryosurgery.** If a lesion is more extensive, cryotherapy may be used provided the colposcopic evaluation has been adequate and the most abnormal areas have been biopsied.

c. **Laser vaporization** can be used in the same manner as cryotherapy and is as effective as cryotherapy although more expensive in most practice situations. It offers an advantage in the treatment of cervices with anatomic distortions and has less of a tendency to drive the S-C junction up the endocervical canal, thus making future evaluations easier.

2. **CIN II (moderate dysplasia)** can be treated in a manner similar to CIN I.
3. **CIN III (severe dysplasia or carcinoma in situ)**
   a. **Hysterectomy.** If the patient does not wish to bear children or has completed her family, CIN III is often treated by hysterectomy, either vaginal or abdominal. Hysterectomy is also indicated if the patient has other uterine or adnexal pathology that requires surgical intervention.
   b. **Conization of the cervix.** If further fertility is desired, or the patient feels strongly against hysterectomy, a conization with endocervical curettage is done. This will be a therapeutic as well as diagnostic procedure if pathologic analysis of the specimen shows only dysplasia whereas further treatment will be needed if invasive carcinoma is discovered.
   c. **Cryosurgery or laser vaporization.** When there is no question that colposcopy is adequate, there is confidence in the competence of the colposcopist and in the pathologist who has read the directed biopsy specimens, the patient has been adequately informed of all the risks, and there is no dysplasia in endocervical glands (where cryosurgery may not destroy abnormal cells), a cryosurgical or laser vaporization procedure may be done rather than cervical conization or hysterectomy. The qualifiers must be rigidly observed, however, because these procedures do not produce a specimen for pathologic evaluation. By following these criteria, the clinician minimizes the chance of inappropriately treating an early invasive carcinoma.

B. **Follow-up of CIN.** One of the most important aspects of CIN treatment is the follow-up process after therapy has been completed. A PAP smear should be repeated every 3 to 4 months during the first year and every 6 months during the second year posttreatment. Some physicians suggest that an endocervical curettage be performed in those patients treated by cervical conization of cryotherapy because there is a tendency for the S-C junction to be inverted in these patients.

C. **Management of invasive cervical carcinoma.** For years the standard therapy for cervical carcinoma was radiation therapy. With increasing availability of trained pelvic surgeons and with the improved anesthesia, antibiotics, and ancillary care facilities in modern medical centers, radical pelvic surgery is now playing a major role in the treatment of early stage disease. Chemotherapy is now also used as adjunctive therapy in the treatment of some cases of advanced cervical carcinoma. The decision of which modalities should be used is individualized, and depends on the patient's age, presentation of the tumor, medical status, and personal preference. When all the other factors are equal, the decision is often based on which department (radiotherapy or gynecology) has the best-trained personnel. In broad terms, appropriate therapy by stage of invasive cervical carcinoma may be generalized as shown in Table 29.1 (see clinical staging of cervical carcinoma section, VII for staging criteria).

## IX. Therapy

A. **Simple hysterectomy.** Extrafascial hysterectomy is sufficient therapy for microinvasive cervical carcinoma because the incidence of lymph node metastasis is negligible.

B. **Radical hysterectomy with node dissection**

1. **Rationale.** The rationale for a radical hysterectomy for stage IB or IIA cervical carcinoma is to remove the uterus and adequate vaginal cuff and the parametria en bloc to ensure removal of all tumor. The dissection is delicate because the ureters run through the parametria. Therefore, they must be dissected out of their paracervical tunnel prior to removal of the specimen. A pelvic lymphadenectomy and a para-aortic node sampling are routinely added to the radical hysterectomy. The para-aortic node sam-

**Table 29.1. Suggested Therapy by Stage of Disease for Cervical Carcinoma**

| STAGE | THERAPY |
|---|---|
| Microinvasive*,† | Simple hysterectomy, or cone biopsy |
| Stage IB‡ or IIA | Radical hysterectomy and node dissection or radiation therapy |
| Stage IIB | Radiation therapy |
| Stage IIIA | Radiation therapy |
| Stage IIIB | Radiation therapy |
| Stage IVA | Primary pelvic exenteration |
| Stage IVB | Individualized therapy: palliative radiation and/or palliative surgery and/or chemotherapy. |

*Increasingly new evidence has accumulated indicating microinvasive carcinoma can be treated adequately with conization only. Definitive clinical trials have not been completed.

†In the case of an endophytic lesion, leading to a barrel-shaped lesion, radiation therapy must be followed by a simple hysterectomy.

‡In stage IB lesions greater than 4 cm in diameter, the recurrence rate after radical hysterectomy is inordinately high. These lesions are probably best treated by radiation. In some selected young patients with large clinically stage IB lesions, a pretreatment extraperitoneal para-aortic node sampling can be done to map the treatment fields for radiation therapy.

pling is done first. The nodes are sent for frozen section. If there is a tumor present, the procedure is terminated and radiation therapy is given.

2. **Complications.** The complications of radical hysterectomy (if there are any) appear early.
    a. **Intraoperatively** the main problem that can arise is excessive bleeding.
    b. **Postoperative.**
        (1) **Fistula formation.** As the ureter is dissected out of its tunnel, it becomes denuded and part of its vascular supply is disrupted. A ureterovaginal fistula may result. Depending on the operator and how radical the procedure, the ureterovaginal fistula rate varies from 1% to 3% of all cases, with the former being the more accepted rate. A vesicovaginal fistula is also a possible complication.
        (2) **Bladder denervation** occurs after a radical hysterectomy, requiring bladder drainage for at least 2 weeks or until it can resume normal function. In some cases this may take months.

C. **Radiation therapy** is effective in cervical carcinoma because, although squamous carcinoma is a relatively radioresistant tumor, the cervix and uterus can tolerate extremely high doses of radiation. Thus, effective radiation doses may be administered to cervical cancers without destruction of the surrounding tissues.

1. **Radiation therapy delivery systems.** There are many different systems of radiation delivery. Broadly, they combine external beam radiation with brachytherapy or intracavitary cesium implants. One of the systems used bases its dosimetry on an imaginary point in the pelvis called point A. It is defined as a point located 2 cm from the midline of the cervical canal and 2 cm superior to the lateral vaginal fornix. There is also point B, defined as 3 cm lateral to point A. This system aims to deliver about 70 Gy to 80 Gy to point A and 50 Gy to 60 Gy to point B. This can be done with 45 Gy to 50 Gy whole pelvic radiation (i.e., every point in the pelvis receives minimum of 45 Gy to 50 Gy) followed by a cesium implant that will deliver a further 20 Gy to 30 Gy to point A. Under such a system, the tumor dose on the cervix may approach 200 Gy.
2. **Complications of radiation therapy** are divided into immediate and delayed problems.
    a. **Immediate complications** are nausea and diarrhea. They can be controlled by a combination of antiemetic and antidiarrheal medications and delay of subsequent radiation treatments.
        (1) **Antidiarrheal medication.** Diphenoxylate (Lomotil), a combination medication containing 2.5

mg diphenoxylate hydrochloride and 0.025 mg atropine sulfate, is an excellent antidiarrheal. It is usually given in an oral adult dosage of 5 mg p.o. t.i.d. or q.i.d. The addition of an antiemetic is helpful.

(2) Antiemetic prochlorperazine (Compazine) is available in the following preparations:
   (a) **Injectable solution** of mg/mL in 2 mL and 10 mL containers, usually given in an adult dose of 5 to 10 mg IM q3–4 h, not to exceed 40 mg/d total dose.
   (b) **Rectal suppositories** of 2.5, 5, and 25 mg sizes, usually given in an adult dose of 25 mg per rectum b.i.d.
   (c) **Tablet form:** 5,10, or 25 mg per tablet.
   (d) **Timed-release capsules:** 10, 15, 30, or 75 mg per capsule.

b. **Long-term complications** appear from 6 to 18 months after completion of radiation therapy. They include rectal ulcers, chronic hemorrhagic proctitis, rectovaginal fistulas, sigmoid obstruction, small bowel (enteroentero) fistulas, hemorrhagic cystitis, and others. Fortunately, when dealing with small tumors, the doses of radiation can be kept low, thus reducing the risk of complications. However, frequently complications can be severe, requiring surgical intervention such as colostomy or bowel resection.

**D. Follow-up care.** Patients are seen every 6 weeks during the first year, every 8 weeks during the second year, every 3 months during the third year and semi-annually thereafter.

1. PAP smear and careful pelvic exam including recto-vaginal assessment are done on each visit.
2. Node-bearing areas including groin and supraclavicular regions are carefully palpated at each visit.
3. Depending on the therapy used, signs and symptoms associated with possible complications are sought.
4. VP is done annually for at least the first 3 years.
5. Chest radiography is done annually for at least the first 5 years.

**E. Management of recurrence**

1. **Local recurrences** are the most commonly encountered recurrences. Treatment depends on the initial treatment of the lesion.
   a. **Radiation.** If the patient was originally treated with surgery, recurrence can be treated with radiation and the 5-year survival is around 25%. If radiation was the original treatment, re-radiation is not possible as the abdominal and pelvic organs have already reached maximum doses.
   b. **Pelvic exenteration.** In carefully selected patients,

pelvic exenteration may be the procedure of choice, carrying a 5-year survival after pelvic exenteration of 35% to 40%. This extensive operation involves removal of the bladder, rectum, uterus, and vagina. A colostomy, ileal conduit, and, in some cases, vaginal reconstruction are part of the procedure. Pelvic exenteration is an extremely morbid procedure.

(1) **Preoperative evaluation.** Prior to its initiation, a thorough evaluation must be done to ensure that the patient is emotionally and physically able to withstand the operation. A metastatic work-up, including liver scan, bone scan, IVP, BE, CT scan, scalene node biopsy, and fine needle aspiration of suspicious retroperitoneal nodes must be done, as patients with such distant metastases almost always die and hence are not candidates for pelvic exenteration.

(2) **Surgical procedure.** If the pelvic side walls are involved with tumor, surgery cannot be done.

(a) On starting an exenteration, peritoneal surfaces in the abdomen are checked first. If there is tumor on any peritoneal surface, the operation is temporarily stopped.

(b) A node dissection is then done and all nodes are sent for frozen section. If any are positive, the operation is stopped.

(c) If the pelvic side walls are involved with tumor, the operation is terminated.

(d) By proper "surgical selection" preoperatively and intraoperatively, the 5-year survival after exenteration is 35% to 40%.

c. **Re-irradiation.** In some centers, patients with late (20 years) local recurrences are being re-irradiated with some success.

2. **Distant recurrence.** In the face of distant recurrence (metastasis), the clinician can only hope for palliation. Rarely does a patient with squamous cell carcinoma metastases survive. If metastatic lesions (e.g., lung, bone) cause discomfort, radiation can be directed to specific areas to attempt to reduce tumor size and thereby decrease discomfort. Chemotherapy may be used, although it is less than satisfactory for even palliation. The most active agent now available is cisplatin. There has been some limited success in terms of tumor response to the use of combinations of bleomycin, methotrexate, vincristine, etoposide, and ifosfamide.

## X. Prognosis

A. **Five-year survival rates.** Although some variation is reported between institutions, radiation therapy and surgery have identical 5-year survival rates (see Table 29.2).

**Table 29.2. Survival by Stage for Cervical Carcinoma**

| STAGE | 5-YEAR SURVIVAL RATE |
|---|---|
| Microinvasive | 98% to 100% |
| Stage IB and IIA | 85%<br>If positive pelvic nodes are discovered on surgery, cure rate drops to 40% |
| Stage IIB | 35% |
| Stage III | 20% |
| Stage IV | 10% |

**B. Factors affecting survival**

1. Rarely does a patient have long-term survival if the para-aortic nodes are found to contain tumor at the start of radical hysterectomy and node dissection, whether or not they are treated with radiation therapy.
2. In stage IB disease, even if nodes are negative for metastasis and margins of resection are free of disease, there is high recurrence rate if the tumor is large, and if the tumor invades deeply into the stroma of the cervix. Whether the prognosis can be improved by adding adjunctive whole pelvic radiation in cases of deep stromal penetration found on pathologic examination is questionable.

## BIBLIOGRAPHY


Baird PF. The role of human papilloma and other viruses. Clin Obstet Gynecol 1985; 12:19–32.

Barber HRK. Relative prognostic significance of preoperative and operative findings in pelvic exenteration. Surg Clin North Am 1969; 49:431.

Beral V. Cancer of the cervix: A sexually transmitted infection? Lancet 1974; 1:1037.

Coppleson M. The diagnosis and treatment of early (preclinical) invasive cancer. Clin Obstet Gynecol 1985; 12:149–68.

Fink DJ. Changes in the American Cancer Society check-up guidelines for the detection of cervical cancer. Cancer 1988; 38:127.

Johnston M, Benrubi G, Nuss R. Age and cervical dysplasia. South Med J 1988; 81:1458.

Lemon K, Nuss R, Benrubi G. Repeat cytology of women with interested atypical Papanicolaou smears. Coloscopy Gynecol Laser Supply 1987; 3:177.

Spanos W, King A, Keeney E, Wagner R, Slater JM. Age as a prognostic factor in carcinoma of the cervix. Gynecol Oncol 1989; 36:66.

# CHAPTER 30

# Carcinoma of the Uterus

**Guy I. Benrubi**

## ADENOCARCINOMA OF THE ENDOMETRIUM

Endometrial carcinoma is the most common gynecologic malignancy. If diagnosed promptly, it is also the most readily curable with therapeutic modalities that are well-tolerated by the patient.

I. **Incidence.** Carcinoma of the endometrium is the most common gynecologic malignancy, with more than 38 000 new cases diagnosed annually. The lifetime risk for developing this disease is 2.2% among whites and 1.1% in blacks. The average age for endometrial carcinoma is 60 years, although 10% of these cancers occur in women under 40. Women between 50 and 60 years of age are at greatest risk. This age distribution is important as there are currently 40 million women in the United States over age 50, a number that should double in the next 15 to 20 years as the baby boom generation reaches maturity. It is therefore obvious that the gynecologist will see more and more of this disease. The incidence rates for endometrial carcinoma rose throughout the early 1970s, although they now appear to be stabilizing. There was a 50% increase (one and one-half-fold) in the incidence of endometrial carcinoma during the 1970s, despite a 30% hysterectomy rate in women under age 70.

II. **Morbidity and mortality.** More than 3000 women die yearly from this disease. Because the average age at diagnosis is 60, there is minimal morbidity to reproductive potential. However, because these patients are older and often obese, they are relatively suboptimal surgical and radiation therapy candidates. Adjuvant radiation therapy is indicated in many patients with this disease. Because this therapy must be given in conjunction with surgical treatment, morbidity to intraabdominal tissues, particularly small bowel, may be significant. Fortunately, neither the operative procedure nor the radiotherapy need be as extensive as that required for the treatment of cervical carcinoma. However, typical patients with uterine cancer are older and they may have medical problems that put them at higher risk for postoperative complications, including myocardial infarction, pulmonary embolus, phlebitis, wound infection and dehiscence, and atelectasis and pneumonia.

III. **Etiology and risk factors.** Adenocarcinoma of the endometrium includes two distinct diseases. The first component of endometrial cancer may be a cancer that is estrogen dependent and results from an endocrinopathy. The second may be a hormonally independent tumor. This concept of two distinct diseases is becoming increasingly important in modern treatment regimens. In any event, certain risk factors are associated with endometrial carcinoma. Obesity, nulliparity, hypertension, late menopause, diabetes, infertility, polycystic ovaries, and postmenopausal estrogen use have all been implicated as risk factors. It is difficult to differentiate between independent risk factor and concomitant ones. Note that, just as cervical carcinoma can be thought of as a venereal disease, most endometrial carcinomas can be seen as due to an endocrinopathy.

A. **Obesity** is the most important risk factor for development of endometrial carcinoma. The increased risk is three times normal for those women 20 to 60 lb overweight and nine times normal for those greater than 50 lb overweight. The presumed mechanism is conversion of androstenedione to estrone by fat cells, with subsequent conversion to estradiol, which has a deleterious effect on the endometrium. Another view is that obesity is just a reflection of a general hormonal imbalance that may have endometrial carcinoma as one of its manifestations.

B. **Nulliparity and infertility.** It has been epidemiologically difficult to decide whether pregnancy bestows protection against endometrial carcinoma or whether the increased incidence of this disease among nulliparous women is an additional manifestation of the previously mentioned general hormonal imbalance — an imbalance that makes those women obese, hypertensive, diabetic, and infertile. One study has shown that married nulliparous women have a higher risk of developing this disease than do unmarried women or married, parous women. This implies that infertility, rather than parity, may be the important factor. However, studies show that the use of oral contraceptives for 1 year bestows a protective effect, possibly indicating that the hormonal changes during pregnancy may be important in preventing this disease.

C. **Early menarche and late menopause.** Women whose menarche occurred before age 12 have been shown to have a 1.6-fold increase in risk for developing endometrial carcinoma compared to women who have menarche after age 12. Women who undergo menopause after age 52 have 2.4 times the risk of developing endometrial carcinoma compared to those women who experience menopause at age 49 or younger.

However, not all studies looking at these questions have confirmed these findings. **Note:** The three risk factors other than postmenopausal estrogen use that are most clearly implicated are obesity, nulliparity, and late menopause. Their effects seem to be additive so that a woman who is nulliparous, is 50 lb overweight, and experienced menopause after age 52 is five times more likely to develop endometrial cancer than a woman who is parous, of normal weight, and who had menopause before age 49.

D. **Postmenopausal estrogens.** Since the middle of the 1970s there have been several retrospective studies showing that postmenopausal estrogen replacement therapy, when estrogen is used alone without a progestational drug, increases the risk of developing endometrial cancer from fourfold to ninefold. The proportional increase in risk is greater for women without other risk factors than it is for women with those risk factors. However, estrogen use imparts an additive risk to those women who are obese and nulliparous. In view of the well-documented deleterious effect of estrogen, the use of postmenopausal estrogen should follow the guidelines discussed in Chapter 22—Menopause and the Climacteric, including the use of a progestational agent. For those endometrial adenocarcinomas that seem to be related to the hormonal milieu, the operant variable may be the total lifetime ratio of estrogen to progesterone exposure. The greater the total lifetime of progesterone exposure either by pregnancy or exogenous medication, the smaller the risk for endometrial adenocarcinoma.

E. **Hypertension.** The association between high blood pressure and endometrial carcinoma has been widely studied. From one-third to three-fourths of patients with endometrial carcinoma have been noted to be hypertensive. It has been difficult to answer whether this is a concomitant factor secondary to obesity. One study concluded that when controlled for obesity, hypertension as a risk factor persisted to some extent.

F. **Polycystic ovary syndrome.** Women with chronic anovulation have been found to develop endometrial carcinoma at a much earlier age than the remainder of the female population. They account for most of the cases diagnosed before age 40. In some series, 25% to 40% of the women with polycystic ovaries were noted to have developed this disease. In these patients, the use of oral contraceptives, in theory, might be helpful in preventing the development of endometrial carcinoma. It remains to be seen, however, whether long-term use of oral contraceptives is indeed protective in this group of women.

G. **Diabetes mellitus.** The association between diabetes and endometrial carcinoma has not been confirmed although it has been clinically touted for many years. There are some studies that show up to 20% incidence of diabetes mellitus in patients with endometrial carcinoma vs. 3% in controls, but its role as an independent risk factor has yet to be clearly defined.

## IV. Pathogenesis

A. **Precursor lesions.** Agreement among cancer specialists is fairly unanimous that cervical dysplasia is a precursor lesion of cervical carcinoma and that both have a high likelihood of being an infectious venereal disease. In contrast, there is still considerable controversy as to what constitutes a comparable precancerous lesion for endometrial cancer and as to what may cause either or both conditions. Many investigators agree there is a spectrum of disease leading from benign to precancerous endometrial changes. They agree that these changes are likely to be associated in some way with the effect of excessive, endogenous, unopposed estrogen. The lesions are classified into two groups: cystic hyperplasia and carcinoma in situ of the endometrium. Some oncologists, however, consider cystic hyperplasia an atrophic change and, therefore, not really part of this spectrum of disease. Others never use the designation "carcinoma in situ." There is further controversy over whether adenomatous hyperplasia without atypia does or does not progress to endometrial carcinoma. Different studies have found various progression rates for the components of the spectrum of disease. These range from 5% to 40% progression to invasion, with the most atypical lesion being the most likely to invade.

B. **Histology**

1. **Adenocarcinoma.** Most endometrial carcinomas are adenocarcinomas. They are graded according to their appearance, with good correlation between grade and prognosis.
   a. **Grade 1** (well-differentiated adenocarcinomas) have a glandular pattern with atypical cells.
   b. **Grade 2** (moderately differentiated adenocarcinomas) show a glandular pattern with some partly solid areas.
   c. **Grade 3** (undifferentiated [poorly differentiated] adenocarcinomas) are characterized by the absence of a glandular pattern that is replaced by sheets of atypical cells.
2. **Clear cell adenocarcinoma.** About 5% of patients with adenocarcinoma have the clear cell variety. Clear cell adenocarcinoma tends to be at a more advanced stage than a comparable adenocarcinoma at the same time of diagnosis.
3. **Adenoacanthoma.** In about 15% of patients there is benign squamous metaplasia associated with an adenocarcinoma. These tumors, called adenoacanthomas, tend to behave somewhat less aggressively than adenocarcinoma as the glandular elements are usually well-differentiated.
4. **Adenosquamous carcinoma.** In about 12% of patients the tumor has both glandular and squamous elements that are malignant, adenosquamous carcinoma. Adenosquamous

carcinoma tends to occur in an older age group and is an aggressive tumor, as the cellular elements are poorly differentiated.

5. **Papillary adenocarcinoma.** Another variant of endometrial adenocarcinoma is the papillary adenocarcinoma that has a histologic appearance similar to a serous cystadenocarcinoma. These tumors tend to be more aggressive in clinical behavior than the glandular tumors.

C. **Spread pattern.** Endometrial carcinoma spreads by local extension to the myometrium, the cervix and the adnexa. Lymphatic spread of this cancer involves the pelvic nodes, primarily the external iliac chain, and the para-aortic area. Distant metastasis of endometrial carcinoma is either by lymphatic or hematogenous routes. When the latter involves metastasis to the lungs, the outcome is usually fatal.

## V. Differential diagnosis

### A. Common problems

1. **Postmenopausal atrophy** of any part or all of the lower genital tract may lead to postmenopausal bleeding and suspicion of cancer.
2. **Endometrial hyperplasia** causing irregular or postmenopausal bleeding.
3. **Dysfunctional uterine bleeding,** especially in women above age 40.

### B. Less common problems

1. Other genital neoplasias, especially endocervical lesions.
2. Genital infections, especially in older women.

## VI. Diagnosis

### A. Signs and symptoms

1. **Vaginal bleeding** is the most frequent historical finding in endometrial carcinoma.
   a. **Postmenopausal bleeding** has an especially high association with endometrial carcinoma, and indeed a postmenopausal woman with vaginal bleeding is presumed to have endometrial carcinoma until further diagnostic evaluation proves or disproves this clinical suspicion.
   b. **Irregular or profuse vaginal bleeding** in perimenopausal or late reproductive-age patients should similarly be regarded with great suspicion for endometrial carcinoma.
2. **Pressure symptoms from a mass lesion.** In more advanced stages, the cancer may present as a pelvic or adnexal mass, or as parametrial induration, although gross extension to the cervix is uncommon. Such involvement may cause pressure symptoms (pelvic pressure from the enlarged uter-

us, pain from the same cause, pressure upon the bladder or ureters or upon the bowel).

B. **Physical examination**

1. **Careful pelvic examination** is performed to help assess the stage of an endometrial carcinoma, including attention to the size and shape of the cervix, uterus, and adnexal structures, and the characteristics of the parametria, uterosacral ligaments, and pelvic side walls.
2. **Rectovaginal examination** is necessary to adequately examine the parametria, uterosacral ligaments, and pelvic side walls.
3. **Examination of the breast and rectum** are essential to evaluate for extension of neoplasia.
4. **General physical examination** is also essential to assess the patient's ability to withstand surgery, with special emphasis on cardiovascular function. Examination of lymph nodes, including those in the groin, axillae, and supraclavicular areas, should be performed.

C. **Laboratory examinations and diagnostic procedures**

1. **Endometrial screening tests.** As in all cancers, the earlier the diagnosis, the more efficacious the treatment. In cervical carcinoma, an excellent screening method in the form of the Papanicolaou (PAP) smear exists, but no similarly easy and accurate method exists for endometrial carcinoma screening.
   a. **Routine screening.** There is much controversy over the frequency and method of endometrial screening.
      (1) **Methods.** Endometrial asperation techniques are generally well-tolerated and preferred. These aspiration techniques (e.g., Vabra, Pipelle) yield an histologic, not a cytologic, sample and in some series have been shown to be as effective as a dilation and curettage (D & C) in identifying the presence of hyperplasia and/or carcinoma. A PAP smear is inadequate as a screening test for endometrial pathology. Four quadrant endometrial biopsy with the Novak or Kevorkian curette is probably 90% effective in diagnosing precursor lesions, but it is too painful a method for routine screening purposes.
      (2) **Frequency.** The frequency of routine endometrial sampling has to be individualized according to the clinical situation of each patient. Those women who demonstrate many risk factors for development of endometrial carcinoma should have endometrium sampling performed by such a screening test once a year. Low-risk women probably do not have to be sampled unless there

is postmenopausal bleeding or an abnormal pelvic examination.

b. **Endometrial sampling in postmenopausal bleeding.** Whether the most common cause of postmenopausal bleeding is atrophy of the endometrium or endometrial hyperplasia and carcinoma is a controversial point. Nevertheless, there is agreement that in the presence of postmenopausal bleeding, the endometrium should be sampled. If office endometrial biopsy does not show carcinoma, some physicians believe a D & C must be done to completely rule out that possibility. However, other investigators believe that endometrial sampling is adequate, and would only perform a D & C if the bleeding were persistent or recurrent, and could not be controlled with hormonal replacement. Because early endometrial carcinoma is symptomatic, this disease is most often diagnosed in stage I and, therefore, is curable in the vast majority of cases. Thus the most important aspect of early diagnosis is the thorough and prompt evaluation of all postmenopausal bleeding.

2. **Metastatic work-up.** If a patient is found to have endometrial carcinoma on endometrial biopsy, a preoperative metastatic work-up should be performed, or, if the cancer is discovered at surgery, performed in the postoperative time. Such a work-up is individualized to the clinical status of the patient based on the clinical experience of the physician.
   a. **Intravenous pyelogram** is performed to rule out side wall or parametrial metastasis as well as assess the urinary tract for possible obstruction and/or involvement with tumor.
   b. **Barium enema.** Patients with endometrial cancer have an increased incidence of bowel carcinoma. A barium enema is needed to rule out concomitant carcinoma of the large bowel or the less common case in which the gynecologic tumor involves the bowel. It is also useful to allow diagnosis of conditions such as diverticulitis, which preclude radiotherapy.
   c. **Chest radiography.** A chest x-ray is important both in determining the cardiovascular status of the patient and in ruling out metastasis. The lungs are the most frequently involved distal organ.
   d. **Computerized tomography (CAT).** A CAT scan with special attention to node-bearing areas has some value but can be dispensed with if time or finances do not permit its use. The value of this test is slowly increasing as experience with its use accumulates.
   e. **Magnetic resonance imaging** in some centers is being

used for preoperative determination of myometrial penetration status.

3. **Other tests.** As most patients with endometrial cancer are elderly and overweight, laboratory tests to assess the patient's ability to withstand therapy are also indicated. In addition to general testing for medical status, such evaluation should include an electrocardiogram and for most patients pulmonary function studies.

## VII. Staging of endometrial carcinoma

The initial step to all cancer therapy is staging. The International Federation of Gynecology and Obstetrics (FIGO) classification of endometrial carcinoma is the most widely used and useful classification of endometrial carcinoma. The new FIGO staging is surgical, and not clinical.

| A. | **Corpus cancer staging** |
|---|---|
| IA G 1,2,3 | Tumor limited to endometrium |
| IB G 1,2,3 | Invasion to $<1/2$ myometrium |
| IC G 1,2,3 | Invasion $>1/2$ myometrium |
| IIA G 1,2,3 | Endocervical glandular involvement only |
| IIB G 1,2,3 | Cervical stromal invasion |
| IIIA G 1,2,3 | Tumor invades serosa and/or adnexae and/or positive peritoneal cytology |
| IIIB G 1,2,3 | Vaginal metastases |
| IIIC G 1,2,3 | Metastases to pelvic and/or para-aortic lymph nodes |
| IVA G 1,2,3 | Tumor invasion bladder and/or bowel mucosa |
| IVB | Distant metastases including intra-abdominal and/or inguinal lymph node |

1. **Special notes on staging histopathology—degree of differentiation.** Cases of carcinoma of the corpus should be grouped with regard to the degree of differentiation of the adenocarcinoma as follows:
   - G1 = 5% or less of a nonsquamous or nonmorular solid growth pattern
   - G2 = 6% to 50% of a nonsquamous or nonmorular solid growth pattern
   - G3 = more than 50% of a nonsquamous or nonmorular solid growth pattern
2. **Pathological grading**
   a. Notable nuclear atypia, inappropriate for the architectural grade, raises the grade of a grade 1 or grade 2 tumor by 1 grade.
   b. In serous adenocarcinomas, clear cell adenocarcinomas, and squamous cell carinomas, nuclear grading takes precedence.

c. Adenocarcinomas with squamous differentiation are graded according to the nuclear grade of the glandular component.

3. **Other rules related to staging**
   a. Since corpus cancer is now surgically staged, procedures previously used for determination of stages are no longer applicable, such as the finding of fractional D & C to differentiate between stage I and stage II.
   b. It is appreciated that there may be a small number of patients with corpus cancer who will be treated primarily with radiation therapy. If that is the case, the clinical staging adopted by FIGO in 1971 would still apply but designation of that staging system would be noted.
   c. Ideally, width of the myometrium should be measured along with the width of tumor invasion.

## VIII. Management

**A. Management of precursor lesions** (endometrial hyperplasia). The management of precursor lesions is controversial. What must be kept in mind, however, is the age of the patient and the histologic appearance of the lesion. The more atypical the lesion histologically and/or the older the patient, the more often surgical rather than conservative therapy is appropriate. Factors influencing the management of precursor lesions include:

1. Patients who desire future fertility can be treated by estrogen–progestin combinations to ensure regular endometrial shedding. Any of the standard 35 or 50 μg estrogen oral contraceptives may be used for this purpose. These patients are anovulatory during the time of treatment, but when pregnancy is desired ovulation can be induced by the use of clomiphene citrate (Clomid) or menotropins (Pergonal).
2. In patients who have completed childbearing or women in the late reproductive years and/or women with more atypical lesions, hysterectomy should be considered.
3. If biopsy reveals moderate or severe atypical hyperplasia, hysterectomy and bilateral salpingo-oophorectomy should be recommended.
4. If biopsy reveals hyperplasia without atypia, progestins can be used (500 mg of medroxyprogesterone acetate suspension [Depo-Provera] IM monthly, medroxyprogesterone acetate [Provera] 20/mg d, or megestral acetate, [Megace] 160 mg/d in divided doses). Hormonal therapy should be continued for 3 to 6 months. Up to 20% of these lesions will progress despite hormonal therapy; up to 60% will remit. The endometrium should be sampled again, preferably by a suction curettage (e.g., Pipelle) or D & C, after 3 months and again at 6 months.

5. **Postmenopausal women.** The recommended treatment has been hysterectomy and bilateral salpingo-oophorectomy for any postmenopausal woman with atypical adenomatous hyperplasia, who is an operative candidate.
6. **Evaluation for coexisting ovarian disease.** In all women with hyperplasia, careful evaluation of the ovaries should be done to rule out coexisting hormone-producing ovarian neoplasia.

B. **Management of invasive endometrial cancer**

1. **General principles of therapy.** What constitutes proper management of invasive endometrial carcinoma is a question without a definitive answer; however certain principles are agreed to by most oncologists:
   a. The mainstay of therapy in stage I cancer is total abdominal hysterectomy and bilateral salpingo-oophorectomy. In more advanced stages of endometrial carcinoma, individualized regimens combining surgery and/or radiation therapy and/or chemotherapy are recommended.
   b. Radiation therapy alone does not cure the disease. In vitro, it is just as sensitive as squamous carcinoma of the cervix. However, in vivo there is no practical way to deliver to the endometrium the dosage necessary for eradication.
   c. The histologic grading of the tumor is a crucial prognostic factor. Size of the uterus is not significant as a prognostic factor, whereas the depth of myometrial invasion and metastasis to pelvic and para-aortic lymph nodes are major determinants of recurrence.
2. **Stage I.** The questions in the treatment of stage I lesions are whether to add radiation therapy to surgery, and, if added, whether to do it before or after surgery and whether to give whole pelvis or vaginal radiation. At the same time, the role of routine lymphadenectomy is also in the process of being defined. A recommended scheme of treatment for stage I lesions, based on tumor grade and for variants of endometrial carcinoma, follows.
   a. **Grade I tumors**
      (1) Because the incidence of lymph node metastasis is only 2% in stage I, grade 1 tumors, a total abdominal hysterectomy, bilateral salpingo-oophorectomy, and peritoneal washing for cytologic evaluation should be done without routine pelvic node sampling.
      (2) If there is no myometrial invasion or if there is only minimal (less than 50% of myometrial thickness) invasion, no further therapy is needed.
      (3) If there is greater than 50% myometrial penetration, 50 Gy whole pelvic radiation is given.

b. **Grade 2 tumors.** The chance of lymph node metastasis is 10% in stage I, Grade 2 tumors.
   (1) A total abdominal hysterectomy and bilateral salpingo-oophorectomy with selective para-aortic and pelvic lymph node dissections are done.
   (2) If the lymph nodes are negative for metastatic tumor and there is no myometrial invasion, no further therapy is given.
   (3) If there is minimal invasion with negative nodes, still no adjuvant therapy is necessary.
   (4) If there is deep myometrial invasion or metastasis to pelvic nodes, whole pelvic radiation is administered.
   (5) If para-aortic nodes are positive, progestational or chemotherapeutic agents are added, depending on the estrogen/progesterone receptor assay of the main tumor. If a receptor assay is unavailable, progestational agents are given.

c. **Grade 3 tumors**
   (1) A total abdominal hysterectomy and bilateral salpingo-oophorectomy with para-aortic and pelvic lymphadenectomy are done.
   (2) Since the incidence of lymph node metastasis is 25% to 30%, radiation therapy is added for the same indication as in grade 2 lesions.

d. **Adenosquamous carcinomas** are treated the same as are grade 2 and 3 lesions.

e. **Positive peritoneal cell washings**
   (1) Patients who have positive peritoneal cell washings are at risk for peritoneal recurrence and can be treated with either progestational agents or chemotherapy.
   (2) If positive cytology is the only adverse risk factor, patients can be treated with intraperitoneal chronic phosphate ($P_{32}$).

**3. Stage II.** For stage II disease with a gross lesion on the cervix, the treatment is similar to that for stage IB carcinoma of the cervix (see Chapter 29—Carcinoma of the Cervix).

   a. If the patient is medically able to withstand extensive surgery, a radical hysterectomy can be done.
   b. If the patient is not able to withstand extensive surgery, 40 Gy to 50 Gy whole pelvic radiation is given, followed by an intracavitary cesium application of approximately 20 Gy to 30 Gy to point A, followed in 6 weeks by an extrafascial hysterectomy.
   c. If there is a sub-clinical stage II, exploratory laparotomy is done and then adjuvant radiation is tailored to the disease.

4. **Stages III and IV.** Therapy for stages III and IV must be individualized under the guidance of a gynecologic oncologist.
   a. If there is disease in the adnexa, surgery may be done first.
   b. If there is parametrial disease, radiotherapy is indicated initially.
5. **Recurrent carcinoma.** In the face of recurrent carcinoma, the decision must be made whether to use progestational agents or chemotherapy. Progestational agents alone cause a remission in approximately one-third of recurrences. There is now some evidence that the combination of progestational agents with chemotherapy may be self-defeating. The tumors that respond to progestins are those that have progesterone receptors. There is some evidence that tumors with estrogen receptors may respond poorly to chemotherapeutic drugs. Furthermore, those tumors that have estrogen receptors may respond best to tamoxifen citrate, an antiestrogenic agent. The distribution of receptors in endometrial carcinoma has been shown to be:

| | |
|---|---|
| Estrogen positive | 70% |
| Estrogen positive/progesterone positive | 50% |
| Estrogen negative/progesterone negative | 30% |
| Estrogen positive/progesterone negative | 20% |
| Estrogen negative/progesterone positive | 0% |

If these figures continue to be valid with the data from further investigational series now in progress, and if the capability of receptor assay becomes widespread, endometrial carcinoma recurrence can be treated as shown.

| **Type** | **Distribution** | **Therapy** |
|---|---|---|
| E−/P− | 30% | Chemotherapy (doxorubicin hydrochloride [Adriamycin] and/or cyclophosphamide [Cytoxan] and/or cisplatin [Platinol]) |
| E+/P+ | 40% to 50% | Medroxyprogesterone (Depo-Provera—1 g IM weekly, or megestrol acetate [Megace] 160 mg p.o. daily) |
| E+/P− | 20% to 30% | Tamoxifen citrate |

6. **Follow-up care of patients with treated endometrial carcinoma**
   a. **Follow-up schedule.** Patients should be followed every 6 weeks for the first year, every 8 weeks for the second, every 3 months for the third, and every 6 months thereafter.

b. **Follow-up examination** should include:
   (1) Careful pelvic examination, including rectovaginal assessment.
   (2) Examination of node-bearing areas and chest.
   (3) Yearly chest x-rays, because the lungs are a primary site of metastasis.
   (4) Yearly mammogram and stool guaiac, because these patients are at higher risk than average women for cancer of the breast or rectum.
   (5) Assessment of possible complications of therapy, especially if radiation has been given (see Chapter 29—Carcinoma of the Cervix).

**Note:** Estrogens should never be given during the first 3 years unless there is a definite benefit to be derived that outweighs the risks of estrogen-associated exacerbation of the carcinoma. In any event, estrogen therapy should be limited to the patient who has an early lesion with no risk factors. After the first 3 years, caution should be used.

## IX. Prognosis

A. **Five-year survival rates** for endometrial carcinoma are:

| Stage | Survival rate |
|---|---|
| Stage I | 70%–75% |
| Stage II | 50% |
| Stage III | 25%–30% |
| Stage IV | 5%–10% |

B. **General considerations**

1. **Prognostic factors** for survival are:
   a. Grade of tumor
   b. Myometrial invasion
   c. Lymph node metastasis
   d. Peritoneal cytology
   e. Cervical involvement
   f. Adnexal involvement
2. The last five factors above are functions of histologic grade, that is, the more undifferentiated the tumor, the more likely it is to have myometrial invasion and/or lymph node metastasis and/or peritoneal cytology positive for malignant cells, and so on.
3. In stage I disease, the patient with a grade 1 tumor with no nodal metastasis and no myometrial invasion has a 95% chance of being alive and disease-free 5 years from the time of diagnosis. A patient with stage I, grade 3 disease with deep myometrial invasion and pelvic node metastasis probably has only a 20% to 30% chance of 5-year survival. If para-aortic nodes are positive, the prognosis is even worse.
4. Between the above two extremes are all the various possible combinations that can exist with stage I disease, such as stage I, grade 1, with deep myometrial invasion and

negative nodes, or stage I, grade 2 with superficial invasion and positive nodes. The important point is that 5-year survival is in inverse proportion to the number of serious risk factors present.

## UTERINE SARCOMAS

**I. Incidence.** Sarcomas of the uterus are uncommon tumors, accounting for approximately 3% to 4% of all uterine malignancies. Women who have been treated with radiation therapy for other pelvic malignancies face an increased risk of developing uterine sarcomas, specifically mixed Müllerian tumors. Sarcomatous degeneration in leiomyomata is an extremely rare event, probably less than 2 per thousand. Approximately 1500 new cases are diagnosed annually. The peak incidence for all sarcomas is age 60, although for leiomyosarcomas it is age 50.

**II. Morbidity and mortality.** Patients with sarcomas face high morbidity and mortality rates. If a sarcoma is confined to the uterus, there is a 50% 5-year mortality. If the sarcoma has spread out of the uterus mortality approaches 100%. In addition, as sarcomas are frequently diagnosed in elderly patients, surgical morbidity is significantly increased.

**III. Etiology.** In most types of sarcomas, the initiating factors are elusive. However, in mixed Müllerian tumors, two risk factors have been suggested: an endocrinological imbalance as in endometrial cancer, and previous pelvic radiation, such as for treatment of cervical cancer.

**IV. Pathogenesis**

**A. Classification of uterine sarcomas.** The nomenclature for sarcomas has been ambiguous in the past, perhaps adding to the confusion of their optimal management. The Kempson modification of Ober's classification is now the accepted nomenclature.

1. **Pure sarcomas**
   a. **Pure homologous**
      (1) Leiomyosarcoma
      (2) Stromal sarcoma
      (3) Angiosarcoma
      (4) Fibrosarcoma
   b. Pure heterologous sarcomas
      (1) Rhabdomyosarcoma
      (2) Chondrosarcoma
      (3) Osteogenic sarcoma
      (4) Liposarcoma
2. **Mixed sarcomas**
   a. Mixed homologous
   b. Mixed heterologous
   c. Mixed combined

3. **Malignant mixed Müllerian tumors (MMT)**
    a. MMT homologous type
    b. MMT heterologous type
4. **Sarcoma unclassified**
5. **Malignant lymphoma**

"Pure" refers to a sarcoma made up of one cell type. "Heterologous" refers to a sarcoma that has cells not normally found in a uterus (e.g., bone, cartilage). These probably arise from totipotential mesenchymal cells. Mixed Müllerian tumors have both sarcomatous and carcinomatous elements and arise probably from totipotential Müllerian cells.

B. **Leiomyosarcomas, endometrial stromal sarcomas, and mixed Müllerian tumors.** The three most common varieties of sarcomas encountered at most referral centers are leiomyosarcomas, endometrial stromal sarcomas, and mixed Müllerian tumors. The remaining sarcomas are rare and their clinical behavior is not sufficiently different from the more common tumors to warrant more detailed discussion.

1. **Leiomyosarcomas** are malignant smooth muscle tumors that can arise in preexisting leiomyomas or in normal myometrium. They account for approximately 1% to 1.5% of all malignancies of the uterus and, in most series, for about 20% to 30% of all uterine sarcomas.
2. **Endometrial stromal sarcomas** are rare lesions and in most series account for approximately 10% of all uterine sarcomas. They are presumed to arise from the endometrial stromal cell. They comprise a continuous spectrum of lesions from relatively benign to malignant. The terms stromatosis and stromal nodule are used to describe the more benign conditions. Endolymphatic stromal myosis is an intermediate entity and is malignant but behaves more indolently. The term stromal sarcoma is used to describe the most malignant varieties.
3. **Mixed Müllerian tumors** are now the most frequently seen sarcomas. They account for 60% of all sarcomas and for 2% to 4% of all uterine malignancies. They have been referred to by a plethora of names, such as mesenchymal tumors, mixed mesodermal tumors, carcinosarcoma, dysontogenic tumors, and many more. It is currently believed that these tumors arise from a totipotential epithelial cell.

C. **Spread pattern of sarcomas** include hematogenous, local invasion, and lymphatic. The tumor has a great affinity for pulmonary metastasis, and death is usually by lung involvement.

## V. Differential diagnosis.

Any process that causes vaginal bleeding may confound the diagnosis, especially as sarcomas are rare lesions and are not of primary consideration. The problems in the differential diagnosis are identical to those outlined for endometrial cancer (see part on Adenocarcinoma of the Endometrium, section V this chapter).

**VI. Diagnosis.** The diagnosis discussion under adenocarcinomas of the uterus is also applicable to uterine sarcomas when they are diagnosed prior to surgery. However, the most frequent method of diagnosis is as an incidental finding at hysterectomy. Possible exceptions are mixed Müllerian tumors. They are frequently present within the endometrial cavity, and D & C can be a useful tool for diagnosis.

**VII. Management.** The most important determinant in the treatment of uterine sarcomas is the stage at the time of diagnosis. The staging system used for uterine sarcomas is the same as that used for endometrial carcinomas (see part on Adenocarcinoma of the Endometrium, section VII this chapter). The histologic type of tumor is not an important variable in choosing treatment, and all of the above-mentioned sarcomas are treated in the same way. However, at the time of diagnosis the vast majority of leiomyosarcomas will be stage I (probably 80%), whereas mixed Müllerian tumors will show a 40% to 60% incidence of tumor outside the uterine corpus.

A. **Surgery.** The mainstay of adequate control of this disease is surgery, specifically total abdominal hysterectomy and bilateral salpingo-oopherectomy. Radiation as a sole mode of therapy has been shown consistently to be inadequate. There are few surgical histologic studies reviewing the incidence of pelvic nodes and para-aortic node involvement in the different stages of this disease. It is therefore difficult to be dogmatic as to the desirability of node sampling in those cases where diagnosis has been made prior to surgery in stage I disease. A possible incidence of nodal metastasis in these cases may be 20% to 25%.

B. **Radiation.** In the treatment of disease limited to the uterus (stages I and II), there is disagreement as to the role of radiation. No good prospective studies have been published to help the clinician choose a management from this controversy. There are some ongoing studies that show clearly that adjuvant radiation therapy does decrease pelvic recurrence but does not significantly alter 5-year survival rates. There may be some benefit to pelvic radiation if the sarcoma is a mixed Müllerian tumor.

C. **Chemotherapy.** The role of adjuvant chemotherapy is still not defined at this time for stage I disease.

D. **Follow-up care** for patients with uterine sarcomas is similar to that described for adenocarcinoma.

E. **Adjuvant therapy** such as radiation or chemotherapy is most appropriate for cases of disease limited to the uterus but with poor prognostic factors. In advanced disease, palliative chemotherapy has some limited success with cisplatin, showing a

20% response rate. Factors related to poor prognosis include:

1. Deep myometrial invasion
2. Involvement of lower uterine segment or cervix
3. Adnexal involvement
4. Histology of mixed Müllerian tumor as opposed to leiomyosarcoma
5. Nodal involvement
6. Extrauterine disease

## VIII. Prognosis

Stage I patients have a 5-year survival of approximately 50% in most series. Those that do have recurrence, do so within the first 24 to 30 months. The most frequent site of recurrence is a combination of pelvis, upper abdomen, and lung (45%), whereas the next most common is recurrence in the lung and upper abdomen with no pelvic recurrence (40%). Isolated pelvic recurrence is much less frequent (10%). For stage III and IV disease, results are uniformly poor. Few authors describe any treatment successes in these patients. The average time of treatment failure is 6 months to 1 year. In diseases such as sarcomas where survival is so dismal, the concept of progression-free interval is more appropriate than survival. Adjuvant therapies may increase the progression-free interval in stage I poor risk factor disease even though the 5-year survival may not be changed.

## BIBLIOGRAPHY

Baltzer J, Lohe KJ. What's new in the prognosis of uterine cancer? Pathol Res Pract 1984; 178:635.

Bonte J, Decoster JM, Ide P, Billiet G. Hormonoprophylaxis and hormonotherapy in the treatment of endometrial adenocarcinoma by means of dioxyprogesterone acetate. Gynecol Oncol 1978; 6:60–75.

Campbell K, Nuss R, Benrubi G. An evaluation of the clinical stagings of endometrial cancer. Reprod Med 1988; 33:8.

Cavanaugh D, Marsden DE, Ruffolo EH. Carcinoma of the endometrium. Obstet Gynecol Ann 1984; 13:211.

Creaseman WT, Weed JC Jr. Screening techniques in endometrial cancer. Cancer 1976; 38:436.

Davies JL, Rosenshein NB, Antones CM, Stolley PD. A review of the risk factors for endometrial carcinoma. Obstet Gynecol Surv 1981; 36:107–116.

Enriori CL, Reforzo-Membrives J. Peripheral aromatization as a risk factor for breast and endometrial cancer in postmenopausal women: A review. Gynecol Oncol 1984; 17:1–21.

Fehr PE, Prem KA. Malignancy of the uterine corpus following irradiation therapy for squamous cell carcinoma of the cervix. Am J Obstet Gynecol 1974; 119:685.

Ferenczy A, Gelfand MM, Tzipris F. The cytodynamics of endometrial hyperplasia and carcinoma. A review. Ann Pathol 1983; 3:189.

Gallup D, Cordray D. Leiomyosarcoma of the uterus. Obstet Gynecol Surv 1979; 34:300.

Gambrell RD Jr, Bagnell CA, Greenblatt RB. Role of estrogens and progesterone in the etiology and prevention of endometrial cancer: A review. Am J Obstet Gynecol 1983; 146:696.

Gordon AN, Fleisher AC, Dudley BS, Drolshagan LF, Kalemeris GC, Partain CL, Jones HW, Burnett LS. Preoperative assessment of myometrial invasion of endometrial adenocarcinoma by sonography and magnetic resonance imaging. Gynecol Oncol 1989; 34:175–179.

Gray LA, Christopherson WH, Hoover RN. Estrogens and endometrial carcinoma. Obstet Gynecol 1977;49:385.

Gusberg SB. Precursors of corpus carcinoma, estrogens and adenomatous hyperplasia. Am J Obstet Gynecol 1947; 54:905.

Kauppila A. Progestin therapy of endometrial, breast and ovarian carcinoma. A review of clinical observations. Acta Obstet Gynecol Scand 1984; 63:441.

Lyon FA, Frisch MJ. Endometrial abnormalities occurring in young women on long-term sequential oral contraception. Obstet Gynecol 1976; 47:639.

MacDonald PC, Siiteri PK. The relationship between extraglandular production of estrone and the occurrence of endometrial neoplasia. Gynecol Oncol 1974; 2:259.

Malkasian GD. Progesterone treatment of recurrent endometrial carcinoma. Am J Obstet Gynecol 1971; 110:15.

Malviya VK, Deppe G, Malone JM, Sundareson AS, Lawrence WD. Reliability of frozen section examination in identifying poor proportic indicators in Stage I endometrial adenocarcinoma. Gynecol Oncol 1989; 34:299–304.

Morrow CP. The benefits of estrogen to the menopausal woman outweigh the risks of developing endometrial cancer. CA 1984; 34:220.

Salazar OM, Bonfiglio TA, Patten SF, Keller BE, Feldstein ML, Dunne ME, Rudolph J. Uterine sarcomas: Analysis of failures with special emphasis on the use of adjuvant radiation therapy. Cancer 1978; 42:1161–70.

Salazar OM, Bonfiglio TA, Patten SF, Keller BE, Feldstein ML, Dunne ME, Rudolph J. Uterine sarcomas: Natural history, treatment and prognosis. Cancer 1978; 1152–60.

Silverberg SG. New aspects of endometrial carcinoma. Clin Obstet Gynecol 1984; 11:189.

# CHAPTER 31

# Carcinoma of the Fallopian Tube

**Guy I. Benrubi**

Most cancers found in the fallopian tube are metastatic, usually arising in the ovary or endometrium. Primary adenocarcinoma of the fallopian tube is the rarest malignancy of the female reproductive tract. Consequently, clear information concerning the natural history and proper management of this disease is lacking. Management decisions are based on the fact that tubal cancers are Müllerian in origin and generally behave like comparable tumors arising in other areas of the genital tract.

I. **Incidence.** Primary carcinoma of the fallopian tube is the rarest gynecologic malignancy, comprising less than 1% of gynecologic cancers. Approximately 1000 cases of primary carcinoma of the fallopian tube have been reported in the entire gynecologic literature. Cancer of the fallopian tube can occur in women of any age, although the mean age is in the sixth decade.

II. **Morbidity and mortality.** The 5-year survival rate for all stages is 30% to 40%, although in early tumors (stage I primarily) it approaches 90%. In advanced tumors, the 5-year survival rate drops to about 10%. Infertility results from definitive therapy, even in early disease.

III. **Etiology and risk factors.** The tubal epithelium is Müllerian in origin. Stimuli such as endocrine abnormalities or talc from surgical gloves are presumed to cause neoplastic change similar to that of other Müllerian epithelium in the reproductive tract. A familial predisposition has not been identified in the small total number of cases available for study.

IV. **Pathology and pathogenesis.** Primary tubal cancers are almost invariably adenocarcinomas. Sarcomas of the fallopian tube are exceedingly rare and, as in uterine cancers, they may exhibit homologous or heterologous elements. Fallopian tube carcinoma is spread by surface extension and by lymphatic infiltration, as in ovarian cancer. Death is most commonly caused by bowel obstruction.

V. **Differential diagnosis.** Any pathological process that leads to an adnexal mass may confound the correct diagnosis of fallopian tube cancer.

VI. **Diagnosis.** Because carcinoma of the fallopian tube is rare, there is a low index of suspicion making its preoperative diagnosis infrequent. The diagnosis of carcinoma of the fallopian tube is usually made as an incidental finding at the time of tubal ligation or at laparotomy for other suspected pathology.

A. **Signs and symptoms.** Abnormal vaginal bleeding is the most common symptom associated with primary tubal carcinoma. As this tumor frequently occurs in postmenopausal women, this symptom may be mistakenly ascribed to the postmenopausal bleeding associated with endometrial carcinoma or with postmenopausal endometrial changes. **Hydrops tubae profluens** is a classically described symptom characterized by pain relieved by profuse watery blood-tinged vaginal discharge. It is caused by blood and fluid accumulation in a tube partially occluded by tumor. This leads to tubal distention and colicky pain. As this collection is released, the pain is relieved and the discharge results. However, because any tubal pathology that leads to such occlusion may yield this sign, it is not pathognomonic for tubal carcinoma.

B. **Physical examination.** Careful pelvic examination, with rectovaginal evaluation, is basic to the investigation of possible fallopian tube carcinoma. The remainder of the examination is similar to that for ovarian carcinoma (see Chapter 32—Carcinoma of the Ovary, diagnosis section, VII).

C. **Laboratory and diagnostic procedures.** Because the diagnosis of tubal cancer is rarely suspected preoperatively, the laboratory and diagnostic procedures consist of those that are used to assess any suspected adnexal neoplasm, in addition to those studies needed for the general preoperative evaluation of the patient (see Chapter 32—Carcinoma of the Ovary, diagnosis section, VII).

VII. **Management.** Although the diagnosis is most often made intraoperatively, the surgeon must be prepared to perform definitive surgery at the time of laparotomy or have a gynecologic oncologist available for intraoperative consultation and assistance.

A. **Staging.** All cancer therapy begins with accurate staging. In tubal cancer, as in ovarian cancers, staging is surgical and it is performed as part of definitive therapy.

1. **Staging classification.** There is no International Federation of Gynecology and Obstetrics (FIGO) staging for tubal cancer. Because tubal cancer behaves somewhat like ovarian cancer in its spread pattern, a consensus staging system

based on the staging of ovarian carcinoma has been devised and is in general use:

**Stage I:** Tumor limited to one, or both tubes

**Stage II:** Tumor with extension to other pelvic organs

**Stage III:** Tumor spread to upper abdomen or retroperitoneal nodes

**Stage IV:** Tumor spread outside of abdomen or to the parenchyma of the liver

2. **Surgical staging** especially for early disease discovered incidentally at the time of laparotomy for other indications, must be aggressive. Microscopic metastasis must be ruled out from all possible tumor spread areas. The techniques of surgical staging are similar to those for ovarian carcinoma (see Chapter 32—Carcinoma of the Ovary).

**B. Therapy for stage I disease**

1. **Initial therapy.** Total abdominal hysterectomy and bilateral salpingo-oophorectomy is the first line of therapy. Most tubal cancers occur in postmenopausal women, or are found incidentally at the time of tubal ligation. Thus, only rarely does a concern about fertility conservation confound treatment decisions. When fertility is an issue, individualized decision-making with consultation from a gynecologic oncologist is mandatory. In theory, both fallopian tubes should be equally susceptible to carcinoma. Therefore, there is no role for conservation in this disease, and both adnexae as well as uterus should be removed.
2. **Adjuvant therapy.** Because of the rarity of this disease, decision-making as to proper adjuvant therapy is based on educated guesses rather than clinical trials.
   a. In small, stage I histologically well-differentiated cancers limited to the tubal mucosa, with no evidence of disease on aggressive staging and negative peritoneal fluid cytology, no further therapy after surgery is indicated.
   b. In similar cases, but with positive peritoneal cytology, intraperitoneal chromic phosphate ($P_{32}$) can be instilled.
   c. For more anaplastic tumors or if the muscularis of the tube is involved, adjuvant chemotherapy is indicated. As most Müllerian tumors seem to respond to cisplatin-based combination chemotherapy regimens, this type of therapy seems appropriate. This consists of cisplatin 50 mg/m$^2$ in addition to cyclophosphamide 1000 mg/m$^2$ every 3 weeks for eight treatments.
3. **Second look laparotomy** after completion of therapy for stage I carcinoma will define further management as described in Chapter 32–Carcinoma of the Ovary.

**C. Therapy for stage II, III, or IV disease.** As in the treatment of stage I disease, total abdominal hysterectomy and bilateral salpingo-oophorectomy are the mainstays of treatment. The best chance of survival is aggressive tumor debulking at the time of initial surgery. It is imperative that the surgeon feels comfortable in performing aggressive abdominal and pelvic surgery, including bowel resection if necessary. Removal of all palpable tumor at the time of initial exploratory laparotomy provides the best chance of cure. Adjuvant therapy is determined by the amount of residual tumor after initial surgery, and may include radiation and/or chemotherapy. Treatment is individualized and should be determined in consultation with a gynecologic oncologist and radiation therapist.

VIII. **Prognosis** for fallopian tube carcinoma is difficult to determine because of the paucity of cases in the literature. It is probably similar to that of ovarian epithelial carcinomas. Five-year survival for all stages is approximately 30% to 40%, although aggressively staged and treated stage I disease probably carries a 5-year survival of 85% to 90%.

## BIBLIOGRAPHY

Denham JW, Meclennan KA. The management of primary carcinoma of the fallopian tube. Cancer 1984; 53:166.

Rosenblatt K, Weiss N, Schwartz S. Incidence of malignant fallopian tube tumors. Gynecol Oncol 1989; 35:236.

Sedlis A. Carcinoma of the fallopian tube. Surg Clin North Am 1978; 58:121.

Yoonessi N. Carcinoma of the fallopian tube. Obstet Gynecol Surg 1979; 34:257.

# CHAPTER 32

# Carcinoma of the Ovary

**Guy I. Benrubi**

Ovarian malignancy presents a perplexing challenge to the clinician. It is often not diagnosed until far advanced because of the lack of symptoms and the difficulties involved in the physical examination of the adnexae. In addition, a lack of specific biochemical or histologic/cytologic screening tests exists. The best hope for cure in ovarian cancer is early diagnosis. Management depends upon an understanding of the pathologic classification and biologic behavior of these tumors and the roles and limitations of cytoreductive surgery, radiation therapy, and chemotherapy.

I. **Incidence.** Ovarian cancer is the second most common malignancy of the female reproductive tract. In excess of 17 000 new cases of ovarian carcinoma are diagnosed yearly in the United States, and approximately 11 000 annual deaths are attributed to this disease. Ovarian cancer accounts for 25% of gynecologic malignancies and 50% of gynecologic cancer deaths. At birth a female's risk of eventually having ovarian cancer is 1.5%. Whites have a higher incidence of ovarian neoplasia than blacks.

II. **Morbidity and mortality.** Ovarian malignancy is the most deadly gynecologic cancer because the diagnosis is so often made after the cancer has spread beyond early stage disease. In cases in which diagnosis occurs in early stage disease, cure may be possible. However, depending on the stage of the disease at the time of diagnosis, the therapeutic intent of the physician may be the prolongation of a progression-free interval rather than cure. Because therapy must necessarily be aggressive, therapeutic morbidity is significant. As cure rates improve, and as progression-free intervals lengthen, long-term effects of treatment are manifested (e.g., the leukemogenic potential of chemotherapeutic drugs). Ovarian cancer in young women frequently leads to infertility, although the newer chemotherapeutic drug combinations allow conservation of reproductive function in some cases.

**III. Etiology and risk factors.** The etiology of ovarian carcinoma is unknown and the risk factors remain unclear.

- A. **Diet** may have a significant role, as populations with high-fat diets have increased incidences of this disease. Complex carbohydrate diets may be protective.
- B. **Environmental factors.** Women living in industrialized countries have a higher incidence of ovarian carcinoma, perhaps due to diet or to environmental irritants. Women in Scandinavian countries have the highest incidence of disease, whereas those in African countries experience the lowest incidence. Japan has a lower rate than the United States, but Japanese-Americans have rates approaching white American women.
- C. **Talc.** Hygienic habits such as use of substances containing talc around the perineum have been implicated.
- D. **Ovulation.** Another theory states that ovulation may be the initiating event for ovarian carcinoma. According to this view, ovulation in some instances may lead to an epithelial inclusion cyst. When this capsular epithelium comes under the influence of stromal hormones, it may progress to epithelial ovarian neoplasia. Recent evidence that birth control pills may protect against ovarian epithelial cancer supports this theory.
- E. **Familial factors.** Although several families with multiple members developing ovarian cancer have been reported, a genetic predisposition for ovarian malignancy has not been documented.

**IV. Pathogenesis and pathology.** Understanding the different types of malignant tumors that can occur in the ovary depends upon knowing the different types of cells that are normally found in that organ. Each of these cells has its associated malignancy. The cell types are:

- A. **Germ cells,** the raison d'etre of the ovary.
- B. **Specialized stromal cells,** which "nurse" the germ cells and also produce hormones; with the germ cells they form the follicles.
- C. **Stromal cells,** which provide the structure of the ovary and the matrix for the germ cells.
- D. **Epithelial cells,** the epithelium of the ovarian capsule, which surrounds the whole structure and is Müllerian in origin.

A. **Germ cell tumors** comprise 20% to 25% of all ovarian neoplasms, and arise from the primitive totipotential germ cell of the embryonic gonad. Most germ cell tumors occur in children and young adults, but some varieties are seen throughout life.

1. **Dysgerminoma.** Accounting for 1% to 2% of all ovarian neoplasms and about 5% of all malignant ovarian tumors, dysgerminomas are unilateral 85% of the time. They are the most common malignant ovarian tumors associated with pregnancy and one of the most common ovarian malignancies in the first 3 decades of life. Dysgerminomas

are made up of undifferentiated germ cells, identical to those seen in seminomas in males. Microscopically, they are composed of islands of tumor cells surrounded by connective tissue infiltrated with lymphocytes. They are unique clinically because they are extremely radiosensitive.

2. **Embryonal cell carcinoma** is an extremely rare ovarian tumor. It is a malignancy of children and young adults and is often seen in combination with other germ cell tumors. Embryonal cell carcinomas are composed of minimally differentiated germ cells and are identical to the tumor seen in the testes in the male. This tumor has an aggressive behavior and a poor prognosis.
3. **Endodermal sinus tumor** is an extremely malignant ovarian neoplasm seen primarily in the first 30 years of life. Also known as yolk sac tumor, mesoblastoma, or Teilum tumor, this malignant neoplasm can be thought of as an embryonal carcinoma that has differentiated toward yolk sac structures. Histologically, some of these tumors exhibit the Schiller–Duval body (endodermal sinus), which is a narrow band of connective tissue with a capillary in the middle lined by cuboidal cells. Endodermal sinus tumor cells secrete alpha-fetoprotein (AFP), which can be used for diagnosis or for assessment of efficacy of treatment or evidence of recurrence.
4. **Choriocarcinoma** is a rare malignant tumor of children and young adults, which usually presents as a unilateral pelvic mass. This is a nongestational, germ cell tumor and can be thought of as an embryonal carcinoma that has differentiated toward trophoblastic structures. It is composed of cytotrophoblast and syncytiotrophoblast, and it secretes human chorionic gonadotropin (hCG), which can be used clinically in the same manner that AFP is used in the endodermal sinus tumor. Because hCG can stimulate the prepubertal ovary, it may be a cause of precocious puberty.
5. **Teratomas** are the most differentiated germ cell tumors. Ninety-five percent of these tumors are benign mature cystic forms, also known as dermoid cysts, whereas the remainder are immature forms.
   a. **Immature teratomas** are tumors of early life and are rarely seen after the reproductive years. They are composed of germ cells that have differentiated into immature elements derived from all three layers (endoderm, mesoderm, ectoderm). If mature elements are seen, the tumor may be hard to distinguish from a mature teratoma with malignant transformation. These tumors have a poor prognosis, although it is better than the prognosis for endodermal sinus tumors.

b. **Mature teratomas** (see Chapter 8—Benign Diseases of the Ovaries and Fallopian Tubes).

6. **Gonadoblastoma** is an uncommon tumor, usually seen in patients with gonadal dysgenesis, the majority of these patients being phenotypic females. Gonadoblastomas usually occur in the first 3 decades of life and are composed of undifferentiated germ cells and sex cord stromal derivatives, such as granulosa cells or Sertoli cells. They are associated with dysgerminomas in 50% of patients. Pure gonadoblastomas are usually benign.

B. **Specialized stromal cell tumors** account for 5% of all ovarian tumors. These neoplasms are derived from specialized stromal cells of the ovary called nurse cells, that surround the germ cells in the embryonic gonad. They may be associated with excessive hormonal release, although the majority are nonfunctioning. Most of these tumors behave in a benign manner. Some, however, recur many years after the original diagnosis. Therefore, diagnosis of malignancy is based on clinical presentation and not histologic appearance.

1. **Granulosa cell tumors** account for 1% to 2% of all ovarian tumors and are unilateral in 90% of patients. They present in various histologic patterns, but the constant characteristic is the presence of granulosa cells. Call-Exner bodies, which are small cavities containing eosinophilic fluid surrounded by granulosa cells, are often seen in the microfollicular histologic pattern of this tumor. These tumors usually occur late in the reproductive years and postmenopausally, but they are also seen in prepubertal children. Those tumors that produce estrogen cause a hyperplasia of the endometrium which may be cystic or adenomatous. Up to a 20% incidence of endometrial carcinoma has been reported in patients with granulosa cell tumors. These tumors have low malignant potential, and if they do recur, they do so several years after the initial diagnosis. Although most functioning granulosa tumors are estrogenic, a small percentage may actually be androgen secreting.
2. **Thecomas** may occur alone or in conjunction with granulosa cell tumors or fibromas. They are almost always benign and unilateral, occur more often in older women than do granulosa tumors, and are frequently estrogenic.
3. **Sertoli-Leydig cell tumors** comprise less than 0.5% of all ovarian neoplasms, occur most frequently in young women, and are unilateral in 95% of patients. Most are not malignant. They are often referred to as arrhenoblastomas or androblastomas. These tumors have varying histologic appearances. Some are composed of only Sertoli cells arranged in tubules, others exhibit both Sertoli and Leydig cells, and still others are made up of pure Leydig cells containing Reinke crystals (hilus cell tumors) composed of

remnant embryologic hilar Leydig cells. Some are undifferentiated and may resemble sarcomas or carcinomas. Although they are commonly associated with masculinization and androgen production, many of these tumors are endocrinologically inert and some may even be estrogen secreting.

4. **Gynandroblastomas** are interesting, rare tumors composed of well-differentiated male and female sex cord stromal cells. Because the cellular elements are well-differentiated, the vast majority of these tumors behave in a benign manner. When they do recur, it is frequently after several years. These tumors may secrete estrogens or androgens.

C. **Stromal cells represented in mesenchymal tumors.** These are tumors that arise from supportive and vascular structures in the ovary, and they are similar to tumors that may arise from these structures in any organ system of the body. Examples include:
   1. Fibromas
   2. Leiomyomas
   3. Lipomas
   4. Lymphomas
   5. Sarcomas

D. **Epithelial tumors** are the most common ovarian neoplasms, representing 60% to 70% of all ovarian tumors. They can be found in all age groups but are most frequently seen in the late reproductive years. They are thought to arise from the coelomic epithelium covering the ovary.
   1. **Serous cystadenocarcinoma** is the most common malignant ovarian tumor, accounting for 40% of all ovarian malignancies and presenting bilaterally in 50% of cases. They exist in different histologic grades from well to poorly differentiated. A borderline malignant variety also exists, microscopically revealing numerous papillary projections covered with two or three cell layers, but distinguished by the lack of stromal invasion. Serous cystadenocarcinomas tend to be in a more advanced stage at the time of diagnosis than do endometroid or mucinous carcinomas. However, stage for stage and grade for grade, the behavior of all three is similar.
   2. **Mucinous cystadenocarcinomas** account for 10% of all malignant ovarian tumors, presenting bilaterally 20% of the time. As with other epithelial malignancies, they range from well to poorly differentiated and demonstrate a borderline malignant form.
   3. **Endometrioid carcinoma** comprises 20% of all ovarian malignancies and may occur bilaterally in up to 50% of patients. Histologically, these tumors are similar to endometrial carcinoma of the uterus. As in other epithelial tumors, they may be well, moderately, or poorly differentiated and are also seen in a borderline malignant variety.

In 20% of patients they are associated with carcinoma of the endometrium.

4. **Clear cell carcinoma.** Once erroneously referred to as "mesonephromas," clear cell carcinomas are now thought to arise from the coelomic epithelium covering the ovary. They are made up of cells with clear cytoplasm and round hyperchromatic nuclei. Careful histologic analysis will, on occasion, reveal areas of serous, mucinous, or endometroid cells.
5. **Brenner tumors** comprise 0.5% of all ovarian tumors and occur bilaterally in 10% of patients. Their peak incidence is between 40 and 50 years of age. Most of these tumors are benign, but a malignant variety exists. Histologically, nests of epithelial cells with "coffee bean" nuclei are seen surrounded by strands of fibrous connective tissue.
6. **Undifferentiated carcinoma.** In 10% of the malignant tumors of the ovary, no differentiation can be made histologically into either serous, mucinous, or endometriotic type. These carcinomas are highly malignant and are usually in an advanced stage at the time of initial diagnosis.
7. **Mixed Müllerian tumors.** Also referred to as mixed epithelial-mesenchymal tumors, it is now believed that mixed Müllerian tumors arise from the multipotential germinal epithelium lining the ovary. Thus, they can be classified as epithelial tumors. There are two varieties, both highly malignant. The **carcinosarcomas** consist of adenocarcinomas with a stroma composed of sarcomatous spindle cells. **Mixed mesodermal tumors** have a sarcomatous component that consists of malignant cartilage, striated muscle, or bone, in addition to spindle cells.

E. **Metastatic neoplasms.** About 10% of ovarian tumors are metastatic from an extraovarian primary site. The most common primary site is the endometrium. Difficulties may arise in deciding whether there is a concomitant endometroid carcinoma of the ovary and endometrial carcinoma of the uterus or a metastasis to the ovary from the uterus. The other two most common primary sites are the gastrointestinal tract and the breast. The Krukenberg tumor is one consisting of epithelial cells filled with mucin, giving a signet-ring appearance. Ninety percent of these tumors arise in the stomach.

## V. Spread pattern and natural history of ovarian carcinoma

A. **Epithelial tumors** spread by surface extension over the peritoneum and serosal surfaces of the abdominal organs. Death from epithelial ovarian carcinoma is usually the result of bowel obstruction, general debility, and infection. Borderline epithelial tumors have the same patterns of spread, but they are extremely slow growing and the patient may live with the tumors for years. Lymphatic spread is also frequently encountered. Hematogenous spread is possible although less common. The liver is the most common distal organ involved with metastasis.

B. **Germ cell tumors, stromal, and specialized stromal malignancies** spread in a similar pattern to that found in epithelial ovarian carcinoma, although lymphatic and hematogenous spread is more frequent in these cancers. Death is more frequently associated with metastasis to the liver and lungs.

## VI. Differential diagnosis

### A. Common problems

1. **Uterine leiomyomata,** especially predunculated subserous myomas, may be confused with solid ovarian tumors. As a result, it is an altogether too frequent occurrence to explore a patient for uterine fibroids and encounter an ovarian malignancy. A high index of suspicion is necessary because the patient must be properly prepared prior to debulking surgery.
2. **Pelvic inflammatory disease,** especially with the formation of tubo-ovarian complexes, is sometimes confused with solid adnexal masses. This is a more common misdiagnosis in younger individuals in whom ovarian cancer may not be suspected.
3. **Endometriosis,** especially an endometrioma of the ovary, may be mistaken for ovarian neoplasia.
4. **Functional ovarian cysts** may be felt as an ovarian mass and hence be confused with ovarian neoplasia.

B. **Less common problems.** Bowel tumors and other diseases of the bowel must be considered, particularly in older people who have a higher incidence of such problems. Diverticular disease and colonic carcinomas are the two most common diseases encountered.

## VII. Diagnosis

A. **Signs and symptoms.** Difficulty in making the diagnosis of ovarian cancer results because symptoms are minimal and vague in both early disease and in more advanced stages. Thus, there is frequently a delay from the onset of symptoms to the patient seeking medical care. This delay often results in the progression of the cancer to a more advanced stage before diagnosis is made. Depending on the degree of progression, symptoms may include:

1. Inability to ingest usual volumes of food or early satiety (probably the earliest symptoms of ovarian carcinoma and the most often missed of symptoms).
2. Bloating.
3. Loss of appetite.
4. Nausea and emesis.
5. Generalized distention from ascites.
6. Abdominal pain.
7. Vaginal bleeding or menstrual irregularity.

**Note:** The classic description of the patient with advanced ovarian carcinoma is a cachectic, middle-aged female with ascites and symptoms of intermittent small bowel obstruction. She is often hungry but can tolerate only minimal quantities of food.

B. **Physical examination.** A thorough physical examination is important in patients suspected of having ovarian carcinoma because of the complexity of its spread patterns and because these patients often require extensive surgical procedures.

1. **Cardiac and pulmonary evaluation** should be meticulous.
2. **Examination of the abdomen and pelvis** must be given special attention. The abdominal examination should include evaluation of the liver, spleen, and general configuration of the abdomen as well as evaluation for abnormal conditions, such as ascites. The size, shape, configuration, mobility, and relationship to other structures must be noted for all abdominal or pelvic masses.

C. **Laboratory and diagnostic procedures**

1. **Routine studies**
   a. Complete blood count
   b. Serum electrolyte evaluation including blood urea nitrogen and creatinine
   c. Liver function tests (including lactic dehydrogenase, which is elevated in ovarian neoplasia)
   d. Coagulation studies
   e. Intravenous pyelogram (IVP)
   f. Chest x-ray
   g. Barium enema
   h. β-hCG
   i. AFP
2. **Imaging studies** are useful to help define the extent of disease and its involvement in nongenital organ systems in preparation for treatment.
   a. An IVP, chest x-ray, and barium enema should be performed.
   b. Liver and bone scans are used by some centers as baseline studies. However, they have limited value.
   c. Ultrasonography and computerized axial tomography have a use commensurate with the expertise of the consulting radiologist.
3. **CA-125 immunologic test.** In many centers the immunologic test, CA-125, which is a marker for epithelial ovarian cancers (with the exception of mucinous tumors), is available, and should be ordered.
4. **Other studies.** Pulmonary function studies and additional cardiac studies are ordered if indicated by history or physical examination findings suggestive of dysfunction or tumor involvement in these systems.

   **Note:** Although the presumptive diagnosis of ovarian cancer is made by the diagnostic maneuvers discussed above, the confirmation of the diagnosis of ovarian cancer is histologic and made from tissue specimens taken at the time of laparotomy (see staging of ovarian carcinoma section, VIII-B).

## VIII. Staging of ovarian carcinoma

A. **Staging of ovarian carcinoma.** The first step in the management of any cancer is accurate staging (see Table 32.1). Ovarian cancers are staged surgically, not clinically.

B. **Intraoperative technique for staging.** Ovarian carcinoma, particularly of epithelial origin, spreads over peritoneal surfaces. An adequate staging laparotomy is simple if there is widespread disease throughout the peritoneum. If, on the other hand, the tumor appears to be limited to the ovary or pelvis, a careful sequence of steps at laparotomy must be followed to assure that metastasis is not overlooked.

1. Fluid samples for cytology (cell washings) must be obtained upon entering the abdomen. A syringe, or syringe with a catheter attached, is used to aspirate fluid from the pelvis proper, both paracolic gutters, and both subdiaphragmatic areas. Each specimen should be marked and sent separately for analysis. If there is little fluid, warm normal saline solution may be washed over the areas mentioned and reaspirated as a "washing procedure."
2. All peritoneal surfaces must be inspected and palpated.
3. The bowel should be thoroughly examined and all mesenteric surfaces examined, with any enlarged mesenteric nodes sampled.
4. If no disease is seen outside the pelvis, random biopsies should be taken from the peritoneum, both paracolic gutters, both diaphragms, and from the bladder serosa.
5. The surface of the liver and spleen should be palpated.
6. The undersurface of the diaphragm should be visualized. This may be aided by the use of a sterile sigmoidoscope or laparoscope.
7. Omentectomy should be performed.
8. If the above steps are completed and still no tumor is identified outside the pelvis, para-aortic, common iliac, and external iliac retroperitoneal nodes should be sampled. About 15% of these would be positive in stage I disease.

## IX. Management.

The treatment of ovarian malignancy varies among clinical centers, depending on the opinions of clinicians about the various treatment modalities, the availability of such modalities, and often the access to clinical research protocols that provide various new treatments. There are general principles, however, that apply in almost all situations. The details of management of patients with ovarian cancer should be decided by a trained gynecologic oncologist.

**Table 32.1. FIGO Classification for Staging of Ovarian Cancer**

| STAGE | DESCRIPTION |
|---|---|
| Stage I | Growth limited to the ovaries |
| Stage IA | Growth limited to one ovary; no ascites; no tumor on the external surfaces; capsules intact |
| Stage IB | Growth limited to both ovaries; no ascites; no tumor on the external surfaces; capsules intact |
| Stage IC | Tumor either stage IA or stage IB but with tumor on the surface of one or both ovaries; or with capsule ruptured; or with ascites present containing malignant cells or with positive peritoneal washings |
| Stage II | Growth involving one or both ovaries with pelvic extension |
| Stage IIA | Extension and/or metastases to the uterus and/or tubes |
| Stage IIB | Extension to other pelvic tissues |
| Stage IIC | Tumor either stage IIA or stage IIB but with tumor on the surface of one or both ovaries; or with capsule(s) ruptured; or with ascites present containing malignant cells or with positive peritoneal washings |
| Stage III | Tumor involving one or both ovaries with peritoneal implants outside the pelvis and/or positive retroperitoneal or inguinal nodes; superficial liver metastasis equals stage III; tumor is limited to the true pelvis but with histologically verified malignant extension to small bowel or omentum |
| Stage IIIA | Tumor grossly limited to the true pelvis with negative nodes but with histologically confirmed microscopic seeding of abdominal peritoneal surfaces |
| Stage IIIB | Tumor of one or both ovaries; histologically confirmed implants of abdominal peritoneal surfaces, none exceeding 2 cm in diameter; nodes negative |
| Stage IIIC | Abdominal implants 2 cm in diameter and/or positive retroperitoneal or inguinal nodes |
| Stage IV | Growth involving one or both ovaries with distant metastasis; if pleural effusion is present, there must be positive cytologic test results to allot a case to stage IV; parenchymal liver metastasis equals stage IV |

FIGO = International Federation of Gynecology and Obstetrics.

A. **Therapy of epithelial ovarian neoplasm demonstrating borderline malignancy**

1. **No preservation of fertility.** If the maintenance of fertility is not an issue, total abdominal hysterectomy and bilateral salpingo-oophorectomy are the treatment of choice. Because of the possibility that what appears to be a borderline malignancy on frozen section may be frankly invasive on review of permanent sections, an aggressive staging, as described, should be done, including multiple peritoneal biopsies and washings. As the prognosis for these lesions is 95% or higher for ultimate cure, most centers now do not add chemotherapy as part of the initial treatment. Even in higher stage disease, the value of adjuvant therapy has not been clearly demonstrated.
2. **Preservation of fertility.** If the maintenance of fertility is desired, the issue is to make as certain as possible that the cancer has not spread beyond the involved ovary, which is usually removed. The presumed uninvolved ovary must be wedge biopsied, because conservative treatment, that is, removal of only one adnexa, should be carried out only if the contralateral tube and ovary are free of pathology.

B. **Therapy of malignant epithelial ovarian tumors** varies from center to center, although some general principles of treatment apply. The first is that surgery (usually total abdominal hysterectomy, bilateral salpingo-oophorectomy, omentectomy, and metastatis evaluation) is the primary mode of therapy. The second is that these tumors, except for the most confined, well-differentiated varieties, must have adjuvant therapy. Most centers rely on chemotherapy for this purpose, although some use pelvic or whole abdominal irradiation. In advanced stages, the prognosis for long-term survival and possible cure is in direct proportion to the completeness of the tumor excision at the time of initial laparotomy. Meticulous cytoreductive surgery, or debulking, is the crucial factor.

1. **Treatment of epithelial cancers of the ovary.** Table 32.2 gives an outline for treatment of epithelial cancers of the ovary. However, treatment in this disease must be highly individualized.
   a. In stages III and IV disease, combination chemotherapy is more effective than use of a single agent.
   b. In early stage disease with no residual tumor after surgery, intraperitoneal $P_{32}$ has been used with success in many centers.
   c. Whole abdominal radiation by open field technique to approximately 30 Gy has been used with success in stage III disease optimally debulked with no residual gross tumor.
   d. The most effective combination chemotherapy regimen has been cyclophosphamide (Cytoxan)–doxorubicin (Adriamycin)–cisplatin (Platinol). New thera-

**Table 32.2 Treatment Outline for Ovarian Epithelial Cancers**

| STAGE | TREATMENT |
|---|---|
| Stage IA; IB, grade 1 | TAH, BSO; staging laparotomy |
| Stage IA, IB, grade 2,3<br>Stage IC<br>Stage IIA | TAH, BSO; staging laparotomy; chemotherapy or whole abdomen radiation 25 Gy to 30 Gy b.i.d. technique |
| Stage IIB | TAH, BSO; staging laparotomy; dubulking of all disease in pelvis, then depending on amount of residual disease, either chemotherapy or whole abdomen radiation 25 Gy to 30 Gy b.i.d. technique |
| Stage III<br>State IV | TAH, BSO; maximal cytoreductive surgery; combination chemotherapy either peripheral or intraperitoneal |

TAH = total abdominal hysterectomy; BSO = bilateral salpingo-oophorectomy.

peutic modalities have focused on using analogues of cisplatin with fewer side effects and eliminating doxorubicin particularly in optimally debulked stage III disease.

e. Carboplatinum, because it can be administered without prehydration, and because of less severe side effects, in replacing cisplatin in many centers.

f. In substantially debulked patients, many centers are initiating intraperitoneal chemotherapy by an indwelling port, using cisplatin and etoposide (VP-16).

**2. Second-look laparotomy**

a. **Indication and preparation.** If after an appropriate course of chemotherapy the patient is clinically free of disease, a decision must be made whether or not to discontinue therapy. To help make this decision, the patient undergoes a repeat metastatic work-up, including intravenous urogram, barium enema, computed tomography scan, bone scan, cystoscopy, and proctoscopy, as well as complete physical examination. If the repeat metastatic work-up is negative, an exploratory laparotomy may be performed. This surgery is commonly referred to as a second-look exploratory laparotomy, as the goal is a "second-look" to see if tumor remains. If no tumor is seen, the maneuvers described for initial staging at laparotomy are repeated.

b. **Laparoscopy** can be used prior to laparotomy, and if tumor is seen, celiotomy can be avoided. However, negative laparoscopy is not sufficient evidence for absence of disease. In some situations, even if tumor is known to be present, laparoscopy and laparotomy can be used to assess the efficacy of the drugs being given and progress being made.

c. **The therapeutic decisions** that must be made after the second-look laparotomy are complex and often controversial. If the laparotomy is negative, should all chemotherapy be stopped or should a maintenance regimen be carried out? No randomized prospective studies exist to answer this. If there is disease found, but less than that left behind at initial surgery, should the same chemotherapeutic drugs be continued or a different regimen devised? If there is a progression of disease, what is the most appropriate next step? Alternative chemotherapy? Radiation therapy? Further cytoreductive surgery? Each case is decided on an individual basis. Because of the complexity of these enzymes, the role of second-look laparotomy itself, is under scrutiny.

**C. Management of specialized stromal tumors.** Stromal tumors are managed in the same basic manner as are epithelial tumors, with some differences depending on the tumor cell type.

1. **Granulosa cell tumors** are of low malignant potential and recurrence may occur several years after initial therapy. When recurrence does occur, it is most often in residual pelvic structures. Therefore, optimal therapy includes total abdominal hysterectomy and bilateral salpingo-oophorectomy. Disseminated or recurrent granulosa tumors respond to doxorubicin, and cisplatin combinations. Many of these tumors are estrogen producing, causing endometrial stimulation and abnormal or postmenopausal bleeding. Endometrial biopsy is often required to rule-out endometrial carcinoma. The 5-year survival rate is 70% to 90%.
2. **Sertoli-Leydig cell tumors.** Optimal therapy for Sertoli-Leydig cell tumors is total abdominal hysterectomy and bilateral salpingo-oophorectomy. However, conservation of the contralateral ovary and the uterus is safe if the tumor is limited to one ovary. These tumors may present with increasing masculinization, including acne, hirsutism, voice change, clitoromegaly, and amenorrhea, although some may present with hyperestrogenic effects. These tumors have a low malignant potential and a 5-year survival rate of 70% to 90%.

**D. Management of germ cell tumors.** Germ cell tumors comprise 15% to 20% of all ovarian neoplasms and are most frequently seen in young women. The discussion of diagnosis, staging, and therapy for epithelial tumors is broadly applicable to these tumors with some specific differences dictated by the unique natures of each germ cell tumor. Malignant germ cell neoplasms tend to enlarge rapidly so that evaluation and management must be done with clarity. Certain tumor markers are associated with these tumors: Endodermal sinus tumor—AFP; choriocarcinoma—hCG; embryonal carcinoma—AFP and hCG. These tumor markers can be used both in making the diagnosis and in determining persistence or recurrence of the disease. Any patient with a suspected germ cell neoplasm should have hCG and AFP assays performed. Many germ cell tumors may contain more than one element. Therapy should be tailored toward successful treatment of the element with the worst prognosis.

1. **Dysgerminoma.** Pure dysgerminomas are exquisitely sensitive to radiation therapy. The initial management decision is difficult when deciding between the use of a conventional therapeutic modality and a more experimental one that would conserve the patient's fertility. Each case must be individualized, with parental and patient input playing a major role. Recurrences of this tumor are also radiosensitive, and 75% show an excellent response.
2. **Endodermal sinus tumors, embryonal carcinomas, and choriocarcinoma** are best treated with surgery, followed by combination chemotherapy. Regimens used include VP-16–bleomycin–cisplatin (VBP), vincristine–actinomycin D–chlorambucil (MAC).
3. **Immature teratomas.** As these are almost always unilateral, oophorectomy followed by VAC or VBP chemotherapeutic regimens has shown considerable success.

## X. Chemotherapeutic agents.

**X. Chemotherapeutic agents.** Chemotherapy for ovarian cancer is a rapidly changing field. New drugs and combinations are constantly being evaluated in multicenter studies. Below is a classification and brief description of those agents most often used in gynecologic oncology at this time.

A. **Alkylating agents** are noncyclodependent cytotoxic agents that work by cross-linking strands of DNA.

1. **Melphalan (Alkeran)**
   a. It is the standard by which efficacy of other chemotherapeutic drugs, or combinations, is measured in the treatment of ovarian epithelial cancers. It is now seldom used.
   b. Usually given orally, although may be given intravenously.
   c. Usually given intermittently over a 4-to-5 day period once every 4 to 6 weeks.
   d. Adverse reactions: bone marrow depression, acute nonlymphocytic leukemia with high cumulative doses.
2. **Cyclophosphamide**
   a. Inhibits DNA synthesis and, therefore, is the only alkylator that is cycloactive.

b. May be given as intermittent intravenous therapy or daily oral dose.
c. Potent immunosuppressant.
d. Platelet sparing.
e. Adverse reactions: alopecia, hemorrhagic cystitis, bone marrow depression.

3. **Chlorambucil (Leukeran)**
a. Given orally.
b. Relatively nontoxic.
c. Adverse reactions: macroglobulinemia, bone marrow depression.

B. **Antimetabolites** are cycloactive and work by inhibiting DNA and RNA synthesis. Their action is usually in the S phase of the cell cycle. Purine and pyrimidine metabolism are primarily affected.

1. **Methotrexate (A-methopterin, MTX)**
a. Inhibits dihydrofolate reductase, thus preventing biosynthesis of thymidylic acid, which is required for DNA and RNA synthesis.
b. Effects can be countered by giving citrovorum factor, which bypasses the enzymatic inhibition.
c. Can be given orally, intramuscularly, or intravenously.
d. Adverse reaction: toxic to bone marrow, causes stomatitis, nausea, and vomiting.
e. Ninety percent of drug excreted unchanged in the urine.

2. **5-fluorouracil (5-FU)**
a. Inhibits thymidylate production needed for DNA synthesis.
b. Competes with uracil at RNA sites.
c. May be given intravenously, orally, or as a topical cream.
d. Adverse reactions: diarrhea, alopecia, stomatitis, bone marrow toxicity, gastrointestinal ulceration.
e. Metabolized primarily by the liver.

C. **Antibiotics** used in cancer chemotherapy are derived mainly from *Streptomyces*. They exert most of their effect on DNA synthesis.

1. **Actinomycin-D (dactinomycin, Cosmegen)**
a. Inhibits DNA-dependent RNA synthesis.
b. Excreted unchanged in bile. Therefore, it can be given even with impaired renal function, but patient must have good hepatic function.
c. Given intravenously only. Can be irritating to the tissue if it extravasates.
d. Has a synergistic effect with radiation on skin.

2. **Bleomycin (Blenoxane)**
a. Acts by causing breaks in DNA strands.
b. Has no bone marrow toxicity.

c. It is broken down by enzymes in all tissues of the body except skin and lungs, and therefore is toxic to skin and lungs and may cause fevers.
d. If total dose administered is greater than 400 U, a high risk of pulmonary fibrosis is encountered.

3. **Doxorubicin (Adriamycin)**
    a. Reacts by forming complexes with DNA that break down helix.
    b. Given intravenously.
    c. May cause necrosis and sloughing of skin if it extravasates into subcutaneous tissue.
    d. If total lifetime dose exceeds 550 mg/m$^2$, patient may develop cardiomyopathy and heart failure unresponsive to cardiotonic drugs.
    e. Other adverse reactions: toxic to hair, bone marrow, and gastrointestinal tract.

D. **Vinca alkaloids** are plant alkaloids that work by arresting cell division in the metaphase of mitosis. They also affect biosynthesis of RNA.

1. **Vinblastine**
    a. Given intravenously, it can cause severe local irritation if it extravasates.
    b. Metabolized in liver.
    c. Adverse reactions: bone marrow depression, alopecia, peripheral neuropathy.
2. **Vincristine**
    a. Given IV, may cause local irritation if it extravasates.
    b. Metabolized by the liver.
    c. Causes minimal bone marrow toxicity.
    d. May cause marked peripheral neurotoxicity, severe constipation, and alopecia.

E. **Miscellaneous agents**

1. **Cisplatin**
    a. Works by creating cross-linkages with DNA.
    b. Must be given only after aggressive hydration. Urinary output must be monitored carefully after treatment.
    c. Adverse reactions: renal, neural, and vestibulocochlear toxicity. Severe nausea and vomiting.

F. **New chemotherapeutic agents and technique**

1. **Carboplatinum**
    a. Same activity as cisplatin.
    b. Much less renal, vestibular, neural, and ototoxicity than cisplatin.
    c. Does not require prehydration for administration.
    d. Has higher myelotoxicity than cisplatin.
    e. Is replacing cisplatin in many centers.
2. **Etoposide (VP-16)**
    a. Has broad spectrum of activity.
    b. Useful in germ cell tumors of the ovary as well as gestational trophoblastic neoplasia.

c. Efficacious combined with cisplatin in intraperitoneal chemotherapy.

3. **Ifosfemide**

a. Causes hemorrhagic cystitis and must be given in conjunction with mesua.

b. Used increasingly as second-line therapy in ovarian, cervical and sarcomatous malignancies.

c. Being used increasingly in combination with etoposide and cisplatin.

4. **Intraperitoneal chemotherapy**

a. Can be used as second-line therapy, or as primary therapy if there is bulky residual disease.

b. It is based on the principle of high level concentration with decreased systemic concentration, therefore causing less side effects.

c. Can be given with systemic protector (e.g., thiosulfate) to minimize side effects at distant organs.

**XI. Follow-up during chemotherapy and other adjuvant therapy.** During adjuvant therapy, the patient must be examined at least monthly or before each treatment course, whichever is more frequent. If there is progression of disease, the treatment must be changed. Once therapy is completed, follow-up should be every 8 weeks for the first 2 years, and semi-annually thereafter.

A. **Evaluation for toxicity of chemotherapy.** Depending on the chemotherapeutic agent used, follow-up should include evaluation for toxicity: doxorubicin–cardiac dysfunction; cisplatin–neurotoxicity, renal toxicity, cochlear damage; bleomycin–interstitial pneumonitis; melphalan–leukemogenic potential.

B. **Psychosocial evaluation.** Ongoing psychosocial evaluation must be conducted to adequately determine the benefit of continued chemotherapy when the therapeutic intent is palliative and noncurative.

C. **Assessment of response to therapy.** The role of CA-125 in assessing response to therapy is useful. However, a negative CA-125 does not guarantee loss of disease.

**XII. Prognosis.** Patients with early stage disease may experience cure, but in most cases, diagnosis is not made until ovarian cancer is at a more advanced stage. In most cases of advanced ovarian cancer, the aim of therapy is palliative. It is important to recognize that the goal is a greater progression-free interval and not necessarily cure. With the advances in new therapeutic modalities on the horizon, especially the use of biologicals such as interleukin-2, interferon, and monoclonal targeting, prolongation of a progression-free interval may prove curative. The most important criterion for survival in epithelial ovarian cancer is whether or not the surgeon who performed the initial exploratory procedure did the necessary aggressive surgery. Adjuvant therapy plays only a secondary role.

A. **Survival statistics for epithelial ovarian cancers**

1. Five-year survival statistics for epithelial ovarian cancers, as well as mean survival time in months, are difficult to determine accurately for the following reasons:
   a. Possible understaging of what appear to be early lesions but which, in reality, are stage III tumors. For example, a grade 3 carcinoma limited to one ovary may have metastasized to the para-aortic nodes, but a retroperitoneal node dissection was not done at the initial laparotomy.
   b. Nonuniformity in the thoroughness of cytoreductive surgery at initial laparotomy.
   c. The use of new drugs and new drug combinations that have not been in use long enough to judge their potency.
2. **Survival statistics**
   a. **For stage I disease,** 5-year survival is quoted as being 70%. However, in those series of patients where aggressive staging was done, survival was 90% in stage IA and IB. In stage IC the usual figure is 50%.
   b. **For stage II and stage III disease,** 5-year survival depends on whether or not the tumor was completely excised.
      (1) In stage II patients with completely excised tumor there is a 35% to 50% 5-year survival. If the tumor is not completely excised, survival drops to 15%.
      (2) In stage III patients where the tumor is completely excised 30% to 40% will survive for 5 years. If the tumor is partially excised, 5-year survival is 5%.
      (3) One other subgroup of stage III includes those patients who are optimally debulked. In these patients tumor is still present, but no individual tumor nodule is greater than 1.5 cm in any dimension. In several centers a 50% 2-year survival has been obtained in these patients.
   c. **For stage IV disease the 5-year survival is 5%**
      **Note:** If mean survival time in months is examined, patients on a single agent who are in stage III and minimally debulked have a survival time of 1 year. Maximally debulked patients in the same category have a mean survival time as high as 3 years. Combination regimens double the mean survival time.

B. **Survival in germ cell ovarian tumors**

1. Dysgerminoma 5-year survival is 70% to 90%.
2. In other germ tumors, especially advanced ones, the prognosis has traditionally been dismal. However, with the recent use of new combination chemotherapy, especially VBP, a drastic reduction in mortality has resulted.

## BIBLIOGRAPHY

Barber HRK, Graber EA. Gynecologic tumors in childhood and adolescence. Obstet Gynecol Surv 1973; 28:357.

Chen S. Survival of ovarian carcinoma with or without lymph node metastasis. Gynecol Oncol 1987; 27:368.

Creasman WT, Fetter BF, Hammon CB, Parker RT. Germ cell malignancies of the ovary. Obstet Gynecol 1979; 53:226.

Dembo AJ, Bush RS, Beale FA, Bean HA, Pringle JF, Sturgeon JF. The Princess Margaret Hospital study of ovarian cancer: Stages I, II and asymptomatic III presentations. Cancer Treat Rep 1979; 63:249–254.

Evans AJ, III, Gaffey TA, Malkasian GD, Jr., Annegers JF. Clinicopathologic review of 118 granulosa and 82 theca cell tumors. Obstet Gynecol 1980; 55:231–238.

Freel JH, Cassir JF, Pierce VK, Woodruff J, Lewis JL, Jr. Dysgerminoma of the ovary. Cancer 1979; 43:798–805.

Granbeys S, Noren H, Friley L. Ovarian cancer stages I and II predictions and 5-year survival in two decades. Gynecol Oncol 1989; 35:204.

Griffiths CT, Parker LM, Fuller AF. Role of cytoreductive surgical treatment in the management of advanced ovarian cancer. Cancer Treat Rep 1979; 63:235.

Knapp RC, Friedman EA. Aortic lymph node metastases in early ovarian cancer. Am J Obstet Gynecol 1974; 119:1013.

McGowan L, Parent L, Lednar W, Norris HJ. The woman at risk for developing ovarian cancer. Gynecol Oncol 1979; 7:325–344.

Omura GA, Morrow CP, Blessing JA, Miller A, Buchsbaum HJ, Homesley HD, Leone L. Randomized trial of melphalan versus melphalan plus hexamethylmelamine versus adriamycin plus cyclophosphamide in advanced ovarian adenocarcinoma. Cancer Res 1983; 51:783–789.

Piver MS. Incidence of subclinical metastasis in Stage I and II ovarian carcinoma. Obstet Gynecol 1978; 52:100.

Scully RE. Ovarian tumors. A review. Am J Pathol 1977; 87:686.

Smith JP, Delgado G, Ruledge F. Second look operation in ovarian carcinoma. Cancer 1976; 38:1738.

Sotrel G, Jafari K, Lash AF, Stepto RC. Acute leukemia in advanced ovarian carcinoma after treatment with alkylating agents. Obstet Gynecol 1976; 47:67S–71S.

Podczaski E, Stevens C, Menetta A. Use of second look laparotomy in the management of patients with ovarian epithelial malignancies. Gynecol Oncol 1987; 28:205.

Zanaboni F, Vergadoro F, Presti M, Gallotti P, Lombardi F, Bolis G. Tumor antigen CA125 as a marker of ovarian epithelial carcinoma. Gynecol Oncol 1987; 28:61–67.

# CHAPTER 33

# Gestational Trophoblastic Disease

**John R. Lurain III**

Gestational trophoblastic disease encompasses four clinical–pathologic forms of growth disturbances of the human trophoblast: hydatidiform mole, invasive mole, choriocarcinoma, and placental site trophoblastic tumor. The term gestational trophoblastic tumor has been applied to the latter three conditions because the diagnosis and decision to institute treatment are often undertaken without knowledge of the precise histology. The overall cure rate in the treatment of gestational trophoblastic tumors now exceeds 90%. This high success rate is the result of: (1) effective use of sensitive assays for the tumor marker human chorionic gonadotropin (hCG); (2) the inherent sensitivity of trophoblastic tumors to chemotherapy; (3) the referral of patients to specialized treatment centers; (4) the identification of high-risk factors that enhance individualization of therapy; and (5) the aggressive use of combination chemotherapy, irradiation, and occasionally surgical intervention in the care of high-risk patients.

## I. Incidence

- A. **Hydatidiform mole.** The incidence of hydatidiform mole in the United States and Europe is approximately 1 in 1500 pregnancies. In other areas, especially the Orient, the incidence has been reported to be more than 1 in 100 pregnancies. However, much of this geographic variation may be due to reporting differences rather than true incidence differences. There is an increased incidence of molar pregnancy for women over the age of 40 and at the lower end of the reproductive range, although there appears to be no significant association with gravidity.
- B. **Invasive mole.** The overall incidence of invasive mole has been estimated to be 1 per 15 000 pregnancies.
- C. **Choriocarcinoma** is reported to occur in 1 in 40 000 pregnancies.

## II. **Morbidity and mortality.** With the advent of effective chemotherapy for the treatment of gestational trophoblastic neoplasia, the

overall cure rate now exceeds 90% and there has been a marked decrease in morbidity. Prior to the use of chemotherapy, results of treatment for gestational trophoblastic neoplasia were poor. The overall mortality from invasive mole was 14% to 35%, with deaths not due to matastatic or malignant disease but rather to hemorrhage, sepsis, embolic phenomena, uterine perforation, or complications from surgery. Choriocarcinoma was a rapidly progressing tumor with a high death rate. The cure rate with hysterectomy when disease was thought to be confined to the uterus was only 40%, and almost all patients with metastatic disease died. The causes of death in the majority of patients with metastatic disease are related to hemorrhage from one or more sites, including the lungs, brain, liver, gastrointestinal tract, and other intraperitoneal structures, and/or pulmonary insufficiency.

**III. Etiology.** The etiology of hydatidiform mole remains unclear, but it appears to be due to abnormal gametogenesis and fertilization. Two main theories have been proposed to explain the sequence of events that produce hydatidiform mole. Hertig and Edmonds considered that the lesion was caused by retention of a blighted ovum, with cessation of development of the villous stromal circulation. They noted that continued secretory activity of the trophoblast, nourished by the maternal blood, resulted in varying degrees of fluid accumulation within the villous stroma and trophoblastic proliferation. Park believed that the primary abnormality lay in the trophoblast, dysplasia, and resultant proliferation of the trophoblast causing an oversecretion of fluid into the villous stroma. Neither theory can completely explain the absence of a fetus or fetal tissues in complete moles, the reasons for varying degrees of hydropic change and trophoblastic proliferation seen in complete moles, partial moles, and abortuses, or the cytogenetic differences between complete and partial moles. No environmental exposure, infectious agents, or nutritional factors have definitely been implicated in the etiology of trophoblastic diseases, although one study suggests a possible link between dietary carotene/vitamin A deficiency and hydatidiform mole.

**IV. Pathogenesis and pathophysiology**

A. **Hydatidiform mole** is characterized by vesicular swelling of placental villi and usually the absence of an intact fetus. Microscopically proliferation of the trophoblast (cytotrophoblast and syncytiotrophoblast), with varying degrees of hyperplasia and dysplasia, is seen. The chorionic villi are fluid-filled and distended and blood vessels are scanty. Two syndromes of hydatidiform mole have been described based on both cytogenetic and morphologic criteria.

1. **Complete or classical hydatidiform moles** undergo early and total hydatidiform enlargement of placental villi in the absence of an ascertainable fetus/embryo, and the trophoblast is consistently hyperplastic. Complete moles usually

give a 46,XX karyotype derived from a paternal haploid set that totally replaces the maternal contribution and reaches the 46,XX status by its own duplication. Occasionally a 46,XY karyote occurs as a result of fertilization of an empty egg. Trophoblastic sequelae (invasive mole or choriocarcinoma) follow complete mole in 15% to 20% of cases and are most commonly associated with heterozygote moles.

2. **Partial hydatidiform moles** are characterized by slowly progressing hydatidiform change in the presence of functioning villus capillaries that affects only some of the villi. These changes are associated with an identifiable fetus/embryo (alive or dead) or fetal membranes or red blood cells. Trophoblastic immaturity is a consistent microscopic finding and there is only focal hyperplasia. Partial moles give a triploid karyotype, usually 69,XXY. The reported incidence of trophoblastic sequelae following partial mole varies between 4% and 11%, with metastases occurring rarely. A histopathologic diagnosis of choriocarcinoma has not been confirmed following a partial mole.

B. **Invasive mole,** a benign tumor arising from a hydatidiform mole, invades the myometrium by direct extension or by way of venous channels and may metastasize to distant sites in about 15% of cases, most commonly to the lung and vagina. The tumor is characterized by swollen villi and accompanying trophoblast with hyperplasia and usually by dysplasia located in sites outside the cavity of the uterus. Invasive mole tends to undergo spontaneous regression.

C. **Choriocarcinoma,** a malignant disease, is characterized by abnormal trophoblastic hyperplasia and anaplasia, absence of chorionic villi, hemorrhage and necrosis, direct invasion of the myometrium, and vascular spread to the myometrium and distant sites, the most common being the lungs, brain, liver, pelvis/vagina, spleen, intestines, and kidney.

D. **Placental-site trophoblastic tumor** was originally described as an exaggerated form of syncytial endomyometritis. Pathologically, the trophoblastic cells infiltrate the myometrium and grow between smooth muscle cells, but unlike syncytial endomyometritis, there is vascular invasion. Placental-site trophoblastic tumor differs from choriocarcinoma primarily because of the absence of an alternating pattern of cytotrophoblast and syncytiotrophoblast, the cells being of one type thought to represent intermediate cells. Hemorrhage and necrosis are less evident in this tumor than in choriocarcinoma. There are no placental villi. Human placental lactogen is present in the tumor cells, whereas immunoperoxidase staining for hCG is positive in only scattered cells and serum hCG levels are relatively low compared with choriocarcinoma. There appears to be a direct correlation between the mitotic activity and the clinical behavior of the tumor. Although most reports have noted a benign course for these tumors, they are relatively resistant to chemotherapy, and surgery has been the mainstay of treatment.

## V. Differential diagnosis

**A. Hydatidiform mole** must be distinguished from:

1. A normal intrauterine pregnancy.
2. A threatened or missed abortion.
3. An intrauterine pregnancy complicated by multiple gestation or diseases associated with an enlarged placenta and elevated hCG levels (e.g., erythroblastosis fetalis and intrauterine infections).
4. An enlarged uterus secondary to uterine leiomyomata with a small normal intrauterine pregnancy.

**B. Gestational trophoblastic tumors** (invasive mole and choriocarcinoma) are usually easily diagnosed following a molar pregnancy. Choriocarcinoma associated with a nonmolar pregnancy, however, must be distinguished from:

1. Retained products of conception or pelvic infection as causes of postpartum uterine bleeding and subinvolution.
2. Primary or metastatic tumors of other organ systems.
3. Another pregnancy occurring shortly after the first.

## VI. Diagnosis

### A. Signs and symptoms

**1. Hydatidiform mole**

a. Uterine bleeding, usually occurring during the 6th to 16th week of gestation in over 95% of patients.
b. Toxemia of pregnancy in the first or second trimester.
c. Hyperemesis.
d. Hyperthyroidism (rare).
e. Trophoblastic emboli with symptoms and signs of congestive heart failure and pulmonary edema (rare).
f. Spontaneous expulsion of typical molar tissue.

**2. Invasive mole and choriocarcinoma**

a. Continued uterine bleeding after molar evacuation or other pregnancy event.
b. Bleeding from metastatic lesions.
c. Uterine perforation.

### B. Physical examination

**1. Hydatidiform mole**

a. Uterine enlargement greater than expected for gestational dates (50% of cases).
b. Bilateral theca lutein cyst enlargement of the ovaries (15% of cases).
c. Fetal heart tones usually absent.

2. **Invasive mole and choriocarcinoma**
   a. Enlarged, irregular uterus.
   b. Persistent bilateral ovarian enlargement.
   c. Detection of a metastatic lesion.

C. **Diagnostic findings**

1. **Hydatidiform mole**
   a. Ultrasonography that demonstrates multiple echoes and holes within the placental mass (the snowstorm pattern) and usually no fetus. Ultrasound has virtually replaced all other means of preoperative diagnosis.
   b. Human chorionic gonadotropin levels usually, but not always, higher than in normal gestation.
2. **Invasive mole and choriocarcinoma**
   a. Human chorionic gonadotropin levels persistently elevated or rising after any pregnancy event.
   b. Metastatic lesions identified by radiologic studies and scans of various organs.
   c. Angiographic identification of intramyometrial lesion.
   d. Pathologic diagnosis can sometimes be made by curettage, biopsy of metastatic lesions, or occasionally by examination of hysterectomy specimens or placentas. However, biopsy of a vaginal lesion is infrequently performed because of the massive and uncontrolled bleeding that may occur.

## VII. Management

A. **Hydatidiform mole**

1. **Preoperative evaluation** consists of the history and physical examination, complete blood count (CBC) and platelet count, coagulation profile, serum chemistries, thyroid panel, blood type and cross match, quantitative hCG level, urinalysis, chest x-ray (posterior–anterior and lateral), pelvic ultrasound, electrocardiogram (ECG).
2. **Surgical evacuation**
   a. Suction curettage followed by sharp curettage is the preferred method of evacuation, independent of uterine size. Intravenous pitocin (20 to 40 U/L of fluid at 6 to 8 h/L rates for most patients) should be infused near the end of evacuation and continued for several hours.
   b. Hysterectomy is an alternative to suction curettage if no further childbearing is desired.
3. **Follow-up hCG levels** should be obtained every 1 to 2 weeks until negative for three consecutive determinations, followed by every 3 months for 1 year.
4. **Postoperative physical examination** should be performed in 1 month.

5. **Contraception** should be maintained during this follow-up period (1 year). Oral contraceptives are acceptable, although any effective method is satisfactory.
6. **Patients at highest risk for postmolar trophoblastic tumors**
   a. Pre-evacuation uterine size larger than expected for gestational duration or greater than 20 weeks size.
   b. Bilateral ovarian enlargement (theca lutein cysts).
   c. Age greater than 40 years.
   d. High hCG levels.
   e. Medical complications of molar pregnancy such as toxemia, hyperthyroidism, and trophoblastic embolization.
   f. Repeat hydatidiform mole.
7. **Indications for treatment of postmolar trophoblastic tumor**
   a. Plateauing hCG levels for three consecutive determinations.
   b. Rising hCG levels for two consecutive determinations.
   c. High hCG levels (> 20,000 mIU/mL) more than 4 weeks after evacuation.
   d. Persistently elevated hCG levels 6 months after evacuation.
   e. Histopathologic diagnosis of choriocarcinoma.

**B. Gestational trophoblastic tumors** (invasive mole or choriocarcinoma)

1. **Pretreatment evaluation.** After a thorough history and physical examination, the following studies should be obtained: chest x-ray (chest computed tomography [CT] scan if negative), abdominopelvic CT scan, brain CT scan or magnetic resonance imaging, CBC and platelet count, serum chemistries, and a quantitative serum hCG.
2. **Staging.** After these initial studies, patients are categorized based on anatomic extent of disease and likelihood of response to various chemotherapy protocols. Based on these classifications, treatment is carried out accordingly.
   a. **International Federation of Gynecology and Obstetrics (FIGO) clinical staging** (Table 33.1). A system based on anatomic criteria and conforming to the staging systems used for all other gynecologic cancer was adopted by the FIGO Cancer Committee in 1982. Most treatment centers in the United States and Europe determine therapy and report results of treatment using prognostic-factor systems rather than an anatomic system alone.
   b. **Prognostic group clinical classification** (Table 33.2). This system is the basis by which most major U.S. trophoblastic disease centers determine treatment and

**Table 33.1. FIGO Clinical Staging**

| STAGE | DESCRIPTION |
|---|---|
| I | Gestational trophoblastic tumor strictly contained to the uterine corpus |
| II | Gestational trophoblastic tumor extends to the adnexae, outside the uterus but is limited to the genital structures |
| III | Gestational trophoblastic tumor extends to the lungs with or without genital tract involvement |
| IV | All other metastatic sites |

FIGO = International Federation of Gynecology and Obstetrics.

**Table 33.2. Prognostic Group Clinical Classification**

I. Nonmetastatic gestational trophoblastic tumor
II. Metastatic gestational trophoblastic tumor
  A. Low-risk
    1. hCG <100 000 IU/24-hour urine or <40 000 mIU/mL serum
    2. Symptoms present for less than 4 months
    3. No brain or liver metastases
    4. No prior chemotherapy
    5. Pregnancy event is not term delivery (i.e., mole, ectopic, or spontaneous abortion)
  B. High-risk
    1. hCG > 100 000 IU/24-hour urine or >40 000 mIU/mL serum
    2. Symptoms present for more than 4 months
    3. Brain or liver metastases
    4. Prior chemotherapeutic failure
    5. Antecedent term pregnancy

hCG = human chorionic gonadotropin.

report results. Patients with gestational trophoblastic tumors are divided into three groups: nonmetastatic, low-risk metastatic, and high-risk metastatic. "High-risk" refers to those patients who are not likely to be cured by single-agent chemotherapy and are at the highest risk for treatment failure.

c. **World Health Organization (WHO) prognostic scoring system** (Table 33.3). In 1983, the WHO adopted a modified prognostic scoring system proposed by Bagshawe based on nine factors. A weighted score was applied to each factor, each was assumed to act as an independent variable, and their effects were assumed to be additive. Patients with a score of four or less are considered to be low risk, those with a score of five to seven are middle-risk, and those with scores of eight or greater are high-risk.

**Table 33.3. Scoring System Based on Prognostic Factors in Gestational Trophoblastic Disease**

| RISK FACTORS | SCORE 0 | 1 | 2 | 4 |
|---|---|---|---|---|
| Age (y) | ≤39 | >39 | | |
| Antecedent pregnancy | Hydatidiform mole | Abortion | Term | |
| Pregnancy event to treatment interval (mo) | <4 | 4–6 | 7–12 | >12 |
| hCG (IU/L) | $<10^3$ | $10^3$–$10^4$ | $10^4$–$10^5$ | $>10^5$ |
| ABO blood groups (female × male) | | O × A<br>A × O | B<br>AB | |
| No. of metastases | | 1–4 | 4–8 | >8 |
| Site of metastases | | Spleen<br>Kidney | GI tract<br>Liver | Brain |
| Largest tumor mass, including uterine (cm) | | 3–5 | >5 | |
| Prior chemotherapy | | | Single drug | Two or more drugs |

The total score for a patient is obtained by adding the individual scores for each prognostic factor. Total score: ≤4 = low risk; 5–7 = middle risk; ≥8 = high risk. hCG = human chorionic gonadotropin; GI = gastrointestinal.

3. **Treatment of nonmetastatic gestational trophoblastic tumors.**
   a. **Hysterectomy** is used as initial treatment if there is no desire for further fertility or if the diagnosis is placental-site trophoblastic tumor. Adjuvant single-agent chemotherapy at the time of operation is indicated to eradicate any occult metastases. Hysterectomy may also be required as secondary treatment if resistance to chemotherapy develops.
   b. **Single-agent chemotherapy** with methotrexate or actinomycin D is the treatment of choice. Several different chemotherapy protocols have been used, all yielding excellent and comparable results (Table 33.4). No course of chemotherapy should be started if the white blood cell (WBC) count is < 3000 or the platelet count is < 100 000. Actinomycin D should be administered as an injection over 5 to 10 minutes through a well-running intravenous infusion because vascular extravasation results in extensive tissue necrosis.
   c. **The most common toxic reactions** to these drugs are oropharyngeal ulcerations (stomatitis), conjunctivitis, pleuritic or peritoneal pain, vulvovaginitis, and skin

rash. Significant hair loss, leukopenia, and thrombocytopenia are rare.

d. **Chemotherapy is changed** to the alternate agent if the hCG level plateaus or if toxicity precludes an adequate dose or frequency of treatment. If there is a significant elevation in hCG level or development of metastases, multi-agent chemotherapy should be started.

e. **Treatment is continued** until three consecutive normal hCG levels have been obtained and two courses of chemotherapy have been given after the first normal hCG level.

4. **Treatment of low-risk metastatic gestational trophoblastic tumors**

   a. **Single-agent chemotherapy** with methotrexate or actinomycin D, as described above in the section on nonmetastatic disease, is the treatment for patients in this category (Table 33.4). When resistance to single-agent chemotherapy develops, combination chemotherapy as for high-risk disease is used.

   b. **Hysterectomy** may be necessary to eradicate persistent, chemotherapy resistant disease in the uterus, or it can be performed as adjuvant treatment coincident with the institution of chemotherapy to shorten the duration of therapy.

5. **Treatment of high-risk metastatic gestational trophoblastic tumors**

   a. **Multi-agent chemotherapy** (MAC). The EMA-CO chemotherapy regimen formulated by Bagshawe is currently the treatment of choice for high-risk patients (Table 33.5). This regimen uses etoposide, high-dose methotrexate infusion with folinic acid rescue, actinomycin D, cyclophosphamide, and vincristine (Oncovin). When brain metastases are detected, the dosage of methotrexate is increased to 1 g/m$^2$ in conjunction with folinic acid 30 mg every 12 hours for 3 days starting 32 hours after the beginning of the infusion. The MAC triple chemotherapy regimen, using methotrexate, actinomycin D, and cyclophosphamide or

**Table 33.4. Chemotherapy Protocols for Nonmetastatic and Low-Risk Metastatic Gestational Trophoblastic Tumors**

1. Methotrexate 0.4 mg/kg IV or IM qd × 5 days; repeat every 12 to 14 days (7–9 day window)
2. Methotrexate 1 mg/kg IM days 1,3,5,7; folinic acid 0.1 mg/kg IM days 2,4,6,8; repeat every 15 to 18 days (7–10 day window)
3. Actinomycin D 10 to 13 μg/kg IV qd × 5 days; repeat every 12 to 14 days (7–9 day window)
4. Actinomycin D 1.25 mg/m$^2$ IV; repeat every 14 days

**Table 33.5. EMA-CO Chemotherapy Regimen for High-Risk Metastatic Gestational Trophoblastic Tumors**

| | |
|---|---|
| Day 1 | Etoposide 100 mg/m$^2$ IV infusion in 250 mL NS over 30 min<br>Actinomycin D 0.5 mg IV push<br>Methotrexate 100 mg/m$^2$ IV push<br>200 mg/m$^2$ IV infusion in 1000 mL $D_5W$ over 12 h |
| Day 2 | Etoposide 100 mg/m$^2$ IV infusion in 250 mL NS over 30 min<br>Actinomycin D 0.5 mg IV push<br>Folinic acid 15 mg IM every 12 h for four doses beginning 24 h after starting methotrexate |
| Day 8 | Vincristine 1.0 mg/m$^2$ IV push<br>Cyclophosphamide 600 mg/m$^2$ IV |

Repeat cycle on days 15, 16, and 22 (every 2 weeks).
NS = normal saline; $D_5W$ = 5% dextrose in water.

chlorambucil, and the modified Bagshawe protocol CHAMOCA are no longer acceptable alternative regimens for treatment of these high-risk patients.

Chemotherapy is continued until three consecutive normal hCG levels are reached and from two to four courses have been given after the first normal hCG. Only rarely should a course of chemotherapy be started if the WBC count is $< 3000$ or the platelet count is $< 100\,000$.

b. **Toxicity** to combination chemotherapy is significantly greater than to single-agent treatment. Toxic reactions are similar to those listed above for methotrexate and actinomycin D, however, complete alopecia occurs and leukopenia and thrombocytopenia can sometimes be severe. Vincristine may cause neurotoxicity and it acts as a vesicant agent if vascular extravasation occurs. Nausea and vomiting can be moderately severe.

c. **Secondary chemotherapy** yields poor results. Cisplatin and bleomycin are other chemotherapeutic agents with proven activity in trophoblastic tumors. Combinations of these agents with etoposide or vinblastine have resulted in cures in some patients who have failed initial combination chemotherapy for high-risk metastatic disease.

d. **Radiation therapy.** If central nervous system metastases are present, whole-brain irradiation (30–40 cGy) is given simultaneously with the initiation of combination chemotherapy using high-dose infusion methotrexate with folinic acid rescue. Approximately 50% to 60% of patients with brain metastases will achieve sustained remission using this treatment plan.

e. **Surgery.** Adjuvant surgical procedures, especially hysterectomy and thoracotomy, may be useful for the purpose of removing known foci of chemotherapy-resistant disease, controlling hemorrhage, relieving bowel or urinary obstruction, treating infection, or dealing with other life-threatening complications.

6. **Follow-up after successful treatment**

a. **Serum quantitative hCG levels** should be obtained monthly for 6 months, every other month for the remainder of the first year, every 3 months during the second year, and at 6-month intervals indefinitely thereafter.

b. **Contraception** should be maintained for 1 year after the completion of chemotherapy. Barrier methods and oral contraceptives are both acceptable forms of contraception; the latter have the advantage of suppressing pituitary luteinizing hormone, which may interfere with the accurate measurement of hCG.

c. **Subsequent pregnancy.** During a subsequent pregnancy, a pelvic ultrasound is recommended in the first trimester to confirm a normal gestation, because these patients are at increased risk for another gestational trophoblastic disease event. Also, the products of conception or placentas from future pregnancies should be carefully examined histopathologically and an hCG level obtained 6 weeks after pregnancy termination.

## VIII. Prognosis

A. **Hydatidiform mole.** Follow-up of patients after evacuation of hydatidiform mole indicates that this therapy alone is curative in over 80% of patients. Repeat hydatidiform moles occur in 0.5% to 2.6% of patients, with a subsequent greater risk of developing invasive mole or choriocarcinoma.

B. **Nonmetastatic trophoblastic tumor.** Cure is anticipated in essentially all patients with nonmetastatic disease. Approximately 85% of patients will be cured by the initial chemotherapy regimen. Most of the remaining patients will be placed into permanent remission with additional chemotherapy. Less than 5% of patients will require hysterectomy for cure.

C. **Low-risk metastatic trophoblastic tumor.** Cure rates should approach 100% in this group of patients if treatment is administered properly. Approximately 40% to 50% of patients in this category will develop resistance to the first chemotherapeutic agent and require alternate treatment. It is, therefore, important to carefully monitor patients undergoing treatment for evidence of drug resistance so that a change to a second agent can be made at the earliest possible time. About 10% to 15% of patients treated for low-risk metastatic disease will require combination chemotherapy with or without surgery to achieve remission.

D. **High-risk metastatic trophoblastic tumor.** Intensive therapy with combination chemotherapy and, where indicated, adjuvant radiotherapy and surgery has resulted in cure rates of 80% to 90% in patients with high-risk metastatic gestational trophoblastic tumors. Factors primarily responsible for treatment failures in these patients are:
   1. Presence of extensive choriocarcinoma at the time of diagnosis.
   2. Lack of appropriately aggressive initial treatment.
   3. Failure of presently used treatment protocols to control advanced disease.

E. **Reproductive performance.** The successful treatment of gestational trophoblastic tumors with chemotherapy has resulted in a large number of women whose reproductive potential has been retained despite exposure to drugs that have teratogenic potential. Many successful pregnancies have been reported in this group of patients. In general, these patients experience no increase in abortions, stillbirths, congenital anomalies, prematurity, or major obstetrical complications. There is no evidence for reactivation of disease due to a subsequent pregnancy. These patients are at greater risk for the development of a second trophoblastic disease episode in a subsequent pregnancy, but this is unrelated to whether or not they have received chemotherapy previously.

## BIBLIOGRAPHY

Bagshawe KD. Risk and prognostic factors in trophoblastic neoplasia. Cancer 1976; 38:1373.

Bagshawe KD. Treatment of high-risk choriocarcinoma. J Reprod Med 1984; 29:813.

Curry SL, Hammond CB, Tyrey L, Creasman WT, Parker RT. Hydatidiform mole. Diagnosis, management and longterm follow-up of 347 patients. Obstet Gynecol 1975; 45:41.

DuBeshter B, Berkowitz RS, Goldstein DP, Cramer DW, Bernstein MR. Metastatic gestational trophoblastic disease; experience at the New England Trophoblastic Disease Center, 1965 to 1985. Obstet Gynecol 1987; 69:390–395.

Hammond CB, Weed JC, Currie JL. The role of operation in the current therapy of gestational trophoblastic disease. Am J Obstet Gynecol 1980; 136:844.

Hertig AT. Human Trophoblast. Springfield, Ill: Charles C Thomas; 1968.

Lurain JR. Chemotherapy of Gestational Trophoblastic Disease. In: Deppe G, ed. Chemotherapy of Gynecologic Cancer, 2nd ed., New York: Alan R. Liss; 1990.

Lurain JR. Causes of treatment failure in gestational trophoblastic disease. J Reprod Med 1987; 32:675.

Lurain JR. The natural history of gestational trophoblastic diseases. In: Szulman AE, Buchsbaum HJ, eds. Gestational Trophoblastic Disease. New York: Springer–Verlag; 1987.

Lurain JR, Brewer JI, Torok EE, Halpern B. Gestational trophoblastic disease. Treatment results at the Brewer Trophoblastic Disease Center. Obstet Gynecol 1982; 60:364–360.

Lurain JR, Brewer JI, Torok EE, Halpern B. Natural history of hydatidiform mole after primary evacuation. Am J Obstet Gynecol 1983; 145:591–595.

Miller DS, Lurain JR. Classification and staging of gestational trophoblastic tumors. Obstet Gynecol Clin North Am 1988; 15:477.

Morrow CP, Kletzky OA, DiSaia PJ, Townsend DE, Mishell DR, Nakamura RM. Clinical and laboratory correlates of molar pregnancy and trophoblastic disease. Am J Obstet Gynecol 1977; 128:424–430.

Park WW. Choriocarcinoma: A Study of Its Pathology. Philadelphia: FA Davis; 1971.

Soper JT, Clarke-Pearson D, Hammond CB. Metastatic gestational trophoblastic disease: Prognostic factors in previously untreated patients. Obstet Gynecol 1988; 71:338.

Weed JC, Woodward KT, Hammond CB. Choriocarcinoma metastatic to the brain: Therapy and prognosis. Semin Oncol 1982; 9:208.

World Health Organization Scientific Group. Gestational Trophoblastic Disease, Technical Report Series #692, Geneva, World Health Organization, 1983.

# Part V

# Ambulatory Gynecology

# CHAPTER 34

# Common Office Gynecologic Procedures

**Robert L. Summitt, Jr.**
**Thomas G. Stovall**
**Charles R. B. Beckmann**

Many gynecologic procedures can be accomplished in the office. This chapter discusses procedures and techniques for the following: (1) culdocentesis, (2) drainage of a Bartholin's duct cyst, (3) endometrial biopsy, (4) vulvar biopsy, (5) colposcopy, and (6) cryotherapy for cervical dysplasia.

## CULDOCENTESIS

### I. Introduction

**A.** Culdocentesis may be indicated when the diagnosis of intraperitoneal bleeding is uncertain. Note that hemoperitoneum is not always symptomatic. Although, more often used in the patient with a suspected ectopic pregnancy, culdocentesis is not a test for ectopic pregnancy, but rather it is a test for the presence of hemoperitoneum. With the advent of laparoscopic surgical techniques and nonsurgical management, the role of culdocentesis has been called into question. It has been shown that 50% to 60% of patients with small, unruptured ectopics will have a small amount of blood in the cul-de-sac. Because this is not a contraindication to laparoscopic or medical treatment, the exact role of culdocentesis is not well-defined.

**B.** Culdocentesis involves the insertion of a needle through the posterior fornix into the cul-de-sac of Douglas and the aspiration of any fluid contained within it. The procedure (Fig. 34.1) is safe, has minimal discomfort, and is easy to perform. Anesthesia, either systemic or local, is of little benefit in culdocentesis. Instead, the operator should rely on a quick and sure performance of the procedure to minimize discomfort.

### II. Steps in the procedure

**A.** Before culdocentesis, a careful bimanual examination is performed to locate the position and shape of the uterus and to identify other structures in the pelvis.

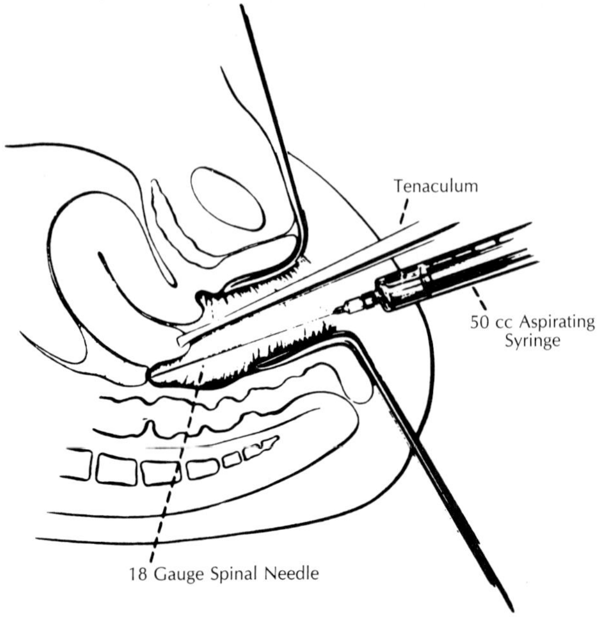


FIGURE 34.1. Culdocentesis. From Mattingly R. Telinde's Operative Gynecology. Philadelphia, Pa: J B Lippincott; 1977. Reprinted with permission.

**B.** Before the procedure, the patient is asked to sit for a few minutes at a 30° to 45° angle so that fluid may accumulate in the cul-de-sac, providing material for sampling as well as further expanding the space to make the likelihood of successful sampling greater.

**C.** The uterus is elevated and the cul-de-sac space "expanded" by traction on the lower lip of the cervix with a tenaculum. To avoid laceration, a vertical rather than horizontal placement of the tenaculum is best.

**D.** A 16-gauge needle, which will not bend and deflect into an unintended site upon insertion, should be used. A 10 or 20 cc syringe is used because it is of sufficient size yet is comfortable to manipulate. The needle should be swiftly and surely inserted into the cul-de-sac, whose position should be carefully visualized in the operator's mind prior to the insertion attempt.

**E.** When the loss of resistance is felt, the needle is in the cul-de-sac. Gentle aspiration will retrieve whatever fluid is in the space.

## III. Interpretation

With good technique, culdocentesis may be considered accurate in about two-thirds of cases of hemoperitoneum, the false-negative rate of about 10% overshadowing the false positive rate of about 2%.

A. **Positive culdocentesis** is defined as easy aspiration of at least 5 cc nonclotting blood. 50% to 60% of patients with an unruptured ectopic will have a positive culdocentesis.
B. **Negative culdocentesis** is defined as aspiration of at least 5 cc clear, serous fluid. Failure to detect hemoperitoneum by a negative culdocentesis usually indicates the absence of intra-abdominal bleeding, but not the absence of an ectopic pregnancy.
C. **Equivocal culdocentesis** is defined as difficult aspiration of less than 5 cc blood-tinged fluid. Equivocal findings may represent the incomplete aspiration of a hemoperitoneum or the aspiration of blood from a vessel in the uterus, ovary, or vaginal wall. Such a finding is not diagnostic of either the presence or absence of hemoperitoneum, and culdocentesis must either be repeated or a diagnosis made on other criteria such as clinical signs and symptoms, physical findings, laboratory evaluation, ultrasonography, or diagnostic laparoscopy.

## DRAINAGE OF A BARTHOLIN'S DUCT CYST

### I. Introduction

A. Obstruction of a Bartholin's duct occurs most commonly near the orifice. The exact etiology is usually unknown, although infection with inflammation probably plays a major role. As a result, the duct becomes closed, while the mucus-secreting glands of the transitional epithelium continue to produce fluid. With acute inflammation, an abscess develops with symptoms of swelling, tenderness, and erythema. Initially, sitz baths may be used to decrease the tenderness and inflammation while at the same time allowing the abscess to "mature" to the point where drainage can be easily accomplished.
B. The incision and drainage of a Bartholin's duct cyst, with Word catheter (Fig. 34.2) placement, will be discussed. This simple procedure will take care of the majority of these cysts. However, if they recur, marsupialization will be required. If the patient has had prior marsupialization, then excision is usually necessary.

### II. Technique of incision and drainage with Word catheter placement

A. The site where the duct opens into the vaginal mucosa is infiltrated with 1% xylocaine. An alternative is to use a spray or topical anesthetic such as ethyl chloride.
B. The wall of the cyst is incised on its medial border, through the vaginal mucosa, outside the hymenal ring. A criss-cross incision, or small linear incision can be made with a #11 blade.
C. A specimen of the discharge should be sent for culture.
D. The cyst cavity is irrigated with normal saline.
E. A Word catheter is placed through the incision and the bulb distended with 2 or 3 cc normal saline.

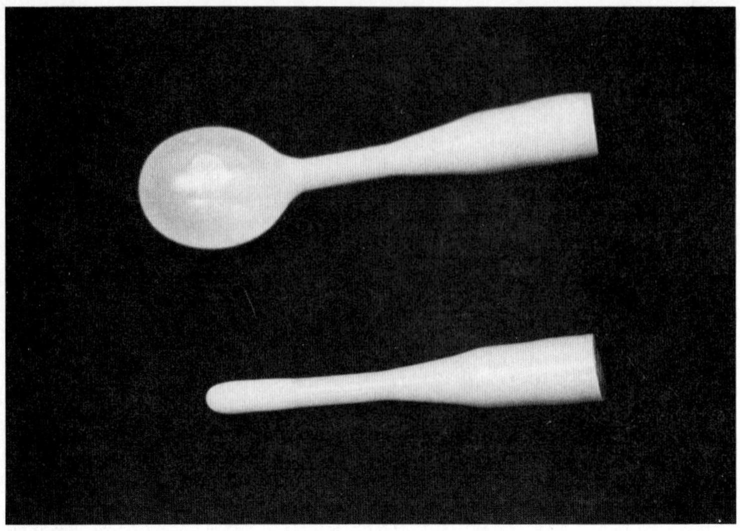

FIGURE 34.2. Word catheter.

F. The nipple of the catheter is inserted into the vagina.
G. Alternatively, the cyst may be packed with iodoform gauze. A pediatric foley may also be used in the place of the Word catheter. The catheter bulb is filled with normal saline and tied with silk suture. The catheter is cut at 2 in.

III. **After-care and follow-up.** The catheter should be left in place for 7 to 14 days to allow for epithelization of the drainage tract that has been created. Twice daily sitz baths will aid in decreasing inflammation and discomfort.

## ENDOMETRIAL BIOPSY

### I. Introduction

A. Endometrial biopsy is one of the diagnostic tests performed most frequently by gynecologists. Indications for endometrial sampling include:
   1. Pre- or postmenopausal abnormal uterine bleeding
   2. Endometrial dating
   3. Documentation of ovulation
   4. The ruling out of endometrial infection

   Many techniques have been described to obtain a sample of endometrial tissue. We will discuss three well-accepted techniques: (1) Pipelle Curette™, (2) Novak Curette, and (3) Vabra™ Aspirator (Fig. 34.3).

B. **General considerations**
   1. The patient should be informed of the risk, benefits, and diagnostic alternatives.

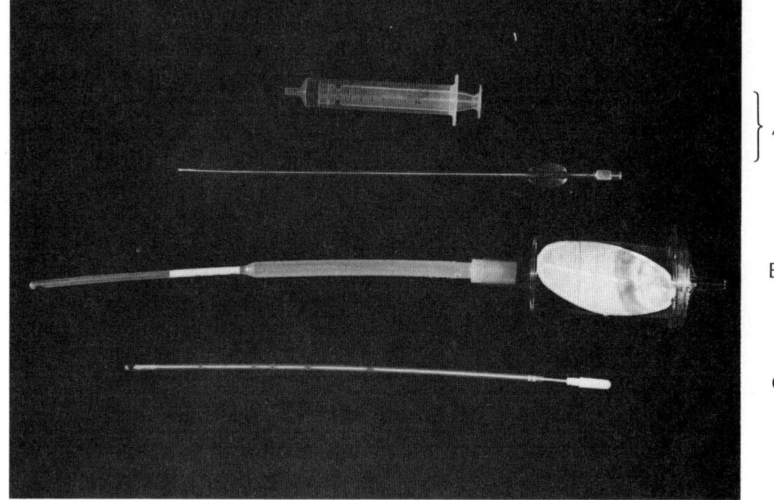


FIGURE 34.3. Endometrial biopsy instruments from top to bottom: (A) Novak Curette and syringe, (B) Vabra Aspirator, and (C) Pipelle Curette.

2. To minimize uterine cramping and patient discomfort, a nonsteroidal anti-inflammatory drug can be given 30 minutes prior to the procedure. Typically, either naproxen-sodium (Anaprox DS) or ibuprofen (Motrin) 800 mg is used.
3. The primary disadvantages to a biopsy procedure is the small sample, which can lead to fear of a missed lesion. However, in several trials, each of the methods discussed have been shown to be reliable.
4. A diagnostic biopsy performed in the cycle of conception, although of concern, does not appear to be associated with pregnancy loss or complication.

## II. Technique

A. After pelvic examination to ascertain uterine size, shape, and position, a speculum is inserted into the vagina and the cervix cleansed with betadine. The anterior lip of the cervix is grasped with a single-toothed tenaculum. Many endometrial biopsies can be accomplished without the use of a tenaculum.

B. **The Pipelle Curette**

1. The Pipelle Curette is inserted into the uterine cavity, and the piston withdrawn, creating negative pressure in the curette.
2. The outer sheath is then rotated and moved from side to side while being slowly withdrawal from the uterus.

3. The plunger is then pushed through the outer sheath and the tissue sample discharged into a 10% formalin solution.
4. The tenaculum is removed, and hemostasis at the site of placement is observed.

C. **The Novak Curette**

1. The Novak Curette is inserted into the uterine cavity and pressed firmly against the anterior wall.
2. Constant suction is applied using a 10 cc plastic or glass syringe as the curette is withdrawn.
3. The specimen is then placed in 10% formalin and the curette rinsed with the formalin.
4. The tenaculum site is checked for bleeding before the speculum is removed.

D. **The Vabra Aspirator**

1. The vacuum pump and hose are checked to be sure they are working properly and create a vacuum.
2. The Vabra cannula is inserted into the uterine cavity.
3. The aspirator is attached and turned on, creating a negative pressure within the cannula.
4. Curettage is performed, covering the entire endometrial surface in a rotating motion.
5. The aspirate is removed and 30 to 40 cc of 10% formalin are suctioned into the aspirator container and sent for histologic analysis.

## III. Complications of endometrial sampling

A. **Perforation.** An instrument may traverse the uterine wall.

1. If the perforation is midline and the peritoneal cavity is entered, the procedure should be discontinued. The patient should be observed for 1 to 2 hours. If stable, the patient should be re-biopsied in no less than 1 week.
2. If the perforation is suspected to be lateral into the broad ligament, the chance of uterine vessel damage is greater. The patient should be observed for signs of blood loss or enlarging broad ligament hematoma.

B. **Infection.** The instrument may introduce bacteria into the uterine cavity leading to infection. The inflammation usually resolves promptly with broad spectrum antibiotics therapy such as doxycycline 100 mg b.i.d. for 10 days.

C. **False channel.** The instrument may dissect through cervical tissue creating a false channel. If this occurs the procedure should be abandoned and repeated at a later date.

# VULVAR BIOPSY

## I. Introduction

A. The ability to evaluate and diagnose vulvar disease is one of the most important aspects of gynecologic practice. Performing an adequate vulvar biopsy lies at the heart of the diagnostic process. This section will address the proper technique for performing vulvar biopsy.

**B.** Prior to performing a vulvar biopsy, thorough evaluation of the vulva should be performed. If a circumscribed lesion has been found, or a diffuse area of disease noted, the remaining vulva should be examined for similar findings. This examination may be assisted by the use of a colposcope and adjunctive staining solutions such as toluidine blue or acetic acid.

## II. Technique

**A.** In general, biopsies of the vulva may be obtained in two ways:

1. **The punch biopsy** is used when representative samples of vulvar skin are desired from a diffuse area of disease. Full thickness skin is obtained as opposed to irregular or inadequate sections that might be obtained with shave biopsies.
2. **Excisional biopsy** is used when a circumscribed lesion is present and complete removal is desired.

**B. Preparation.** No specific skin preparation is necessary prior to vulvar biopsy, although if desired, the area may be swabbed with alcohol or a betadine solution. Hair clipping or shaving is unnecessary.

**C. Anesthesia.** For patient comfort, adequate anesthesia is paramount prior to performing the biopsy. Local infiltration usually suffices for most office biopsies. This is performed with a 1% lidocaine solution, injected subepidermally with a 25 or 26 gauge needle. Lidocaine with epinephrine may be desired to prolong anesthesia and provide hemostasis from vasoconstriction. An adequate amount of anesthesia should be used. This will vary with the size of the area to be removed. For punch biopsies, a single injection of 3 to 4 mL of anesthetic may suffice. However, for excisional biopsies, several injections around the lesion may be required.

**D. Punch biopsy**

1. **Instruments needed**
   a. The **Keyes cutaneous punch** is the biopsy instrument used (Fig. 34.4). It provides a core of tissue for examination. Various diameters exist, but a 4 to 5 mm is best for vulvar use.
   b. Adson forceps
   c. Small tissue scissors
   d. Needle holder
   e. 3.0 chromic suture
2. **Procedure**
   a. After an anesthetic has been injected, the area to be biopsied is grasped between finger and thumb and lifted slightly.
   b. Using a twisting motion, the punch is used to make a circular incision through the epidermis to the level of the dermis. Care should be taken to avoid going too

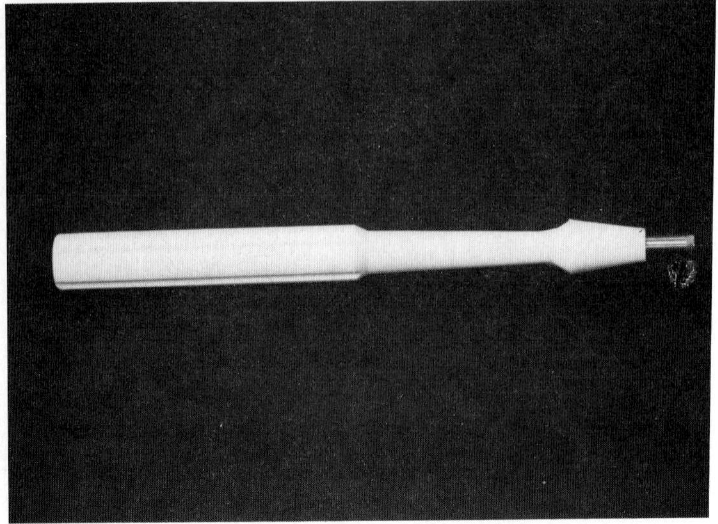

FIGURE 34.4. The Keyes punch.

deep, but too shallow of a specimen may also be a problem.

c. The punch is laid aside and Adson forceps are used to grasp the specimen and lift. The base of the specimen is then cut with the scissors.
d. If bleeding is minimal, hemostasis can be achieved with Monsel's solution or silver nitrate. However, for larger biopsies associated with more bleeding, a single interrupted stitch of 3-0 chromic suture may be necessary.
e. The biopsy specimen should be oriented epidermal-side-up on tissue paper, a sponge or absorbant cardboard prior to submission to the pathologist.

**E. Excisional biopsy**

**1. Instruments needed**

a. No. 15 knife blade
b. Tissue forceps
c. Small tissue scissors
d. Needle holder
e. 3-0 chromic suture

**2. Procedure**

a. The incision should include the entire lesion. The blade makes the incision at right angles to the skin in an ellipse around the lesion. The ellipse axis should be made in accord with its orientation to the introitus (vertical), labia (vertical), or perineum (horizontal).

b. Once the incision is made, the specimen edges may be grasped with forceps and the lesion cut free with either the knife or scissors.
c. Hemostasis and closure of the site may be obtained with interrupted figure-of-8 stitches of 3-0 chromic.
d. Tissue handling should be performed in the same fashion that the punch biopsy is prepared for submission to pathology.

## III. After-care and follow-up

A. **Analgesics** are rarely necessary after vulvar biopsy. If needed, acetaminophen or nonsteroidal anti-inflammatory agents suffice.

B. **Local care** consisting of warm sitz baths should be performed for the first week to assure healing and absorption of sutures. Ice packs to the biopsy site may reduce swelling.

# COLPOSCOPY

## I. Introduction

A. **Colposcopy** is the magnification and evaluation of the stratified squamous epithelium of the cervix, vagina, and vulva by means of a low-powered binocular microscope combined with bright illumination. Magnification of 10X or greater is used to image and determine changes in the surface epithelium and also alterations in the vascular arrangement within the connective tissue stroma.

B. **Indications.** The majority of colposcopic examinations performed are for the purpose of evaluating the presence and extent of cervical intraepithelial neoplasia (CIN). In general, indications for colposcopy include:

1. Abnormal cervical cytology.
2. Genital condyloma.
3. Any abnormal lesion of the cervix seen on gross examination.

## II. Criteria for evaluation.

To perform an accurate colposcopic examination, specific diagnostic criteria must be evaluated and met. The following is a list of these criteria and an explanation of the terminology.

A. **Squamocolumnar (S-C) junction and transformation zone**

1. **Original S-C junction.** This is the original interface between the squamous and columnar epithelium. When visualized in the neonate, this junction lies towards the portio of the cervix.
2. **New S-C junction.** Under the influence of estrogen, the acidity of the vagina changes with the presence of lactobacilli. When exposed to an acid pH, reserve cells emerge, producing a multilayered epithelium and lifting off the columnar epithelium. The result of this metaplastic process

is new stratified squamous epithelium. A new S-C junction is established, closer to the cervical os.

3. **Transformation zone.** The region of the cervix lying between the original and new S-C junctions is the transformation zone. This zone is the site for initiation of neoplastic changes of the cervix.

B. **Vascular and epithelial changes.** When evaluating the cervix for abnormal changes, specific vascular and epithelial characteristics should be noted.

1. **Vascular pattern.** This is best seen with the green filter.
   a. **Normal changes** include hairpin capillaries, network and tree-like branching. Hairpin capillaries consist of an ascending and descending branch. When branching is seen, dichotomous division is noted from larger to smaller capillaries.
   b. **Abnormal changes**
      1. **Punctation** appears as red dots. This is due to proliferation of dividing cells that compress capillaries vertically, producing tortuosity and dilation.
      2. **Mosaicism** results from further proliferation of dysplastic cells causing compression of a capillary network into basket-like structures.
      3. **Atypical vessels** are seen in advanced disease. Resulting from stimulation of new, but abnormal, capillary growth, the appearance can be characterized by aberrant shapes, sizes, and patterns.

2. **Intercapillary distance** refers to the space between corresponding parts of adjacent vessels. The normal intercapillary distance ranged from 50 to 250 μm (mean 100 μm). As dysplastic tissue expands and compresses capillaries, the intercapillary distance will increase.

3. **Epithelial color and response to acetic acid.** Normal squamous epithelium maintains a pink tone due to transmission of the vascular content beneath. Rapidly proliferating cells have an increased protein content and therefore do not transmit light as well. Therefore, a gray or white color may be noted. This opacity may be accentuated by the application of acetic acid, which denatures and condenses protein. Metaplastic epithelium usually presents a gray appearance. Dysplastic epithelium usually produces an acetowhite change. The amount of white change is directly proportional to the degree of dysplasia. Leukoplakia presents as a white lesion, not requiring acetic acid to produce its appearance.

4. **Surface contour.** Normal squamous epithelium has a smooth, glistening appearance. Normal columnar epithelium appears as a papillary, grape-like surface. Dysplastic epithelium and invasive cancer may produce an uneven, elevated, or eroded surface. Flat condyloma can demonstrate a cobble-stone pattern.

5. **Demarcation of border between normal and abnormal epithelium.** The border between squamous metaplasia, or mild dysplasia, and normal epithelium may be diffuse. The border demarcation of normal epithelium and more severe dysplasia is usually sharp.

C. **Satisfactory colposcopic examination**
   1. To accurately evaluate the cervix colposcopically, the examination must be considered satisfactory. The following criteria must be met.
      a. The new S-C junction and transition zone must be entirely visualized.
      b. The lesion must be seen in its entirety.
   2. If these criteria cannot be met, the examination must be classified unsatisfactory.

## III. Colposcopic equipment

A. **The colposcope** is essentially a binocular microscope used for examination of the cervix, vagina, and vulva. Magnification can range from 6 to 40X, but the standard magnification used is 10X. The colposcope should contain a green filter, used for enhancement of vascular changes. Mountings for colposcopes vary to some degree. A mobile mounting, either on a stationary stand or wheels, allows the colposcope to be moved from room to room. Other mounts include those that are attached to the wall or the examination table. These allow easy manipulation of the scope but do not allow mobility. Other accessories that are important to teaching include an observation tube and a camera.

B. **Specula.** The standard bivalve speculum is the most commonly used. A large Graves speculum is desired in that it allows full retraction of the vaginal sidewalls and good visualization of the cervix. In nulliparous patients, a Pederson speculum may be all that can be accommodated.

C. **The endocervical speculum** is an instrument that allows visualization of the cervical canal. Placed at the end of long handles, it can be inserted transversely into the canal and opened, allowing adequate visibility.

D. **Staining solutions.** These may be applied directly to the cervix with large cotton swabs or sponges.
   1. **Acetic acid** used in a 3% to 5% concentration, denatures protein in cells, producing a white change in dysplastic or rapidly proliferating epithelium.
   2. **Lugol's solution** is taken up by glycogen-rich epithelium of the cervix and vagina. Dysplastic epithelium does not stain and can be viewed easily. Lugol's solution is not commonly used today for colposcopy.

E. **Biopsy instruments**
   1. **Punch biopsy forceps** are required to obtain directed biopsies. The most commonly used is the Kevorkian biopsy instrument. Biopsy instruments have a pistol type grip and a scissor-like action at the tip of the forceps. The jaws should

meet completely so that a clean cut of tissue may be obtained.

2. **An endocervical curette,** with narrow grooves on the end, is required for obtaining an endocervical curettage (ECC).

F. **Hemostatic solutions and equipment**

1. **Monsel's solution** may be applied with a cotton swab to obtain hemostasis. Several applications may be required.
2. **Silver nitrate,** usually on the end of a wooden stick, may be used to stop bleeding in small biopsy sites.
3. **Suture** usually of 3-0 chromic, may be necessary to stop persistent bleeding from the cervix when the above solutions have failed.

G. **Miscellaneous**

1. **A single tooth tenaculum** may be necessary to stabilize the cervix when directed biopsies are taken.
2. **Ring forceps** are helpful to aid in removing the mucus and cellular debris obtained during endocervical curettage.
3. Glass slides, a wooden spatula, cotton swabs, or brushes will be needed to obtain pap smears.

## IV. The procedure

A. **Positioning the patient.** Examination is performed in the lithotomy position as if for routine pelvic examination. The patient's buttocks should be placed at the end of the examining table. Stirrups are preferred, rather than under-the-thigh supports, as they allow adequate separation of the knees.

B. **Initial exposure and visualization of the cervix.**

1. Insert the speculum and open the blades as widely as possible to obtain full visualization of the cervix.
2. Observe cervical and vaginal secretions. A wet mount may be obtained.
3. Papanicolaou (PAP) smear is performed at this time. If excessive cervical secretion is present, it may first be gently removed with a swab.
4. Initial observation of the cervix, through the colposcope, is then performed, once secretions are removed. A magnification of 10X is preferred. Differences in color, contour, and margins of normal epithelium and lesions are observed. Blood vessel patterns are then observed, using the green filter to enhance vascular changes. Vascular patterns are best demonstrated without the application of acetic acid.

C. **Acetic acid** is then gently swabbed over the entire cervix. Not only will this produce acetowhite epithelial change, but it will coagulate and remove excess mucus. Care should be taken not to wipe with acetic acid as this may traumatize the epithelium. Swabs may be held against the epithelium for 1 to 2 minutes to obtain maximal acetowhite change. Excess acetic acid should be removed with dry swabs. Once staining has been performed, a **second examination** of the cervix is performed to observe acetowhite epithelium, contour changes, and demarcation of margins between normal and abnormal epithelium.

D. **Biopsies**

1. **Endocervical curettage** should be performed in all patients undergoing colposcopic examination for abnormal cervical cytology except when the patient is pregnant. By performing ECC prior to directed biopsies, pick-up of epithelial debris from the biopsies may be avoided. The patient should be warned that she may experience cramping. The curette is placed into the cervix and with pressure applied directly to the canal wall, the endocervix is scraped throughout its entire circumference. The curette is then spun several times, depressed and then withdrawn to remove a maximal amount of tissue. If excessive tissue remains, it may be removed with ring or tissue forceps. Consistency of the canal wall should be noted during the curettage because a firm regular surface is unlikely to represent invasive cancer.
2. **Directed biopsies.** All areas of abnormal vasculature and atypical epithelial change (e.g., acetowhite epithelium) should be biopsied. Once these sites are mentally noted, the colposcope can be moved out of the way to facilitate manipulation of biopsy forceps. Again, the patient should be warned of the possibility of mild-to-moderate sharp pain. The biopsy forceps should be firmly applied to the tissue and this pressure should be maintained during the actual biopsy process. If the cervix moves excessively, it may be stabilized with a tenaculum. The specimen should be placed epithelium-side-up on a sponge, tissue paper or cardboard square prior to sending to pathology. Each biopsy specimen should be labeled as to its location of removal from the cervix (e.g., 3 o'clock).

E. **Hemostasis** at biopsy sites can be obtained with Monsel's solution. This is applied directly to the site of bleeding with a cotton swab. Several applications may be needed. For large biopsy sites, or for persistent bleeding, a single or figure-of-8 stitch of 3-0 chromic suture may be necessary.

F. **Documentation of findings.** All colposcopic findings should be accurately recorded after the examination. This is best done on a preprinted form with a schematic picture of the cervix. All epithelial and vascular abnormalities should be drawn and labeled. Record whether the examination was satisfactory or not. Mark all areas that biopsies were taken from. Last of all, record the colposcopic impression of the disease.

G. **After-care and follow-up**

1. Rarely is any pain medication required after the examination.
2. The patient should be informed that she may have vaginal spotting for several days and may experience a dark vaginal discharge if Monsel's solution is used.

3. A return appointment with the patient should be scheduled soon after the examination to review the results and establish a care plan. The early return appointment also serves to reduce anxiety that the patient may have related to fear of cervical cancer.

H. **Review of histopathology.** The histopathologic specimens are reviewed with the pathologist in a conference-type setting. The PAP smear obtained at the time of examination is correlated with the findings of the pathologist. By meeting as a group, the histopathologic, cytologic, and clinical findings can be reviewed, thus allowing a comprehensive diagnosis and treatment plan to be derived.

## CRYOTHERAPY OF THE CERVIX

### I. Introduction

A. **Indications.** Cryotherapy of the cervix is indicated for the treatment of CIN and cervical condyloma. Data exists to suggest that cryotherapy is inferior to laser surgery in eradicating extensive cervical lesions (>3 cm) and severe grades of CIN (CIN III).

B. **General considerations.** Cryotherapy is a safe and simple procedure, routinely performed in an office setting. No anesthesia and no vaginal prep are necessary. No sterilization of equipment is necessary, although probe tips should be cleansed with cidex before and after a procedure.

### II. Steps in the procedure

A. Prior to performing cryotherapy, the patient must have undergone a proper colposcopic examination including directed biopsies and endocervical curettage. The full extent of the lesion must be visualized.

B. A metal or plastic speculum is inserted into the vagina. The largest size that the vagina will accommodate is used to allow full visualization of the cervix and to prevent freezing of the vaginal side walls.

C. A solution of 3% acetic acid may be used to remove excess mucus from the cervix.

D. After assessing the shape of the cervix and extent of the lesion, the proper probe tip is selected (Fig. 34.5).

  1. A flat probe is preferred if disease is confined to the ectocervix.
  2. A more conical probe may be desired if the fully visualized lesion extends to the endocervix.

E. Lubricating jelly is spread over the probe tip to facilitate temperature transfer.

F. **Freezing technique.** A gun-type cryosurgery unit can be used for the procedure. The refrigerant is usually either nitrous oxide or carbon dioxide. It is important that the tank pressure be adequate prior to freezing.

  1. The lubricated probe is gently applied to the cervix and the refrigerant flow is begun.

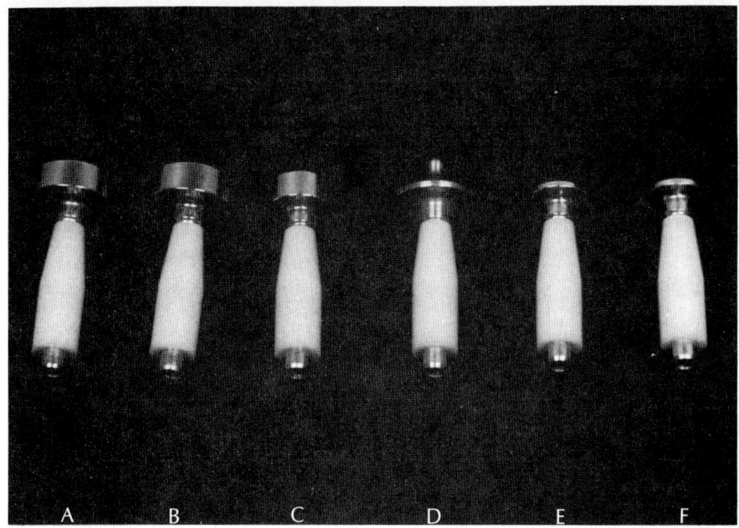


FIGURE 34.5. Cryosurgery probes: (A–C) flat probes; (D–F) conical probes.

2. A double-freeze technique is preferred, usually consisting of a 3-minute freeze, 5-minute thaw and 3-minute freeze.
3. It is important that the iceball extend at least 5 mm beyond the edge of the lesion.
4. For extensive disease, the cervix may be subdivided into quadrants and each section frozen separately.

**G.** Once freezing is completed, the probe and speculum are removed. It may be advisable to have the patient remain supine for 5 to 10 minutes because some patients may experience mild cramping, lightheadedness, and headache during or after the procedure.

## III. After-care and follow-up

**A.** The patient should be informed that she may experience a profuse watery discharge for 1 to 2 weeks requiring several sanitary napkins per day. The patient should avoid sexual intercourse for at least 2 weeks.

**B.** A mild analgesic may be necessary for those few patients who experience cramping after the procedure. Acetaminophen or a nonsteroidal anti-inflammatory agent are sufficient.

**C.** A routine follow-up examination is scheduled 6 weeks after the procedure to assess healing and provide the patient with informational support.

**D.** PAP smears are not routinely performed until 3 to 4 months after cryotherapy to avoid a false positive cytologic smear resulting from the healing process. When performed correctly, cryotherapy should provide a cure rate of 80% to 90%.

## BIBLIOGRAPHY

Burghardt E, ed. Colposcopy cervical pathology. New York: Thieme-Stratton Inc; 1984:121–127.

Friedrich EG, ed. Vulvar disease. 2nd ed. Philadelphia: Pa. WB Saunders Co; 1983:62–68.

Hatch KD, ed. Handbook of Colposcopy: Diagnosis and Treatment of Lower Genital Tract Neoplasia and HPV Infections. Boston: Little, Brown and Co. 1989:39–50.

Mattingly RF, Thompson JD, eds. Te Linde's Operative Gynecology. 6th ed. Philadelphia, Pa: JB Lippincott Co; 1985:435.

# CHAPTER 35

# Differential Diagnosis by Presentation

**W. Kirkland Ruffin**
**Thomas G. Stovall**
**Frank W. Ling**
**Robert L. Summitt, Jr.**

## BREAST MASS

Eighty percent of all breast masses are benign. For patients under 30, the most common diagnosis of a solitary mass is a fibroadenoma. For patients over 30, fibrocystic disease becomes the most common diagnosis, however cancer becomes increasingly likely. For the 20% of patients with a malignant mass, early detection remains crucial to provide the greatest likelihood for cure. Many potential diagnoses are indicated when a breast mass is first palpated.

### I. General considerations

**A. The potential diagnoses of a palpable breast mass include:**

1. Breast cancer
2. Fibroadenoma
3. Fibrocystic disease
   a. Sclerosing adenosis
   b. Apocrine metaplasia
   c. Duct ectasia
   d. Macro- or microcysts
   e. Fibrosis
   f. Hyperplasia with or without atypia
4. Mastitis/abscess
5. Other lipoma, epidermal cyst, lymph node

**B. Age.** Increasing age and female sex are the two largest risk factors for the development of breast cancer. Although less likely at a young age, breast cancer can occur at any age.

**C. Risk.** The overall lifetime risk for a woman to develop breast cancer is 8%, with a lifetime mortality risk of 2.7%. In addition to age and female sex, the following are risk factors for the development of breast cancer:

1. **Family history.** The history of breast cancer in a first degree relative (mother, sister, or daughter), particularly if that cancer occurred at a premenopausal age, or was bilateral, increases a patient's risk threefold, or to about 25%.

2. **Benign breast disease.** The overall risk for patients with fibrocystic disease is slightly increased over those without it, however it is important to define the histologic type of the fibrocystic disease to accurately assess the risk.
   a. No increased risk
      (1) Sclerosing adenosis
      (2) Apocrine metaplasia
      (3) Duct ectasia
      (4) Macro- or microcysts
      (5) Fibroadenoma
      (6) Mild hyperplasia
   b. Slightly increased risk (1.5–2X)
      (1) Moderate hyperplasia without atypia
      (2) Intraductal papilloma
   c. Moderately increased risk (5X)
      (1) Ductal or lobular hyperplasia with atypia
3. **Reproductive and endocrine factors.** Early menarche, late menopause, nulliparity, or first pregnancy after age 35 all increase a patient's risk for breast cancer. The risk of the use of oral contraceptives is controversial, although most studies show no increase in the risk of breast cancer from their use.
4. **Radiation.** Modern film-screen mammography exposes the breast to 0.001 Gy for each of the two films taken of each breast in a standard mammogram. Although radiation is a known etiologic factor in breast cancer, the low dose received by the breast during the course of a standard mammogram is unlikely to result in a malignancy, especially when mammography is begun between ages 35 to 40. The benefits obtained from a dedicated mammography program outweigh the risks involved.
5. **History and physical examination**
   a. The history should include an assessment of:
      (1) Length of time the breast mass has been present.
      (2) Any changes or growth in the mass, particularly in relation to the menstrual cycle. Breast cancer tends to grow slowly and progressively, whereas fibrocystic disease tends to worsen just prior to the menses and regress after the menses when the levels of estrogen and progesterone decrease. For this reason, an exam is most accurate just after a menstrual cycle.
      (3) The presence of pain or tenderness. Breast cancer and fibroadenomas tend to be painless whereas fibrocystic disease may be quite painful and tender.
      (4) The presence of nipple discharge.
      (5) The patient's risk factors for breast cancer.
   b. The physical examination should include:

(1) Inspection of the breasts to assess for any skin or nipple dimpling, retraction, or edema.
(2) Palpation of the breasts to assess for the presence of a mass. Note should be made of the size, shape, mobility, texture, and tenderness of the mass. Examination should determine if there is symmetry regarding any nodularity in the breasts.
(3) Palpation of the nipples to assess for discharge.
(4) Palpation of the axilla to assess for lymphadenopathy.

## II. Management (Fig. 35.1)

**A.** All discrete breast masses must have a definite diagnosis, either by excisional biopsy, aspiration cytology, or aspiration of a cyst with full resolution of the mass.

**B.** Although breast cancer risk increases with increasing age, all patients must be considered as possibly having cancer in the presence of a palpable mass, regardless of age.

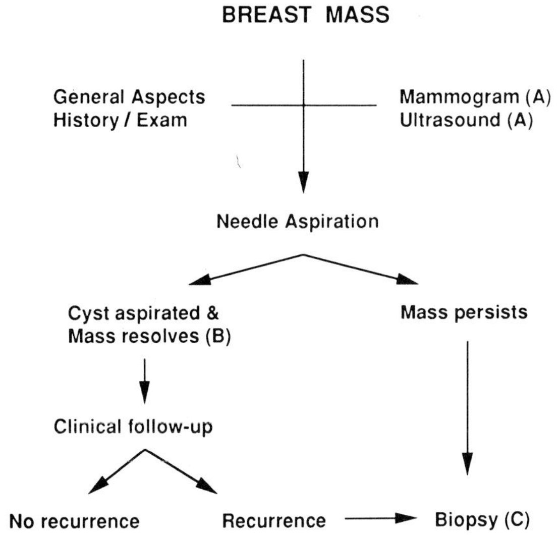

BREAST MASS

General Aspects
History / Exam
Mammogram (A)
Ultrasound (A)
Needle Aspiration
Cyst aspirated &
Mass resolves (B)
Mass persists
Clinical follow-up
No recurrence
Recurrence
Biopsy (C)

FIGURE 35.1. Algorithm for the diagnosis of breast mass. (A) Mammography is not indicated for patients less than 30 years old; for patients older than 30 it is used to characterize the mass and examine the remainder of the breasts. Ultrasonography is useful in younger patients or to characterize a mass as cystic or solid. (B) Fluid cytology is generally not indicated for routine green-gray cyst fluid. However, blood in the aspirate makes cytologic examination mandatory. (C) Biopsy may be excisional or by aspiration. Excisional biopsy with frozen section is preferred as it allows for complete mass removal, eliminates sampling error, and allows for hormone receptor analysis if malignant.

**C.** In the presence of a palpable mass, a normal mammogram should not deter a biopsy. The sensitivity rate for mammography is only about 80%, and particularly in young patients, the normal dense breast parenchyma may obscure a malignancy.

**D.** Biopsy may be performed under local or general anesthesia. Excisional biopsy with frozen section pathologic analysis is preferred as it allows for complete removal of the mass, eliminates sampling error, and allows for hormone receptor analysis if the mass proves to be malignant. The tissue must be frozen within 30 minutes; warm ischemia greater than 30 minutes results in loss of hormone receptors and a false negative receptor analysis.

**E.** The incision for the biopsy should be placed in a position where it can be easily included in a mastectomy incision if the mass proves to be malignant. An incision at the edge of the areola is both cosmetic and satisfies this requirement.

## NIPPLE DISCHARGE

### I. General considerations

**A. Differential diagnosis.** The potential diagnoses for a patient with nipple discharge include:

1. Breast cancer
2. Intraductal papilloma
3. Galactorrhea
    a. Postpartum
    b. Hyperprolactinemia
4. Fibrocystic disease
5. Physiologic
6. Pseudodischarge
7. Drug therapy

**B. Age.** The risk for breast cancer increases with age. Benign conditions more likely in the younger patient.

**C. Spontaneous or manually expressed.** Clinically significant lesions that present with nipple discharge will have spontaneous, recurrent, and nonlactational discharge. Nipple discharge that is elicited only by palpation or squeezing of the nipple is generally of no clinical importance.

**D. Single or multiple ducts.** A significant lesion will usually result in discharge from a single duct only, which is often identifiable by the patient. The most common cause of nipple discharge from a single duct is an intraductal papilloma. Discharge from multiple ducts, or bilateral discharge, usually indicates a diffuse or systemic condition, and is less likely to be the result of malignancy.

**E. Character of fluid**

1. Milky—galactorrhea
2. Green, grey, sticky—fibrocystic disease (generally cystic mastitis or duct ectasia)
3. Clear, serosanguineous, or bloody—cancer, intraductal papilloma

F. **The following medications** may cause nipple discharge
   1. Oral contraceptives and other hormone preparations
   2. Phenothiazines
   3. Tricyclic antidepressants
   4. $\alpha$-methyldopa

G. **History and physical examination**
   1. The history should include an assessment of:
      a. Pattern of discharge (i.e., spontaneous or manually expressed).
      b. Frequency of discharge and relationship to the menstrual cycle.
      c. Number of ducts from which the discharge occurs.
      d. Color and consistency of the discharge.
      e. Recent pregnancy or lactation.
      f. Risk factors for breast cancer.
      g. Drug use.
   2. The physical examination should include:
      a. Complete inspection and palpation of the breasts and axilla.
      b. Careful inspection of the nipple to assess for irritation, excoriation, edema, or other primary nipple pathology.
      c. Palpation of the nipple and surrounding breast to check for a subareolar mass.
      d. Squeezing of the nipple to determine which duct(s) is (are) involved.

## II. Management (Fig. 35.2)

A. **A careful history, physical examination and mammogram** (age >30) will often lead to a likely diagnosis.

B. **Cytologic examination of the nipple discharge** may be of help for clear, serosanguineous or bloody discharge.

C. Patients with clear, serosanguineous, or bloody nipple discharge require **subareolar duct excision** even in the presence of a normal exam, mammogram, and cytologic examination.

D. **Nonlactational galactorrhea should be evaluated** with a prolactin level.

E. **Discharge** that is green, grey, black, or otherwise dark (nonbloody), and usually arising from multiple ducts, arises from fibrocystic disease. If there is no palpable mass or abnormality on mammogram, reassurance of the patient and treatment of the fibrocystic disease is indicated.

# ABNORMAL MAMMOGRAM

## I. General considerations

A. For patients without clinically evident breast disease, **routine screening mammography should be performed** in accordance with the recommendations of the American Cancer Society, the American College of Surgeons, and the American College of

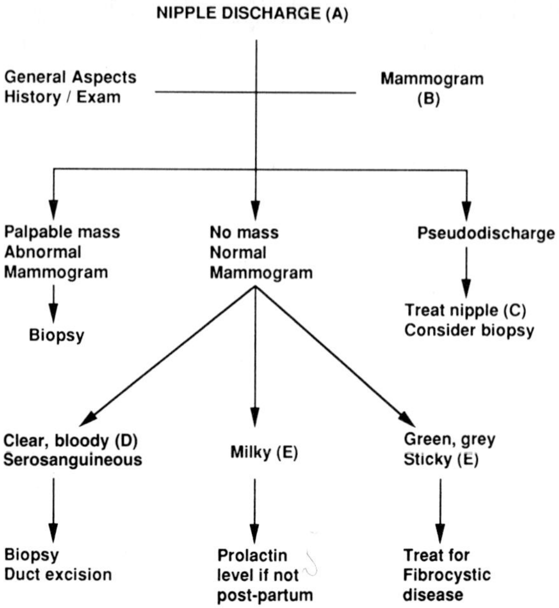

NIPPLE DISCHARGE (A)

General Aspects History / Exam — Mammogram (B)

| Palpable mass Abnormal Mammogram | No mass Normal Mammogram | Pseudodischarge |
|---|---|---|
| → Biopsy | | → Treat nipple (C) Consider biopsy |

No mass / Normal Mammogram →

| Clear, bloody (D) Serosanguineous | Milky (E) | Green, grey Sticky (E) |
|---|---|---|
| → Biopsy Duct excision | → Prolactin level if not post-partum | → Treat for Fibrocystic disease |

FIGURE 35.2. Algorithm for the diagnosis of nipple discharge. (A) Discharge should be spontaneous and recurrent. Discharge elicited only by palpation or squeezing of the nipple is of no clinical importance. (B) Age over 30. (C) Paget's disease of the nipple often presents as an irritated appearing nipple. Diagnosis is made only by biopsy. (D) Generally from a single duct. (E) Generally multiple ducts.

Radiology, as follows:

1. Age 35 to 39—baseline mammogram
2. Age 40 to 49—mammogram every 1 to 2 years
3. Age 50 or over—mammogram every year.

B. **A mammogram should be performed** with craniocaudal and mediolateral projections of each breast. Each film should be examined for the following abnormalities:

1. **Soft tissue density, mass, or nodule.** In addition to its presence, each soft tissue abnormality should be characterized according to size, shape, regularity of its margins, and presence or absence of any architectural distortion.
2. **Clustered microcalcifications** (defined as calcifications each less than 1 mm and grouped within 1 cm). Note the following:
   a. Number of calcifications.
   b. Size of calcifications.
   c. Morphologic characteristics, such as round, curvilinear, or branched.

d. Degree of pleomorphism among the individual calcifications.

3. Asymmetry between opposite breasts examined in the same projection.
4. Skin or nipple thickening or retraction.
5. Any change from prior mammogram.

C. **Abnormal mammograms can be classified as follows:**
(The clinical relevance of each classification is noted, and assumes that there is no palpable mass to go with the abnormality.)

1. **Soft tissue density without microcalcifications**
   a. Asymmetric density—almost certainly benign and of limited clinical importance.
   b. Smooth nodule—generally a benign cyst or fibroadenoma.
   c. Slightly irregular or poorly visualized nodule—an irregular margin increases the likelihood of a malignancy, but still more likely to be benign.
   d. Irregular or stellate mass—much more likely to be malignant.
2. **Clustered microcalcifications without a mass**
   a. Less than five—more likely benign, in particular sclerosing adenosis.
   b. Five or more—more likely malignant.
3. **Soft tissue density or mass with associated microcalcifications.** This group in general has a much higher likelihood of being malignant. Here the number of calcifications is not as important as when there is no mass.
   a. Asymmetric density—possibly malignant.
   b. Smooth nodule—may be degenerating fibroadenoma but still must be considered suspicious.
   c. Slightly irregular nodule—more likely malignant.
   d. Very irregular or stellate mass—almost certainly malignant.

   In addition, for any of the above, the presence of architectural distortion of the breast, skin retraction, or a change from a prior mammogram, makes any abnormality a suspicious finding.

## II. Management (Fig. 35.3)

A. In general, **a biopsy should routinely be performed** for all of the above abnormalities except:

1. Asymmetric density without calcifications.
2. Smooth, solid nodule without calcifications and less than 1 cm in size.
3. Less than five microcalcifications without an associated mass.

For findings such as these, consider biopsy for high-risk patients or if there has been a change in the mammogram.

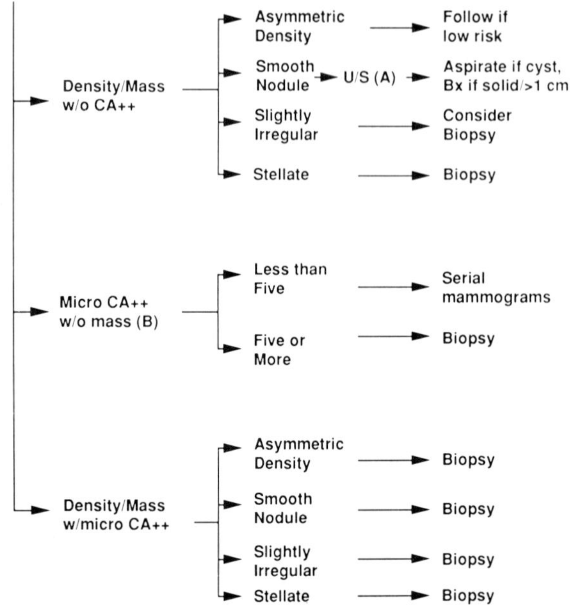


FIGURE 35.3. Algorithm for the diagnosis of abnormal mammogram. (A) U/S—ultrasound useful for determining if smooth nodule is cystic or solid. If cystic, the ultrasound may be used to guide aspiration. (B) In addition to number of calcifications (CAtt), consider the shape and appearance of the calcifications. Bx = biopsy.

B. **Biopsies for nonpalpable abnormalities** must be done with preoperative mammographic localization, generally with a needle or hook-wire technique.
C. **During needle-localized biopsies,** specimen radiography should be performed in most cases, particularly if calcifications are present. Alternatively, a follow-up mammogram must be obtained to ensure the lesion in question was successfully removed.

## VULVOVAGINAL DISCHARGE

### I. General considerations

A. **Vulvovaginal discharge** is one of the most common reasons that outpatient therapy is instituted in the gynecologic patient. Excessive, noticeable discharge is usually vaginal in origin but, in rare instances, may arise from the vulva only.
B. **For proper evaluation and treatment of vulvovaginal discharge, an understanding of normal vaginal physiology is necessary.**

1. **Vaginal secretions arise from:**
    a. Vulvar secretions of sweat, sebaceous, Bartholin's, and Skene's glands
    b. Vaginal wall transudate
    c. Exfoliated cells
    d. Cervical mucus
    e. Endometrial and tubal fluids
    f. By-products of vaginal microflora
2. **Normal vaginal biology is dependent on:**
    a. Resident microflora
        (1) *Lactobacillus*
        (2) *Bacteroides*
        (3) *Corynebacterium*
        (4) *Peptostreptococcus*
        (5) *Staphylococcus epidermidis*
        (6) Small numbers of *Candida* species
    b. Epithelial make-up and integrity.
        (1) Squamous cells of superficial type are rich in glycogen and predominate in the reproductive years. They are estrogen dependent, thick, and protective.
        (2) Parabasal cells, low in glycogen, predominate in premenarche and postmenopause. They are thin, less protective, and estrogen responsive.
    c. Hormonal status
    d. Glycogen content
        (1) Converted to lactic acid by normal flora, maintaining low pH
    e. Vaginal pH (normal—3.5–4.5)
    f. Medications and inert foreign substances

C. **Predisposing factors to vulvovaginitis include:**

1. Epithelial changes
    a. Premenarche and menopause predispose to changes in vaginal epithelium.
    b. Thinning secondary to hypoestrogenism leads to a lack of glycogen and an alkaline pH.
2. Alterations in pH
    a. Low pH allows normal flora to predominate.
    b. Factors raising pH allow pathogen overgrowth.
        (1) Menstrual blood
        (2) Semen (pH 6–7)
        (3) Excessive cervical mucus
3. Alterations in vaginal flora
    a. Loss of normal flora allow suppressed or newly infective pathogens to predominate.
    b. Factors changing flora include:
        (1) Broad-spectrum antibiotics
        (2) Large inoculum of pathogenic organisms
        (3) Douching

**D. Potential causes for vulvovaginal discharge include:**

1. Vaginitis syndromes
   a. *Trichomonas vaginalis*
   b. *Gardnerella vaginalis*
   c. *Candida*
2. Atrophic vaginitis
3. Physiologic discharge and *Lactobacillus* overgrowth
4. Cervicitis
   a. *Chlamydia*
   b. Gonorrhea
   c. Herpes simplex II
5. Vulvovaginal condyloma
6. Syphilis
7. Foreign body
8. Allergens
9. Genital tract neoplasm

**E. History and clinical examinations**

1. History
   a. History should be directed towards potential causes or precursors of vulvovaginal discharge
      (1) Exposure to or history of sexually transmitted diseases
      (2) Methods of contraception (oral contraceptives, diaphragm, foam, sponge)
      (3) Hygiene (douching, tampon use)
      (4) Medication use (recent antibiotics, hormonal preparations)
   b. Associated symptoms should be noted
      (1) Vulvar pruritis
      (2) Vulvar lesions
      (3) Color and odor of discharge
2. Physical examination (Fig. 35.4):
   a. Vulvar inspection is initially performed to assess the presence of
      1. Erythema *(Candida)*
      2. Accuminate wart (condyloma)
      3. Ulceration (herpes, syphilis)
   b. Speculum examination is the most important part of the assessment process and allows the following:
      1. Inspection of vagina to rule out foreign body or allergic irritation.
      2. Inspection of vaginal mucosa for ulceration (herpes, syphilis), condyloma, neoplasm, estrogen status.
      3. Inspection of cervix for gross neoplasia. Obtain Papanicolaou (PAP) smear.
      4. Obtainment of cervical cultures for gonorrhea and *Chlamydia* in the presence of mucopurulent discharge or ectropion.

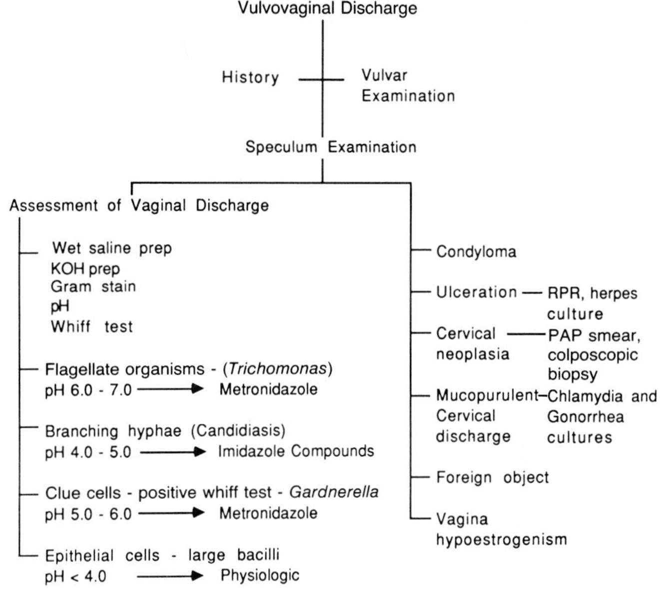


FIGURE 35.4. Algorithm for diagnosis of vulvovaginal discharge. RPR = rapid plasma reagent; KOH = potassium hydroxide.

5. Obtainment of vaginal discharge for clinical and laboratory testing.

**3.** Assessment of vaginal discharge
   a. Wet saline mount—look for presence of trichomonads, clue cells, white blood cells.
   b. Potassium hydroxide (KOH) preparation—look for presence of branching hyphae or budding yeast.
   c. Gram stain—allows visualization of *G. vaginalis* and intracellular diplococci (gonorrhea).
   d. Whiff test—"fishy" odor released when KOH interacts with amines produced by *Gardnerella* organisms.
   e. Vaginal pH
      (1) pH 4.0 to 5.0—*Candida*
      (2) pH 5.0 to 6.0—*Gardnerella*
      (3) pH 6.0 to 7.0—*Trichomonas*

**II. Management** (Fig. 35.4). The following is an abbreviated list of treatment methods for the most common adult vulvovaginitis syndromes.

**A. Candidiasis**

1. Initial infections
    a. Imidazole compounds
        (1) Miconazole or clotrimazole cream one applicatorful or 100 mg suppository every night for 7 days
        (2) Butaconazole, one prefilled applicatorful every night for 3 days
    b. Gentian violet dye
2. Recurrent infections
    a. Gentian violet dye weekly.
    b. Miconazole or clotrimazole intravaginally and to vulva for 14 to 21 days.
    c. Oral nystatin 1 000 000 units t.i.d. for 7 days.
    d. If associated with menses, use imidazole compound for 3 nights prior to each menses; continue for 6 months.

**B. Trichomoniasis**

1. Metronidazole is the drug of choice (two different dosing regimens).
    a. 2 g p.o. stat.
    b. 250 mg p.o. t.i.d. for 7 days.
2. Treat sexual partner.

**C. *G. vaginalis***

1. Metronidazole is the drug of choice (500 mg po b.i.d. for 7 days).
2. Treat sexual partner.
3. Other treatment options such as ampicillin, tetracycline, and triple-sulfa cream have been used with limited success.

## ABNORMAL UTERINE BLEEDING

**I. Definition.** Abnormal uterine bleeding is any bleeding that occurs outside of the normal menstrual cycle or menstrual bleeding that is either abnormally prolonged or increased in amount. Dysfunctional uterine bleeding (DUB) is abnormal uterine bleeding for which a specific organic etiology cannot be identified. Therefore, the clinician must rule out all possible organic causes of menstrual dysfunction before treating DUB (Table 35.1).

**II. Age considerations**

**A. Prepubertal.** Bleeding that occurs prior to the age of 9 years of age.

1. **History.** Consider the character of the bleeding, the possibility of maternal diethylstilbestrol use during pregnancy, ingestion of steroid-containing substances, and a family history of blood dyscrasias.
2. **Physical examination.** All children in this age group should have a height/weight determination to screen for precosity. If an adequate vaginal exam cannot be performed in the office, vaginoscopy should be performed.

**Table 35.1. Etiologies for Abnormal and Dysfunctional Uterine Bleeding**

I. Extragenital
  A. Urinary tract
  B. Gastrointestinal tract

II. Pregnancy
  A. Trophoblastic disease
  B. Ectopic pregnancy
  C. Threatened abortion
  D. Incomplete abortion

III. Tumor
  A. Vulva
    1. Varices
    2. Condyloma
    3. Malignancy
  B. Vagina
    1. Vaginal adenosis
    2. Condyloma
    3. Malignancy
    4. Sarcoma botryoides
  C. Cervix
    1. Polyp
    2. Cervical ectopy
    3. Condyloma
    4. Malignancy
  D. Uterine
    1. Leiomyomata
    2. Sarcoma
    3. Endometrial polyp
    4. Endometrial malignancy
    5. Endometrial hyperplasia
  E. Fallopian tube
    1. Neoplasm
    2. Ectopic pregnancy
  F. Ovary
    1. Granulosa cell tumor
    2. Theca cell tumor

IV. Infection
  A. Vaginitis
  B. Cervicitis
  C. Endometritis
  D. Salpingitis

V. Systemic medical conditions
  A. Thyroid
  B. Liver
  C. Adrenal gland
  D. Kidney
  E. Diabetes
  F. Malnutrition
  G. Congestive heart failure

VI. Blood dyscrasias
  A. Idiopathic thrombocytopenia purpura
  B. Leukemia
  C. Aplastic anemia
  D. Von Willebrand's disease

VII. Iatrogenic
  A. Oral contraceptives
  B. Intrauterine devices
  C. Medications
    1. Androgens
    2. Steroids
    3. Psychotropic drugs
    4. Anticholinergic agents
    5. Anticoagulants

VIII. Trauma
  A. Foreign body
  B. Coital injury
  C. Tampon
  D. Pessaries

3. **Most common conditions**
   a. Vulvovaginitis
   b. Vaginal foreign body
   c. Perineal trauma
   d. Urethral prolapse
   e. Benign and malignant vaginal tumors

**B. Reproductive years**

1. **History**
   a. Irregular menstrual cycles are common up to 2 years after menarche.
   b. Menstrual history should include time of menarche, regularity, duration, intermenstrual bleeding, and amount of flow.
   c. Associated symptoms of anemia, thyroid, or liver disease and symptoms associated with pregnancy should be determined.
2. **Physical examination**
   a. **General physical.** A physical examination must be done to rule out extragenital problems, signs of anemia, and other medical conditions that might present as abnormal bleeding.
   b. **Pelvic examination** will reveal uterine size, shape, position, consistency, and the presence or absence of tenderness. The adnexa can be accessed for size and tenderness.
3. **Investigative procedures**
   a. **PAP smear.** Cytologic examination of any suspicious lesion as well as biopsy of any gross exophytic lesion is mandatory.
   b. **Occult blood.** Stool should be obtained from rectal examination.
   c. **Complete blood count** should be done especially in the patient with prolonged or heavy menses. A screen platelet count will also access for thrombocytopenia.
   d. **Urinalysis.** A clean voided urine specimen or catheterized specimen if bleeding is profuse should be collected and examined for hemoglobin.
   e. **Pregnancy test.** With the newer, more sensitive pregnancy test, a negative pregnancy test essentially rules out pregnancy-associated causes of abnormal uterine bleeding.
4. **Etiology specific for age group**
   a. Pregnancy associated
   b. Oral contraceptive associated
5. **Acute management**
   a. Estrogen and progesterone (outpatient)
      (1) Oral contraceptives beginning with four pills per day, then three pills per day, then two per day, then one daily until the 21-day pack is completed.

(2) Lack of proper response (24 hours) requires further investigation.

b. Intravenous estrogen (prolonged bleeding or hypoestrogenic conditions)

(1) Conjugated estrogen 20 to 25 mg IV every 4 to 6 hours until the bleeding stops.

(2) Dilation and curettage (D & C) should be used if the bleeding has not stopped within 24 hours.

c. Sequential estrogen and progestin

(1) Conjugated estrogen (Premarin) 10 mg daily for 21 days followed by medroxyprogesterone acetate (Provera) 10 mg daily on days 17 through 21.

(2) If bleeding persists beyond the first 2 days, double the Premarin dose, then continue for 21 days with Provera added on days 17 through 21.

(3) If no response, D & C.

6. **Chronic management**

a. Oral contraceptives, if fertility is not a concern.

b. Periodic withdrawal using Provera 10 mg on days 1 to 5, or 1 to 10 each month for the anovulatory patient.

c. D & C for repeated episodes.

d. Hysteroscopy for repeated episodes.

e. Hysterectomy/endometrial ablation would be used only in those patients resistant to conservative management including hormonal therapy, D & C, and hysteroscopy.

C. **Postmenopausal bleeding.** Bleeding, regardless of the amount, that occurs after a 12-month cessation of regular menstrual flow.

1. **History.** A thorough history should be taken for systemic disease, especially diabetes, hypertension, liver disease, or obesity. A history of estrogen replacement therapy should also be sought.

2. **Physical examination** includes both a general and pelvic examination.

3. **Investigative procedures**

a. PAP smear

b. Complete blood count (CBC)

c. Endometrial sampling

4. **Etiology specific for age group**

a. Atrophic vaginitis

b. Endometrial carcinoma

5. **Management**

a. **Endometrial sampling** may be done as an in-office procedure. D & C must be done for those patients with persistent bleeding despite a negative biopsy.

b. **Observation,** once cancer has been ruled out, perimenopausal bleeding may be self-limited by the impending menopause.

c. **Hormonal therapy** with estrogen replacement therapy and cyclic or continuous medroxyprogesterone acetate.
d. **Hysterectomy** is used only when conservative management has failed.

## ADNEXAL MASS

### I. General considerations

A. **Differential diagnosis** varies according to patient age.
1. In the premenarchal and postmenopausal woman, an adnexal mass must be considered highly abnormal, and immediately investigated.
2. In the menstruating patient, the differential diagnosis is varied, with both benign and malignant processes present.
3. Extragenital lesions may also be encountered, and found on pelvic or abdominal examination.
a. Pelvic masses of nongynecologic origin
(1) Bowel
(2) Bladder distention
(3) Urachal cyst
(4) Abdominal wall
b. Miscellaneous etiologies
(1) Pelvic kidney
(2) Retroperitoneal neoplasm

B. **Clinical work-up**
1. **History and physical examination.** The approach to the patient depends on her age, and the acuteness of the situation. As a rule, a thorough physical examination, bimanual rectal and vaginal examination should be performed with prior emptying of the rectum and bladder. The best time to evaluate ovarian size is just following menses.
2. **Ultrasound.** When bimanual exam is difficult, such as in the obese woman, pelvic sonography may be helpful. However, the sonogram should never replace the physical examination in the work-up of an adnexal mass. The sonogram may be confusing, because of the inability to distinguish between benign and malignant masses. Also, exophytic masses and pedunculated masses of the uterus, mesentery, omentum, and small bowel may all be misinterpreted sonographically as an adnexal mass.
3. **Computerized axial tomography (CAT)** scan for pelvic mass evaluation will provide basically the same information as ultrasound. Advantages to the CAT scan include the detection of preclinical ascites, detection of metastases, and it's superiority in the evaluation of the retroperitoneum.
4. **Magnetic resonance imagery (MRI)** offers advantages over the CAT scan in terms of resolution. However, in general,

there are few indications at the present time in gynecology for MRI.

5. **Barium enema** contrast studies of the gastrointestinal tract should be used liberally, especially when there is any suspicion that the mass is gastrointestinal in origin. Also, patients with hemepositive stools and those over the age of 40 should have a gastrointestinal evaluation prior to laparotomy to exclude colonic causes. A study of the upper portion of the gastrointestinal tract may be indicated in this group of patients, because gastric cancer often metastasizes to the ovaries, especially in the postmenopausal patient.
6. **Intravenous pyelogram (IVP)** may be helpful in that it outlines ureteral displacement and distortion of the bladder contour. In addition, renal function and position can be assessed. If ultrasound examination has been performed and reveals the kidneys to be in the proper location, IVP in and of itself is of limited clinical value.
7. **Mammography** should be performed on all patients who are over the age of 35. Although uncommon, a primary breast carcinoma can become metastatic to the ovary. If a breast mass is found, this will further direct the patient's diagnostic evaluation, and if breast biopsy is indicated, this can be performed at the time of surgical exploration for the pelvic mass.
8. **Chest x-ray** is used to discover the presence of any metastatic disease and/or pleural effusions. Information regarding heart size, can also be obtained.
9. **CA-125.** Several investigators have sought to determine the role of serum CA-125 in the preoperative evaluation of patients with a pelvic mass. In general, an elevated CA-125 occurs in approximately 90% of nonmucinous epithelial ovarian carcinomas. In addition, elevated CA-125 levels have been reported in other nonovarian gynecologic malignancies, and are known to be elevated by smoking and in patients with endometriosis. Its current role remains somewhat controversial, but it is probably helpful when correlated to the physical examination and ultrasound findings, especially in the perimenopausal and postmenopausal patient with a 3 to 4 cm cystic ovarian mass.
10. **KUB.** A flat radiograph of the abdomen may reveal the outline of a pelvic mass, and the finding of "teeth" indicates a benign teratoma. However, all calcifications are not teeth, and psammoma bodies in serous adenocarcinomas of the ovary are commonly found radiopaque entities noted on roentgenologic examination. Other findings on KUB include a radiolucent shadow cast by the lipidic fluid filling the cyst, and the "capsule sign" (rim of radiodensity circumscribing the cyst).

11. **Laparoscopy.** Diagnostic laparoscopy may be helpful in the evaluation of a patient with a pelvic mass (distinguishing a uterine myoma from an ovarian neoplasm). Laparoscopy is helpful in the situation where the source of a pelvic mass is uncertain, and the source will determine whether the treatment is surgical or nonsurgical. Laparoscopic removal is also proposed by some; thus, avoiding the risk of laparotomy.

    Laparoscopy may reveal an incidental cystic enlargement of the ovary. Some physicians advise puncture of these cysts, with cytologic analysis of the cystic contents. However, most of these cysts will disappear on their own or reform. Therefore, no treatment at all or surgical removal is indicated. In retrospect, laparotomy could be avoided in the patient with hydrosalpinx, endometriosis, postoperative adhesion formation, or when small serosal uterine fibroids are present.

## II. Management approach

A. **The approach to the patient must be individualized** based on the patient's age, history, and physical examination findings, as well as the findings of any diagnostic test that is obtained.

B. **Benign tumors** are usually smooth walled, cystic, mobile, unilateral, and less than 8 cm in diameter. **Malignant tumors** are usually solid or semisolid, bilateral, irregular, fixed, and associated with nodules in the cul-de-sac. Ascites is frequently present.

C. **There are no "mandatory rules"** regarding preoperative evaluation. This is where **clinical judgement and experience** is important.

D. **Functional neoplasms** of the ovary are rarely larger than 7.0 cm, and are usually unilateral and freely mobile. Thus, a unilateral cystic mass smaller than 8.0 cm in an ovulating woman should be followed for 4 to 8 weeks to determine if regression occurs.

E. **Ovarian suppression** for the adnexal mass that does not meet the criteria for immediate laparotomy has proven effective in suppressing the functional cyst. This cyst will spontaneously resolve while oral contraceptives prevent the occurrence of a second physiologic cyst by suppressing the pituitary–gonadal axis.

F. **All persistent adnexal enlargements must be considered malignant until proven otherwise.**

G. **Indications for surgical intervention include:**

1. A palpable tumor in a premenarchal patient.
2. A palpable tumor in a postmenopausal patient.
3. An ovarian mass in a premenopausal patient measuring 5.0 cm or more in diameter that has been followed through at least two menstrual cycles.
4. Any solid ovarian tumor.
5. An ovarian mass larger than 7.0 to 8.0 cm in diameter.

6. Signs or symptoms suggesting adnexal torsion.
7. Ovarian enlargement causing sufficient pain to interfere with the patient's activities.
8. Unexplained ascites with malignant cells in the peritoneal fluid and/or malignant cells identifiable on PAP smear, for which an etiology cannot be found.

**III. Surgical considerations**

**A. Type of incision.** As a general rule, a vertical skin incision is the incision of choice. A Pfannenstiel incision or DeCherney incision may be used but offer less exposure and the inability to extend the incision into the upper abdomen if a malignant process is encountered. These incisions should be reserved when there is an unequivocal diagnosis of benign disease. For example, such a patient might have had a dermoid documented by roentgenogram or endometriosis confirmed by previous laparoscopy.

**B. Peritoneal cytology** should always be collected as should any ascites that are present. This can be done by using 50 to 75 cc of saline and by irrigating and collecting the washing from the pelvis, pericolic gutters, and upper abdomen.

**C. Abdominal exploration.** The upper abdomen, diaphragms, and liver should be palpated for evidence of tumor spread. In addition, the pelvis, retroperitoneal spaces, and aorta bifurcation should be palpated for evidence of enlarged nodal tissue. The contralateral ovary must always be examined, even with a benign neoplasm, as these may be bilateral.

**D. Cystectomy.** With a benign neoplasm, ovarian tissue should always be conserved in the reproductive-aged woman desiring future fertility. In the perimenopausal patient (age >40 years) consideration should be given to oophorectomy with hysterectomy. For the young patient with a small unilateral malignant tumor, without spread (stage IA), consideration should be given to conservation of the contralateral ovary.

## ACUTE PELVIC PAIN

For a diagrammatic representation of the following text, see Figure 35.5.

**I.** Patients presenting with acute pelvic pain should be managed in an efficient, relatively focused fashion to avoid delay of appropriate management. The patient's age will determine the likelihood and appropriateness of some of the diagnostic possibilities. Menstrual history, contraceptive technique used, and sexual activity can be used to determine whether to focus on a possible pregnancy or its complications. Gastrointestinal and urinary symptoms are also important.

**II.** In addition to the requisite vital signs, focused evaluation of the abdomen and pelvis should help identify localized tenderness, rebound tenderness, and voluntary guarding to determine likely sources of

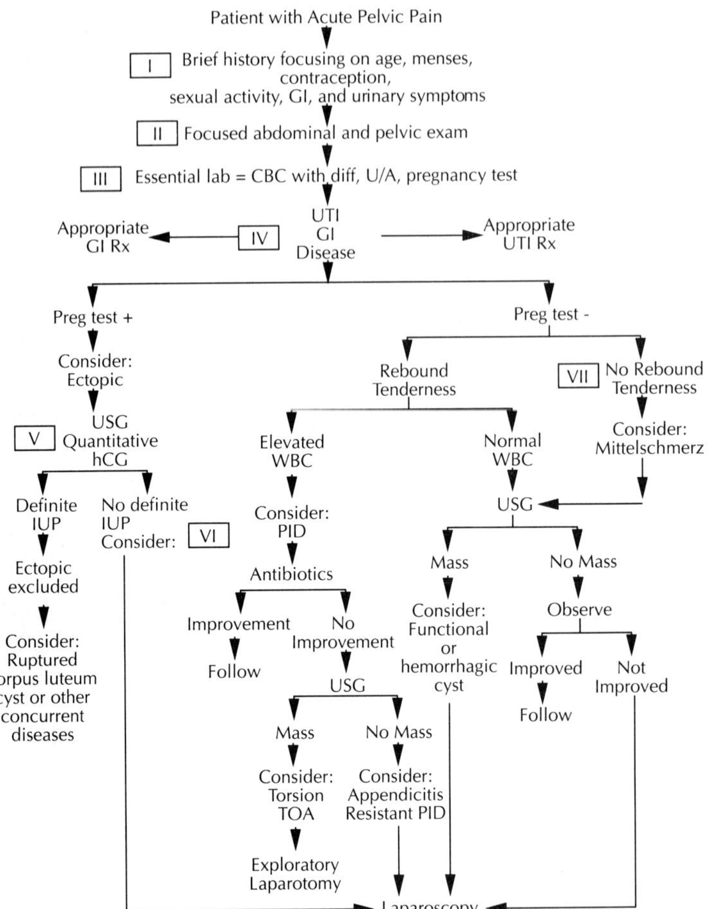


FIGURE 35.5. Algorithm for diagnosis of acute pelvic pain. U/A = urinalysis; hCG = human chorionic gonadotropin; UTI = urinary tract infections; WBC = white blood count; IUP = intrauterine pregnancy; GI = gastrointestinal; CBC = complete blood count; USG = ultrasound; PID = pelvic inflammatory disease; TOA = tubo-ovarian accesses. (*Note:* Roman numerals refer to corresponding text sections.)

acute pain, as well as the need for potential emergent surgical intervention.

**III.** A CBC with differential, urinalysis, and pregnancy test are readily available in a rapid fashion. Erythrocyte sedimentation rate is recommended by some in cases of possible pelvic inflammatory disease.

**IV.** If an obvious urinary tract infection is apparent on urinalysis and symptoms are compatible, appropriate therapy should be instituted with the possibility that this might be concurrent with other conditions. Similarly, obvious gastrointestinal symptoms should be managed but other diagnostic possibilities should not be eliminated without due consideration.

**V.** When ectopic pregnancy is considered, quantitative human chorionic gonadotropin (hCG) levels should be correlated with pelvic ultrasound, either transvaginal or transabdominal. An intrauterine pregnancy is typically expected to be seen on transabdominal ultrasound when the hCG level has reached 6500, whereas the corresponding hCG level for transvaginal ultrasound is 2000 to 2500.

**VI.** If no intrauterine pregnancy is visualized, the clinician must consider diagnoses such as an intrauterine pregnancy too early to be visualized by ultrasound, missed abortion, incomplete abortion, or completed abortion. Of greatest concern, however, is the potential of an ectopic pregnancy. For this reason, laparoscopy should be considered. Evacuation of the uterine contents may reveal placental villi, which would rule out ectopic pregnancy. Evacuation of the uterus can, however, only be done in circumstances when termination of a potentially viable pregnancy is considered acceptable.

**VII.** In cases where the pregnancy test is negative, reproductive-aged women not on oral contraceptives can have midcycle pain due to ovulation, otherwise known as Mittelschmerz. If the timing or circumstances for this diagnosis are not correct, the work-up should then proceed to ultrasonography to rule out the presence of a possible adnexal mass, with possible rupture or torsion.

## CHRONIC PELVIC PAIN

For a diagrammatic representation of the following text, see Figure 35.6.

**I. Initial evaluation.** Once it is determined that the pain is not an acute episode and that it does not fall under the category of either dysmenorrhea or premenstrual syndrome, the history should scrutinize both gynecologic as well as nongynecologic etiologies. Environmental stressors are of particular importance, because it is on this background that the chronic pain is superimposed. Therefore, insight into the patient's day-to-day life-style is important. Questions regarding the following topics are appropriate: marital relationship, financial status, job problems, and family interpersonal relationships.

**II. Urinary symptoms.** Significant urinary symptoms in conjunction with physical findings suggestive of pathology of the urinary tract suggest pain that is nongynecologic, but potentially of urologic etiology. A thorough evaluation of these symptoms and physical find-is within the purview of an experienced gynecologist, but certainly may be referred to a urologist with interest in this area and/or a urogynecologist with special training.

**III. Musculoskeletal pain.** It is not unusual for musculoskeletal dysfunction to present as pelvic pain. There is often a precipitating event, although it is not uncommon for life-style factors such as a particular job or sleeping position to come into play. Superficial palpation of the back and abdomen may elicit the same pain as the patient's chief

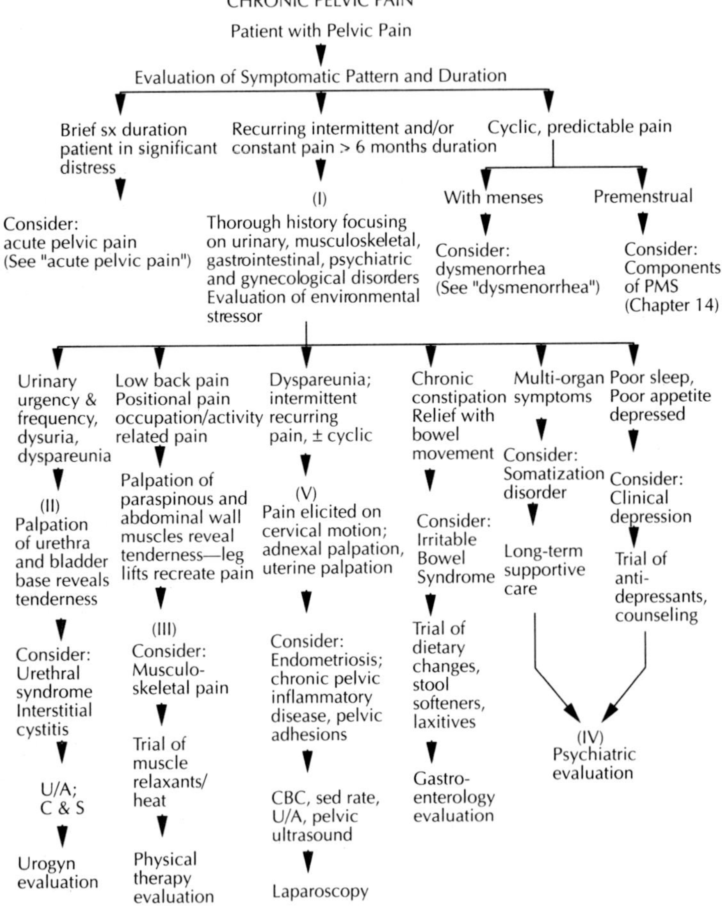


FIGURE 35.6. Algorithm for diagnosis of chronic pelvic pain. U/A = urinalysis; C&S = culture and sensitivity; CBC = complete blood count; Sed Rate = erythrocyte sedimentation rate; PMS = premenstrual syndrome; Sx = symptoms. (*Note:* Roman numerals refer to corresponding text sections.)

complaint. Having the patient raise her head as if sitting up or asking her to perform a leg lift can recreate low abdominal pain that otherwise is perceived as pelvic etiology. Such patients can often find symptomatic improvement with muscle relaxants and/or local moist heat but often require ongoing physical therapy treatment.

IV. **Psychiatric component.** Patients may have an underlying psychiatric condition that presents with physical complaints. There may also be underlying clinical depression of which early symptoms might include disturbed sleep, change in appetite, or loss of energy.

Somatization is a process in which emotional problems are converted into physical complaints. In these cases, there tends to be multiple complaints for which there is no organic cause or that appear to be out of proportion to identifiable medical or surgical disease. Symptoms appear in association with stress and there may be dramatic descriptions of distress.

Patients in both categories can be handled by the primary care provider if desired, but certainly can benefit from psychiatric evaluation and consultation.

V. **Dyspareunia.** Chronic, recurring intermittent or constant pain associated with dyspareunia is often a history elicited due to a myriad of other confounding symptoms. A thorough history should attempt to rule out other organ symptoms, but associated findings of cervical motion tenderness, tenderness of adnexa, and/or uterus would strongly point to a pelvic etiology. Laboratory tests including a CBC, sedimentation rate, and urinalysis are typically needed as preoperative evaluation but can help in ruling out intercurrent acute disease. Pelvic ultrasound is helpful in those patients in whom the examination is difficult or in which there are equivocal findings. The ultimate technique in ruling out pelvic pathology is diagnostic laparoscopy. Laparoscopy can also be used for therapy should significant pathology be found.

## DYSMENORRHEA

For a diagrammatic representation of the following text, see Figure 35.7.

I. **Primary dysmenorrhea** is painful menstruation that does not have a demonstrable etiology. Typically, it occurs in ovulatory women and often has its onset when an adolescent female first starts having regular periods. It is felt that dysmenorrhea is caused by an increase in circulating levels of prostaglandins that increase uterine contractions.

II. **Secondary dysmenorrhea** is typically later in onset than primary dysmenorrhea and is due to a specific organic etiology. The most common causes include: endometriosis, uterine leiomyomata, adenomyosis, cervical stenosis, uterine polyps, and presence of an intrauterine device.

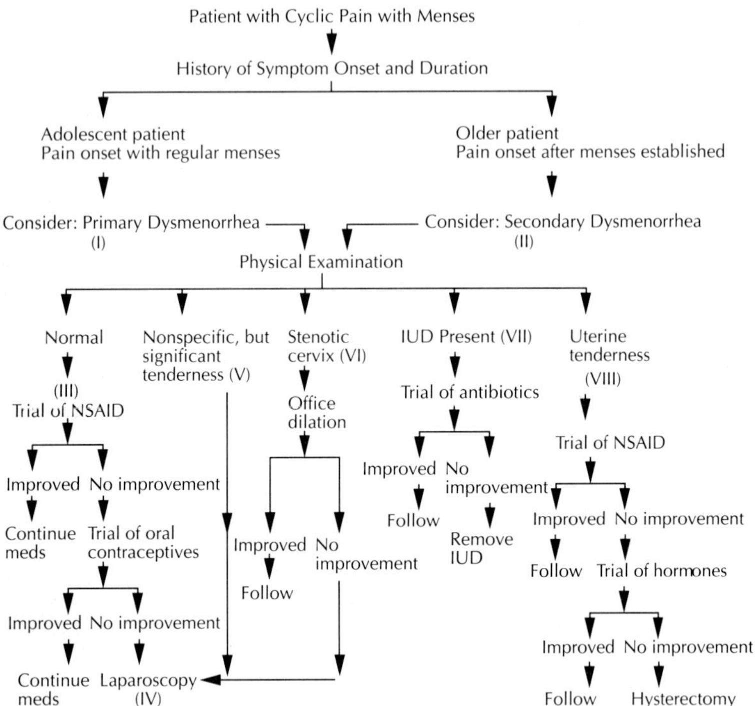


FIGURE 35.7. Algorithm for diagnosis of dysmenorrhea. NSAID = nonsteroidal anti-inflammatory medication; IUD = intrauterine device. (*Note:* Roman numerals refer to corresponding text sections.)

**III.** **Nonsteroidal anti-inflammatory drugs** are frequently effective for the treatment of both primary and secondary dysmenorrhea by preventing production of prostaglandins and/or counteracting their action. These medications are most appropriate as a first-line therapy in face of a normal examination, but are certainly appropriate in any case of dysmenorrhea to provide the patient symptomatic relief.

**IV.** **Laparoscopy** to evaluate pelvic structures should be considered any time the patient has not responded to conservative measures or in patients who have a suspicious examination. Diagnostic laparoscopy may also be accompanied by hysteroscopy and/or D & C to evaluate intrauterine causes of pain. Laparoscopy allows the physician to identify conditions such as endometriosis, pelvic inflammatory disease, pelvic adhesions, and other pathology of the uterus, tubes and ovaries that are otherwise not appreciated on physical examination or diagnostic radiologic imaging. Claims have been made for uterosacral nerve ablation at the time of laparoscopy for relief of dysmenorrhea.

V. **Conservative treatment.** In patients with nonspecific yet significant tenderness on pelvic examination, reasonable conservative measures include nonsteroidals and oral contraceptives. It is not unusual, however, to expect that these patients will ultimately have to undergo laparoscopy.

VI. **Cervical stenosis** is not a common finding, but should be looked for in any patient with dysmenorrhea. Patients will sometimes give a prior history of cervical trauma, for example, related to an elective pregnancy termination. If relieving the cervical stenosis does not help the dysmenorrhea, consideration should be given to possible intrapelvic pathology.

VII. **An intrauterine device** (IUD) causes dysmenorrhea much as a uterine polyp would. The uterus contracts excessively in an attempt to expel the intrauterine contents. The presence of endometritis caused by an IUD can cause dysmenorrhea, such that a trial of antibiotics is appropriate prior to removal of the IUD.

VIII. **Uterine tenderness** in the presence of a history of significant dysmenorrhea, particularly in a multigravid patient, may be suggestive of adenomyosis. The index of suspicion is raised for this condition if there is no adnexal pain and the uterus feels globular, mildly enlarged, and boggy. As in all cases of dysmenorrhea, conservative forms of therapy with nonsteroidals as well as hormones is appropriate prior to considering operative intervention. If adenomyosis is considered the likely etiology, hysterectomy is the definitive operative procedure. Laparoscopy will not reveal any abnormality except a mildly enlarged uterus with a normal exterior appearance. It is for this reason, that surgery and particularly hysterectomy should be considered only as a last resort.

## DYSPAREUNIA

For a diagrammatic representation of the following text, see Figure 35.8.

I. If a patient complains of pain on sexual intercourse, all efforts should be made to differentiate the location of the pain as well as the pattern of painful intercourse. Patients can typically say that the pain is on entrance, or on deep thrusting ("feels like he is bumping into something"). Also, it is important to note whether or not the painful intercourse is on every coital attempt, or if it is periodic. If it does not occur with every coital attempt, circumstances surrounding those situations in which it has occurred would be important. For example, the most common cause of entrance dyspareunia is lack of lubrication because of inadequate arousal.

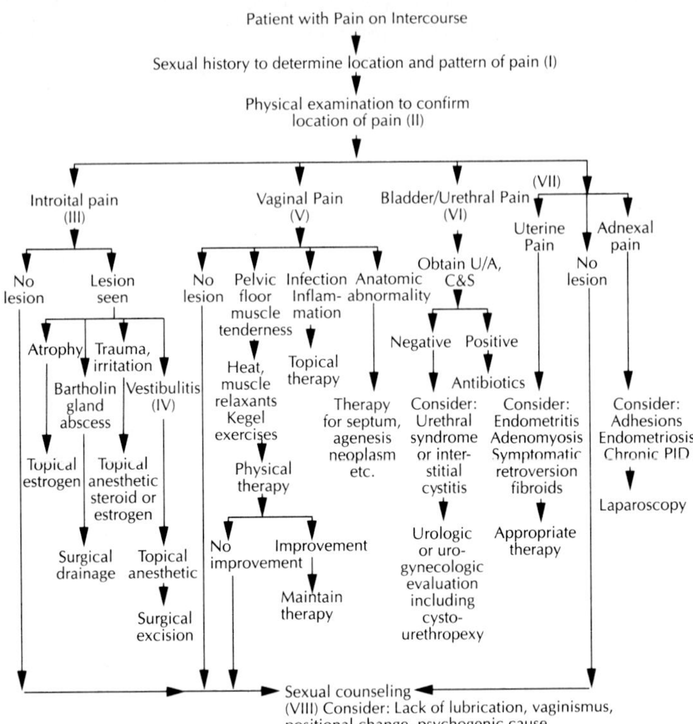


FIGURE 35.8. Algorithm for diagnosis of dyspareunia. U/A = urinalysis; C&S = culture and sensitivity; PID = pelvic inflammatory disease. (*Note:* Roman numerals refer to corresponding text sections.)

**II.** The physical examination should attempt to confirm the patient's history of the location of the pain. In those cases in which the location has not been identified by the history, a gentle pelvic examination can do a great deal to help the patient gain insight into the source of her pain.

**III.** Note that the most common cause of introital pain is because of lack of lubrication. This can be resolved by either increasing the amount of endogenous lubrication through more pleasuring for the female prior to penile insertion, or through exogenous lubrication in the form of a water-soluble lubricant.

**IV.** Close inspection of the introitus is necessary to rule out vestibulitis (also referred to as vestibular adenitis). It is a condition of chronic inflammation of unknown etiology that affects the entire vestibular area from just beneath the clitoral hood, around both labia minora to the posterior fourchette, just outside the hymenal ring. Gentle palpation with a cotton swab can confirm the location of pain in these instances. Symptomatic relief is sometimes obtained with topical anesthetics or steroids. Surgery to remove the affected area has been reported to be successful in approximately 75% of cases. This therapy should only be considered as a last resort because approximately 50% of cases resolve by themselves.

**V.** If an obvious anatomic abnormality or inflammation is not appreciated, gentle palpation of the posterior vagina to identify muscular pain should be carried out. Asking the patient to contract her pelvic floor muscles, as if she were trying to stop her urine stream, can sometimes also illicit pain, recreating her chief complaint.

**VI.** Consideration should be given to urologic causes of dyspareunia. When performing a pelvic examination, attempts should be made to differentiate vaginal barrel pain caused by posterior causes (such as muscular pain) from anterior causes (such as urethral or bladder tenderness). Gentle massaging of the urethra and the bladder base with the forefinger can often elicit the pain the patient has experienced. If no obvious infection is found, urologic or urogynecologic evaluation to rule out urethral syndrome or interstitial cystitis would be appropriate.

**VII.** It is unlikely that deep dyspareunia can be identified by visualization. Palpation of uterine tenderness would imply conditions such as endometritis, adenomyosis, symptomatic uterine retroversion, and uterine leiomyomata, each of which requires separate therapy. Adnexal discomfort would suggest a need for laparoscopy to rule out conditions such as pelvic adhesions, chronic pelvic inflammatory disease, or laparoscopy.

**VIII.** Sexual counseling is within the purview of any health-care provider who routinely investigates gynecologic problems such as dyspareunia. The primary focus of sexual counseling is behavior modification. For example, in cases where a lack of lubrication due to inadequate sexual arousal is the cause of entrance dyspareunia, providing techniques to increase endogenous lubrication or to simply provide exogenous lubrication is a first-line form of therapy rather than investigating what may potentially be deep-seated etiologies for the lack of arousal. Patients may need to be treated for other conditions such as vaginismus, anatomic abnormalities requiring positional change when coitus is attempted, or psychogenic causes.

## BIBLIOGRAPHY

Cunanan RG, Courey NG, Lippes J. Laparoscopic findings in patients with pelvic pain. Am J Obstet Gynecol 1983; 146:589.

Early TK, Norton LW. Nipple discharge. In: Norton LW, Eiseman B, eds. Surgical Decision Making. Philadelphia, PA: W B Saunders Co; 1986; 202–203.

Friedrich EG. Vulvar vestibulitis syndrome. J Reprod Med 1987; 32:110.

Hanid MA, Levi AJ. Medical causes of pain in the lower abdomen. Clin Obstet Gynecol 1981; 8:15.

Is fibrocystic disease of the breast precancerous? Consensus Meeting of the Cancer Committee of the College of American Pathologists. Arch Path Lab Med, 1986; 110:171–173.

Mettlin C. Breast cancer risk factors. In: Ariel IM, Cleary JB, eds. Breast Cancer. New York: McGraw-Hill; 1987: 35–44.

Owen PR. Prostaglandin synthetase inhibitors in the treatment of primary dysmenorrhea. Outcome trials reviewed. Am J Obstet Gynecol 1984; 148:96.

Renaer M. ed. Chronic Pelvic Pain in Women. New York: Springer–Verlag; 1981.

Skinner MA, Swain M, Simmons R, McCarty KS, JR., Sullivan DC, Iglehart JD. Nonpalpable breast lesions at biopsy: A detailed analysis of radiographic features. Ann Surg 1988; 208:203–208.

Steege JF. Dyspareunia and vaginismus. Clin Obstet Gynecol 1984; 27:750.

The Centers for Disease Control Cancer and Steroid Hormone Study. Long term oral contraceptive use and the risk of breast cancer. JAMA 1983; 249:1591.

# Appendix A

# Drug Therapy in Gynecology

Rebecca Rogers

## DRUGS IN GYNECOLOGY: USES AND CORRESPONDING DOSE*

| GENERIC (TRADE) NAME | INDICATION | COMMENTS |
| --- | --- | --- |
| Acetaminophen-codeine (Tylenol #3, Phenaphen #3) | Moderate pain: 1 or 2 tablets p.o. every 4–6 hours as needed, up to 12 tablets per day. | See morphine comments. Each tablet contains: acetaminophen 325 mg, codeine 30 mg. |
| Acetaminophen-oxycodone (Tylox, Percocet) | Moderate–severe pain: 1 or 2 tablets p.o. every 6 hours as needed. | Tylox contains oxycodone hydrochloride (HCl) 4.5 mg, oxycodone terephthalate 0.38 mg, acetaminophen 500 mg. Percocet contains oxycodone HCl 5 mg, acetaminophen 325 mg. |
| Alprazolam (Xanax) | Anxiety disorders or short-term relief of symptoms of anxiety: 0.25–0.5 mg t.i.d. as a starting dose. Titrate to patient needs to a maximum of 4 mg/day. | When reducing dose or ending therapy, reduce no more than 0.5 mg every 3 days. |
| Aminophylline (various) | Asthma, other pulmonary conditions requiring bronchodilation: Oral loading dose: 6–10 mg/kg ideal body weight (IBW). IV loading dose: 6 mg/kg IBW over 20 minutes. IV loading dose with history of theophylline or aminophylline ingestion within last 24 hours:<br>Dose = (0.5) (desired level minus actual level) (IBW in kg)<br>Oral maintenance dose: 4 mg/kg IBW every 6 hours.<br>IV maintenance dose: 0.5 mg/kg/hour. | For oral loading dose, use rapid-release tablets or liquid formulation. IBW = 45 kg + 2.3 kg (height in inches–60). See theophylline comments. |
| Amitriptyline (Elavil) | Endogenous depression: initially begin with 75 mg/day in divided doses, progressing to a maximum of 150 mg/day. Maintenance consists of 50–100 mg/day. | Amitriptyline has been recommended for the treatment of interstitial cystitis, maximum dosing of 75 mg every night. |

| | | |
|---|---|---|
| Bethanechol (Duvoid, Urecholine) | Postoperative bladder atony: 10 mg p.o. 3–4 times daily, increasing to 50 mg per dose as needed. Subcutaneous dose: 2.5–5 mg SC 3–4 times daily. | May cause lacrimation, flushing, sweating, gastrointestinal disturbances. |
| Bleomycin (Blenoxane) | Cervical or vulvar carcinoma, embryonal cell carcinoma, choriocarcinoma: 0.25–0.5 units per kg IM or IV 1–2 times weekly. May be given IV push. | Maximum lifetime dose limited to 400 mg due to risk of pulmonary fibrosis. Causes stomatitis. 1 mg = 1 unit. Reduce dose in renal compromise:<br>Serum creatinine: Reduce dose by:<br>2.5–4 mg/dL 75%<br>4.0–6 mg/dL 80%<br>6–10 mg/dL 90% |
| Bromocriptine (Parlodel) | Hyperprolactinemia: 1.25–2.5 mg p.o. daily for 3–7 days, increasing to a maximum of 2.5 mg three times daily. | Side effects: nausea, dizziness, headache, fatigue. Take with snack. Very expensive. |
| Buspirone (BUSPAR) | Anxiety disorders or short-term relief of symptoms of anxiety: begin with 5 mg t.i.d. and increase dose as needed for relief of symptoms (maximum 60 mg/day). | In research protocols, buspirone has been used for the treatment of premenstrual syndrome with good success. |
| Calcitonin (Calcimar) | Postmenopausal osteoporosis: 100 IU SC or IM daily. | May decrease rate of bone loss. Does not appear to decrease incidence of fractures. May cause skin rash. Patients should also receive supplemental calcium and vitamin D. |
| Calcium carbonate (Os Cal, various) | Nutritional supplement: 600–1600 mg p.o. daily. | Any calcium supplement that can be tolerated by an individual's gastrointestinal system is acceptable (e.g., TUMS 2–3/day). |

*(Continued)*

**Drugs in Gynecology: Uses and Corresponding Dose *(Continued)***

| GENERIC (TRADE) NAME | INDICATION | COMMENTS |
|---|---|---|
| Carboplatin (Paraplatin) | Ovarian carcinoma: 360 mg/$m^2$ IV every 4 weeks. | Hydration or forced diuresis not required. Less toxic than cisplatin. Reduce dose in renal compromise: Creatinine clearance 41–59 mL/min: 250 mg/$m^2$. 16–40 mL/min: 200 mg/$m^2$. |
| Chloral hydrate | Sedative: 250 mg p.o. three times daily. Hypnotic: 500 mg–1 g p.o. 30 minutes before bedtime. | |
| Chlorambucil (Leukeran) | Epithelial ovarian carcinoma, Stage 1A: 0.1–0.2 mg/kg p.o. daily. | Available as 2 mg tablets. White blood cell (WBC) nadir: 7–14 days. |
| Cimetidine (Tagamet) | Preoperatively: 300 mg IM or diluted in 20–100 mL for IV. Peptic ulcer disease: 300 mg p.o. 30 minutes before meals and at bedtime for 6 weeks, then 400 mg at bedtime. Prophylaxis against stress ulcers: 300 mg IV every 6 hours. | Can induce galactorrhea with chronic dosing. Can increase theophylline serum concentration by 30%. |
| Cisplatin (Platinol) | Metastatic ovarian tumors, combination therapy: 50 mg/$m^2$. IV over 6–8 hours every 3 weeks. Single agent therapy: 100 mg/$m^2$ IV every 4 weeks. | Nausea and vomiting may be severe. Pretreat with metoclopramide, dexamethasone, diphenhydramine. Monitor renal function. Hydrate with 1–2 liters of fluid, administer mannitol 12.5 g prior to therapy. Reduce dose in renal impairment, specific guidelines have not been established. WBC nadir: 7–10 days. Extravasation antidote: sodium thiosulfate 10%–4 mL diluted to 10 mL with sterile water, administered IV. |

| | | |
|---|---|---|
| Clomiphene citrate (Clomid) | Ovulation induction: 50 mg p.o. for 5 days, starting on fifth day of menses. | Expect ovulation 5–11 days after last dose. May increase in 50 mg increments on successive cycles, up to 200 mg. Risk of ovarian enlargement: $< 10\%$. Risk of multiple gestation: $< 4\%$ to 9%. May cause vasomotor symptoms, bloating, nausea, vomiting, visual disturbance. |
| Clonidine (Catapres) | Hypertension: 0.1 mg p.o. twice daily, increased by 0.1–0.2 mg/day until control is achieved. Hypertensive emergency: 0.2 mg p.o. followed by 0.1 mg p.o. every hour up to 0.7 mg, or until 20 mm Hg reduction in diastolic pressure has been achieved. Vasomotor symptoms: 0.1 mg p.o. twice daily, increasing to control symptoms. | Upon discontinuation, taper dose over 1 week to avoid rebound hypertension. Maximum daily dose: 2.4 mg. |
| Codeine (various) | Postoperative pain or moderate–severe pain: 15–60 mg p.o. or IM every 6 hours as needed. Antitussive: 5–15 mg p.o. every 4 hours. | See morphine comments. |
| Cyclophosphamide (Cytoxan) | Cervical, ovarian, endometrial carcinoma, breast carcinoma: 500–1500 mg/m$^2$ as a single IV infusion every 3 weeks, or 60–120 mg/m$^2$ p.o. daily. | Pretreat with antiemetics. Maintain adequate hydration due to risk of hemorrhagic cystitis. WBC nadir: 8–14 days. WBC recovery: 18–25 days. Protocols may vary. |
| Danazol (Danocrine) | Endometriosis: 600–800 mg p.o. daily for 1 month, then decrease to 200 — 400 mg daily, using the lowest dose that maintains amenorrhea. Also indicated for fibrocystic breast disease. | Pain relief begins within 1–2 months. Androgenic side effects. |

(Continued)

**Drugs in Gynecology: Uses and Corresponding Dose *(Continued)***

| GENERIC (TRADE) NAME | INDICATION | COMMENTS |
|---|---|---|
| Dantroline (Dantrium) | Malignant hyperthermia: Discontinue anesthesia. Administer 1 mg/kg rapid IV push. Repeat as needed until symptoms subside or a cumulative dose of 10 mg/kg is reached. Oral follow-up: 1–2 mg/kg every 6 hours for 1–3 days. | Incidence of malignant hyperthermia in anesthetized patients: 1:20 000. May cause drowsiness, dizziness, fatigue, weakness, malaise, diarrhea. Capsules: 25 or 50 mg. |
| Dexamethasone (Decadron, Hexadrol) | Induction of follicular maturation in congenital adrenal hyperplasia: < 70 kg: 0.5 mg p.o. at bedtime. > 70 kg: 0.75 mg p.o. at bedtime. Antiemetic: 20 mg IV push prior to chemotherapy. | Compatible with metoclopramide and diphenhydramine when used prior to chemotherapy. |
| Dicyclomine (Bentyl) | To inhibit involuntary detrusor contractions: 10–20 mg p.o. three to four times daily. | Anticholinergic side effects may be less than with propantheline. |
| Dienestrol (OrthoDienestrol cream, suppositories) | Atrophic vaginitis: 1 suppository or 1 applicatorful one to two times daily for 1–3 weeks. Decrease to 1 to 3 times weekly after restoration of vaginal mucosa. | Suppositories contain tartrazine. |
| Diethylstilbestrol | Postcoital contraception: 25 mg p.o. twice daily for 5 days, beginning within 72 hours of unprotected intercourse. Vasomotor symptoms: 0.25–1 mg p.o. daily for 21–25 days per month. Dysfunctional uterine bleeding: 2 mg p.o. every 2 hours until bleeding stops. Breast cancer: 10–20 mg p.o. daily. | Postcoital contraceptive use of diethylstilbestrol (DES) is associated with a high frequency of nausea and vomiting. Pretreat with an antiemetic. DES dephosphate 1.6 mg is equivalent to 1 mg of DES. Use should be limited due to association with adenosis and clear cell carcinoma of the vagina. |
| Digoxin (Lanoxin) | Atrial fibrillation, congestive heart failure: Loading dose: 0.01 mg/kg IV or 0.015 mg/kg p.o. divided into 3–4 doses over 24 hours. Maintenance dose: 0.125–0.5 mg daily in one dose. | Time to steady state: 8 days. Desired serum concentration: 0.9–2.1 ng/mL. Obtain serum concentration 8–24 hours after dose. |

| | | |
|---|---|---|
| Diphenhydramine (Benadryl) | Hypnotic: 50–100 mg p.o. or IM 30 minutes before bedtime. Antiemetic: 50 mg IV 30 minutes prior to chemotherapy. Anaphylaxis, allergic reactions: 50 mg p.o., IM, or IV, depending on severity. May repeat every 4–6 hours as needed. | Compatible when mixed with metoclopramide and dexamethasone prior to chemotherapy. |
| Doxorubicin (Adriamycin) | Adenocarcinoma of the endometrium, tube, ovary, vagina; uterine sarcoma: 60–100 mg/m$^2$ IV every 3 weeks. | Cumulative dose should not exceed 660 mg/m$^2$ (or 400 mg/m$^2$, with prior irradiation therapy) due to risk of cardiomyopathy. Reduce dose in severe hepatic failure:<br>Serum bilirubin: Reduce dose by:<br>$<$ 1.2 mg/dL No reduction<br>1.2–3 mg/dL 50%<br>$>$ 3 mg/dL 75%<br>Discolors urine, causes stomatitis. Administer IV push through running IV. Treat extravasation with an ice compress for 30–40 minutes. WBC nadir: 14 days. WBC recovery: 22–25 days. |
| Estradiol (Estrace) | Vasomotor symptoms: 1–2 mg p.o. daily for 25 days per month. | Available as a vaginal cream also. See estrogens, conjugated. |
| Estradiol transdermal (Estraderm) | Vasomotor symptoms: One patch (0.05 or 0.1) to clean, dry skin on body trunk. Change patch twice weekly. | Should not be applied to the breast. Rotate site of application. |
| Estradiol valerate (Delestrogen, various) | Vasomotor symptoms: 10–20 mg IM every 4 weeks. | Response will vary. Adjust dose and interval accordingly. See estrogens, conjugated. |

*(Continued)*

**Drugs in Gynecology: Uses and Corresponding Dose *(Continued)***

| GENERIC (TRADE) NAME | INDICATION | COMMENTS |
|---|---|---|
| Estrogens, conjugated (Premarin) | Vasomotor symptoms: 0.3–2.5 mg p.o. daily for 25 days per month, adjust dose according to response. Vaginal atrophy: 0.3–1.25 mg p.o. daily for 25 days per month, or ½–1 applicatorful, adjust dose per response. Osteoporosis: 0.625–1.25 mg p.o. daily. Castration: 0.625–1.25 mg p.o. daily. Dysfunctional uterine bleeding: 25 mg IV Push every 4 hours for 24 hours. | Cycle with progestin in patients with an intact uterus. Vaginal cream is absorbed systemically: each gram contains 0.625 mg of conjugated estrogens.<br>Estrogen equivalents:<br>Chlorotrianisene 12.0 mg<br>Estrone sulfate, piperazine 1.25 mg<br>Micronized estradiol 1.0 mg<br>Conjugated estrogens 0.625 mg<br>Diethylstilbestrol 0.25 mg<br>Mestranol 0.02 mg<br>Ethinyl estradiol 0.015 mg<br>Quinestrol 0.00014 mg |
| Estrone sulfate, piperazine (Ogen) | Vasomotor symptoms: 0.625–5 mg p.o. daily for 25 days per month, adjust dose according to response. Vaginal atrophy: ½–1 applicatorful daily for 25 days, adjust dose per response. Castration, primary ovarian failure: 1.25–7.5 mg p.o. daily. | See estrogens, conjugated. |
| Famotidine (Pepcid) | Active duodenal ulcer: 40 mg p.o. once daily, or 20 mg IV every 12 hours. Maintenance dose: 20 mg p.o. once daily. | Also available as oral suspension 40 mg/5 mL. |
| Ferrous sulfate (various) | Iron deficiency anemia: 1 tablet (325 mg) p.o. two to three times daily with meals. | Elemental iron content: Ferrous sulfate: 20%<br>Ferrous gluconate: 11%<br>Ferrous fumarate 33%<br>May cause black stools, which does not interfere with guiac test. Incidence of constipation: 10%. Incidence of nausea/diarrhea: 5% |

| | | |
|---|---|---|
| Flavoxate (Urispas) | Bladder antispasmotic: 100–200 mg p.o. three to four times daily. | Also has local anesthetizing properties. |
| Flurazepam (Dalmane) | Insomnia: 15–30 mg p.o. 30 minutes prior to bedtime. | Long half-life. May cause prolonged drowsiness with repeated doses. |
| Flurouracil (Efudex) | Ovarian, endometrial carcinoma, cervical adenocarcinoma: 12 mg/kg IV daily for 4 days, then 6 mg/kg IV every other day for 4 doses. Repeat monthly. Condyloma accuminata: application and dosing vary according to individual research protocols. | Maximum daily dose: 800 mg. Base dose on actual body weight except in extreme obesity. Causes stomatitis, alopecia. WBC nadir: 7–14 days. WBC recovery: 20–30 days. |
| Furosemide (Lasix) | Diuresis in mild–moderate hypertension: 20–40 mg p.o. daily initially then titrate dose to desired effect. Acute pulmonary edema: 40 mg IV over 1–2 minutes, repeat with 80 mg as needed. | |
| Heparin (various) | Deep vein thrombosis: 70 U/kg IV bolus, then 15 U/kg/h. Continue for 7 days. Pulmonary embolus: 100 U/kg IV bolus, then 25 U/kg/h. Continue for 7–10 days. Prophylaxis: 5000 SC 30–60 minutes prior to surgery, then q 8–12 hours postoperatively until ambulatory. | Evaluate activated partial thromboplastin time (APTT) 8 hours after initiation of therapy, then once daily, adjusting infusion rate to maintain APTT 1.5–2 times control value. |
| Human chorionic gonadotropin (Profasi, various) | To effect ovulation: 10 000 units IM 1 day after last dose of menotropins. | Monitor for hyperstimulation syndrome 7–10 days after ovulation. |
| Hydroxyprogesterone (various) | Amenorrhea: 375 mg IM, given at any time. Advanced adenocarcinoma of the endometrium: 1000 mg IM twice weekly for 12 weeks, or until relapse. Protocols may vary. | May affect liver function tests. |

*(Continued)*

**Drugs in Gynecology: Uses and Corresponding Dose *(Continued)***

| GENERIC (TRADE) NAME | INDICATION | COMMENTS |
|---|---|---|
| Hydroxyurea (Hydrea) | Cervical or ovarian carcinoma: 80 mg/kg p.o. every 3 days or 20 mg/kg p.o. daily. Protocols may vary. | Available as 500 mg capsules. Causes anorexia and nausea. |
| Ibuprofen (Motrin, Rufen, Advil, Nuprin) | Dysmenorrhea, procedures producing uterine cramping, mild postoperative pain: 400–800 mg p.o. four times daily, or as needed. | Avoid in true aspirin allergy. Take with food or milk. Over-the-counter tablets are 200 mg each. |
| Imipramine (Tofranil, various) | Detrusor instability, Stress urinary incontinence: 25–150 mg p.o. every night. Mild–moderate depression: 75 mg p.o. initially in 1–3 daily doses, increasing to 200 mg/d as needed. | Side effects: drowsiness, anticholinergic. |
| Indomethacin (Indocin) | Dysmenorrhea, procedures producing uterine cramping, mild postoperative pain: 25–50 mg p.o. every 6 hours. | Avoid in true aspirin allergy. Take with food or milk. |
| Leucovorin calcium (Wellcovorin) | Leucovorin rescue with methotrexate chemotherapy: 10 mg/m$^2$ p.o., IM, or IV every 6 hours for 72 hours, beginning within 24–36 hours of methotrexate. | Protocols may vary. |
| Lidocaine (Xylocaine) | Ventricular tachycardia or fibrillation: 200 mg IV over 2 minutes followed by 2 g in 500 mL, continuous infusion of 1.5–4 mg/min. | Adjust infusion rate to control arrythmia. Desired serum concentrations: 2–4 mg/L. Evaluate serum level 12 hours after initiation. |
| Lorazepam (Ativan) | Anxiety: 0.5–2 mg p.o. or IM every 8 hours. Insomnia, preoperative sedation: 2–4 mg IM or p.o. | No metabolites; excreted unchanged. |

| | | |
|---|---|---|
| Medroxyprogesterone acetate (Provera, Amen, Depo-Provera) | Vasomotor symptoms: 150 mg IM monthly. Endometrial hyperplasia: 10 mg p.o. daily on days 16–25. Amenorrhea: 10 mg p.o. daily for 5–7 days. Contraception: 150 mg IM every 3 months. Dysfunctional uterine bleeding: 10 mg p.o. daily, beginning on day 16. Endometrial carcinoma: 400–800 mg p.o. or IM weekly. | Dosing regimens may vary. |
| Mefanamic acid (Ponstel) | Dysmenorrhea: 500 mg p.o. initially, then 250 mg p.o. every 6 hours as needed. | Avoid in true aspirin allergy. Take with food or milk. |
| Megestrol (Megace) | Breast cancer: 40 mg p.o. 4 times daily. Endometrial hyperplasia: 20–40 mg p.o. twice daily. Endometrial carcinoma: 40–80 mg p.o. four times daily. Protocols may vary. | May affect liver function tests. Individualize initial dose empirically based on body size. |
| Melphalan (Alkeran) | Carcinoma of the cervix, ovary, endometrium, fallopian tube: 0.2 mg/kg p.o. daily for 4 days. Repeat at 4–6 week intervals. | Available as 5 mg tablets. WBC nadir: 10–12 days. |
| Menotropins (Pergonal) | Follicular growth and maturation: Contents of one ampule IM daily for 9–12 days, followed by human chorionic gonadotropin (hCG). Dosing will vary based on ultrasound findings and serum estradiol. | Each vial contains luteinizing hormone 75 IU, follicle-stimulating hormone 75 IU. Dissolve ampule contents in 2 mL sterile water. |
| Meperidine (Demerol) | Postoperative or severe pain: 25–50 mg IV, 50–100 mg IM or 50–100 mg p.o. Repeat every 3–4 hours as needed. | See morphine comments. |

(Continued)

**Drugs in Gynecology: Uses and Corresponding Dose *(Continued)***

| GENERIC (TRADE) NAME | INDICATION | COMMENTS |
|---|---|---|
| Metaproterenol (Alupent) | Asthma, other conditions requiring bronchodilation: 0.3 mg in 2.5 mL normal saline by hand nebulizer or intermittent positive pressure breathing every 3–4 hours. Metered-dose inhaler: 2–3 inhalations every 3–4 hours, up to 12 inhalations per day. | Side effects: tachycardia, nervousness, tremor, insomnia. |
| Methotrexate | Choriocarcinoma: 10–30 mg IV daily for 5 days. Ovarian or cervical carcinoma: 200–2000 $mg/m^2$ IV with leucovorin rescue. Mixed germ cell tumor: 0.3 mg/kg IM or IV daily for 5 days, repeat once monthly. | WBC nadir: 7–14 days. WBC recovery: 14–21 days. Causes stomatitis, diarrhea. Protocols may vary. |
| Midazolam (Versed) | Preoperative sedation, induction of general anesthesia: 0.07–0.08 mg/kg (5–10 mg) IM or IV over 60–90 seconds. | Administer slow IV push to minimize risk of respiratory depression or arrest. |
| Methyldopa (Aldomet) | Chronic or acute hypertension: 250–750 mg p.o. or IV 2, 3, or 4 times daily. | May improve vasomotor symptoms. |
| Methylergonovine (Methergine) | Uterine involution: 0.1 mg IV or 0.2 mg IM immediately postpregnancy termination followed by 0.2 mg p.o. 3–4 times daily for 1–7 days. | May cause nausea and vomiting. |
| Methyltestosterone (Metandren, Oreton methyl) | Endometriosis: 5–mg p.o. daily for a minimum of 6–12 weeks. Breast cancer: 200 mg p.o. or 100 mg buccally daily. | Discontinue use if menses are delayed until pregnancy is ruled out. Side effects: virilization, acne, menstrual irregularities; hepatocellular jaundice associated with oral form. |

| | | |
|---|---|---|
| Metoclopramide (Reglan) | Antiemetic: 2 mg/kg IV in 50 mL $D_5W$. Administer 30 minutes prior to chemotherapy and 2, 4, and 6 hours after chemotherapy. Gastric stimulant: 10 mg p.o. or IV four times daily. | May cause drowsiness. May be mixed with dexamethasone and diphenhydramine. |
| Morphine | Postoperative or severe pain: 2–5 mg IV or 5–10 mg IM, repeat every 4–6 hours as needed. | Equivalent parenteral analgesic doses:<br>Alphaprodine 45 mg<br>Butorphanol 27 mg<br>Codeine 120 mg<br>Hydromorphone 1.5 mg<br>Meperidine 100 mg<br>Morphine 10 mg |
| Naloxone (Narcan) | Reversal of narcotic overdose: 0.4 mg IV initially. May repeat every 2–3 minutes for three doses. | May be given SQ or IM also. Duration: 1–2 hours. |
| Naproxen (Naprosyn) | Dysmenorrhea, procedures inducing uterine cramping, mild postoperative pain: 500 mg p.o. initially, followed by 250 mg p.o. every 4–6 hours. Anaprox DS: 550 mg | Avoid in true aspirin allergy. Take with food or milk. |
| Naproxen sodium (Anaprox) | Dysmenorrhea: 2 tablets (550 mg) p.o. initially, followed by 1 tablet (275 mg) every 6–8 hours. | Avoid in true aspirin allergy. Take with food or milk. |
| Nizatidine (Axid) | Active duodenal ulcer: 300 mg p.o. at bedtime. Maintenance dose: 150 mg p.o. at bedtime. | |
| Norethindrone (Micronor, Nor-QD, Norlutin) | Contraception: 0.35 mg p.o. daily, continously. Endometriosis: 10 mg p.o. daily for 2 weeks, increase by 5 mg/day each week to 30 mg, continue for 6–9 months. Amenorrhea: 5–20 mg p.o. on days 5–25. | May affect liver function tests. A nonhormonal method of contraception should be used during the first 14 days. |

(Continued)

**Drugs in Gynecology: Uses and Corresponding Dose** ***(Continued)***

| GENERIC (TRADE) NAME | INDICATION | COMMENTS |
|---|---|---|
| Norethindrone acetate (Norlutate) | Amenorrhea: 2.5–10 mg p.o. daily on days 5–25. Endometriosis: 5 mg p.o. daily for 2 weeks, increase by 2.5 mg/day each week to 15 mg, continue for 6–9 months. | See norethindrone comments. |
| Norgestrel (Ovrette) | Contraception: 1 tablet (0.075 mg) p.o. daily, continuously. | Contains tartrazine. See norethindrone comments. |
| Oxybutynin chloride (Ditropan) | To inhibit involuntary detrusor contractions, bladder antispasmotic: 5 mg p.o. 2–4 times daily. | Side effects: anticholinergia. |
| Pentazocine (Talwin, Talwin NX) | Moderate–severe pain: 1 tablet p.o. or 30 mg IM every 3–4 hours as needed, up to 12 tablets or 360 mg IM daily. | Tablets contain 50 mg pentazocine, 0.5 mg naloxone HCl. Causes CNS depression. |
| Phenzaopyridine (Pyridium) | Pain, burning, urgency from irritation of the lower urinary tract as a result of infection, trauma, endoscopy, or surgery: 100–200 mg p.o. t.i.d. after meals. | Avoid use in patients with renal insufficiency. Warn patient that urine will turn orange in color. |
| Phenoxybenzamine (Dibenzyline) | Postoperative urethral spasm: 10 mg p.o. 1–3 times daily | May be given with bethanechol. Side effects: postural hypotension, miosis, nasal stuffiness, dry mouth, tachycardia. |
| Prochlorperazine (Compazine) | Postoperative nausea, vomiting: 5–10 mg IM every 4–6 hours or 25 mg rectally every 12 hours as needed. | May cause false positive or false negative pregnancy tests. Side effects: sedation, anticholinergia. |

| | | |
|---|---|---|
| Progesterone | Amenorrhea: 150 mg IM. Dysfunctional uterine bleeding: 5–10 mg IM for 6 days. Inadequate luteal phase: 12.5 IM daily or 25 mg vaginally twice daily, beginning on the second day of basal body temperture rise, and continuing for 6 weeks or until menstruation. Premenstrual syndrome: 200 mg vaginally or rectally twice daily from ovulation to menses. | IM is irritating and painful. Risk of female fetal masculinization when used in pregnancy. The vaginal or rectal suppository must be prepared extemporaneously. |
| Promethazine (Phenergan) | Postoperative nausea, vomiting: 25 mg IM or rectally every 4–6 hours as needed. | Side effects: sedation, anticholinergia. |
| Propranolol (Inderal) | Hypertension, supraventricular arrythmias: 10–60 mg p.o. divided into 2, 3, or 4 daily doses. Maximum daily dose: 240 mg. | Side effects: Bradycardia, depression, bronchospasm. Avoid in patients with pulmonary disorders. |
| Protamine sulfate | Hemorrhage associated with heparin therapy, immediately postheparin: 1 mg per 100 units of heparin, IV push over 2–3 minutes. 60 minutes postheparin: 0.5 mg per 100 units. 120 minutes postheparin: 0.25 mg per 100 units. | May cause hypotension, further anticoagulation. Risk of anaphylaxis. |
| Quinestrol (Estrovis) | Vasomotor symptoms, vaginal atrophy, female castration, primary ovarian failure: 1 tablet p.o. daily for 7 days, then one tablet once weekly. Increase to two weekly tablets if needed. | Metabolized to ethinyl estradiol. Each tablet contains 100 μg of quinestrol. See estrogens, conjugated. |
| Ranitidine (Zantac) | Active duodenal ulcer: 150 mg twice daily for 4 weeks. Stress ulcer prophylaxis: 50 mg IV every 8 hours. | Note difference in oral and parenteral dosing. Widen dosage interval in renal compromise. |
| Simethicone (Mylicon) | Antiflatulant: 1–2 tablets (40–80 mg) chewed thoroughly four times daily after meals and at bedtime. | |

(Continued)

**Drugs in Gynecology: Uses and Corresponding Dose *(Continued)***

| GENERIC (TRADE) NAME | INDICATION | COMMENTS |
| --- | --- | --- |
| Spironolactone (Aldactone) | Mild–moderate hypertension: 25 mg p.o. four times daily, increasing as needed to control blood pressure. Hirsuitism: 100–150 mg p.o. on days 4–21 of menstrual cycle, using lowest possible dose. Premenstrual syndrome: 25 mg p.o. 2–5 times daily from ovulation to menses. | Monitor serum potassium. May cause gynecomastia, irregular menses, amenorrhea, postmenopausal bleeding. |
| Tamoxifen (Nolvadex) | Palliative treatment of advanced breast cancer: 10–20 mg p.o. every 12 hours. | May cause hypercalcemia, vasomotor symptoms, menstrual irregularities. |
| Testosterone (various) | Breast carcinoma: 100 mg IM three times weekly, continuing for as long as improvement is maintained. | Response should occur within 3 months. May cause virilization. |
| Theophylline (Theodur, Resbid, Slo-bid, Theolair) | Asthma, other conditions requiring bronchodilation: Loading dose: 5–7.5 mg/kg IBW. Use rapid release or liquid formulations. Initial oral maintenance dose: 6.5 mg/kg IBW p.o. every 12 hours, sustained release formulation. | Monitor serum levels. Time to steady state approximately 2 days. Smoking and phenobarbital increase drug elimination. Cardiac disease, erythromycin, cimetidine, ciprofloxacin, and liver disease may decrease drug elimination. May cause nausea, vomiting, insomnia, headache, tremor. These often do not precede life-threatening seizures and should not be relied upon as warning signs or a dosing endpoint. Guidelines for dosage adjustment at steady state:<br>5–7.9 μg/mL: Increase daily dose by 50% Consider trial off drug if asymptomatic.<br>8.9 μg/mL: Increase daily dose of 20% if clinically needed. |

| | | |
|---|---|---|
| | | 10–13.9 μg/mL: Increase daily dose by 10% if clinically indicated.<br>14–19.9 μg/mL: No adjustment needed.<br>20–24.9 μg/mL: Decrease daily dose by 10% even if side effects are absent.<br>25–30 μg/mL: Hold next dose, decrease daily dose by 30%.<br>> 30 μg/mL: Hold next two doses, decrease daily dose by 50%. |
| Triazolam (Halcion) | Insomnia, preoperative sedation: 0.25–0.5 mg p.o. at bedtime.<br>Elderly patients: 0.125–0.25 mg p.o. at bedtime. | |
| Thiotepa | Carcinoma of the cervix, ovary, endometrium, and fallopian tube: 0.2 mg/kg IV daily for 5 days per month. | WBC nadir: 14–28 days. |
| Warfarin (Coumadin) | Anticoagulation: 10 mg p.o. daily for 3 days, beginning on day 1 or 2 of heparin therapy. Check prothrombin time (PT) on day 4. Adjust to maintain PT 1.5–2 times the control value. | Small body size, malnourishment, or cancer may increase sensitivity to warfarin. |

* Note: For information on oral contraceptives refer to Chapter 17—Contraception and Sterilization, Table 17.2.

# Appendix B

# Antibiotic Therapy in Gynecology

Rebecca Rogers

## ANTIBIOTICS IN GYNECOLOGY: USES AND CORRESPONDING DOSE

| GENERIC (TRADE) NAME | INDICATION | COMMENTS* |
|---|---|---|
| Acyclovir (Zovirax) | Severe primary episode of herpes simplex virus (HSV) II: 5 mg/kg IV every 8 hours for 5 days. Moderate primary episode of HSV II: 200 mg p.o. five times daily for 10 days. Recurrent episodes: 200 mg p.o. five times daily for 5 days. Chronic suppression: 200 mg p.o. 2–5 times daily. Topical ointment: Apply generously with gloved hand every 3 hours for 7 days. | Treatment of recurrent episodes has not been shown to decrease time to lesion healing, but may decrease viral shedding by 1–2 days. Chronic use for longer than 6 months has not been studied. (a) |
| Amikacin (Amikin) | Abdominal/pelvic infections: Loading dose: 7.5 mg/kg IV, followed by 5 mg/kg IV every 8 hours. Urinary tract infection (UTI): 3–5 mg/kg IV or IM every 8–12 hours. | See gentamicin comments for guidelines, alternative dosing chart, and recommendations for dosing in renal insufficiency. Desired serum peak: 15–30 μg/mL. Desired serum trough: < 10 μg/mL |
| Amoxicillin (Amoxil, Polymox, Trimox) | Uncomplicated gonococcal infections: 3 g p.o. with 1 g probenecid taken 30 minutes prior. | |
| Ampicillin (Polycillin-N, various) | Subacute bacterial endocarditis (SBE) prophylaxis: 2 g IV or IM 0.5–1 hour prior to procedure, repeat in 8 hours. Abdominal/pelvic infections: 1–2 g IV every 6 hours. UTI: 500 mg p.o. four times daily for 7–10 days. Uncomplicated gonococcal infections: 3.5 g p.o. with 1 g probenecid taken 30 minutes prior. | Drug of choice for group D streptococci (enterococci). Ten percent incidence of rash. |
| Ampicillin/sulbactam (Unasyn) | Abdominal/pelvic infections: 1.5–3 g IV every 6 hours. | Each 1.5 g vial contains ampicillin 1 g, sulbactam 0.5 g. Do not exceed 4 g sulbactam per day. Activity against enterococci no greater than ampicillin alone. |

| | | |
|---|---|---|
| Aztreonam (Azactam) | Gram-negative aerobic infections: 1 g IV every 8 hours. | Can be used in penicillin allergy. (a) |
| Carbenicillin (Geopen) | Abdominal/pelvic infections: 5 g IV every 4 hours. UTI: 2 g IV or IM every 6 hours. Uncomplicated gonococcal infections: 2 g IM in each hip, one dose only, with 1 g probenecid taken 30 minutes prior. | Use in combination with an aminoglycoside in severe infections or until identification of infecting organism is confirmed. (a) |
| Carbenicillin (Geocillin) | UTI: 1–2 tablets p.o. every 6 hours. | Each tablet contains carbenicillin indanyl sodium equivalent to 382 mg of carbenicillin. |
| Cefaclor (Ceclor) | UTI, pyelonephritis, cystitis: 250 mg p.o. every 8 hours. | (b) (c) |
| Cefamandole (Mandol) | Abdominal/pelvic infections: 1 g IV every 6 hours. UTI: 500 mg IV or IM every 6 hours. | (a) (b) (c) (d) |
| Cefazolin (Ancef, Kefzol) | Surgical prophylaxis: 1–2 g IV or IM 30 minutes prior to procedure. UTI, upper respiratory infection (URI): 0.5–1 g IV every 8 hours. | (a) (b) (c) (d) |
| Cefonicid (Monocid) | Surgical prophylaxis: 1 g IV or IM 30 minutes prior to procedure. | (b) (c) (d) |
| Cefoperazone (Cefobid) | Abdominal/pelvic infections: 2 g IV every 12 hours. | (b) (c) (d) |
| Ceforanide (Precef) | Surgical prophylaxis: 1 g IV or IM 30 minutes prior to procedure. | (b) (c) (d) |
| Cefotaxime (Claforan) | Uncomplicated gonococcal infections: 1 g IM. Abdominal/pelvic infections: 1–2 g IV every 6 hours. | (b) (c) (d) |

*(Continued)*

**Antibiotics in Gynecology: Uses and Corresponding Dose *(Continued)***

| GENERIC (TRADE) NAME | INDICATION | COMMENTS* |
|---|---|---|
| Cefotetan (Cefotan) | Abdominal/pelvic infections: 2 g IV every 12 hours. Surgical prophylaxis: 2 g IV or IM 30 minutes prior to procedure | (b) (c) (d) |
| Cefoxitin (Mefoxin) | Uncomplicated gonococcal infections: 2 g IM with 1 g probenecid p.o. 30 minutes prior. Abdominal/pelvic infections: 2 g IV every 6 hours. | (a) (b) (c) (d) |
| Ceftazidime (Fortaz, Tazicef, Tazidime) | Abdominal/pelvic infections: 2 g IV every 8 hours. Complicated UTI: 500 mg IM or IV every 8–12 hours. | Reserve for when *Pseudomonas aeruginosa* is suspect. |
| Ceftizoxime (Cefizox) | Abdominal/pelvic infections: 2 g IV every 8–12 hours. UTI: 500 mg IV or IM every 12 hours. Uncomplicated gonococcal infection: 1 g IM. | (a) (b) (c) (d) |
| Ceftriaxone (Rocephin) | Uncomplicated gonococcal infections: 250 mg IM. Abdominal/pelvic infections: 2 g IV every 24 hours. | Centers for Disease Control recommends for areas with high incidence of resistant *Neisseria gonorrhea*. (b) (c) (d) |
| Cefuroxime (Kerfurox, Zinacef) | Skin/skin structure infections, UTI: .75–1.5 g IV every 8 hours. Uncomplicated gonococcal infections: 1.5 g IM. Surgical prophylaxis: 1.5 g IM or IV 30 minutes prior to procedure. | (b) (c) (d) |
| Cephalexin (Keflex) | UTI, URI: 250 mg p.o. every 6 hours. | (b) (c) (d) |

| | | |
|---|---|---|
| Cephalothin (Keflin) | Surgical prophylaxis: 1 g IV or IM 30 minutes prior to procedure, repeated at 6, 12, 18, and 24 hours. UTI: 0.5–1 g IV every 6 hours. | (a) (b) (c) (d) |
| Cephradine (Velosef) | UTI: 250 mg p.o. every 6 hours for 7–10 days. | (b) (c) (d) |
| Chloramphenicol (Chloromycetin) | Abdominal/pelvic infections: 50–100 mg/kg IV daily divided into four doses. | Risk of reversible bone marrow suppression: 14% Risk of aplastic anemia: 1:40 000. |
| Cinoxacin (Cinobac) | UTI: 500 mg p.o. every 12 hours. | (b) (c) (d) |
| Ciprofloxacin (Cipro) | UTI, lower respiratory, skin and skin structure, infectious diarrhea: 250–500 mg p.o. twice daily. | Administer 1 hour before or 2 hours after meals. Avoid concomitant ingestion of antacids. (a) |
| Clindamycin (Cleocin) | Abdominal/pelvic infections: 600 mg IV every 6 hours or 900 mg IV every 8 hours. Oral follow-up: 450 mg p.o. every 6 hours. | May be mixed together with gentamicin or tobramycin in the same small volume parenteral. (c) |
| Clotrimazole (Mycelex G, Gynelotrimen) (Mycelex Oral troches) | Vulvovaginal candidiasis: one applicatorful or one 100 mg tablet per vagina at bedtime for 7–14 days. Three-day treatment: two 100 mg suppositories per vagina at bedtime for 3 days. One-day regimen: one 500 mg suppository per vagina, single dose. Oropharyngeal candidiasis: one 10 mg troche dissolved slowly in mouth five times daily for 14 days. | One-day course marketed for use in physician's office; melt time is approximately 20 minutes. Three-day course is not effective in pregnancy. |
| Dicloxacillin (Dynapen, various) | Postoperative wound breakdown, skin and soft tissue infection associated with penicillinase-producing staphylococci: 250–500 mg p.o. every 6 hours. | Available as oral capsules and suspension only. |

(Continued)

**Antibiotics in Gynecology: Uses and Corresponding Dose *(Continued)***

| GENERIC (TRADE) NAME | INDICATION | COMMENTS* |
|---|---|---|
| Doxycycline (Vibramycin, various) | Surgical prophylaxis in pencillin allergic patients: 100 mg IV 30 minutes prior to procedure, followed by 100 mg IV in 12 hours. *Chlamydia trachomatis:* 100 mg p.o. twice daily for 7 days. Abdominal/pelvic infections: 100 mg IV every 12 hours | Avoid concomitant ingestion of calcium-containing products or antacids. Avoid direct exposure to sunlight. |
| Erythromycin (various) | Syphilis (penicillin allergy): 500 mg p.o. four times daily for 15 days. *Chlamydia trachomatis:* 500 mg p.o. four times daily for 7 days. Surgical prophylaxis, bowel preparation: 1 g p.o. at 1 PM, 2 PM, and 11 PM on the day prior to surgery, with neomycin. | Salt forms include free base, stearate, estolate, and ethylsuccinate. Estolate and ethylsuccinate forms are associated with rare intrahepatic jaundice, seen mostly in adults. May increase theophylline serum concentrations. |
| Gentamicin (Garamycin) | SBE prophylaxis: 1.5 mg/kg IM or IV 30 minutes prior to procedure, repeat in 8 hours. Abdominal/pelvic infections, pyelonephritis: 2 mg/kg IV loading dose, followed by 1.5 mg/kg IV every 8 hours. UTI: 1 mg/kg every 8 hours. Alternative dosing recommendations: see Tables B.1 and B.2. | Evaluate serum peak and trough concentrations with third maintenance dose. Desired peak: 4–10 μg/mL. Desired trough: $< 2$ μg/mL. Monitor serum creatinine before and every 2–3 days during therapy. Increase or decrease dose as indicated clinically with laboratory back-up. Risk of ototoxicity and nephrotoxicity increases with prolonged use, and with concomitant vancomycin. |
| Ketoconazole (Nizoral) | Systemic fungal infections: 200 mg p.o. daily before meals. Vaginal candidiasis: 400 mg p.o. daily for 5 days, or 200 mg p.o. daily for 10 days. | H-2 antagonists and antacids decrease absorption. Use in vaginal candidiasis usually reserved for cases failing standard topical regimens. |

**Table B.1. DOSING RECOMMENDATIONS**

| AMINO-GLYCOSIDE | USUAL LOADING DOSES | EXPECTED PEAK SERUM LEVELS |
|---|---|---|
| Tobramycin<br>Gentamycin | 1.5 to 2.0 mg/kg | 4 to 10 μg/mL |
| Amikacin<br>Kanamycin | 5.0 to 7.5 mg/kg | 15 to 30 μg/ml |

1. Select loading dose in mg/kg (ideal weight) to provide peak serum levels in range listed above for desired aminoglycoside.

Calculate ideal body weight:
Males: 50 kg + 2.3 (inches over 5 ft)
Females: 45.5 kg + 2.3 (inches over 5 ft)

2. Select maintenance dose (as percentage of chosen loading dose) to continue peak serum levels indicated above according to desired dosing interval and the patient's corrected creatinine clearance.

Estimate creatinine clearance:
Males: (140 − age) + serum creatinine
Females: males (.85)

**Table B.2. PERCENTAGE OF LOADING DOSES REQUIRED FOR DOSAGE INTERVAL SELECTED**

| CREATININE CLEARANCE (mL/min) | HALF LIFE* (h) | 8 h | 12 h | 24 h |
|---|---|---|---|---|
| 90 | 3.1 | 84 | – | – |
| 80 | 3.4 | 80 | 91 | – |
| 70 | 3.9 | 76 | 88 | – |
| 60 | 4.5 | 71 | 84 | – |
| 50 | 5.3 | 65 | 79 | – |
| 40 | 6.5 | 57 | 72 | 92 |
| 30 | 8.4 | 48 | 63 | 86 |
| 25 | 9.9 | 43 | 57 | 81 |
| 20 | 11.9 | 37 | 50 | 75 |
| 17 | 13.6 | 33 | 46 | 70 |
| 15 | 15.1 | 31 | 42 | 67 |
| 12 | 17.9 | 27 | 37 | 61 |
| 10† | 20.4 | 24 | 34 | 56 |
| 7 | 25.9 | 19 | 28 | 47 |
| 5 | 31.5 | 16 | 23 | 41 |
| 2 | 46.8 | 11 | 16 | 30 |
| 0 | 69.3 | 8 | 11 | 21 |

* Alternatively, one-half of the chosen leading dose may be given at an interval equal to the estimated half-life.
† Dosing for patients with creatinine clearance ≤ 10 mL/min should be assisted by measured serum levels.
From Sarubbi FA, Hull JH. Ann Intern Med 89 (Pt 1:1978; 612–618). Reprinted with permission.

*(Continued)*

**Antibiotics in Gynecology: Uses and Corresponding Dose *(Continued)***

| GENERIC (TRADE) NAME | INDICATION | COMMENTS* |
|---|---|---|
| Metronidazole (Flagyl, various) | Symptomatic trichomoniasis: 250 mg p.o. three times daily for 7 days or 2 g p.o. single dose for both partners. *Gardnerella vaginalis:* 500 mg p.o. twice daily for 7 days. Pseudomembranous enterocolitis caused by *Clostridium difficile* endotoxin: 500 mg p.o. every 12 hours for 10 days. Abdominal/pelvic infections: 1 g IV loading dose, followed by 500 mg IV every 6 hours. | Avoid alcohol ingestion during therapy and for 1 day afterward |
| Mezlocillin (Mezlin) | Abdominal/pelvic infections: 4 g IV every 6 hours. | (a) (d) |
| Miconazole (Monistat-3, Monistat 7) | Vulvovaginal candidiasis: One 200 mg suppository per vagina at bedtime for 3 days; or one 100 mg suppository or one applicatorful per vagina at bedtime for 7 days. | |
| Moxalactam (Moxam) | Abdominal/pelvic infections: 2 g IV every 8 hours. | Evaluate baseline bleeding status. Administer vitamin K 10 mg per week during therapy. (a) (b) (c) (d) |
| Nafcillin (Nafcil, Unipen) | Postoperative wound breakdown: 0.5–1 g IV every 6 hours. Oral follow-up: 250–500 mg p.o. four times daily. | (c) (d) |
| Nalidixic acid (Neg Gram) | UTI: 1 g p.o. four times daily for 7–10 days | |

| | | |
|---|---|---|
| Neomycin | Surgical phophylaxis, bowel preparation: 1 g p.o. at 1 PM, 2 PM, and 11 PM, on day prior to surgery, with erythromycin. | |
| Netilmicin (Netromycin) | Abdominal/pelvic infections: 2 mg/kg IV loading dose, followed by 1.5 mg/kg IV every 8 hours. UTI: 1 mg/kg IV every 8 hours. | See gentamicin comments for guidelines and alternative dosing chart. Desired serum peak: 4–10 μg/mL. Desired serum trough: < 2 μg/mL. |
| Nitrofurantoin (Furadantin, Macrodantin) | UTI: 100 mg p.o. four times daily for 7–10 days. | (e) |
| Nystatin (Nilstat, Mycostatin) | Vulvovaginal candidiasis: One suppository per vagina at bedtime for 15 days. Oral candidiasis: 4–6 mL p.o. four times daily. Intestinal candidiasis: One or two tablets p.o. three times daily, continuing for 48 hours post clinical cure. | Oral suspension should be swished in mouth and retained as long as possible before swallowing. Each mL contains 100 000 U. Each tablet contains 500 000 U. |
| Norfloxacin (Noroxin) | UTI: 400 mg p.o. twice daily for 7–10 days. | Maximum daily dose should not exceed 800 mg/d. Administer 1 hour before or 2 hours after meals. Avoid concomitant ingestion of antacids. |
| Oxacillin (Prostaphlin) | Postoperative wound breakdown: 0.5–1 g IV every 4–6 hours. Oral follow-up: 250–500 mg p.o. 4 times daily. | (c) (d) |
| Penicillin G (Various) | UTI, including pyelonephritis: 1 million U IV every 4 hours. Abdominal/pelvic infections: 2–3 million U IV every 4 hours. Neurosyphilis: 2–4 million U IV every 4 hours for 10 days. | Allergy incidence to penicillins is approximately 10%. Anaphylaxis incidence is approximately 0.04%. 250 mg = 400 000 U. |

(Continued)

**Antibiotics in Gynecology: Uses and Corresponding Dose *(Continued)***

| GENERIC (TRADE) NAME | INDICATION | COMMENTS* |
|---|---|---|
| Pencillin G, benzathine (Bicillin) | Primary or secondary syphilis, latent syphilis of less than one year: 1.2 million U in each hip, one dose only. Latent syphilis of greater than one year: 1.2 million U in each hip once weekly for 3 weeks. | See penicillin G. |
| Penicillin G, aqueous Procaine (Wycillin) | Uncomplicated gonococcal infections: 2.4 million U in each hip, one dose only, with probenecid 1 g p.o. | See pencillin G. |
| Penicillin VK (Pen Vee K, V Cillin K, various) | UTI, other mild–moderate infections: 250–500 mg p.o. four times daily for 10–14 days. | See penicillin G. |
| Phenazopyridine (Pyridium, Urogesic, various) | Symptomatic relief of bladder pain, burning, urgency, frequency, and other discomforts associated with infection, trauma, or surgery: 200 mg p.o. three times daily. | Do not exceed 600 mg/d. Contraindicated in renal insufficiency. No antimicrobial activity. (e) |
| Piperacillin (Pipracil) | Abdominal/pelvic infections: 4 g IV every 6 hours. | (a) (d) |
| Spectinomycin (Trobicin) | Uncomplicated gonococcal infections: 2 g IM, one dose only. | For use in penicillin allergy. |
| Sulfamethoxazole (Gantanol, Gantanol DS) | UTI: 2 g p.o., followed by 1 g p.o. twice daily for 7–10 days. | (e) |
| Sulfamethoxazole-phenazopyridine (Azogantanol) | UTI: 4 tablets p.o., followed by 2 tablets twice daily for 2 days. Continue treatment beyond 2 days with sulfamethoxazole alone. | (e) |

| | | |
|---|---|---|
| Sulfasoxazole (Gantrisin) | UTI: 2–4 g p.o., followed by 1–2 g four times daily for 7–10 days. | (e) |
| Sulfasoxazole-phenazopyridine (Azogantrisin) | UTI: 4–6 tablets p.o., followed by 2 tablets four times daily for 2 days. Continue treatment beyond 2 days with sulfasoxazole alone. | (e) |
| Tetracycline (Achromycin, Sumycin, various) | Oral follow-up in PID: 500 mg p.o. four times daily to complete a 14 day course. Uncomplicated gonococcal infections: 500 mg p.o. four times daily for 7 days. Primary or secondary syphilis in penicillin allergy: 500 mg p.o. four times daily for 15 days. Latent syphilis, penicillin allergy: 500 mg p.o. four times daily for 30 days. *Chlamydia trachomatis* infections: 500 mg p.o. four times daily for 7 days. | Avoid IV use due to extreme venous irritation (see doxycycline). Avoid calcium containing products and antacids for 2 hours before and after medication ingestion. |
| Ticarcillin (Ticar) | Abdominal/pelvic infections: 3 g IV every 4 hours. | (a) (d) |
| Ticarcillin-clavulanate (Timentin) | Abdominal/pelvic infections, wound breakdown: 3.1 g IV every 6 hours. | More active against staphylococcus and anaerobes than ticarcillin alone. |
| Tobramycin (Nebcin) | Abdominal/pelvic infections: 2 mg/kg IV loading dose, followed by 1.5 mg/kg IV every 8 hours. UTI: 1 mg/kg IV every 8 hours. | See gentamicin comments for guidelines, recommendations in renal insufficiency, and alternative dosing chart. Desired serum peak: 4–10 μg/mL. Desired serum trough: < 2 μg/mL. |

(Continued)

**Antibiotics in Gynecology: Uses and Corresponding Dose *(Continued)***

| GENERIC (TRADE) NAME | INDICATION | COMMENTS* |
|---|---|---|
| Trimethoprim-sulfamethoxazole, (Bactrim, Septra) | UTI: 2 regular-strength or 1 double-strength tablet every 12 hours for 10–14 days. | (e) |
| Vancomycin (Vancocin) | Infections with methicillin-resistant staphylococci or streptococci: 500 mg IV every 6 hours, or 1 g IV every 12 hours. SBE prophylaxis in penicillin allergy: 1 g IV 30 minutes prior to procedure, repeat in 8 hours. Pseudomembranous enterocolitis caused by *C. difficile* endotoxin: 250 mg p.o. four times daily for 7–10 days. | Not absorbed orally. Monitor serum peak and trough with IV therapy if possible. Desired serum peak: 20–40 μg/mL. Desired trough: < 10 μg/mL. Drug of choice for enterococcal infections in penicillin allergy. Increased risk of otoxicity or nephrotoxicity when administered with an aminoglycoside. |

* LEGEND: (a) Widen dosage interval when creatinine clearance is less than 50 mL/min; (b) 10% cross-sensitivity with penicillins; (c) Not active against enterococci (group D streptococci); (d) Not active against *Chlamydia trachomatis;* (e) May cause hemolysis in patients with G6PD deficiency.

# Index


Abdomen
  acute, 447
  examination of, 189, 223
  pain, 188
  as pregnancy site, 185, 203
  x-ray of, 36
Abdominal hysterectomy, 105, 111, 113–114
Abdominal pregnancy, 185, 203
Abnormal uterine bleeding, 586–590
Abortion
  classification, 164–165
  complete, 165
  and contraceptives, 286
  definition, 164
  and dysfunctional uterine bleeding, 351
  failed, 182
  first trimester
    complications of, 180–182
    criminal, 175–176
    curettage, 176–180
    definition, 164
    dilation, 176–180
    elective, 164, 175
    etiology, 168–169
    incomplete, 165, 171–173, 180
    inevitable, 165, 171
    missed, 165, 173–174
    prevalence, 168
    recurrent spontaneous 165, 174–175
    septic, 165
    suction, 176–180
    threatened, 165, 169–171
  morbidity, 165, 168
  mortality, 168
  second trimester, 182–183
  and sexual assault, 310
Abuse, sexual (*see* Sexual assault)
Acanthosis nigricans, 389
Acetic acid
  biochloracetic acid, 520
  trichloroacetic acid (TCA), 72, 320
Acne, 388
Actinomycin-D, 538
Actinomycosis infection, 126
Acute pelvic pain
  diagnosis, 222–224
  differential diagnosis, 219–222, 593–595
  and ectopic pregnancy, 220, 595
  etiology, 218
  and leiomyoma uteri diagnosis, 96
  management, 224
  pathophysiology, 218
  prognosis, 224
Acyclovir, 324–325
Adenoacanthoma, 505
Adenocarcinoma, 474–475, 478, 505, 506
Adenoma, 280, 336, 346, 382
Adenomyosis, 226, 226
Adenosquamous carcinoma, 505
Adhesions, 213, 228, 338
Adnexa
  and acute pelvic pain differential diagnosis, 219
  examination, 11, 189
  mass of, 95, 189, 590–593
Adrenal cortical adenoma, 382
Adrenal enzyme defects, 346
Adrenal glands
  and amenorrhea, 341
  and androgens, 363
  carcinoma of, 382
  and heterosexual pseudoprecocity, 418
  and hyperandrogenemia, diseases associated with, 381–382
  neoplasms of, 382, 417
  tumors of, 341, 417
Adrenal hyperplasia, 341
Adriamycin (*see* Doxorobicin)
Affective disorders, 243
Alkeran, 537
Alkylating agents, 537–538
Alpha-adrenergic agonists, 374
Alpha-feto protein, 122
Alprazolam, 249
Amenorrhea
  and adrenal glands, 341
  and anovulation, 346
  diagnosis, 335, 341–344
  differential diagnosis, 338–341

Amenorrhea continued
  and ectopic pregnancy diagnosis, 188
  end organ causes of, 338–339, 343–344
  hypothalamic, 338
  incidence, 335
  and interstitial ectopic pregnancy, 202
  management, 344–348
  morbidity, 336
  and ovary, 339–340, 344
  and pill, clinical problem of, 278
  and polycystic ovarian disease, 338
  pituitary/hypothalamic causes of, 340–341, 344
  post-pill, 278
  and pregnancy, 338
  prognosis, 348–349
Aminoglycoside, 331
Amoxicillin, 309, 323
Amphotericin B, 39
Analgesics, 21, 233, 567
Androgens
  and adrenal glands, 363
  in endometriosis management, 454
  end-organ insensitivity to, 411–412
  and estrogens, conversion to, 363
  exogenous, 417–418
  and hirsutism pathophysiology, 378–379
  metabolism, 378–379
  and oophorectomy, 112
  and ovarian tumors, 339
  and ovary, 363
  and pill, 279
3 β-Androstanediol, 378
Anesthesia, 565
Aneurysm, aortic, 222
Anorexia nervosa, 340, 382
Anorgasmia, 256
Anovulation (*see also* Dysfunctional uterine bleeding)
  abnormalities of, 426–427
  and amenorrhea, 346
  chronic, 379
  definition, 350
  and endometriosis, 446
  etiology, 426
  and infertility evaluation, 426–427
Anterior colporrhaphy, 142
Antibiotics
  in Bartholin's duct abscess management, 74
  in criminal abortion, 175
  in granuloma inguinale, 70
  in incomplete abortion, 173
  in lymphogranuloma venereum management, 71
  in mycoplasmas, 328
  in ovarian carcinoma chemotherapy, 538–539
  in septic shock management, 39–40
  in sexually transmitted disease treatment, 309–310
  in syphilis treatment, 327
  in vulvovaginitis in children, 210
Antibodies, 436
Antidepressants, 249
Antifungal preparations, 68
Antihistamines, 77
Antimetabolites, 538
Antimicrobial therapy, 160
Anti-Müllerian duct hormone (AMH), 402
Antiprogesterone drugs, 201
Antishock garment, 27–29, 37–38
Anxiolytics, 248–249
Aortic aneurysm, 222
Arias-Stella, 187
Arrhenoblastoma, 406
Arterial catheter, 37
Arterial embolization, 29
Asherman's syndrome, 180, 338
Aspiration, 56–58, 564
Atrophic vaginitis, 254
Autoimmune diseases, 362, 371

Bacterial vaginosis (BV), 83–84, 87
Barium enema (BE)
  in adnexal mass diagnosis, 591
  in cervical carcinoma diagnosis, 494
  as hysterectomy preoperative radiographic study, 109
  in ovarian benign disease diagnosis, 122
  in ovarian carcinoma diagnosis, 531
  in uterine carcinoma diagnosis, 508
Barrier methods of contraception
  condoms, 267
  diaphragms, 267–268
  intrauterine devices, 268–272
  investigative, 287
  spermacides, 266

and sexually transmitted diseases, 329
vaginal sponges, 266
Bartholin's duct, 73–74, 561–562
Basal body temperature (BBT), 356, 425
Basal cell carcinoma, 462, 471
Benzathine penicillin, 327
Bichloracetic acid, 520
Bimanual examination, 10–11, 208
Biochemical disorders, 222
Biofeedback, 158
Biopsy
and abnormal mammogram, 581–582
endocervical, 480
endometrial, 98, 369, 426, 480, 562–563
excisional, 465, 495, 565, 566–567
incisional, 465–466
of macroscopic lesions, 320
open, 58
punch, 465, 565–566
testicular, 430
vaginal, 98, 369, 426, 480, 562-563
vulvar, 76, 563–565
Bladder, 18, 37, 95, 158, 160
Bleeding (*see also* Dysfunctional uterine bleeding; Uterine bleeding; Vaginal bleeding)
breakthrough, 278
irregular, 366
postmenopausal, 4, 506, 589–590
Blenoxane, 538–539
Bleomycin, 538–539
Blighted ovum, 192
Blood transfusion, 26
Bone scan, 531
Boric acid, 86
Botryoid sarcoma, 215–216, 477, 478, 484
Breakthrough bleeding, 278
Breast
abscess of, 64
aspiration of, 56–56
asymmetry, 54
benign diseases of, 62–63, 576
carcinoma of
diagnosis, 53–58
and diet, 61
etiology, 51–52
incidence, 49–51
and menopause, 374
morbidity, 51
mortality, 51
pathophysiology, 53
and pregnancy, 52, 61–62
prognosis, 61
treatment, 58–61
examination, 5–7, 54–56
fibrocystic, 62–63
and hyperandrogenemia diagnosis, 389
lesions of, 56
mass of, 53, 575–578
neoplasms of, 280
physiology of, 49
Breast-feeding, 256
Breast self-examination (BSE), 6–7, 54–56
Brenner tumors, 119, 529
Bromocriptine, 345–346, 437–438
Burch procedure, 143, 155
Burow's solution, 77
Buspirone, 248–249
Butoconazole, 68

CA-125 immunologic test, 122, 531, 591
Caffeine, 248
CAH (*see* Congenital adrenal hyperplasia)
Calcium replacement therapy, 374
Calendar method of contraception, 264
Cancer screening, 369
Candida vaginitis, 84–86, 87
Candidiasis, 67–69, 586
Carbohydrate metabolism, 279–280
Carbon dioxide laser, 468
Carboplatinum, 539
Carboxylates, 235–236
Carcinoid syndrome, 365
Carcinoma
of adrenal glands, 382
basal cell, 462, 471
of breast
diagnosis, 53–58
and diet, 61
etiology, 51–52
incidence, 49–51
and menopause, 374
morbidity, 51

Carcinoma continued
  of breast continued
    mortality, 51
    pathophysiology, 53
    and pregnancy, 52, 61–62
    prognosis, 61
    treatment, 58–61
  of cervix
    diagnosis, 490–494
    differential diagnosis, 490
    and dysfunctional uterine bleeding, 352
    etiology, 487–488
    incidence, 486
    management, 495–497
    morbidity, 486–487
    mortality, 486–487
    pathogenesis, 488–490
    pathophysiology, 488–490
    prognosis, 500–501
    staging, 494–495
    therapy, 497–500
    vaginal bleeding, 491
  and condyloma acuminata, 319
  and dysfunctional uterine bleeding, 352–353
  embryonal cell, 215–216, 526, 537
  endometrioid, 528–529
  of fallopian tube, 520–523
  medullary thyroid, 365–366
  and menopause, 374
  of ovary
    chemotherapeutic agents, 537–540
    diagnosis, 530–532
    differential diagnosis, 530
    and dysfunctional uterine bleeding, 352–353
    etiology, 525
    follow-up, 540
    and hysterectomy, 112
    incidence, 524
    management, 532–537
    morbidity, 524
    mortality, 524
    pathogenesis, 525–529
    pathophysiology, 525–529
    prognosis, 540–541
    spread pattern, 529–530
    staging, 532
    teratomas, 526–527, 537
  of perineum, 352
  undifferentiated, 529
  of uterus
    diagnosis, 506–509
    differential diagnosis, 506
    and dysfunctional uterine bleeding, 352
    etiology, 503–504
    incidence, 502
    and infertility, 503
    management, 510–514
    morbidity, 502–503
    mortality, 502–503
    pathogenesis, 505–506
    prognosis, 514–515
    staging, 509–510
  of vagina
    diagnosis, 478–481
    differential diagnosis, 478
    and dysfunctional uterine bleeding, 352
    embryonic, 215–216
    etiology, 476–477
    incidence, 474–475
    management, 481–484
    morbidity, 475
    mortality, 475–476
    pathogenesis, 477–478
    pathophysiology, 477–478
    prognosis, 484–485
    staging, 481
  of vulva
    diagnosis, 463–466
    differential diagnosis, 462–463
    and dysfunctional uterine bleeding, 352
    etiology, 460–461
    incidence, 459–460
    management, 466–471
    morbidity, 460
    mortality, 460
    pathophysiology, 461–462
    prognosis, 472–473
    recurrent, 471
    staging, 466
Carcinoma in situ
  vaginal, 474, 475, 476, 478–479, 481–482
  vulvar, 461, 464
Carcinosarcoma, 529
Cardiovascular disease, 326, 360–361, 371, 375
Catheterization, 37, 396
Cefoxitin, 331
Ceftriaxone, 309

Cellular leiomyomata, 93
Central nervous system (CNS) drugs, 354
Central venous pressure (CVP), 27
Cervical conization, 482–483, 492–493, 496
Cervical culture, 223–224
Cervical incompetence, 180
Cervical intraepithelial neoplasia (CIN), 489, 495–496
Cervical leiomyomata, 91
Cervical mucus method (of contraception), 264
Cervical pregnancy, 204
Cervicitis, 353–354
Cervix
  anomalies of, 89
  benign diseases of, 89–90
  carcinoma of
    diagnosis, 490–494
    differential diagnosis, 490
    and dysfunctional uterine bleeding, 352
    dysplasia, 418
    etiology, 487–488
    incidence, 486
    management, 495–497
    morbidity, 486–487
    mortality, 486–487
    pathogenesis, 488–490
    pathophysiology, 488–490
    prognosis, 500–501
    staging, 494–495
    therapy, 497–500
    vaginal bleeding, 491
  cryotherapy of, 572–573
  and ectopic pregnancy diagnosis, 189
  examination, 10, 172
  and gamete transport, 433, 440
  lacerations of, 90, 180–181
  lesions of, 89–90
  neoplasms of, 280
  polyps of, 89
  pregnancy, 204
  scarring of, 180
  stenosis of, 180, 227, 599
  visualization of, 8–10, 208
Chancre, 325
Chancroid, 67–70
Chemotherapy
  in breast carcinoma treatment, 60
  in embryonic carcinoma treatment, 216
  in gestational trophoblastic tumor treatment, 550–551
  in menopause etiology, 362
  multi-agent, 551–552
  in ovarian carcinoma treatment, 537–540
  in uterine sarcoma management, 517
Chest radiograph (CXR), 109, 508, 531, 591
Childbirth, 131 (*see also* Vaginal delivery)
Children
  anatomic considerations, 206–207
  congenital malformation of genital tract, 208–209
  embryonic carcinoma of vagina, 215–216
  foreign bodies, 211
  labial adhesions, 213
  lichen sclerosus, 212
  physical examination, 207–208
  pinworms, 211–212
  sexual assault, 306–307
  sexually transmitted diseases, 309–310
  urethral prolapse, 213–214
  vaginal bleeding, 214–215
  vulvovaginitis, 209–211
Child welfare authorities, 306–307
Chlamydia trachomatis, 314–318
Chloasma, 278
Chlorambucil, 538
Chorioamnionitis, 328
Choriocarcinoma, 351, 417, 526, 537, 543, 545
Chronic pelvic pain
  and adhesions, 228
  diagnosis, 229–230
  differential diagnosis, 225–229, 595–597
  etiology, 225
  incidence, 225
  and leiomyoma uteri, 96, 226
  morbidity, 225
  mortality, 225
  prognosis, 230
Cisplatin, 539
Clear cell adenocarcinoma, 475–476, 477, 483, 505, 529
Climacteric, 4, 359, 363
Clindamycin, 328, 331
Clitoris, 389, 401

Clomiphene citrate, 347, 399, 436–437
Clotrimazole, 68, 86
Clotting disorders, 354
CNS drugs (*see* Central nervous system drugs)
Coagulation cascade, 31
Coitus interruptus, 265
Colporrhaphy
  anterior, 142
  posterior, 140
Colposcopy
  in cervical carcinoma diagnosis, 492
  definition, 567
  equipment, 569–570
  evaluation criteria, 567–569
  procedure, 570–572
  in sexually transmitted disease diagnosis, 320
  in vaginal carcinoma diagnosis, 479, 480
  in vulvar carcinoma diagnosis, 464
Colpotomy, 284
Combination oral contraceptives
  administration, 277–278
  clinical problems, 278–279
  and dysfunctional uterine bleeding, 356
  effectiveness, 272
  in endometriosis management, 452
  estrogens as, 273
  and hirsutism, 397–398
  indications and contraindications, 273, 277
  and isosexual pseudoprecocity, 417
  mechanism of action, 272–273
  postpartum, 280
  and pregnancy, 280
  and primary dysmenorrhea, 233–234
  progestins as, 273
  side effects, 279–281
Complement cascade, 31, 33
Complete abortion, 165
Complete blood count (CBC), 97, 189, 223
Computerized axial tomography (CAT), 123, 508, 531, 590
Computerized tomography (CT), 37, 98, 394, 494
Condoms, 87, 267
Condyloma acuminata
  and carcinoma, 319
  and cervical lesions, benign, 90
  clinical manifestations, 319–320
  diagnosis, 71–72, 320
  epidemiology, 318–319
  etiology, 71
  incidence, 318–319
  management, 72–73, 320–321
  viral characteristics, 318
Congenital abnormalities, 254
Congenital adrenal hyperplasia (CAH)
  and female pseudohermaphroditism, 403
  heredity factors, 388
  and hyperandrogenemia, diseases associated with, 381
  and polycystic ovarian disease, 390–391, 393
Congenital lipoid adrenal hyperplasia, 408
Congenital malformation of genital tract, 208–209
Conjunctivitis, 316, 317
Consent, 17–18, 286, 306
Constitutional delay of adolescence, 419
Continence, 144–145
Contraceptives (*see also* specific types of)
  and abortion, 286
  barrier methods
    condoms, 267
    diaphragms, 267–268
    intrauterine devices, 268–272
    spermicides, 266
    vaginal sponges, 266
  counseling about, 263
  effectiveness of, 263
  in gestational trophoblastic disease management, 548
  in gestational trophoblastic tumor treatment, 553
  history, 4–5
  investigative methods of, 286–287
  and leiomyoma uteri, 103
  "natural," 264–265
  and pelvic inflammatory disease, 328–329
  postcoital, 310
  during puerperium, 265
  surgical methods of, 283–286
  withdrawal, 265
Corpus luteum cysts, 118
Cornual resection, 202

Corticosteroids, 40–41, 76–77, 78, 396
Cosmegen, 538
Cough stress test, 149
Counseling
  in breast carcinoma treatment, 61
  contraceptive, 263
  incomplete abortion, 173, 174
  sensory urgency, 160
  sexual, 255
  sexual assault, 312
  in sexual problem management, 259–260
  threatened abortion, 170–171
Craniopharyngioma, 337
Criminal abortion, 175–176
Crohn's disease, 126
Crossmatching blood, 26
Cryoprecipitate, 42
Cryosurgery, 321, 495, 496
Cryotherapy, 482, 572–573
Culdocentesis, 193, 195, 224, 559–561
Culdoscopy, 284
Cultures
  in bacterial vaginosis diagnosis, 84
  in pelvic inflammatory disease diagnosis, 329
  in septic shock diagnosis, 36
  in sexually transmitted disease diagnosis, 317, 322, 324
  in trichomonas vaginitis diagnosis, 87
Curettage, 176–180 (*see also* Dilation and curettage)
Cushing's syndrome
  and amenorrhea, adrenal causes of, 341
  and hirsutism, 381–382, 393–394, 396
Cyclophosphamide, 537–538
Cystic degeneration, 93
Cystic masses, 220
Cystocele, 134–135, 140
Cystometry, 148–149, 151, 155, 152, 157
Cystoscopy, 160, 494
Cysts
  aspiration of, 57–58
  corpus luteum, 118
  of fallopian tubes, benign, 126–127
  follicular, 118, 530
  functional, 118
  Nabothian, 89
  ovarian, functional, 530
Cytology, 318

Dactinomycin, 538
Danazol, 451–452
Darkfield microscopy, 326, 326
Decidual cast, 187, 189, 193
Defeminization, 376 (*see also* Hirsutism)
Dehydroepiandrosterone (DHEA), 403, 418
Dehydroepiandrosterone sulfate (DHEAS), 343, 403, 418, 427
Delayed adolescence, 419–423
Depomedroxyprogesterone acetate (DMPA), 281–282
Depo-Provera, 281–282
Depression, 242, 257, 279, 361
17–20 Desmolase deficiency, 410
20–22 Desmolase deficiency, 408–409
Detrusor instability, 155–158
Dexamethasone, 437
Dexamethasone suppression test, 394
DHEA (*see* Dehydroepiandrosterone)
DHEAS (*see* Dehydroepiandrosterone sulfate)
DHT (*see* Dihydrotestosterone)
Diabetes mellitus, 361, 375, 504
Diaphragms, 267–268
DIC (*see* Disseminated intravascular coagulation)
Diet
  and breast carcinoma, 61
  of hospitalized patient, 15
  in ovarian carcinoma etiology, 525
  of postoperational patient, 20
  in premenstrual syndrome treatment, 245, 248
  of preoperational patient, 18
Diethylstilbestrol (DES), 4, 89, 310
Digitalization, 38
Dihydrotestosterone (DHT), 378, 402
Dilation, 176–180, 182
Dilation and curettage (D & C), 98, 195, 356, 493
Direct immunofluorescent staining, 324
Disseminated intravascular coagulation (DIC), 41–42
Disseminated peritoneal leiomyomatosis, 94
Diuretics, 248

DMPA (*see* Depomedroxyprogesterone)
Dobutamine, 38
Dopamine, 38
Doxorubicin, 539
Doxycycline, 309, 318, 327, 328, 331
Drugs (*see also* specific names of)
  and admission to hospital, 15
  and hirsutism, 385
  in hyperprolactinemia etiology, 336
  in menopause management, 372–374
  postoperative, 21
  preoperative, 18–19
  in sexual dysfunction, 255
  sleeping, 310
  therapeutic, 19
  viralizing, 406
Dysfunctional uterine bleeding (DUB)
  and abortion, 351
  and carcinoma, 352–353
  definition, 350
  diagnosis, 355–356
  differential diagnosis, 351–355
  and ectopic pregnancy, 352
  etiology, 350
  incidence, 350
  and infectious diseases, 353–354
  and intrauterine devices, 354
  management, 356–358
  morbidity, 350
  mortality, 350
  pathogenesis, 350–351
  pathophysiology, 350–351
  and pregnancy, 351–352, 357–358
  prognosis, 358
  in uterine carcinoma differential diagnosis, 506
Dysgerminoma, 525–526, 537
Dysmenorrhea
  differential diagnosis, 597–599
  and endometriosis, 447
  and intrauterine devices, 272, 599
  and premenstrual syndrome diagnosis, 243
  primary, 231–237, 597
  psychogeniç, 228
  secondary, 225–230, 597
Dyspareunia, 597, 599–601

Eating disorders, 243
Ectopic pregnancy
  as abortion complication, 180
  and acute pelvic pain, 220, 595
  definition, 185
  diagnosis, 187–195
  differential diagnosis, 187
  and dysfunctional uterine bleeding, 352
  etiology, 186
  future directions, 204
  incidence, 185
  interstitial, 202
  and intrauterine devices, 186, 271
  morbidity, 185–186
  mortality, 185–186
  natural history, 187
  nonsurgical treatment, 200–201
  occurrence sites, 185
  pathogenesis, 186–187
  prognosis, 201–202
  rare types, 202–204
  surgical treatment, 195–200
  tubal, 201–202
Ectropin, 90
Efudex, 72, 321, 468, 481–482
Elective abortion, 164, 175
Electrocardiography, 37
Electron microscopy, 216
Embryonal carcinomas, 215–216, 526, 537
Empty sella syndrome, 337–338, 340–341
Endocervical biopsy, 480
Endocrinopathies, 254–255, 354–355
Endodermal sinus tumors, 526, 537
Endometrial biopsy, 98, 369, 426, 480, 562–563
Endometrial carcinoma (*see* Uterus, carcinoma of)
Endometrial hyperplasia, 506
Endometrial stromal sarcoma, 516
Endometriosis
  and anovulation, 446
  and chronic pelvic pain differential diagnosis, 227
  definition, 444
  diagnosis, 447–449
  differential diagnosis, 446–447
  and dysmenorrhea, 447
  etiology, 444–445
  and gamete transport, 434
  and infertility, 441, 446–447
  management
    concepts, general, 449–451
    endocrine therapy, 451–454

observant, 451
prophylaxis, 449
surgery, 454–455
morbidity, 444
in ovarian carcinoma differential diagnosis, 530
pathogenesis, 445–446
pathophysiology, 445–446
prognosis, 455–456
and sexual dysfunction, 254
staging, 449
and uterine bleeding, 447–448
Endometritis, 315–316, 327, 354
Endometrioid carcinoma, 528–529
Endotoxemia, 33–35
Endotoxin, 33–35
Enolic acids, 235
Enterocele, 136, 140–141
Environmental toxins, 362, 525
Enzyme deficiencies, 383
Enzyme immunoassay (EIA) methods, 317
Enzyme-linked immunosorbent assay (ELISA) tests, 322, 324
Epithelial cell tumors, 118–119, 528–529
Epithelioid leiomyomata, 93
Erythromycin, 309, 318, 328
Estrogen
and androgens, conversion from, 363
as combination oral contraceptive, 273
deficiency, 254
and dysfunctional uterine bleeding management, 356, 357
exogenous sources of, 417
and lichen sclerosus, 212
and oophorectomy, 112
postmenopausal, 504
and precocious thelarche, 418
receptor analysis, 58
and vulvovaginitis in children, 211
Estrogen progestin therapy, 344–345
Estrogen replacement therapy, 137
Ethinyl estradiol, 273, 310
Etoposide, 539–540
Exercise, 248, 340
Exocervical specimen, 11
Fallopian tubes
benign diseases of, 126–127
carcinoma of, 520–523
cysts of, benign, 126–127
as ectopic pregnancy occurrence site, 185
tumors of, benign, 127
False channel, 564
Familial constitutional true precocious puberty, 415–416
Fat necrosis, 64
Fatty degeneration, 93
Febrile morbidity, 105
Female differentiation, normal, 401 (*see also* Sexual differentiation and development)
Female pseudohermaphroditism, 383, 403–407
Female sexual arousal disorders, 258
Fertility, 385, 388
Fetal testicular formation abnormalities, 413–414
Fibroadenoma, 63, 575
Fibrocystic breast, 62–63
First trimester abortion (*see* Abortion)
Fitz-Hugh–Curtis syndrome, 316
Flouroscopy, 152
Fluid imbalances, 240
Fluid resuscitation, 25–26, 37
5-Fluorouracil
in condyloma acuminata treatment, 72, 321
as ovarian carcinoma chemotherapeutic agent, 538
in vaginal carcinoma management, 481–482
in vulvar carcinoma management, 468
in vulvodynia treatment, 79
Follicle-stimulating hormone (FSH), 344, 369, 379–380, 402–403
Follicular cysts, 118
Foreign bodies, 87, 211
Fresh frozen plasma, 42
Fresh whole blood, 42
Functional cysts, 118
Functional dyspareunia, 258
Functional vaginismus, 258, 260–261

*Gardnerella vaginalis,* 584–586
Galactosemia, 362
Gallbladder disease, 280
Gamete transport
and cervix, 433

Gamete transport continued
  defect, 440–441
  and endometriosis, 434
  and ovary, 434
  and pelvis, 433–434, 440–441
  as pregnancy requirement, 430–434
Gastrointestinal tract, 221–222, 447
Germ cell tumors
  in ovarian benign disease pathogenesis, 120–121
  in ovarian carcinoma, 525–527, 536–537
Gestational trophoblastic disease
  definition, 543
  diagnosis, 546–547
  differential diagnosis, 546
  in dysfunctional uterine bleeding differential diagnosis, 351
  etiology, 544
  incidence, 543
  management, 547–553
  morbidity, 543–544
  mortality, 543–544
  pathogenesis, 544–546
  pathophysiology, 544–546
  prognosis, 553–554
Gestational trophoblastic tumors, 548–553
Glucocorticoid, 400, 401, 409, 410
Gonadal dysfunction, 421–422
Gonadal dysgenesis, 339–340, 384–385
Gonadoblastoma, 121, 527
Gonadotropin-releasing hormone agonists, 103, 249, 438, 452–453
Gonorrhea, 321–323
Gram stain, 223–224, 322
Granuloma inguinale, 70
Granulomatous disease, 340
Granulomatous salpingitis, 126
Granulosa cell tumors, 119, 417, 527, 536
Growth hormone deficiency, 421
Gynandroblastoma, 120, 528
Gynecologic history, 4–5

Hageman Factor, 31
Hair removal, 399
Head injuries, 340
Hemodynamic monitoring, 26–27, 37
Hemorrhage (*see also* Hemorrhagic shock)
  as abortion complication, 180
  classes of, 24–25
  and hysterectomy mortality, 105–106
  and leiomyoma uteri pathology, 93
Hemorrhagic shock
  definition, 23
  etiology, 23–24
  management, 25–30
  pathophysiology, 24–25
  surgery, 29–30
Hermaphroditism, true, 407–408
Herpes simplex virus (HSV), 323–325
Heterosexual precocious puberty, 415
Heterosexual pseudoprecocity, 417–418
Heterotopic pregnancy, 185
Hirsutism (*see also* Hyperandrogenemia)
  and combination oral contraceptives, 397–398
  and Cushing's syndrome, 381–382, 393–394, 396
  definition, 376
  diagnosis
    history, 385, 388
    laboratory studies, 389–391, 393–394, 396
    physical findings, 388–389
  diseases associated with
    adrenal gland, 381–382
    other, 382–385
    ovary, 379–381
  drugs associated with, 385
  etiology, 378
  and fertility, 385, 388
  management, 396–399
  and menstruation, 385
  neoplasms with, 399
  pathophysiology, 378–379
  prevalence, 376–378
  prognosis, 399–400
History, 3–5
Hormonal methods of contraception
  combination oral contraceptives
    administration, 277–278
    clinical problems, 278–279
    effectiveness of, 272
    indications and contraindications, 273, 277
    mechanisms of action, 272–273
    side effects, 279–281

depomedroxyprogesterone, 281–282
investigative, 287
postcoital, 282–283
progestin-only pills, 281
Hormonal therapy, 60, 103
Hospitalized patient
admission orders, 14–16
diet of, 15
postoperative considerations, 19–22
preoperative considerations, 16–19
Hot flush, 366, 367
HPV (*see* Human papillomavirus)
HPV-induced papular lesions, 319
HSG (*see* Hysterosalpingography)
HSV (*see* Herpes simplex virus)
Human chorionic gonadotropin (hCG), 122, 402, 412
Human menopausal gonadotropin, 347–348, 438
Human papillomavirus (HPV), 71–73, 314, 318
Hyaline degeneration, 93
Hydatidiform mole, 351, 543, 544–545, 547
Hydrops tubae profluens, 521, 521
11-Hydroxylase deficiency, 405
17-Hydroxylase deficiency, 340
17-α-Hydroxylase deficiency, 409–410
21-Hydroxylase deficiency, 403–405
17-Hydroxyprogesterone (17-OHP), 405
3-β-Hydroxysteroid dehydrogenase deficiency, 405–406, 409
17-β-Hydroxysteroid dehydrogenase deficiency, 410–411
Hymen, 253–254, 339
Hyperandrogenemia
definition, 376
diseases associated with
adrenal gland, 381–382
other, 382–385
ovary, 379–381
Hyperandrogenism, 343, 346
Hyperhidrosis, 388–389
Hyperprolactinemia
definition, 335
diagnosis, 335, 341–344
differential diagnosis, 338–341
etiology, 336–338
incidence, 335
management, 345–348
morbidity, 336
pathogenesis, 335–336
pathophysiology, 335–336
prognosis, 348–349
and sexual dysfunction, 254–255
Hypertension, 280, 504
Hypertrichosis, 376 (*see also* Hyperandrogenemia)
Hypnotics, 18
Hypoactive sexual desire, 257
Hypogastric artery ligation, 29
Hypopituitarism, 340
Hypothalamic amenorrhea (HA), 338
Hypothalamic dysfunction, 420
Hypothalamic-pituitary tumors, 337
Hypothyroidism
in hirsutism diagnosis, 388
and hyperandrogenemia, diseases associated with, 382–383
and hyperprolactinemia etiology, 336, 337
and precocious puberty, 416
and sexual dysfunction, 254
Hysterectomy
abdominal, 105, 111, 113–114
in cervical carcinoma therapy, 497–498
in ectopic pregnancy treatment, 199
in gestational trophoblastic tumor treatment, 550, 551
in hemorrhagic shock management, 29–30
incidence, 104–105
in incomplete abortion, 173
indications, 108
in interstitial ectopic pregnancy management, 202
in leiomyoma uteri management, 100
morbidity, 105–106
mortality, 106–108
in ovarian carcinoma surgical approach, 112
preoperative patient education, 110–111
preoperative radiographic studies, 109–110
racial differentiation, 105
in second trimester abortion, 183
sexual changes after, 257
surgical approach, 111–114
unnecessary, 108–109
vaginal, 105, 111–113

Hysterectomy continued
  in vaginal carcinoma management, 483
Hysterosalpingography (HSG), 98, 432
Hysteroscopy, 98, 285
Hysterotomy, 173, 183

Idiopathic nonadrenal female pseudohermaphroditism, 407
Ifosfemide, 540
Immunotherapy, 72, 321
Imperforate hymen, 339
Incisional biopsy, 465–466
Incomplete abortion, 165, 171–173, 180
Incomplete masculinization of genetic male, 408–414
Incomplete sexual precocity, 419
Incomplete testicular feminization, 412
Incontinence (*see also* Urinary tract)
  clinical examination, 146–149
  and components of continence, 144–145
  detrusor instability, 155–158
  history, 145–146
  other causes, 158–159
  stress incontinence
    definition, 149–150
    history, 150
    incidence, 150
    in pelvic relaxation diagnosis, 133–134
    physical examination, 150
    surgery for, 142–143
    treatment, 142–143, 152–155
    urodynamic assessment, 151–152
Indirect immunoperoxidase staining, 324
Induced abortion, 164, 175
Inevitable abortion, 165, 171
Infections
  antibiotics in treatment of, 39- 40
  of bladder, 160
  and endometrial biopsy, 564
  in leiomyoma uteri pathology, 93
  maternal, 171
  and menopause etiology, 362
  of pelvis, 227
  and precocious puberty, 416
  of urethra, 160
  urinary tract, 149, 221
  of uterus, 221
Infectious diseases (*see also* Vulvar infectious disease)
  in cervical carcinoma etiology, 487–488
  and dysfunctional uterine bleeding, 353–354
  history, 4
  and infertility, 435
  and intrauterine devices, 271
Infertility
  and anovulation, 426–427
  definition, 424
  and endometriosis, 441, 446–447
  etiology
    egg availability, 425–428
    gamete transport, 430–434
    history, 424–425
    other causes, 434–436
    sperm availability, 428–430
  evaluation, 424
  future trends, 442–443
  history, 4
  incidence, 424
  and infectious diseases, 435
  and leiomyoma uteri, 96–97, 100
  male factor, 428–430, 439–446
  management, 436–442
  morbidity, 424
  mortality, 424
  and mycoplasmas, 328
  and polycystic ovarian disease, 427
  and sexually transmitted diseases, 317
  unexplained, 441–442
  and uterine carcinoma, 503
Inhibited female orgasm, 258
Initial interaction with patient, 3
Insemination, intrauterine, 439
Intercourse, 256, 281, 310, 487
Intersexuality
  female pseudohermaphroditism, 383, 403–407
  incomplete masculinization of genetic male, 408–414
  male pseudohermaphroditism, 383–385
  true hermaphroditism, 407–408
Interstitial ectopic pregnancy, 202
Intra-aortic balloon counterpulsation, 38–39
Intraductal papilloma, 63
Intraepithelial neoplasia, 459
Intraligamentous leiomyomata, 92
Intraperitoneal chemotherapy, 540
Intrauterine adhesions, 338

Intrauterine devices (IUDs)
in acute pelvic pain differential diagnosis, 227
complications of, 271–272
as contraceptive, 268–272
copper bearing, 269
and dysfunctional uterine bleeding, 354
and dysmenorrhea, 272, 599
and ectopic pregnancy, 186, 271
effectiveness of, 269
and infectious diseases, 271
insertion of, 269–270
introduction of, 268–269
investigative, 287
lost, 271
and painful orgasm, 257
and pelvic inflammatory disease, 328–329
types of, 269
and vaginal bleeding, 272
Intrauterine fetal demise, 165, 173–174
Intrauterine insemination, 439
Intrauterine pregnancy, 272
Intravenous fluids, 15, 21
Intravenous leiomyomatosis, 94
Intravenous pyelogram (IVP)
in adnexal mass diagnosis, 591
in cervical carcinoma diagnosis, 494
as hysterectomy preoperative radiographic study, 109
in leiomyoma uteri diagnosis, 98
in ovarian benign disease diagnosis, 122
in ovarian carcinoma diagnosis, 531
in septic shock diagnosis, 37
in uterine carcinoma diagnosis, 508
Invasive carcinoma
cervical, 489–490, 496–497
uterine, 511–514
vaginal, 474–475, 478, 482–483, 484
vulvar, 459–460, 461–462, 469, 472
Invasive mole, 351, 543, 545
In vitro fertilization (IVF), 439–440
In vitro fertilization/embryo transfer (IVF/ET), 441
Irradiation, 482
Isosexual precocious puberty, 414–415
Isosexual pseudoprecocity, 417

Kallmann's syndrome, 340, 420
Karyotype assessment, 370
Kegel's exercises, 137–138
17-Ketosteroid reductase deficiency, 410–411

Labial adhesions, 213
Labia majora, 401
Labia minora, 401
Laboratory studies (*see also* specific types of)
in abdominal pregnancy, 203
in admission into hospital, 15
in acute pelvic pain diagnosis, 223–224
in amenorrhea diagnosis, 342–344
in cervical carcinoma diagnosis, 493–494
in chronic pelvic pain diagnosis, 230
in criminal abortion, 175
in detrusor instability diagnosis, 157
in dysfunctional uterine bleeding diagnosis, 355–356
in ectopic pregnancy diagnosis, 189–195
in endometriosis diagnosis, 449
in evitable abortion, 171
in fallopian tube carcinoma diagnosis, 521
in hyperandrogenemia diagnosis, 389
in incomplete abortion, 172
in leiomyoma uteri diagnosis, 97–98
in menopause diagnosis, 369–371
in missed abortion, 174
in mycoplasma diagnosis, 328
in ovarian benign disease diagnosis, 122–123
in ovarian carcinoma diagnosis, 531–532
postoperative, 21
preoperative, 16–17, 19
in primary dysmenorrhea diagnosis, 233
in sensory urgency diagnosis, 160
in septic shock diagnosis, 36, 36
in threatened abortion, 169–170
in urethral diverticula diagnosis, 161
in uterine carcinoma diagnosis, 506–507
Lacerations, cervical, 90, 180–181

Lactate dehydrogenase (LDH), 122
Laminaria, 183
Laparoscopic myomectomy, 102
Laparoscopy
in adnexal mass diagnosis, 592
in cervical carcinoma diagnosis, 493
in chronic pelvic pain diagnosis, 230
in dysmenorrhea evaluation, 432–433
in ectopic pregnancy diagnosis, 195
in endometriosis diagnosis, 448
in endometriosis management, 451
in hyperandrogenemia diagnosis, 396
in infertility evaluation, 432–433
in infertility management, 440–441
in leiomyoma uteri diagnosis, 98
in pelvic inflammatory disease diagnosis, 329
in sterilization of female, 284
Laparotomy
in endometriosis diagnosis, 448
in infertility management, 440–441
in ovarian benign disease management, 125
in ovarian carcinoma management, 535–536
in sterilization, 283–284
Laryngeal papillomatosis, 320
Laser surgery, 321
Laser vaporization, 496
Laurence-Moon-Biedl syndrome, 420
LDH (*see* Lactate dehydrogenase)
Leiomyomata uteri, 93–94, 353
and acute pelvic pain, 96
anatomic classification, 91–92
benign metastasizing, 94
cellular, 93
and chronic pelvic pain, 96, 226
and contraceptives, 103
definition, 91
diagnosis, 95–98
differential diagnosis, 95
etiology, 92
incidence, 91
and infertility, 96–97, 100
management, 98–103
and menopause, 104
morbidity, 92
mortality, 92
in ovarian carcinoma differential diagnosis, 530
parasitic, 91
pathology, 92–95
and pregnancy, 95, 97, 102, 104
prognosis, 103–104
Leiomyosarcoma, 94, 484, 516
LH (*see* Luteinizing hormone)
Lichen sclerosus, 77–78, 212
Lincomycin, 328
Lipid metabolism, 279
Lipid profile, 369
Lippes Loop, 269
Liver adenomas, 280
Liver diseases, 355, 388
Liver scans, 531
Luteal phase defect, 435
Luteinizing hormone (LH)
in gonadal development, 402–403
and ovarian failure, 344, 369
and polycystic ovarian disease, 379–380
testicular unresponsiveness to, 412–413
Luteoma, 380, 417
Lymphangiography, 494
Lymphogranuloma venereum (LGV), 70–71, 316–317

Magnetic resonance imaging (MRI)
in adnexal mass, 590–591
in hyperandrogenemia diagnosis, 396
in leiomyoma uteri diagnosis, 98
in uterine carcinoma diagnosis, 508–509
Male differentiation, normal, 401–402 (*see also* Sexual differentiation and development)
Male pseudohermaphroditism, 383–385
Mammary duct ectasia, 64
Mammography
abnormal, 579–582
in adnexal mass, 591
in breast carcinoma diagnosis, 56
as hysterectomy preoperative radiographic study, 109
in menopause diagnosis, 369
Marijuana, 420
Marshall-Marchetti-Krantz procedure, 142–143, 154–155
Marsupialization, 74, 162
Mastodynia, 243
McCune-Albright syndrome, 417
Mebendazole, 211

Medications (*see* Drugs)
Medroxyprogesterone acetate (MPA), 398
Medullary thyroid carcinoma, 365–366
Melanoma
of vagina, 475, 476, 483
of vulva, 462, 465, 471, 473
Melphalan, 537
Menarche, 3, 503
Meningovascular disease, 326
Menopause
and carcinoma, 374
definition, 359
and depression, 361
diagnosis, 366–371
differential diagnosis, 364–366
etiology, 361
idiopathic, 362
incidence, 359
late, 503–504
and leiomyoma uteri, 104
management, 371–374
morbidity, 359–361
mortality, 359–361
natural, 362, 364–365, 366
pathogenesis, 363–364
pathophysiology, 363–364
and pelvic inflammatory disease, 362
and pelvic relaxation, 131–132, 360
premature, 362, 365, 370–371
prognosis, 374–375
and sexual dysfunction, 360
surgical, 362
Menstrual history, 3–4, 52
Menstruation, 385
Mesenchymal tumors, 528
Mestranol, 273
α-Methopterin, 538
Methotrexate (MTX), 200–201, 538
Metronidazole, 84, 87
Miconazole, 39, 68, 85
Micropapillary plaques, 319
Mineralocorticoid, 401, 409
Mini-pills, 281
Mixed gonadal dysgenesis, 414
Mixed Müllerian tumors, 516, 529
Moles, 351, 543, 544–545, 547
Monilia vaginitis, 84–86
Monoclonal fluorescent antibody test, 317
Morbidity (*see* specific diseases)
Mortality (*see* specific diseases)
Mucinous cystadenocarcinomas, 528
Mucinous cystadenomas, 118
Mucoid degeneration, 93
Mucopurulent cervicitis (MPC), 315
Müllerian agenesis, 338–339
Müllerian defects, 346
Müllerian duct derivatives, 413
Müllerian duct regression, 402
Multi-agent chemotherapy (MAC), 551–552
Muscular disorders, 222
Musculoskeletal pain, 229, 368, 596–597
Mycoplasmas, 327–328
Myocardial contractility impairment, 33–34
Myomectomy, 100–102
Myxomatous degeneration, 93

Nabothian cysts, 89
Naloxone, 38
Natural family planning technique of contraception, 264–265
*Neisseria gonorrhea,* 321–323
Neonates, 321–322
Neoplasms
of adrenal glands, 382, 417
of breast, 280
of cervix, 280
with hirsutism, 399
metastatic, 529
of ovary, 380–381, 534
of uterus, 280
Neuroendocrine alterations, 241
Neurologic disorders, 222, 326
Neurosyphilis, 327
Nipple discharge, 53–54, 58, 578–579
Nonadrenal female pseudohermaphroditism, 407
Nonconsent, 290
Nongonococcal urethritis, 317
Nongynecological disorders, 229
Nonmalignant diseases (*see* Benign diseases)
Nonpenicillin-resistant gonorrhea, 323
Nonsteroidal anti-inflammatory (NSAI) drugs, 234–237
Nonsteroidal inflammatory drugs, 598
Nontreponemal-specific tests, 326
19-Nortestosterone, 273
Novak Curette, 564
Nutrition
and delayed adolescence, 419–420
in hirsutism diagnosis, 388

Nutrition continued
  in premenstrual syndrome etiology, 240–241
  in sexual differentiation and development, 403
Nystatin, 68, 86

Obesity, 52, 355, 388, 503
17-OHP (*see* 17-Hydroxyprogesterone)
One hour pad test, 149
Oophorectomy, 112, 199
Oral contraceptives (*see* Combination oral contraceptives; Pill)
Orgasms, 256, 257, 258
Osteoporosis, 361, 371, 375
Ovarian hyperthecosis, 380
Ovarian pregnancy, 185, 203–204
Ovarian vessel ligation, 29
Ovary
  and amenorrhea, 339–340, 344
  and androgens, 363
  benign diseases of
    diagnosis, 121–123
    differential diagnosis, 121
    etiology, 117
    incidence, 116
    management, 123–126
    morbidity, 116–117
    mortality, 116–117
    pathogenesis, 118–121
    prognosis, 126
    teratomas, 120–121
    tumors, 118–121
  carcinoma of
    chemotherapeutic agents, 537–540
    diagnosis, 530–532
    differential diagnosis, 530
    and dysfunctional uterine bleeding, 352–353
    etiology, 525
    follow-up, 540
    and hysterectomy, 112
    incidence, 524
    management, 532–537
    morbidity, 524
    mortality, 524
    pathogenesis, 525–529
    pathophysiology, 525–529
    prognosis, 540–541
    spread pattern, 529–530
    staging, 532
    teratomas, 526–527, 537
  cysts of, functional, 530
  development of normal, 401
  donation, 439
  as ectopic pregnancy occurrence site, 185
  and gamete transport, 434
  and heterosexual pseudoprecocity, 418
  and hyperandrogenemia
    diagnosis, 389
    diseases associated with, 379–381
  mass of, 95
  neoplasms of, 380–381, 534
  pain, 220
  as pregnancy site, 203–204
  tumors of, 118–121, 339, 417, 534–535
Ovulation
  defects, 436–439
  induction, 346–348
  and ovarian carcinoma etiology, 525
  as pregnancy requirement, 425–428
Ovulatory pain, 220

Packed red blood cells, 26
Paget's disease, 461, 463, 464–465
Pain (*see* also Acute pelvic pain; Chronic pelvic pain)
  abdominal, 188
  in leiomyoma uteri surgical treatment, 99
  mechanism, 232
  medications, 21
  musculoskeletal, 229, 368, 596–597
  ovulatory, 220
  pelvic, 171, 188
  from urinary calculi, 221
  vagina, 169
Panhypopituitarism, 421
Papanicolaou smear (*see* PAP smear)
Papillary carcinoma, 506
Papillomatosis, 79
PAP smear
  in cervical carcinoma diagnosis, 491–492
  in leiomyoma uteri diagnosis, 97
  in physical examination, 11–13
  in sexually transmitted disease diagnosis, 320

in vaginal carcinoma diagnosis, 479–480
Parenchymatous disease, 326
Parlodel, 437–438
Pediculosis pubis, 74–75
Pedunculated submucous leiomyomata, 91
Pedunculated subserous leiomyomata, 91
Pelvic congestive syndrome, 228–229
Pelvic inflammatory disease (PID)
diagnosis, 329–330
in ectopic pregnancy etiology, 186
epidemiology, 328
incidence, 328
and intrauterine devices, 328–329
and menopause, 362
and mycoplasmas, 327
in ovarian carcinoma differential diagnosis, 530
risk factors, 328–329
sequelae, 331
treatment, 330–331
Pelvic lymphadenectomy, 470
Pelvic pain (*see* Acute pelvic pain; Chronic pelvic pain)
Pelvic relaxation
and childbirth, 131
definition, 128
diagnosis, 132–137
etiology, 131–132
incidence, 129–130
and menopause, 131–132, 360
morbidity, 130
organs involved in, 128–129
pathophysiology, 131–132
and pregnancy, 131
prognosis, 143
supportive anatomic structures, 128
treatment, 137–143
Pelvis
examination
in acute pelvic pain diagnosis, 223
in ectopic pregnancy diagnosis, 189
in incontinence, 147
in menopause diagnosis, 368
in physical examination, 7–11
and gamete transport, 433–434, 440–441
infection of, 180, 227
pain, 171, 188
mass of, 220
surgery, 186
Penicillin allergies, 327
allergy, 327
benzathine, 327
Percutaneous needle biopsy, 494
Pereyra procedure, 142, 154
Pergonal, 438
Perianal warts, 319
Perihepatitis, 316
Perineal support, loss of, 137, 140
Perineum carcinoma, 352
Pessary, 138
Pharyngeal gonorrheal infection, 323
Pharyngitis, 316
Physical contact, 289–290
Physical examination
in abdominal pregnancy, 203
in abnormal uterine bleeding diagnosis, 586, 588
in acute pelvic pain diagnosis, 222–223
in adnexal mass diagnosis, 590
in amenorrhea diagnosis, 341–342
bimanual examination, 10–11
breast examination, 5–7
in breast mass diagnosis, 576–577
in cervical carcinoma diagnosis, 493
of children, 207–208
in chronic pelvic pain diagnosis, 229
in criminal abortion, 175
in cystocele diagnosis, 134–135
in detrusor instability diagnosis, 157
in dysfunctional uterine bleeding diagnosis, 355
in ectopic pregnancy diagnosis, 188–189
in endometriosis diagnosis, 448
in enterocele diagnosis, 136
in fallopian tube carcinoma diagnosis, 521
history, 3–5
in incomplete abortion, 172
in inevitable abortion, 171
in infertility evaluation, 424
initial interaction, 3
in leiomyoma uteri diagnosis, 97
in menopause diagnosis, 368
in missed abortion, 174
in nipple discharge, 579
in ovarian benign disease diagnosis, 122

Physical examination continued
in ovarian carcinoma diagnosis, 531
PAP smear, 11–13
pelvic examination, 7–11
in pelvic relaxation diagnosis, 133
in premenstrual syndrome diagnosis, 243
in primary dysmenorrhea diagnosis, 233
principles, 5
in rectocele diagnosis, 136–137
rectovaginal examination, 11
in sensory urgency diagnosis, 159
in septic shock clinical manifestations, 35
in sexual assault initial evaluation and management, 307–309
in sexual problem diagnosis, 258
speculum examination, 8–10
in stress incontinence diagnosis, 134, 150
in threatened abortion, 169
in urethral diverticula, 161
in uterine carcinoma diagnosis, 506
in uterine prolapse diagnosis, 135
in vaginal carcinoma diagnosis, 479
in vulvar carcinoma diagnosis, 463–465
in vulvovaginal discharge diagnosis, 584–585
written report format, 5
Pill, contraceptive
administration, 277–278
clinical problems, 278–279
depomedroxyprogesterone acetate, 281–282
effectiveness, 272
indications and contraindications, 273, 277
mechanisms of action, 272–273
progestin-only, 281
and sexually transmitted diseases, 329
side effects, 279–281
Pinworms, 87, 211–212
Pipelle Curette, 563–564
Pituitary gland
adenoma, 336
dysfunction, 421
in sexual development, 402–403
tumors of, 346
Placental-site trophoblastic tumor, 545–546
Pneumatic antishock garment, 27–29, 37–38
*Pneumocystis carinii* infection, 39–40
Pneumonia, 317
Podophyllin, 72, 321
Polycystic ovarian disease (PCOD)
and amenorrhea, 338
and congenital adrenal hyperplasia, 390–391, 393
and hyperandrogenemia, 379–380, 388
and infertility, 427
management, 396–399
in uterine carcinoma etiology, 504
Polymicrobial infection, 330
Polyps, 89, 226–227, 353
Postabortal syndrome, 180–181
Postabortion endometritis, 327
Postcoital contraception, 282–283, 310
Postcoital test (PCT), 432
Posthysterectomy sexual changes, 257
Postmenopausal atrophy, 506
Postmenopausal bleeding, 4, 589–590
Postmenopausal vaginitis, 88
Postoperative considerations, 19–22
Postpartum endometritis, 316
Postpartum fever, 327–328
Postpartum oral contraceptives, 280
Prader-Willi syndrome, 420
Precocious adrenarche, 418–419
Precocious puberty, 414–416
Precocious thelarche, 418
Prednisone, 398, 398
Pregnancy (*see also* Ectopic pregnancy)
abdominal, 185, 203
and amenorrhea, 338
and breast carcinoma, 52, 61–62
cervical, 204
and combination oral contraceptives, 280
combined, 202
and dysfunctional uterine bleeding, 351–352, 357–358
and failed abortion, 182
and gestational trophoblastic tumor treatment, 553
heterotopic, 185
intercourse during, 256
intrauterine, 272
and leiomyoma uteri, 95, 97, 102, 104
luteoma of, 380

orgasm during, 256
ovarian, 185, 203–204
and pelvic relaxation, 131
and pill, 277, 280
and rape, 310
recurrent loss, 328
requirements for
gamete transport, 430–434
ovulation, 425–428
sperm availability, 428–430
and sexual assault, 290, 309, 310
and sexually transmitted diseases, 309
and sulfa allergy, 69–70
uterine, 185
and viralizing medication, 406
Pregnancy test, 169, 189–190, 224, 342
Premature adrenarch, 415
Premature menopause, 362, 365, 370–371
Premature thelarche, 415
Prematurity, 328
Premenarchal girls, 123 (*see also* Children)
Premenstrual syndrome (PMS)
classification, 238–239
definition, 238
diagnosis, 242–245
differential diagnosis, 242
and dysmenorrhea, 243
etiology, 240–241
incidence, 238–239
morbidity, 239–240
mortality, 239–240
pathophysiology, 240–241
prognosis, 249
symptomatology questionnaire, 243
treatment, 245–249
Preoperative considerations, 16–19
Prepubertal vaginitis, 87–88
Primary dysmenorrhea
and combination oral contraceptives, 233–234
diagnosis, 233–237
differential diagnosis, 232, 597
etiology, 231
incidence, 231
morbidity, 231
pathogenesis, 231–232
pathophysiology, 231–232
prognosis, 237
Probenecid, 309
Prochlorperazine, 310
Proctitis, 316
Proctoscopy, 494
Progestasert, 269
Progesterone, 58, 212, 249
in ectopic pregnancy, 170–171, 190
Progestin, 273, 356, 374, 453–454
Progestin challenge test, 343, 369, 370
Progestin-only pills, 281
Prolactin, 241, 336, 342–343
Prolactin-secreting pituitary
ectopic production of, 338
pituitary adenoma, 346
Prophylaxis, 19, 449
Prostaglandin
induction, 182–183
inhibitors, 248
injection, 201
levels, 240
in primary dysmenorrhea pathogenesis, 231
Pseudohermaphroditism
female, 383, 403–407
idiopathic nonadrenal female, 407
male, 383–385
nonadrenal female, 407
*Pseudomonas* infection, 39
Pseudoprecocious puberty, 414
Psychiatric evaluation, 245
Psychogenic dysmenorrhea, 228
Puberty, precocious, 414–416
Puerperium, 265
Pulmonary capillary wedge pressure, 27
Pulmonary dysfunction, 34
Pulsatile gonadotropin-releasing hormone therapy, 347
Punch biopsy, 465, 565–566
Pyelogram (*see* Intravenous pyelogram)

Q-tip test, 147–148, 151

Radiation therapy
in breast carcinoma treatment, 60
in breast mass management, 576
in cervical carcinoma therapy, 498–499
in gestational trophoblastic tumor treatment, 552
in menopause etiology, 362
in uterine sarcoma management, 517

Radiation therapy continued
  in vulvar carcinoma management, 470–471
Radiographs, 98 (*see also* specific types of)
Rape, 310
Rectal examination, 223
Rectocele, 136–137, 140
Rectovaginal examination, 11
Recurrent spontaneous abortion, 165, 174–175
5-α-Reductase deficiency, 383–384, 411
Reifenstein syndrome, 411, 412
Renal failure, 338
Resistant ovary syndrome, 340, 366
Respiratory system, 40
Rh immunoglobulin, 183
Rh isoimmunization prophylaxis, 173, 173
RhoGAM, 174, 176
Rhythm methods, 264–265
Right heart catheterization, 37
Rokitansky syndrome, 422–423

Saf-T-Coil, 269
Salpingitis (*see also* Pelvic inflammatory disease), 315
Salpingitis isthmica nodosa, 126
Sarcoma
  botryoid, 215–216, 477, 478, 484
  of uterus, 515–518
  of vagina, 477
Scabies, 75
Secondary dysmenorrhea
  and adhesions, 228
  diagnosis, 229–230
  differential diagnosis, 225–229, 597
  etiology, 225
  incidence, 225
  and leiomyoma uteri, 226
  management, 230
  morbidity, 225
  mortality, 225
  prognosis, 230
Sedatives, 19, 171
Semen analysis, 429–430
Sensory urgency, 159–160
Septic abortion, 165
Septic shock
  clinical manifestations, 35
  definition, 30
  diagnosis, 36–37
  differential diagnosis, 35–36
  and disseminated intravascular coagulation, 41–42
  management, 37–41
  microbiology, 31
  mortality, 30–31
  pathophysiology, 31–35
  predisposing factors, 30
  surgery for, 40
  and toxic shock syndrome, 42–45
Serologic testing, 318, 326
Serous cystadenocarcinoma, 528
Serous cystadenoma, 118
Sertoli-Leydig cell tumors, 119–120, 527–528, 536
Serum progesterone, 170, 190, 425–426
Sexological examination, 252–259
Sex steroids, 363–364
Sexual apathy, 257
Sexual assault
  and abortion, 310
  of children, 306–307
  counseling in, 312
  definition, 289–290
  emotional impact, 290–294
  follow-up, evaluation and management, 312
  history, 5
  initial evaluation and management
    discharge and follow-up, 310–311
    first activities, 294, 305–307
    history, 307
    medical management, 209–310
    physical examination, 307–309
  legal issues, 311–312
  and pregnancy, 290, 309, 310
  prevalence, 290
  and sexually transmitted diseases, 309–310
  statistics on, 289
Sexual aversion disorder, 258
Sexual differentiation and development (see also Hirsutism)
  delayed adolescence, 419–423
  heterosexual pseudoprecocity, 417–418
  incomplete sexual precocity, 419
  intersexuality
    female pseudohermaphroditism, 403–407

incomplete masculinization of genetic male, 408–414
true hermaphroditism, 407–408
isosexual pseudoprecocity, 417
normal, 401–403
and nutrition, 423
precocious adrenarche, 418–419
precocious puberty, 414–416
precocious thelarche, 418
Sexual dysfunction, 253–256, 360
Sexual expression, 257
Sexual history, 4
Sexually transmitted diseases (STDs)
and antibiotics, 309–310
and barrier method of contraception, 329
and children, 309–310
*Chlamydia trachomatis,* 314–318
condyloma acuminata, 318–321
herpes simplex virus, 323–325
incidence, 314
and infertility, 317
mycoplasmas, 327–328
*Neisseria gonorrhea,* 321–323
pelvic inflammatory disease, 328–331
and pill, 329
and pregnancy, 309
and sexual assault, 309–310
syphilis, 325–327
Sexual physiology, normal, 251, 253
Sexual problems
diagnosis, 257–259
management, 259–261
and normal sexual physiology and response, 251, 253
physician's help sought in, 256–257
prognosis, 261
and sexual dysfunction, 253–256
Sexual response, normal, 251, 253
Shaving, preoperative, 18
Sheehan's syndrome, 340
Shock, 23 (*see also* Hemorrhagic shock; Septic shock)
Silver's syndrome, 416
Situational depression, 242
Sitz baths, 73–74
"Skinning vulvectomy", 468, 469
Sleep, 15, 21, 256, 367
Sleeping medications, 310
Sling procedure, 155
Sonography, 193
Speculum examination, 8–10
Sperm, carcinogenic, 488
Spermicides, 266
Sperm availability, 428–430, 439–440
Sperm penetration assay, 430
Spironolactone, 398–399
Spontaneous abortion, 164, 174–175, 220–221
Squamous cell carcinoma
vaginal, 475, 476–477, 479, 482–485
vulvar, 459–460, 463
Squamous metaplasia, 488, 488
Staging
cervical carcinoma, 494–495
endometriosis, 449
fallopian tube carcinoma, 521–522
gestational trophoblastic tumors, 548, 548–549
ovarian carcinoma, 532
uterine carcinoma, 509–510
vaginal carcinoma, 481
vulvar carcinoma, 466
Stamey procedure, 154
*Staphylococcus aureus* infection, 39
Starvation, 382
Sterilization, 283–287
Steroid imbalance, 241
Steroids, 354
Stress urinary incontinence
definition, 149–150
history, 150
incidence, 150
physical examination, 150
in pelvic inflammatory disease diagnosis, 133–134
surgery for, 142–143
treatment, 142–143, 152–155
urodynamic assessment, 151–152
Stress urethral pressure profile, 152
Stromal cell tumors
in ovarian benign disease pathogenesis, 119–120, 121
in ovarian carcinoma pathogenesis, 527–529, 536
Stromal luteoma, 380
Subclinical human papillomavirus infection, 319–320
Submucous leiomyomata, 91
Subserous leiomyomata, 91
Suction, 176–180
Sugar, refined, 248

Sulfa, 69–70
Sulfa allergy, 69–70
Sulfisoxizole, 318
Surgery
  in adnexal mass management, 593
  in amenorrhea treatment, 348
  in breast carcinoma treatment, 59–60
  in condyloma acuminata management, 73
  in ectopic pregnancy treatment, 195–200
  in embryonic carcinoma treatment, 216
  in endometriosis management, 454–455
  in end-organ insensitivity to androgens, 412
  in gestational trophoblastic disease management, 547
  in gestational trophoblastic tumor treatment, 553
  in hemorrhagic shock management, 29–30
  history, 4
  hysterectomy, 111–114
  in idiopathic nonadrenal female pseudohermaphroditism, 407
  in infection treatment, 40
  laser, 321
  in leiomyoma uteri management, 99–100
  in lymphogranuloma venereum management, 71
  in nonadrenal female pseudohermaphroditism, 407
  in ovarian benign disease management, 124
  pelvic, 186
  and pelvic inflammatory disease treatment, 331
  in pelvic relaxation management, 139–143
  in polycystic ovarian disease treatment, 399
  in stress incontinence treatment, 142–143, 152, 154–155
  tubal reconstructive, 186
  in uterine sarcoma management, 517
  in virilizing maternal tumor, 406
  in virilizing medication ingested during pregnancy, 406
Surgical methods of contraception, 283–286
Sympathetic nervous system, 33
Symplastic leiomyoma, 93
Symptothermal method of contraception, 264
Syphilis, 325–327
Systemic diseases, 354–355, 416, 419
Systemic fungal infections, 39

Talc, 525
Temperature method of contraception, 264
Teratomas
  and isosexual pseudoprecocity, 417
  in ovarian benign diseases, 120–121
  in ovarian carcinoma, 526–527, 537
Terconazole, 68, 86
Testes, 401, 430
Testicular biopsy, 430
Testicular feminization, 339, 383, 411–412
Testis determining factor (TDF), 401
Testosterone
  and amenorrhea diagnosis, 343
  inborn errors of, 408, 411
  and lichen sclerosus, 78, 212
  and Wolffian duct differentiation, 402
Testosterone-receptor abnormalities, 383
Tetanus toxoid, 310
Tetracycline
  in *Chlamydia trachomatis* managment, 318
  in granuloma inguinale management, 70
  in mycoplasma treatment, 328
  in pelvic inflammatory disease treatment, 331
  in sexually transmitted disease management, 309, 327
Thecoma, 119, 417, 527
Therapeutic abortion, 164–165
Therapeutic medications, 19
Thermocoagulation by laparoscopy, 284
Threatened abortion, 165, 169–171
Thyroid stimulating hormone (TSH), 336, 343
Thyrotropin-releasing hormone (TRH), 336
Toluidine blue, 464
Topical hemostatic agents, 30

Topical hydrocortisone, 210
Topical podophyllin, 72
Toxic shock syndrome, 42–45
Toxins, environmental, 362, 525
Trachoma, 316
Tranquilizers, 77, 310
Transcervical catheterization, 441
Transfusion, blood, 26
Transport system of egg and sperm, 430–434
Transsexuals, 385
Trauma, 290, 305–306, 416
Treponemal-specific tests, 326
Trichloroacetic acid (TCA), 72, 320
Trichomonas vaginitis, 86–87
Trichomoniasis, 586
True hermaphroditism, 407–408
True precocious puberty, 414–415
Tubal ligation, 186
Tubal ligation reversal, 441
Tubal reconstructive surgery, 186
Tuberculosis, 339, 365
Tuberculous salpingitis, 126
Tumor markers, 122
Tumors
- of adrenal glands, 341, 417
- benign, 592
- Brenner, 529
- and chronic pelvic pain differential diagnosis, 228
- endodermal sinus, 526, 537
- epithelial cell, 118–119, 528–529
- of fallopian tube, benign, 127
- fibroid, 221
- germ cell, 120–121, 525–527, 536–537
- gestational trophoblastic, 548–553
- granulosa cell, 119, 417, 527, 536
- hypothalamic-pituitary, 337
- malignant, 592
- mesenchymal, 528
- mixed Müllerian, 516, 529
- of ovary, 118–121, 339, 417, 534–535
- of pituitary gland, 346
- placental-site trophoblastic, 545–546
- and precocious puberty, 416
- Sertoli-Leydig cell, 119–120, 527–528, 536
- stromal cell, 119–120, 121, 527–528, 536
- of urinary tract, 221
- of uterus, benign, 353
- virilizing maternal, 406

Turner's syndrome, 422

Ultrasonography
- in acute pelvic pain diagnosis, 224
- in adnexal mass diagnosis, 590
- in chronic pelvic pain diagnosis, 230
- in ectopic pregnancy diagnosis, 191–192, 193
- in hyperandrogenemia diagnosis, 394
- as hysterectomy preoperative radiographic study, 110
- in infertility evaluation, 426
- in leiomyoma uteri diagnosis, 98
- in ovarian benign disease diagnosis, 123
- in ovarian carcinoma diagnosis, 531
- in primary dysmenorrhea diagnosis, 233
- in septic shock diagnosis, 37
- in stress incontinence assessment, 152
- in threatened abortion, 169–170

Undifferentiated carcinoma, 529
Uninhibited detrusor contractions, 155–158
Unipolar electrical cautery by laparoscopy, 284
Urethra
- calibration, 148, 148
- culture, 160
- dilation and massage, 160
- infection, 160
- obstruction, 96

Urethral diverticula, 160–162
Urethral pressure profile, 162
Urethral prolapse, 213–214
Urethral syndrome, 315
Urethritis, 315
Urethrocystoscopy, 149, 151
Urethrography, 162
Urethroscopy, 160, 161–162
Urinalysis, 170, 223
Urinary (LH) kits, 426
Urinary calculi, 221
Urinary continence (*see* Continence)
Urinary incontinence (*see* Incontinence)
Urinary tract
- disease, 447
- evaluation
  - clinical examination, 146–149
  - history, 145–146

Urinary tract continued
  and menopause diagnosis, 367
  sensory urgency, 159–160
  tumors of, 221
  urethral diverticula, 160–162
Urinary tract infection (UTI), 149, 221
Urine culture, 147, 160, 170
Urine cytology, 160
Urine loss, 149
Urodynamics, 151
Urofollitropin, 438
Urology
  complaints, 144
  continence, 144–146
  lower urinary tract
    conditions, 149–162
    evaluation, 146–149
Uterine artery ligation, 29
Uterine bleeding (*see also* Dysfunctional uterine bleeding)
  abnormal, 586–590
  and endometriosis, 447–448
  and leiomyoma uteri, 95–96, 99
Uterine leiomyomata (*see* Leiomyoma uteri)
Uterine perforation, 180, 271
Uterine pregnancy, 185
Uterine prolapse, 135, 140
Uterus (*see also* Uterine bleeding)
  benign diseases of
    hysterectomy, 104–114
    leiomyoma uteri, 91–104
  carcinoma of
    diagnosis, 506–509
    differential diagnosis, 506
    and dysfunctional uterine bleeding, 352
    etiology, 503–504
    incidence, 502
    and infertility, 503
    management, 510–514
    and menopause, 374
    mortality, 502–503
    pathogenesis, 505–506
    prognosis, 514–515
    staging, 509–510
  as ectopic pregnancy occurrence site, 185
  enlarged, 100
  examination of, 11, 172
  and gamete transport, 433, 441
  neoplasms of, 280
  perforation of, 180, 271, 564
  retroflexed, 95
  sarcomas of, 515–518
  sharply antiflexed, 95
  tumors of, benign, 353

Vabra aspiration, 564
Vaccines, contraceptive, 287
Vagina
  agenesis of, 254
  anomalies of, 88–89
  benign diseases of
    lesions, 88–89
    vulvovaginitis, 80–88
  carcinoma of
    diagnosis, 478–481
    differential diagnosis, 478
    and dysfunctional uterine bleeding, 352
    embryonic, 215–216
    etiology, 476–477
    incidence, 474–475
    management, 481–484
    morbidity, 475
    mortality, 475–476
    pathogenesis, 477–478
    pathophysiology, 477–478
    prognosis, 484–485
    staging, 481
  examination of, 10
  foreign bodies in, 87, 211
  infection, 170
  irradiation of, 482
  lesions of, 88–89, 478, 481, 482–483
  melanoma of, 475, 476, 483
  pain, 169
  preoperative preparation, 18
  sarcoma of, 477
  squamous cell carcinoma of, 475, 476–477, 479, 482–485
  visualization of, 208
  wet prep microscopic examination of, 329–330
Vaginal biopsy, 98, 369, 426, 480, 562–563
Vaginal bleeding
  abnormal, in menopause, 359
  in cervical carcinoma diagnosis, 490
  in children, 214–215
  in ectopic pregnancy diagnosis, 188
  in incomplete abortion, 171
  and intrauterine devices, 272
  irregular, 506

in threatened abortion, 169
Vaginal delivery, 102, 256
Vaginal discharge, 80–83, 490
Vaginal duplication, 89
Vaginal hysterectomy, 105, 111–113
Vaginal mucosal atrophy, 367
Vaginal myomectomy, 102
Vaginal specimen, 12
Vaginal sponge, 266
Vaginal thrush, 84–86
Vaginal vault prolapse, 141–142
Vaginectomy, 482
Vaginitis
atrophic, 254
Candida, 84–86
infectious, 254
and mycoplasmas, 327
prepubertal, 87–88
and sexual dysfunction, 254
trichomonas, 86–87
Vaginoscopy, 210
Vascular thrombosis, 279
Vasectomy, 286
Vasectomy reversal, 439
Vasomotor instability, 366
Vasopressors, 38
Venereal warts, 319
Vestibular gland, 79
Vestibular warts, 319
Vinblastine, 539
Vinca alkaloids, 539
Vincristine, 539
Violence, 290
Virilization, 376, 403 (*see also* Hirsutism)
Virilizing maternal tumor, 406
Virilizing medication, 406
Vital signs, 14, 20
Vitamin $B_6$, 248
VP-16, 539–540
Vulva
benign diseases of
vulvar dystrophies, 75–78
vulvodynia, 78–79
carcinoma of
diagnosis, 463–466
differential diagnosis, 462–463
and dysfunctional uterine bleeding, 352
etiology, 460–461
incidence, 459–460
management, 466–471
morbidity, 460
mortality, 460
pathophysiology, 461–462
prognosis, 472–473
recurrent, 471
staging, 466
lesions of, 77–78, 462–463, 466–467
melanoma of, 462, 465, 471, 473
squamous cell carcinoma of, 459–460, 463
Vulvar biopsy, 76, 563–565
Vulvar dystrophies, 75–78
Vulvar infectious disease
Bartholin's duct abscess, 73–74
candidiasis, 67–69
chancroid, 69–70
condyloma acuminata, 71–73
granuloma inguinale, 70
incidence, 66–67
lymphogranuloma venereum, 70–71
morbidity, 67
mortality, 67
pediculosis pubis, 74–75
scabies, 75
Vulvectomy, 468, 469–470
Vulvodynia, 78–79
Vulvovaginal discharge, 582–586
Vulvovaginitis
bacterial vaginosis, 83–84
candida vaginitis, 84–86
in children, 209–211
definition, 80
postmenopausal vaginitis, 88
predisposing factors, 583
prepubertal vaginitis, 87–88
trichomonas vaginitis, 86–87
vaginal discharge, 80–83

Warts, 319
Weight change, 278, 346
"Wet prep" sample, 83, 329–330
Withdrawal, 265
Wolffian duct differentiation, 402

X chromosomes, 401
X-rays, 36, 37, 224, 233 (*see also* Radiographs)
46,XY gonadal dysgenesis, 422
46,XY pure gonadal dysgenesis, 413–414, 422

Y chromosome, 346, 401
Y chromosome abnormalities, 414
Yeast vaginitis, 84–86